MEDICAL ABBREVIATIONS:

7000 Conveniences at the Expense of Communications and Safety

Fifth Edition, Revised

Neil M. Davis, M.S., Pharm.D., FASHP
Professor of Pharmacy, Temple University
School of Pharmacy, Philadelphia, PA,
Editor-in-Chief, Hospital Pharmacy

published by

Neil M. Davis Associates
1143 Wright Drive
Huntingdon Valley, PA 19006
Phone (215) 947-1752
FAX (215) 938-1937

Preface

Listed are 7000 current acronyms, symbols, and other abbreviations and over 11,000 of their possible meanings. This list has been compiled to assist individuals in reading medical records, medically related communications, and prescriptions. The list, although current and comprehensive, represents only a portion of abbreviations in use and their many possible meanings as new ones are being coined every day.

Abbreviations are a convenience, a time saver, a space saver, and a way of avoiding the possibility of misspelling words. However, a price can be paid for their use. Abbreviations are sometimes not understood or are interpreted incorrectly. Their use may lengthen the time needed to train individuals in the health fields, at times delays the patient's care, and occasionally results in patient harm.

The publication of this list of abbreviations is not an endorsement of their legitimacy. It is not a guarantee that the intended meaning has been correctly captured, or an indication that they are in common use. Where uncertainty exists, the one who wrote the abbreviation must be contacted for clarification.

There are many variations in how an abbreviation can be expressed. Anterior-posterior has been written as AP, A.P., ap, and A/P. Since there are few standards and those who use abbreviations do not necessarily follow these standards, this book only shows Anterior-posterior as AP. This is done to make it easier to find the meaning of an abbreviation as all the meanings of APs are listed together. This elimination of unnecessary duplication also keeps the book at a convenient size thus enabling it to be sold at a reasonable price.

The Council of Biology Editors (CBE), in their CBE Style Manual[1], lists about 600 abbreviations gathered from 15 internationally recognized authorities and organizations. The majority of these symbols and abbreviations tend to be more scientifically oriented than those which would appear in medical records. In the few situations where the CBE abbreviations differ from what is presented in this book, the CBE abbreviation has been placed in parenthesis after the meaning. As is the practice in the United States, mL has been used rather than ml and the spelling of liter, meter, etc. is used rather than litre and metre, even though ml, litre, and metre are listed in the CBE Style Manual.

The abbreviation AP, is listed as meaning doxorubicin and cisplatin. The reason for this apparent disparity is that the official generic names, (United States Adopted Names) are shown, rather than the trade names Adriamycin® and Platinol®. In the case of LSD, the official name, lysergide is given, rather than the chemical name, lysergic acid diethylamide. The Latin derivations for older medical and pharmaceutical abbreviations, (TID, *ter in die,* three times daily) may be found in Remington.[2]

Healthcare organizations are wisely required by the Joint Commission on Accreditation of Healthcare Organizations to formulate an approved list of abbreviations. Every attempt should be made to restrict this list to common abbreviations that are understood by all health professionals who must work with medical records. There are certain dangerous abbreviations that should not be approved, and a warning should be issued about their use (See Table 1 as well as notes in the text).

Many inherent problems associated with abbreviations contribute to or cause errors. Reports of such errors have been published routinely.[3-5]

Abbreviations and symbols can also easily be misread or interpreted in a manner not intended. For example:

(1) "HCT250 mg" was intended to mean hydrocortisone 250 mg but was interpreted as hydrochlorothiazide 50 mg (HCTZ50 mg).

(2) Flucytosine was improperly abbreviated as 5 FU causing it to be read as fluorouracil. Flucytosine is abbreviated 5 FC and fluorouracil is 5 FU.

(3) Floxuridine was improperly abbreviated as 5 FU causing it to be read as fluorouracil. Flucytosine is abbreviated FUDR and fluorouracil is 5 FU.

(4) MTX was thought to be mustargen. MTX is methotrexate and mustargen is abbreviated HN_2.

Table 1. Some dangerous abbreviations

Problem term	Reason	Suggested term
O.D. for once daily	Interpreted as right eye	Write "once daily"
q.o.d. for every other day	Interpreted as meaning once daily or read as q.i.d.	Write "every other day"
q.d. for once daily	Read or interpreted as q.i.d.	Write "once daily"
q.n. for every night	Read as every hour	Write "every night," "H.S." or nightly
q hs for every night	Read as every hour	Use "HS" or "at bedtime"
U for Unit	Read as 0, 4, 6 or cc.	Write "unit"
O.J. for orange juice	Read as OD or OS	Write "orange juice"
µg (microgram)	When handwritten, misread as mg	Write "mcg"
sq or sub q for subcutaneous	The q is read as every	Use "subcut"
Chemical symbols	Not understood or misunderstood	Write full name
Lettered abbreviations for drug names	Not understood or misunderstood	Use generic or trade name
Apothecary symbols or terms	Not understood or misunderstood	Use metric system
per os for by mouth	OS read as left eye	Use "by mouth," "orally," or "P.O."
D/C for discharge	Interpreted as discontinue (orders for discharge medications result in premature discontinuance of current medication)	Write "discharge"
T/d for one per day	Read as T.I.D.	Use "once daily"
/ (a slash mark) for with, and, or per	read as a one	use, "and", "with", or "per"

(5) **The abbreviation "U" for unit is the most dangerous one in the book, having caused numerous 10 fold insulin overdoses. The word unit should never be abbreviated.** The handwritten U for unit has been mistaken for a zero, causing tenfold errors. The handwritten U has also been read as the number four and as "cc".

(6) OD meant to signify once daily has caused Lugol's solution to be given in the right eye.

(7) OJ meant to signify orange juice, looked like OS and caused Saturated Solution of Potassium Iodide to be given in the left eye.

(8) Na Warfarin (Sodium Warfarin) was read as "No Warfarin."

(9) The abbreviation "s̄" for without has been thought to mean "with" (c̄).

(10) The order for PT, intended to signify a laboratory test order for prothrombin time, resulted in the ordering of a physical therapy consultation.

(11) The abbreviation, "TAB", meant to signify Triple Antibiotic, (a coined name for a hospital sterile topical antibiotic mixture), caused patients to have their wound irrigated with a diet soda.

(12) a slash mark (/) has been mistaken for a one causing a patient to receive a 100 unit overdose of NPH insulin when the slash was used to separate an order for two insulin doses.

    6 units regular insulin/20 units NPH insulin

A prescription could be written with directions as follows: "OD OD OD," to mean one drop in the right eye once daily!

Abbreviations should not be used for drug names as they are particularly dangerous. As previously illustrated there is the possibility that the writer may, through mental error, confuse two abbreviations and use the wrong one. Similarly, the reader may attribute the wrong meaning to an abbreviation. To further confound the problem, some drug name abbreviations have multiple meanings (see CPM, CPZ and PBZ in table 2). The abbreviation AC has been used for three different cancer chemotherapy

4

Table 2. Example of abbreviations which have several meanings.

CPM	=	cyclophosphamide; chlorpheniramine maleate; continuous passive motion; continue present management; central pontine myelinolysis; counts per minute and clinical practice model
PBZ	=	phenylbutazone; pyribenzamine; phenoxybenzamine
CPZ	=	chlorpromazine; Compazine®
DW	=	dextrose in water; distilled water; deionized water
MS	=	morphine sulfate; multiple sclerosis; mitral stenosis; musculoskeletal; medical student; minimal support; muscle strength; mental status; milk shake; mitral sound and morning stiffness
CF	=	cystic fibrosis; Caucasian female; calcium leucovorin (citrovorum factor); complement fixation; cancer-free; cardiac failure; coronary flow; contractile force; cephalothin; Christmas factor; count fingers and cisplatin and fluorouracil
NBM	=	no bowel movement; normal bowel movement; nothing by mouth; normal bone marrow

combinations to mean, Adriamycin® and either cyclophosphamide, carmustine, or cisplatin. Beside causing medication errors and incorrect interpretation of medical records, abbreviations can create problems because treatment is delayed while a health professional seeks clarification for the meaning of the abbreviation used. Abbreviations should not be used to designate drugs or combinations of drugs.

Certain abbreviations in the book are followed by a warning, "this is a dangerous abbreviation". This warning could be placed after most abbreviations, but was reserved for situations where errors have been published because these abbreviations were used or where the meaning is critical and not likely to be known. Such warning statements should also appear after every abbreviation for a drug or drug combination.

Abbreviations for medical facility names create problems as they are usually not recognized by the reader in another geographic area. A clue to the fact that one is dealing with such an abbreviation is when it ends with MC, for Medical Center: MH, for Memorial Hospital: CH, for Community Hospital: UH, for University Hospital: and H, for Hospital.

When an abbreviation can not be found in the book or when the listed meaning(s) do not make sense, there is a possibility that the abbreviation has been misread. As an example, a reader could not find the meaning of HHTS. On closer examination it really was +HTS, not HHTS.

An examination of the following list is a testimonial to the problems and dangers associated with most undefined abbreviations.

The assistance of Aphirudee Poshakrishma Hemachudha, former teaching assistant, Temple University School of Pharmacy, Philadelphia, PA; Michael R. Cohen, Director of Pharmacy Service, Quakertown Community Hospital, Quakertown, PA; Ann Sandt Kishbaugh, Merchantville, NJ and all the others that helped is gratefully acknowledged.

A

A	accommodation
	age
	alive
	ambulatory
	angioplasty
	anterior
	apical
	arterial
	artery
	assessment
(a)	axillary temperature
ā	before
A_2	aortic second sound
A250	5% albumin 250 mL
A1000	5% albumin 1000 mL
A II	angiotensin II
AA	acetic acid
	achievement age
	active assistive
	Alcoholics Anonymous
	alcohol abuse
	alveolar-arterial gradient
	amino acid
	antiarrhythmic agent
	aortic aneurysm
	aplastic anemia
	arm ankle (pulse ratio)
	ascending aorta
	audiologic assessment
	authorized absence
	automobile accident
	cytarabine and doxorubicin
aa	of each
A&A	arthroscopy and arthrotomy
	awake and aware
AAA	abdominal aortic aneurysmectomy (aneurysm)
	acute anxiety attack
AAC	antimicrobial agent-associated colitis
AACG	acute angle closure glaucoma
AAD	acid-ash diet
	antibiotic associated diarrhea

AAE	active assistance exercise
	acute allergic encephalitis
A/AEX	active assistive exercise
AAG	alpha-1-acid glycoprotein
AAL	anterior axillary line
AAMS	acute aseptic meningitis syndrome
AAN	analgesic abuse nephropathy
	analgesic-associated nephropathy
	attending's admission notes
AAO	alert, awake, & oriented
AAO × 3	awake and oriented to time, place, and person
AAP	assessment adjustment pass
AAPC	antibiotic acquired pseudomembranous colitis
AAPMC	antibiotic-associated pseudomembranous colitis
AAROM	active assistive range of motion
AAS	atlantoaxis subluxation
	atypical absence seizure
AASCRN	amino acid screen
AAU	acute anterior uveitis
AAV	adeno-associated virus
AAVV	accumulated alveolar ventilatory volume
AB	abortion
	ace bandage
	antibiotic
	antibody
A/B	acid-base ratio
	apnea/bradycardia
A > B	air greater than bone (conduction)
A & B	apnea and bradycardia
ABC	absolute band counts
	absolute basophil count
	apnea, bradycardia, and cyanosis
	aspiration, biopsy and cytology
	artificial beta cells

ABCDE	botulism toxoid pentavalent	A/B SS	apnea/bradycardia self-stimulation
ABD	after bronchodilator	ABT	aminopyrine breath test
ABd	plain gauze dressing, type of	ABVD	adriamycin, bleomycin, vinblastine, and dacarbazine (DTIC)
Abd	abdomen		
	abdominal	ABW	actual body weight
	abductor	ABx	antibiotics
ABDCT	atrial bolus dynamic computer tomography	AC	abdominal circumference acetate
ABE	acute bacterial endocarditis		acromioclavicular acute
	adult basic education		air conditioned
	botulism equine trivalent antitoxin		air conduction anchored catheter
ABEP	auditory brainstem-evoked potentials		antecubital anticoagulant
ABG	aortoiliac bypass graft		assist control
	arterial blood gases		before meals
	axiobuccogingival	A/C	anterior chamber of the eye
ABI	atherothrombotic brain infarction		assist/control
ABID	antibody identification	5-AC	azacitidine
ABK	aphakic bullous keratopathy	ACA	acyclovir adenocarcinoma
ABL	allograft bound lymphocytes		aminocaproic acid anterior cerebral artery
ABLB	alternate binaural loudness balance		anterior communicating artery
A/B Mods	apnea/bradycardia moderate stimulation	AC/A	accommodation convergence–accommo-
A/B MS	apnea/bradycardia mild stimulation		dation (ratio)
ABMT	autologous bone marrow transplantation	ACB	alveolar-capillary block antibody-coated bacteria
		AC & BC	air and bone conduction
ABN	abnormality(ies)	ACBE	air contrast barium enema
A.B.N.M.	American Board of Nuclear Medicine	ACC	accident accommodation
abnor.	abnormal		adenoid cystic carcinomas
ABO	blood group system (A, AB B, and O)		administrative control center
ABP	arterial blood pressure		ambulatory care center
ABR	absolute bed rest	AcCoA	acetyl-coenzyme A
	auditory brain (evoked) responses	ACCR	amylase creatinine clearance ratio
ABS	absent	ACD	absolute cardiac dullness
	absorbed		acid-citrate-dextrose
	absorption		anterior chamber diameter
	acute brain syndrome		anterior chest diameter
	admitting blood sugar		dactinomycin
	at bedside	ACDs	anticonvulsant drugs

ACE	angiotensin-converting enzyme	AD	accident dispensary
			admitting diagnosis
ACF	accessory clinical findings		alternating days (this is a
	acute care facility		dangerous abbreviation)
ACG	angiocardiography		Alzheimer's disease
ACH	adrenal cortical hormone		axis deviation
	aftercoming head		right ear
	arm girth, chest depth,	A&D	alcohol and drug
	and hip width		ascending and descending
ACh	acetylcholine		vitamins A and D
AChE	acetylcholinesterase	ADA	adenosine deaminase
AC & HS	before meals and at		American Diabetes
	bedtime		Association
ACI	adrenal cortical		anterior descending artery
	insufficiency	ADAU	adolescent drug abuse
	aftercare instructions		unit
ACL	anterior cruciate ligament	ADC	Aid to Dependent
ACLS	advanced cardiac life		Children
	support		anxiety disorder clinic
ACMV	assist-controlled	ADCC	antibody-dependent
	mechanical ventilation		cellular cytotoxicity
ACN	acute conditioned neurosis	ADD	adduction
ACP	acid phosphatase		attention deficit disorder
ACPA	anticytoplasmic antibodies		average daily dose
AC-PH	acid phosphatase	ADDH	attention deficit disorder
ACPP	adrenocorticopolypeptide		with hyperactivity
ACPP PF	acid phosphatase prostatic	ADDU	alcohol and drug
	fluid		dependence unit
ACR	adenomatosis of the colon	ADE	acute disseminated
	and rectum		encephalitis
	anticonstipation regimen	ADEM	acute disseminating
ACS	American Cancer Society		encephalomyelitis
	anodal-closing sound	ADFU	agar diffusion for fungus
ACSVBG	aortocoronary saphenous	ADG	atrial diastolic gallop
	vein bypass graft	ADH	antidiuretic hormone
ACSW	Academy of Certified	ADI	allowable daily intake
	Social Workers	A-DIC	doxorubicin and
ACT	activated clotting time		dacarbazine
	allergen challenge test	ADL	activities of daily living
	anticoagulant therapy	*ad lib*	as desired
ACT-D	dactinomycin		at liberty
Act Ex	active exercise	ADM	admission
ACTH	corticotropin		doxorubicin
	(adrenocorticotrophic	Ad-OAP	doxorubicin, vincristine,
	hormone)		cytarabine, and
ACTSEB	anterior chamber tube		prednisone
	shunt encircling band	adol	adolescent
ACV	acyclovir	ADP	arterial demand pacing
	atrial/carotid/ventricular		adenosine diphosphate
ACVD	acute cardiovascular	ADPKD	autosomal dominant
	disease		

	polycystic kidney disease	AES	anti-embolic stockings
		AET	atrial ectopic tachycardia
ADQ	abductor digiti quinti	AF	acid-fast
	adequate		amniotic fluid
ADR	acute dystonic reaction		anterior fontanel
	adverse drug reaction		antifibrinogen
	doxorubicin (Adriamycin®)		aortofemoral
			atrial fibrillation
ADRIA	doxorubicin (Adriamycin®)	AFB	acid-fast bacilli
			aorto-femoral bypass
ADS	anatomical dead space		aspirated foreign body
	anonymous donor's sperm	AFBG	aortofemoral bypass graft
	antibody deficiency syndrome	AFC	adult foster care
			air filled cushions
ADSU	ambulatory diagnostic surgery unit	AFDC	Aid to Family and Dependent Children
ADT	alternate-day therapy	AFE	amniotic fluid embolization
	anticipate discharge tomorrow	AFEB	afebrile
	Auditory Discrimination Test	AFI	amniotic fluid index
		A fib	atrial fibrillation
ADTP	Adolescent Day Treatment Program	AFIP	Armed Forces Institute of Pathology
A5D5W	alcohol 5%, dextrose 5% in water for injection	AFL	atrial flutter
		AFLP	acute fatty liver of pregnancy
AE	above elbow (amputation)	AFO	ankle-foot orthosis
	accident and emergency (department)	AFP	alpha-fetoprotein
		AFRD	acute febrile respiratory disease
	air entry		
	aryepiglottic (fold)	AFV	amniotic fluid volume
A&E	accident and emergency (department)	AFVSS	afebrile, vital signs stable
		AFX	air-fluid exchange
AEA	above elbow amputation	Ag	antigen
AEB	as evidenced by	AG	abdominal girth
AEC	at earliest convenience		aminoglycoside
AED	antiepileptic drug		anion gap
	automated external defibrillator		anti-gravity
			atrial gallop
AEDP	automated external defibrillator pacemaker	A/G	albumin to globulin ratio
		AGA	accelerated growth area
AEEU	admission entrance and evaluation unit		acute gonococcal arthritis
			appropriate for gestational age
AEG	air encephalogram		
AEM	ambulatory electrogram monitor		average gestational age
		AGD	agar gel diffusion
AEq	age equivalent	AGE	acute gastroenteritis
AER	acoustic evoked response		angle of greatest extension
	auditory evoked response		
Aer. M.	aerosol mask		
Aer. T.	aerosol tent	AGF	angle of greatest flexion

AGG	agammaglobulinemia		allergy index
aggl.	agglutination		aortic insufficiency
AGL	acute granulocytic leukemia		artificial insemination
		A & I	Allergy and Immunology (department)
A GLAC-TO-LK	alpha galactoside leukocytes		
		AIA	anti-insulin antibody
AGN	acute glomerulonephritis		aspirin-induced asthma
$AgNO_3$	silver nitrate	AI-Ab	anti-insulin antibody
AGPT	agar-gel precipitation test	AIBF	anterior interbody fusion
AGS	adrenogenital syndrome	AICA	anterior inferior cerebellar artery
AGTT	abnormal glucose tolerance test		anterior inferior communicating artery
AH	abdominal hysterectomy		
	amenorrhea-hyperprolactinemia	AICD	automatic implantable cardioverter/defibrillator
	antihyaluronidase		
A&H	accident and health (insurance)	AID	acute infectious disease
			artificial insemination donor
AHA	acetohydroxamic acid		
	acquired hemolytic anemia		automatic implantable defibrillator
	autoimmune hemolytic anemia	AIDKS	acquired immune deficiency syndrome with Kaposi's sarcoma
AHC	acute hemorrhagic conjunctivitis		
		AIDS	acquired immune deficiency syndrome
	acute hemorrhagic cystitis		
AHD	autoimmune hemolytic disease	AIE	acute inclusion body encephalitis
AHE	acute hemorrhagic encephalomyelitis	AIF	aortic-iliac-femoral
		AIH	artificial insemination with husband's sperm
AHEC	Area Health Education Center		
		AIHA	autoimmune hemolytic anemia
AHF	antihemophilic factor		
AHFS	American Hospital Formulary Service	AIHD	acquired immune hemolytic disease
AHG	antihemophilic globulin		
AHGS	acute herpetic gingival stomatitis	AIIS	anterior inferior iliac spine
AHL	apparent half-life	AILD	angioimmunoblastic lymphadenopathy (with dysproteinemia)
AHM	ambulatory Holter monitoring		
AHN	adenomatous hyperplastic nodule	AIMS	Abnormal Involuntary Movement Scale
	Assistant Head Nurse		Arthritis Impact Measurement Scales
AHP	acute hemorrhagic pancreatitis	AIN	acute interstitial nephritis
AHS	adaptive hand skills		anal intraepithelial neoplasia
AHT	autoantibodies to human thyroglobulin	AINS	anti-inflammatory non-steroidal
AI	accidentally incurred		

11

AION	anterior ischemic optic neuropathy		alternate lifestyle checklist
AIP	acute infectious polyneuritis	ALC R	alcohol rub
	acute intermittent porphyria	ALD	adrenoleukodystrophy alcoholic liver disease aldolase
AIR	accelerated idioventricular rhythm	ALDOST	aldosterone
AIS	Abbreviated Injury Score anti-insulin serum	ALFT	abnormal liver function tests
AIS/ISS	Abbreviated Injury Scale/Injury Severity Score	ALG ALI alk	antilymphocyte globulin argon laser iridotomy alkaline
AITP	autoimmune thrombocytopenia purpura	ALK ISO	alkaline phosphatase isoenzymes
AIU	absolute iodine uptake	ALK-P ALL	alkaline phosphatase acute lymphoblastic
AIVR	accelerated idioventricular rhythm		leukemia acute lymphocytic
AJ	ankle jerk		leukemia
AJR	abnormal jugular reflex		allergy
AK	above knee (amputation) actinic keratosis	ALM	acral lentiginous melanoma
	artificial kidney	ALMI	anterolateral myocardial infarction
AKA	above-knee amputation alcoholic ketoacidosis	ALN	anterior lymph node
	all known allergies	Al(OH)$_3$	aluminum hydroxide
	also known as	ALP	argon laser photocoagula-
AL	acute leukemia		tion
	argon laser		Alupent®
	arterial line	ALPZ	alprazolam
	axial length	ALS	acute lateral sclerosis
	left ear		advanced life support
ALA	aminolevulinic acid		amyotrophic lateral sclerosis
ALAC	antibiotic-loaded acrylic cement	ALT	alanine transaminase (SGPT)
ALAD	abnormal left axis deviation	2 alt	Argon laser trabeculo- plasty
ALARA	as low as reasonably achievable		every other day (this is a dangerous abbreviation)
ALAT	alanine transaminase (alanine aminotrans- ferase; SGPT)	ALTB	acute laryngotracheobron- chitis
		ALVAD	abdominal left ventricular assist device
Alb	albumin	ALWMI	anterolateral wall
ALC	acute lethal catatonia		myocardial infarct
	alcohol	AM	adult male
	allogeneic lymphocyte cytotoxicity		amalgam morning (a.m.)
	alternate level of care		myopic astigmatism

AMA	against medical advice	AMPT	alphamethylpara tyrosine
	American Medical Association	AMR	alternating motor rates
	antimitochondrial antibody	AMS	acute mountain sickness
AMAD	morning admission		aggravated in military service
AMAG	adrenal medullary autograft		amylase
			auditory memory span
AMAL	amalgam	m-AMSA	acridinyl anisidide
AMAP	as much as possible	AMSIT	portion of the mental status examination: A—appearance, M—mood, S—sensorium, I—intelligence, T—thought process
AMAT	anti-malignant antibody test		
A-MAT	amorphous material		
AMB	ambulate		
	ambulatory		
	amphotericin B	amt.	amount
AMC	arm muscle circumference	AMV	assisted mechanical ventilation
AM/CR	amylase to creatinine ratio		
AMD	age-related macular degeneration	AMY	amylase
		AN	anorexia nervosa
	methyldopa (alpha methyldopa)		Associate Nurse
		ANA	antinuclear antibody
AMegL	acute megokaryoblastic leukemia	ANAD	anorexia nervosa and associated disorders
AMES-LAN	American sign language	ANC	absolute neutrophil count
		anch	anchored
AMF	autocrine motility factor	ANCOVA	analysis of covariance
AMG	acoustic myography	AND	anterior nasal discharge
	aminoglycoside	ANDA	Abbreviated New Drug Application
AMI	acute myocardial infarction	anes	anesthesia
	amitriptyline	ANF	antinuclear factor
AML	acute myelogenous leukemia		atrial natriuretic factor
		ANG	angiogram
AMM	agnogenic myeloid metaplasia	ANISO	anisocytosis
		ANLL	acute nonlymphoblastic leukemia
AMML	acute myelomonocytic leukemia		
		ANOVA	analysis of variance
AMMOL	acute myelomonoblastic leukemia	ANP	atrial natriuretic peptide
		ANS	answer
AMN	adrenomyeloneuropathy		autonomic nervous system
amnio	amniocentesis	ANT	anterior
AMN SC	amniotic fluid scan		enpheptin (2-amino-5-nitrothiazol)
AMOL	acute monoblastic leukemia	ante	before
AMP	adenosine monophosphate	ANTI A:AGT	anti blood group A antiglobulin test
	ampicillin		
	ampul	Anti bx	antibiotic
	amputation	ant sag D	anterior sagittal diameter
A-M pr	Austin-Moore prosthesis	ANTU	alpha naphthylthiourea

ANUG	acute necrotizing ulcerative gingivitis			auscultation and percussion
ANX	anxiety	A/P		ascites/plasma ratio
	anxious	$A_2 > P_2$		second aortic sound greater than second pulmonic sound
AO	anterior oblique			
	aorta			
	aortic opening	APACHE		Acute Physiology and Chronic Health Evaluation
	plate, screw (orthopedics)			
	right ear			
A & O	alert and oriented	APAP		acetaminophen
A&O × 3	awake and oriented to person, place, and time	APB		abductor pollicis brevis atrial premature beat
A&O × 4	awake and oriented to person, place, time, and date	APC		adenoidal-pharyngeal-conjunctival adenomatous polyposis of the colon and rectum
AOAP	as often as possible			
AOB	alcohol on breath			aspirin, phenacetin, and caffeine
AOC	anode opening contraction antacid of choice area of concern			atrial premature contraction
AOCD	anemia of chronic disease	APCD		adult polycystic disease
AOD	alleged onset date	APD		afferent pupillary defect
	arterial occlusive disease Assistant-Officer-of-the-Day			aminohydroxypropylidene diphosphate anterior-posterior diameter
AODA	alcohol and other drug abuse			atrial premature depolarization
AODM	adult onset diabetes mellitus			automated peritoneal dialysis
ao-il	aorta-iliac	APDC		Anxiety and Panic Disorder Clinic
AOM	acute otitis media			
AOO	continuous arterial asynchronous pacing	APE		acute psychotic episode acute pulmonary edema
AOP	aortic pressure	APG		Apgar (score)
AOSD	adult-onset Still's disease	APH		adult psychiatric hospital
AP	acute pancreatitis			alcohol-positive history antepartum hemorrhage
	alkaline phosphatase			
	angina pectoris antepartum	APIVR		artificial pacemaker-induced ventricular rhythm
	anterior-posterior (x-ray)			
	arterial pressure	APKD		adult polycystic kidney disease
	apical pulse			
	appendicitis			adult-onset polycystic kidney disease
	atrial pacing			
	attending physician	APL		abductor pollicis longus
	doxorubicin and cisplatin			accelerated painless labor
A&P	active and present			acute promyelocytic leukemia
	anterior and posterior			
	assessment and plans			anterior pituitary-like

	(hormone)	ARC	anomalous retinal correspondence
	chorionic gonadotropin		
AP & L	anteroposterior and lateral		AIDS related complex
APN	acute pyelonephritis		American Red Cross
APO	doxorubicin, prednisone, and vincristine	ARCBS	American Red Cross Blood Services
apo E	apolipoprotein E	ARD	acute respiratory disease
APPG	aqueous procaine penicillin G (dangerous terminology; for intramuscular use only, write as penicillin G procaine)		adult respiratory distress
			antibiotic removal device
			aphakic retinal detachment
		ARDS	adult respiratory distress syndrome
appr.	approximate	ARE	active-resistive exercises
appt.	appointment	ARF	acute renal failure
APPY	appendectomy		acute respiratory failure
APR	abdominoperineal resection		acute rheumatic fever
		ARG	arginine
APS	Adult Psychiatric Service	ARI	aldose reductase inhibitor
APSAC	anistreplase (anisoylated plasminogen streptokinase activator complex)	ARLD	alcohol related liver disease
		ARM	anxiety reaction, mild
			artificial rupture of membranes
APSD	Alzheimer's presenile dementia	ARMS	amplification refractory mutation system
aPTT	activated partial thromboplastin time	ARN	acute retinal necrosis
APVR	aortic pulmonary valve replacement	AROM	active range of motion
			artifical rupture of membranes
aq	water		
AQ	accomplishment quotient	ARP	alcohol rehabilitation program
aq dest	distilled water		
AR	active resistance	arr	arrive
	airway resistance	A.R.R.T.	American Registry of Radiologic Technologists
	alcohol related		
	aortic regurgitation		
	aural rehabilitation	ARS	antirabies serum
	autorefractor	ART	Accredited Record Technician
Ar	argon		
A&R	adenoidectomy with radium		Achilles (tendon) reflex test
	advised and released		acoustic reflex threshold(s)
A-R	apical-radial (pulses)		
ARA-A	vidarabine		arterial
ARA-AC	fazarabine		automated reagin test (for syphilis)
ARA-C	cytarabine		
ARB	any reliable brand	ARTIC	articulation
ARBOR	arthorpod-borne virus	Art T	art therapy
ARBOW	artificial rupture of bag of water	ARV	AIDS related virus

ARW	Accredited Rehabilitation Worker	
ARWY	airway	
AS	activated sleep	
	anal sphincter	
	ankylosingspondylitis	
	aortic stenosis	
	doctor called through answering service	
	atropine sulfate	
	left ear	
ASA	aspirin (acetylsalicyclic acid)	
	American Society of Anesthesiologists	
	argininosuccinate	
ASA I	Healthy patient with localized pathological process	
ASA II	A patient with mild to moderate systemic disease	
ASA III	A patient with severe systemic disease limiting activity but not incapacitating	
ASA IV	A patient with incapacitating systemic disease	
ASA V	Moribund patient not expected to live. (These are American Society of Anesthesiologists' patient classifications. Emergency operations are designated by "E" after the classification).	
ASAA	acquired severe aplastic anemia	
ASACL	American Society of Anesthesiologists Classification	
AS/AI	aortic stenosis/aortic insufficiency	
ASAP	as soon as possible	
ASAT	aspartate transaminase (aspartate aminotrans-ferase) (SGOT)	
ASB	anesthesia standby	

		asymptomatic bacteriuria
ASC		altered state of consciousness
		ambulatory surgery center
		anterior subcapsular cataract
		antimony sulfur colloid
		ascorbic acid
ASCVD		arteriosclerotic cardiovascular disease
ASD		atrial septal defect
ASDH		acute subdural hematoma
ASE		acute stress erosion
ASH		asymmetric septal hypertrophy
AsH		hypermetropic astigmatism
ASHD		arteriosclerotic heart disease
ASI		Anxiety Status Inventory
ASIS		anterior superior iliac spine
ASK		antistreptokinase
ASL		antistreptolysin (titer)
ASLO		antistreptolysin-O
AsM		myopic astigmatism
ASMA		anti-smooth muscle antibody
ASMI		anteroseptal myocardial infarction
ASO		aldicarb sulfoxide
		antistreptolysin-O titer
		arteriosclerosis obliterans
		automatic stop order
ASOT		antistreptolysin-O titer
ASP		acute suppurative parotitis
		acute symmetric polyarthritis
		aspartic acid
ASPVD		arteriosclerotic peripheral vascular disease
ASS		anterior superior supine
		assessment
asst		assistant
AST		aspartate transaminase (SGOT)
		astemizole
		astigmatism
AS TOL		as tolerated
ASTIG		astigmatism

ASTZ	antistreptozyme test	ATS	antitetanic serum (tetanus antitoxin)
ASU	acute stroke unit		
	ambulatory surgical unit		anxiety tension state
ASV	antisnake venom	ATSO4	atropine sulfate
ASVD	arteriosclerotic vessel disease	ATT	arginine tolerance test
		at. wt	atomic weight
ASYM	asymmetric (al)	AU	allergenic units
AT	activity therapy (therapist)		both ears
	antithrombin	Au	gold
	applanation tonometry	198_{Au}	radioactive gold
	atraumatic	AUB	abnormal uterine bleeding
AT 10	dihydrotachysterol	AUC	area under the curve
ATB	antibiotic	AUD	auditory comprehension
ATC	alcoholism therapy classes	COMP	
	around the clock	AUGIB	acute upper gastrointestinal bleeding
ATD	antithyroid drug(s)		
	autoimmune thyroid disease	AUL	acute undifferentiated leukemia
At Fib	atrial fibrillation	AUR	acute urinary retention
AT III FUN	antithrombin III functional	AUS	acute urethral syndrome
			auscultation
ATG	antithymocyte globulin	AV	arteriovenous
ATHR	angina threshold heart rate		atrioventricular
			auditory visual
ATL	Achilles tendon lengthening	AVA	aortic valve atresia
			arteriovenous anastomosis
	adult T-cell leukemia	AVD	aortic valve disease
	anterior tricuspid leaflet		apparent volume of distribution
	atypical lymphocytes		
ATLS	advanced trauma life support	AVDP	asparaginase, vincristine daunorubicin, and prednisone
ATM	acute transverse myelitis		
At ma	atrial milliamp		avoirdupois
	atmosphere	$AVDO_2$	arteriovenous oxygen difference
ATN	acute tubular necrosis		
ATNC	atraumatic normocephalic	AVF	arteriovenous fistula
aTNM	autopsy staging of cancer		augmented unipolar foot (left leg)
ATNR	asymmetrical tonic neck reflux		
		avg	average
ATP	addiction treatment program	AVGs	ambulatory visit groups
		AVH	acute viral hepatitis
	adenosine triphosphate	AVJR	atrioventricular junctional rhythm
ATPase	adenosine triphosphatase		
ATPS	ambient temperature & pressure, saturated with water vapor	AVL	augmented unipolar left (left arm)
ATR	Achilles tendon reflex	AVM	atriovenous malformation
	atrial	AVN	arteriovenous nicking
atr fib	atrial fibrillation		atrioventricular node
ATRO	atropine		avascular necrosis

AVNRT	AV nodal reentry tachycardia	B$_2$	riboflavin
AVOC	avocation	B$_6$	pyridoxine HCl
AVP	arginine vasopressin	B$_7$	biotin
AVR	aortic valve replacement	B$_8$	adenosine phosphate
	augmented unipolar right (right arm)	B$_{12}$	cyanocobalamin
		Ba	barium
AVS	atriovenous shunt	BA	backache
AVSS	afebrile, vital signs stable		benzyl alcohol
AVT	atrioventricular tachycardia		bile acid
			blood alcohol
	atypical ventricular tachycardia		bone age
			Bourns assist
AW	abdominal wall		branchial artery
	abnormal wave		bronchial asthma
A/W	able to work	B > A	bone greater than air
A&W	alive and well	B & A	brisk and active
AWA	as well as	B&B	bowel and bladder
A waves	atrial contraction waves	Bab	Babinski
AWDW	assault with a deadly weapon	BAC	benzalkonium chloride
			blood alcohol concentration
AWI	anterior wall infarct		buccoaxiocervical
AWMI	anterior wall myocardial infarction	BACON	bleomycin, doxorubicin, lomustine, vincristine, and mechlorethamine
AWO	airway obstruction		
AWOL	absent without leave	BACOP	bleomycin, adriamycin, cyclophosphamide, vincristine, and prednisone
ax	axillary		
AXR	abdomen x-ray		
AXT	alternating exotropia		
AZA	azathioprine	BACT	bacteria
5 AZA	azacitidine	BAD	dipolar affective disorder
AZQ	diaziquone	BaE	barium enema
AZT	zidovudine (azidothymidine)	BAE	bronchial artery embolization
A-Z test	Ascheim-Zondek test	BAEP	brain stem auditory evoked potential
	diagnostic test for pregnancy		
		BAERs	brain stem auditory evoked responses
		BAL	balance
			blood alcohol level
			British antilewisite (dimercaprol)
B			bronchoalveolar lavage
B	bacillus	BALB	binaural alternate loudness balance
	bands		
B	bilateral	BaM	barium meal
	black	BAND	band neutrophil (stab)
	bloody	BANS	back, arm, neck and scalp
	both	BAO	basal acid output
	buccal	BAP	blood agar plate
B$_1$	thiamine HCl		

Barb	barbiturate	B/C	because	
BARN	bilateral acute retinal necrosis		blood urea nitrogen/ creatinine ratio	
BAS	boric acid solution	B&C	bed and chair	
BaS	barium swallow		biopsy and curettage	
BASK	basket cells		board and care	
baso.	basophil		breathed and cried	
BASO STIP	basophilic stippling	BC/BS	Blue Cross/Blue Shield	
batt	battery	BCA	balloon catheter angioplasty	
BAVP	balloon aortic valvuloplasty		basal cell atypia brachiocephalic artery	
BAW	bronchoalveolar washing	BCAA	branched-chain amino acids	
BB	baby boy			
	backboard	B. cat	Branhamella catarrhalis	
	bad breath	B-CAVe	bleomycin, lomustine, doxorubicin, and vinblastine	
	bed bath			
	bed board			
	beta blocker	BCC	basal cell carcinoma	
	blanket bath		birth control clinic	
	blood bank	BCCa	basal cell carcinoma	
	blow bottle	BCD	basal cell dysplasia	
	blue bloaters	BCE	basal cell epithelioma	
	body belts	B cell	large lymphocyte	
	both bones	BCG	bacillus Calmette-Guérin vaccine	
	bowel or bladder			
	breakthrough bleeding		bicolor guaiac	
	breast biopsy	BCL	basic cycle length	
	buffer base	BCM	birth control medication	
B/B	backward bending	BCNP	Board Certified Nuclear Pharmacist	
BBA	born before arrival			
BBB	blood-brain barrier	BCNU	carmustine	
	bundle branch block	BCP	birth control pills	
BBBB	bilateral bundle branch block		carmustine, cyclophos- phamide, and prednisone	
BBD	before bronchodilator			
	benign breast disease	BCS	battered child syndrome	
BBM	banked breast milk		Budd-Chiari syndrome	
BBS	bilateral breath sounds	BCU	burn care unit	
BBT	basal body temperature	BD	band neutrophil	
BB to MM	belly button to medial malleolus		base down	
			bile duct	
B Bx	breast biopsy		birth date	
BC	back care		birth defect	
	bed and chair		blood donor	
	birth control		brain dead	
	blood culture		bronchial drainage	
	Blue Cross	BDAE	Boston Diagnostic Aphasia Examination	
	bone conduction			
	Bourn control			

BDBS	Bonnet-Dechaume-Blanc Syndrome	BFP	biologic false positive
BDC	burn-dressing change	*B. frag*	*Bacillus fragilis*
BDE	bile duct exploration	BFT	bentonite flocculation test
BDF	black divorced female		biofeedback training
BDI SF	Beck's Depression Index-Short Form	BFU$_e$	erythroid burst-forming unit
BDL	below detectable limits	BG	baby girl
	bile duct ligation		blood glucose
BDM	black divorced male		bone graft
B-DOPA	bleomycin, dacarbazine, vincristine, prednisone, and doxorubicin	B-G	Bender-Gestalt (test)
		B-GA-LACTO	beta galactosidase
BDP	beclomethasone diproprionate	BGC	basal-ganglion calcification
BDR	background diabetic retinopathy	BGDC	Bartholin gland duct cyst
		BGL	blood glucose level
BE	bacterial endocarditis	BH	breath holding
	barium enema	BHC	benzene hexachloride
	base excess	BHD	carmustine, hydroxyurea, and dacarbazine
	below elbow		
	bread equivalent	B-HEXOS-A-LK	beta hexosaminidase A leukocytes
	breast examination		
B↑E	both upper extremities	BHI	biosynthetic human insulin
B↓E	both lower extremities	BHN	bridging hepatic necrosis
B & E	brisk and equal	BHS	beta-hemolytic streptococci
BEA	below elbow amputation		
BEAM	brain electrical activity mapping		breath-holding spell
		BHT	breath hydrogen test
BEC	bacterial endocarditis	BI	base in
BEE	basal energy expenditure		brain injury
BEF	bronchoesophageal fistula		bowel impaction
Beh Sp	behavior specialist	BIB	brought in by
BEI	butanol-extractable iodine	BIC	brain injury center
BEP	bleomycin, etoposide, and cisplatin	Bicarb	bicarbonate
		BICROS	bilateral contralateral routing of signals
	brain stem evoked potentials	BID	brought in dead
BEV	billion electron volts		twice daily
	bleeding esophageal varices	BIF	bifocal
		BIG 6	analysis of 6 serum components (see SMA 6)
BF	black female		
	boyfriend		
	breakfast fed	BIH	benign intracranial hypertension
	breast-feed		
BFA	baby for adoption		bilateral inguinal hernia
	bifemoral arteriogram	BIL	bilateral
BFC	benign febrile convulsion		brother-in-law
BFL	breast firm and lactating	BILAT SLC	bilateral short leg case
BFM	black married female		

BILAT SXO	bilateral salpingo-oophorectomy	BLESS	bath, laxative, enema, shampoo, and shower
Bili	bilirubin	BLL	bilateral lower lobe
BILI-C	conjugated bilirubin	BLM	bleomycin sulfate
BIMA	bilateral internal mammary arteries	BLOBS	bladder obstruction
BIN	twice a night (this is a dangerous abbreviation)	BLPO	beta-lactamase-producing organism
		BLQ	both lower quadrants
BIOF	biofeedback	BLR	blood flow rate
BiPD	biparietal diameter	BLS	basic life support
bisp	bispinous diameter	B.L. unit	Bessey-Lowry units
B.I.W.	twice a week (this is a dangerous abbreviation)	BM	black male
			bone marrow
BIZ-PLT	bizarre platelets		bowel movement
BJ	Bence-Jones		breast milk
	biceps jerk	BMA	bone marrow aspirate
	bone and joint	BMC	bone marrow cells
BJE	bone and joint examination	BMD	Becker muscular dystrophy
BJM	bones, joints, and muscles		bone marrow depression
			bone mineral density
BJP	Bence-Jones protein	BME	brief maximal effort
BK	below knee (amputation)	BMI	body mass index
	bradykinin	BMJ	bones, muscles, joints
	bullous keratopathy	BMK	birthmark
BKA	below knee amputation	BMM	black married male
BKC	blepharokerato-conjunctivitis	BMP	behavior management plan
bkft	breakfast	BMR	basal metabolic rate
Bkg	background		best motor response
BKU	base up	BMT	bilateral myringotomy and tubes
BKWP	below-knee walking plaster (cast)		bone marrow transplant
BL	baseline (fetal heart rate)	BMTT	bilateral myringotomy with tympanic tubes
	bland		
	blast cells	BMTU	bone marrow transplant unit
	blood level		
	blood loss	BNC	bladder neck contracture
	bronchial lavage	BNCT	boron neutron capture therapy
	Burkitt's lymphoma		
BLB	Boothby-Lovelace-Bulbulian (oxygen mask)	BNO	bladder neck obstruction
		BNR	bladder neck retraction
BLBK	blood bank	BO	behavior objective
BL = BS	bilateral equal breath sounds		body odor
			bowel obstruction
bl cult	blood culture	B & O	belladonna & opium (suppositories)
bldg	bleeding		
bld tm	bleeding time	BOA	born on arrival
BLE	both lower extremities		born out of asepsis
BLEO	bleomycin sulfate	BOB	ball on back

21

BOD	bilateral orbital decompression	BPs	systolic blood pressure	
Bod Units	Bodansky units	BPSD	bronchopulmonary segmental drainage	
BOE	bilateral otitis externa	BPV	benign paroxysmal vertigo	
BOLD	bleomycin, vincristine, (Oncovin) lomustine, and dacarbazine		bovine papilloma virus	
BOM	bilateral otitis media	Bq	becquerel	
BOMA	bilateral otitis media, acute	BR	bathroom	
			bedrest	
BOO	bladder outlet obstruction		Benzing retrograde	
BOOP	bronchitis obliterans with organized pneumonia		blink reflex	
			bowel rest	
BOT	base of tongue		bridge	
BOW	bag of water		brown	
BP	bathroom privileges	Br	bromide	
	bed pan	BRA	brain	
	benzoyl peroxide	BRADY	bradycardia	
	bipolar	BRAO	branch retinal artery occlusion	
	birthplace			
	blood pressure	BRAT	bananas, rice cereal, applesauce, and toast	
	bypass			
	British Pharmacopeia	BRATT	bananas, rice, cereal, applesauce, tea, & toast	
BPI	bipolar affective disorder, Type I			
BPD	biparietal diameter	BRB	blood-retinal barrier	
	borderline personality disorder		bright red blood	
		BRBR	bright red blood per rectum	
	bronchopulmonary dysplasia			
		BRBPR	bright red blood per rectum	
BPd	diastolic blood pressure			
BPF	bronchopleural fistula	BRCM	below right costal margin	
BPH	benign prostatic hypertrophy	BRJ	brachial radialis jerk	
		BRM	biological response modifiers	
BPG	bypass graft			
BPL	benzylpenicilloylpoly-lysine	BRO	brother	
		BRP	bathroom privileges	
BPLA	blood pressure, left arm	BR RAO	branch retinal artery occlusion	
BPM	beats per minute			
	breaths per minute	BR RVO	branch retinal vein occlusion	
BPN	bacitracin, polymyxin B, and neomycin sulfate			
		BRVO	branch retinal vein occlusion	
BPPP	bilateral pedal pulses present			
		BS	bedside	
BPR	blood per rectum		before sleep	
	blood pressure recorder		Bennett seal	
BPRS	Brief Psychiatric Rating Scale		blood sugar	
			Blue Shield	
BPS	bilateral partial salpingectomy		bowel sounds	
			breath sounds	

B & S	Bartholin & Skene (glands)	BST	bedside testing
			brief stimulus therapy
BSA	body surface area	BSU	Bartholin, Skene's, urethra
	bowel sounds active		
BSAB	Balthazar Scales of Adaptive Behavior	BSW	Bachelor of Social Work
		BT	bedtime
BSB	bedside bag		bleeding time
	body surface burned		bituberous
BSC	bedside care		bladder tumor
	bedside commode		blood type
	burn scar contracture		blood transfusion
BSD	baby soft diet		brain tumor
	bedside drainage		breast tumor
BSE	breast self-examination	BTB	break-through bleeding
BSepF	black separated female	BTBV	beat to beat variability
BSepM	black separated male	BTC	bladder tumor check
BSER	brain stem evoked responses		by the clock
		BTE	behind-the-ear (hearing aid)
BSF	black single female		
	busulfan	BTF	blenderized tube feeding
BSGA	beta Streptococcus group A	BTFS	breast tumor frozen section
BSI	body substance isolation	BTG	beta thromboglobulin
	brainstem injury	BTL	bilateral tubal ligation
BSL	blood sugar level	BTPS	body temperature pressure saturated
BSM	black single male		
BSN	Bachelor of Science in Nursing	BTR	bladder tumor recheck
		BU	below umbilicus
BS L base	breath sounds diminished, left base		Bodansky units
			burn unit
BSN	bowel sounds normal	BUdR	bromodeoxyuridine
BSNA	bowel sounds normal and active	BUE	both upper extremities
		BUFA	baby up for adoption
BSNT	breast soft and nontender	BUN	blood urea nitrogen
BSO	bilateral salpingo-oophorectomy		bunion
		BUR	back-up rate (ventilator)
BSOM	bilateral serous otitis media	Burd	Burdick suction
		BUS	Bartholin, urethral, and Skene's glands
BSP	bromsulphalein		
BSPA	bowel sounds present and active	BV	bacterial vaginitis
			biological value
BSPM	body surface potential mapping		blood volume
		BVAD	bi-ventricular assist device
BSS	bedside scale		
	bismuth subsalicylate	BVE	blood volume expander
BSS®	balanced salt solution	BVL	bilateral vas ligation
	black silk sutures	BVO	branch vein occlusion
BSSG	sitogluside	BVRT	Benton Visual Retention Test
BSSS	benign sporadic sleep spikes		
		BW	birth weight

	bite-wing (radiograph)	C&A	Clinitest® and Acetest®
	body water	CAA	crystalline amino acids
	body weight	CAB	catheter-associated
B & W	Black and White (milk of		bacteriuria
	magnesia & aromatic		coronary artery bypass
	cascara fluidextract)	CABG	coronary artery bypass
BWA	bed wetter admission		graft
BWCS	bagged white cell study	CaBI	calcium bone index
BWFI	bacteriostatic water for	CABS	coronary artery bypass
	injection		surgery
BWidF	black widowed female	CACI	computer assisted
BWidM	black widowed male		continuous infusion
BWS	battered woman syndrome	CaCO₃	calcium carbonate
ΦBZ	phenylbutazone	CACP	cisplatin
Bx	biopsy	CAD	coronary artery disease
BX BS	Blue Cross and Blue	CAE	cellulose acetate
	Shield		electrophoresis
BXM	B cell crossmatch		cyclophosphamide,
BZDZ	benzodiazepine		doxorubicin, and
			etoposide
		CAEC	cardiac arrhythmia
			evaluation center

C

C	ascorbic acid	CaEDTA	calcium disodium edetate
	carbohydrate	CAF	cyclophosphamide,
	Catholic		doxorubicin, and
	Caucasian		fluorouracil
	Celsius	CAFT	Clinitron air fluidized
	centigrade		therapy
	clubbing	CAG	continuous ambulatory
	cyanosis		gamma globin
	hundred		(infusion)
c̄	with	CaG	calcium gluconate
C₁...C₇	cervical nerve 1 through 7	CAH	chronic active hepatitis
	cervical vertebra 1		chronic aggressive
	through 7		hepatitis
C₁ to C₉	precursor molecules of		congenital adrenal
	the complement system		hyperplasia
CII	controlled substance,	CAL	callus
	class 2		calories (cal)
C_II	second cranial nerve		chronic airflow limitation
CA	carcinoma	cal ct	calorie count
	cardiac arrest	CALD	chronic active liver
	carotid artery		disease
	celiac artery	CALGB	Cancer and Leukemia
	chronologic age		Group B
	Cocaine Anonymous	CALLA	common acute
	compressed air		lymphoblastic leukemia
	coronary angioplasty		antigen
	coronary artery	CAM	Caucasian adult male
Ca	calcium	CAMF	cyclophosphamide,

		CAVB	complete atrioventricular block
	adriamycin, methotrexate, and fluorouracil		
CAMP	cyclophosphamide, doxorubicin, methotrexate, and procarbazine	CAVC	common arterioventricular canal
		CAVH	continuous ateriovenous hemofiltration
CAN	cord around neck	CAV-P-VP	cyclophosphamide, doxorubicin, vincristine, cisplatin, and etoposide
CA/N	child abuse and neglect		
CANC	cancelled		
CAO	chronic airway (airflow) obstruction	CB	cesarean birth
			chair and bed
CAP	capsule		chronic bronchitis
	chloramphenicol		code blue
	community-acquired pneumonia	C & B	chair and bed
			crown and bridge
	compound action potentials	CBA	chronic bronchitis and asthma
	cyclophosphamide, doxorubicin, and cisplatin	CBC	carbenicillin
			complete blood count
CaP	carcinoma of the prostate	CBD	closed bladder drainage
Ca/P	calcium to phosphorus ratio		common bile duct
		CBDE	common bile duct exploration
CAPB	central auditory processing battery	CBF	cerebral blood blow
CAPD	chronic ambulatory peritoneal dialysis	CBFS	cerebral blood flow studies
CAR	cardiac ambulation routine	CBFV	cerebral blood flow velocity
CARB	carbohydrate	CBG	capillary blood glucose
CAS	carotid artery stenosis	CBI	continuous bladder irrigation
CASHD	coronary arteriosclerotic heart disease	CBN	chronic benign neutropenia
CASP	Child Analytic Study Program	CBP	chronic benign pain
		CBPS	coronary bypass surgery
CASS	computer aided sleep system	CBR	carotid bodies resected
			chronic bedrest
CAT	cataract		complete bedrest
	children's apperception test	CBRAM	controlled partial rebreathing-anesthesia method
	computed axial tomography	CBS	chronic brain syndrome
cath.	catheter		Cruveilhier-Baumgarten syndrome
	catheterization		
CAV	computer-aided ventilation	CBZ	carbamazepine
		CC	cardiac catheterization
	cyclophosphamide, doxorubicin, and vincristine		cerebral concussion
			chief complaint
			chronic complainer

	circulatory collapse	CCHD	cyanotic congenital heart disease
	clean catch (urine)		
	coracoclavicular	CCI	chronic coronary insufficiency
	cord compression		
	corpus collosum	CCK	cholecystokinin
	creatinine clearance	CCK-OP	cholecystokinin octapeptide
	critical condition		
	cubic centimeter (cc), (mL)	CCK-PZ	cholecystokininpancreozymin
	with correction (with glasses)	CCL	cardiac catheterization laboratory
C/C	cholecystectomy and operative cholangiogram		critical condition list
		CCl$_4$	carbon tetrachloride
	complete upper and lower dentures	CCM	cyclophosphamide, lomustine, and methotrexate
C & C	cold and clammy	CCMSU	clean catch midstream urine
CCA	circumflex coronary artery	CCMU	critical care medicine unit
	common carotid artery	CCNU	lomustine
	concentrated care area	C-collar	cervical collar
CCAP	capsule cartilage articular preservation	CCPD	continuous cycling (cyclical) peritoneal dialysis
CCB	calcium channel blocker(s)	CCR	cardiac catheterization recovery
CCC	Cancer Care Center		continuous complete remission
	child care clinic		
	Comprehensive Cancer Center	C$_{cr}$	creatinine clearance
CC & C	colony count and culture	CCRC	continuing care residential community
CCC-A	Certificate of Clinical Competence in Audiology	CCRN	Certified Critical Care Registered Nurse
CCC-SP	Certificate of Clinical Competence in Speech-Language Pathology	CCRU	critical care recovery unit
		CCT	calcitriol
			closed cerebral trauma
CCD	childhood celiac disease		congenitally corrected transposition (of the great vessels)
CCE	clubbing, cyanosis, and edema		crude coal tar
	countercurrent electrophoresis	CCTGA	congenitally corrected transposition of the great arteries
CCF	compound comminuted fracture	CCT in PET	crude coal tar in petroleum
	crystal-induced chemotactic factor	CCTV	closed circuit television
CCFE	cyclophosphamide, cisplatin, fluorouracil, and estramustine	CCU	coronary care unit
			critical care unit
		CCUA	clean catch urinalysis
		CCUP	colpocystourethropexy

CCW	childcare worker counterclockwise			congenital dislocation of hip
CCX	complications			congenital dysplasia of the hip
CD	cadaver donor	CDK	climatic droplet keratopathy	
	cesarean delivery childhood disease	CDLE	chronic discoid lupus erythematosus	
	character disorder common duct	CDP	Child Development Program	
	communication disorders complicated delivery	CDQ	corrected development quotient	
	continuous drainage convulsive disorder	CDR	continuing disability review	
	Crohn's Disease cytarabine and daunorubicin	CDR(H)	cup-to-disc ratio horizontal	
C/D	cigarettes per day cup to disc ratio	CDR(V)	cup-to-disc ratio vertical	
C&D	curettage and desiccation cytoscopy and dilatation	CDU CDV	chemical dependency unit canine distemper virus	
CDA	chenodeoxycholic acid (chenodiol)	CDX cdyn	chlordiazepoxide dynamic compliance	
	congenital dyserythropoietic anemia	CE	California encephalitis cardiac enlargement	
CDAI	Crohn's Disease Activity Index		cardioesophageal cataract extraction	
CDAK	Cordis Dow Artificial Kidney		central episiotomy community education	
CDB	cough, and deep breath		continuing education	
CDC	calculated day of confinement	C&E	contrast echocardiology consultation and examination	
	cancer detection center carboplatin, doxorubicin, and cyclophosphamide		cough and exercise curettage and electrodesiccation	
	Centers for Disease Control	CEA	carcinoembryonic antigen carotid endarterectomy	
CDCA	chenodeoxycholic acid chenodeoxycholic acid (chenodiol)	CEC	Council for Exceptional Children	
CDD	Certificate of Disability for Discharge	CECT	contrast enhancement computed tomography	
CDDP	cisplatin	CEI	continuous extravascular infusion	
CDE	canine distemper encephalitis	CEL	cardiac exercise laboratory	
	Certified Diabetes Educator	CEO	chief executive officer	
	common duct exploration	CEP	cognitive evoked potential	
CDH	chronic daily headache congenital diaphragmatic hernia		congenital erythropoietic porphyria countercurrent electrophoresis	

CEPH	cephalic		prednisone, and
	cephalosporin		tamoxifen
CEPH FLOC	cephalin flocculation	CFS	cancer family syndrome
			Child and Family Service
CER	conditioned emotional		chronic fatigue syndrome
	response	CFT	complement fixation test
CE&R	central episiotomy &	CF test	complement fixation test
	repair	CFU	colony forming units
CERA	cortical evoked response	CFU-S	colony forming
	audiometry		unit—spleen
CERD	chronic end-stage renal	CG	cholecystogram
	disease		contact guarding
CERULO	ceruloplasmin	CGB	chronic gastrointestinal
CERV	cervical		(tract) bleeding
CES	cognitive environmental	CGD	chronic granulomatous
	stimulation		disease
CEV	cyclophosphamide,	CGI	Clinical Global
	etoposide, and		Impressions (scale)
	vincristine	CGL	chronic granulocytic
CF	calcium leucovorin		leukemia
	(citrovorum factor)		with correction/with
	cancer-free		glasses
	cardiac failure	CGN	chronic glomerulonephri-
	Caucasian female		tis
	cephalothin	CGTT	cortisol glucose tolerance
	Christmas factor		test
	cisplatin and fluorouracil	CH	chest
	complement fixation		chief
	contractile force		child (children)
	count fingers		chronic
	cystic fibrosis		cluster headache
CFA	common femoral artery		congenital hypothyroidism
	complete Freund's		convalescent hospital
	adjuvant		crown-heal
CFAC	complement-fixing	c̄ hold	withhold
	antibody consumption	ch[1]	Christ Church
C-factor	cleverness factor		chromosone
CFF	critical fusion (flicker)	CHAD	cyclophosphamide,
	frequency		adriamycin, cisplatin,
CFL	cisplatin, fluorouracil,		and hexamethyl-
	and leucovorin calcium		melamine
CFM	close fitting mask	CHAI	continuous hepatic artery
	cyclophosphamide,		infusion
	fluorouracil, and	CHAM-OCA	cyclophosphamide,
	citoxantrone		hydroxyurea,
CFNS	chills, fever, and night		dactinomycin,
	sweats		methotrexate,
CFP	cystic fibrosis protein		vincristine, leucovorin,
CFPT	cyclophosphamide,		and doxorubicin
	fluorouracil,	CHAP	child health associate

	practitioner		Breakfast
	cyclophosphamide, hexamethylmelamine, doxorubicin, and cisplatin		crying-induced bronchospasm
			cytomegalic inclusion bodies
CHB	complete heart block	CIBD	chronic inflammatory bowel disease
CH_3- CCNU	semustine	CIBP	chronic intractable benign pain
CHD	center hemodialysis	CIC	circulating immune complexes
	childhood diseases		
	chronic hemodialysis		coronary intensive care
	common hepatic duct	CICE	combined intracapsular cataract extraction
	congenital heart disease		
	coordinate home care		
ChemoRx	chemotherapy	CICU	cardiac intensive care unit
CHF	congestive heart failure	CID	cervical immobilization device
	Crimean hemorrhagic fever		
			cytomegalic inclusion disease
CHFV	combined high frequency of ventilation	CIDP	chronic inflammatory demyelinating polyradineuropathy
CHG	change		
CHI	closed head injury		
	creatinine-height index	CIDS	cellular immunodeficiency syndrome
CHIP	iproplatin		
Chix	chickenpox		continuous insulin delivery system
CHO	carbohydrate		
chol	cholesterol	CIE	counterimmunoelectro-phoresis
CHOP	cyclophosphamide, doxorubicin, vincristine, prednisone		
			crossed immunoelectro-phoresis
CHPX	chickenpox	CIEA	continuous infusion epidural analgesia
chr.	chronic		
CHRS	congenital hereditary retinoschisis	CIEP	counterimmunoelectro-phoresis
CHS	Chediak-Higashi syndrome	CIG	cigarettes
		CIHD	chronic ischemic heart disease
CHU	closed head unit		
CI	cardiac index	CIIA	common internal iliac artery
	cesium implant		
	cochlear implant	CIN	cervical intraepithelial neoplasia
	complete iridectomy		
	coronary insufficiency		chronic interstitial nephritis
Ci	curie(s)		
CIA	chronic idiopathic anhidrosis	CINE	chemotherapy-induced nausea and emesis
			cineangiogram
CIAA	competitive insulin autoantibodies	CIP	Cardiac Injury Panel
CIAED	collagen induced autoimmune ear disease	CIPD	chronic intermittent peritoneal dialysis
CIB	Carnation Instant	Circ	circulation

	circumcision	CLLE	columnar-lined lower esophagus
	circumference	cl liq	clear liquid
circ. & sen.	circulation and sensation	CLO	close
CIS	carcinoma in situ		cod liver oil
CISCA	cisplatin, cyclophospha-mide, and doxorubicin	CL & P	cleft lip & palate
Cis-DDP	cisplatin	CLRO	community leave for reorientation
CIT	conventional immunosuppressive therapy	CLT	chronic lymphocytic thyroiditis
	conventional insulin therapy	CL VOID	clean voided specimen
		clysis	hypodermoclysis
CIU	chronic idiopathic urticaria	cm	centimeter
		CM	capreomycin
CJD	Creutzfeldt-Jakob Disease		cardiac monitor
CK	check		Caucasian male
	creatine kinase		centimeter (cm)
CK-BB	creatine kinase BB band		chondromalacia
CKC	cold knife conization		cochlear microphonics
CK-ISO	creatine kinase isoenzyme		common migraine
CK-MB	creatine kinase MB band		continuous murmur
CK MM	creatine kinase MM band		contrast media
CKW	clockwise		costal margin
Cl	chloride		cow's milk
CL	clear liquid		culture media
	cleft lip		cystic mesothelioma
	cloudy		tomorrow morning (this is a danger abbreviation)
	critical list		
	lung compliance	cm³	cubic centimeter
C_L	compliance of the lungs	CMA	compound myopic astigmatism
CLA	community living arrangements	CMAF	centrifuged microaggre-gate filter
Clav	clavicle	CMBBT	cervical mucous basal body temperature
CLB	chlorambucil		
CLBBB	complete left bundle branch block	CMC	carpal metacarpal (joint)
CLC	cork leather and celastic (orthotic)		carboxymethylcellulose
			chloramphenicol
CL/CP	cleft lip and cleft palate		chronic mucocutaneous candidosis
CLD	chronic liver disease	CMD	cytomegalic disease
	chronic lung disease	CME	cervicomediastinal exploration (examination)
CLE	continuous lumbar epidural (anesthetic)		
CLF	cholesterol-lecithin flocculation		continuing medical education
			cystoid macular edema
CLH	chronic lobular hepatitis	CMER	current medical evidence of record
CLL	chronic lymphocytic leukemia		

CMF	cyclophosphamide, methotrexate and fluorouracil		and vinblastine controlled mechanical ventilation
CMFP	cyclophosphamide, methotrexate, fluorouracil, and prednisone		cool mist vaporizer cytomegalovirus
		CN	cranial nerve tomorrow night (this is a dangerous abbreviation)
CMFVP	cyclophosphamide, methotrexate, fluorouracil, vincristine, and prednisone	Cn	cyanide
		C/N	contrast-to-noise ratio
		CN II–XII	cranial nerves 2–12
		CNA	chart not available
CMG	cystometrogram	CNAG	chronic narrow angle glaucoma
CMGN	chronic membranous glomerulonephritis	CNCbl	cyanocobalamin
CMHC	community mental health center	CND	canned cannot determine
CMHN	Community Mental Health Nurse	CNDC	chronic nonspecific diarrhea of childhood
CMI	cell-mediated immunity Cornell Medical Index	CNE	chronic nervous exhaustion
CMIR	cell-mediated immune response	CNF	cyclophosphamide, mitoxantrone, and fluorouracil
CMJ	carpometacarpal joint		
CMK	congenital multicystic kidney	CNH	central neurogenic hypernea
CML	cell-mediated lympholysis chronic myelogenous leukemia	CNM	certified nurse midwife
		CNN	congenital nevocytic nevus
CMM	cutaneous malignant melanoma	CNOR	Certified Nurse, Operating Room
CMML	chronic myelomacrocytic leukemia	CNRN	Certified Neurosurgical Registered Nurse
CMO	Chief Medical Officer	CNS	central nervous system Clinical Nurse Specialist
CMP	cardiomyopathy chondromalacia patellae	CNT	could not test
CMR	cerebral metabolic rate	CO	carbon monoxide cardiac output castor oil centric occlusion cervical orthosis court order
CMRNG	chromosomally mediated resistant *Neisseria gonorrhoeae*		
$CMRO_2$	cerebral metabolic rate for oxygen	Co	cobalt
CMS	circulation motion sensation	C/O	check out complained of complaints under care of
CMSUA	clean midstream urinalysis		
CMT	cutis marmorata telangiectasia	CO_2	carbon dioxide
CMV	cisplatin, methotrexate,	CoA	coarctation of the aorta

COAD	chronic obstructive airway disease		cyclophosphamide, vincristine, methotrexate, and prednisone
	chronic obstructive arterial disease		
COAG	chronic open angle glaucoma	COMT	catechol-o-methyl transferase
COAGSC	coagulation screen	CON A	concanavalin A
COAP	cyclophosphamide, vincristine, cytarabine, and prednisone	conc.	concentrated
		CONG	congenital
			gallon
COB	cisplatin, vincristine, and bleomycin	CONPA-DRI I	cyclophosphamide, vincristine, doxorubicin, and melphalan
COBS	chronic organic brain syndrome		
COBT	chronic obstruction of biliary tract	CONPA-DRI II	conpadri I plus high-dose methotrexate
COCCIO	coccideimycosis	CONPA-DRI III	conpadri I plus intensified doxorubicin
COD	cause of death		
	codeine	cont	continuous
	condition on discharge		contusions
COD-MD	cerebro-ocular-dysplasia-muscular dystrophy	CONTU	contusion
		COP	cicatricial ocular pemphigoid
CODO	codocytes		colloid osmotic pressure
COEPS	cortically originating extrapyramidal symptoms		cycophosphamide, vincristine, and prednisone
COG	Central Oncology Group		
	cognitive function tests	COPD	chronic obstructive pulmonary disease
COGN	cognition		
COH	carbohydrate	COPE	chronic obstructive pulmonary emphysema
COHB	carboxyhemoglobin		
Coke	Coca-Cola®	COPP	cyclophosphamide, vincristine, procarbazine, and prednisone
	cocaine		
COLD	chronic obstructive lung disease		
COLD A	cold agglutin titer	cor	coronary
Collyr	eye wash	CORT	Certified Operating Room Technician
col/ml	colonies per milliliter		
colp	colporrhaphy	COS	clinically observed seizure
COM	chronic otitis media	COT	content of thought
COMF	comfortable	COTA	Certified Occupational Therapy Assistant
COMLA	cyclophosphamide, vincristine, methotrexate, calcium leucovorin, and cytarabine		
		COTX	cast off to x-ray
		COU	cardiac observation unit
		COX	Coxsackie virus
		CP	centric position
COMP	complications		cerebral palsy
	compound		Certified Paramedic
	compress		chest pain

	chloroquine-primaquine combination tablets
	chondromalacia patella
	chronic pain
	cleft palate
	convenience package
	creatine phosphokinase
	cyclophosphamide and cisplatin
C&P	complete and pushing
	cystoscopy and pyelography
CPA	cardiopulmonary arrest
	carotid photoangiography
	cerebellar pontile angle
	conditioned play audiometry
	costophrenic angle
	cyclophosphamide
CPAF	chlorpropamide-alcohol flush
CPAP	continuous positive airway pressure
CPB	cardiopulmonary bypass
	competitive protein binding
CPBA	competitive protein-binding assay
CPC	cerebral palsy clinic
	chronic passive congestion
	clinicopathologic conference
CPCR	cardiopulmonary-cerebral resuscitation
CPCS	clinical pharmacokinetics consulting service
CPD	cephalopelvic disproportion
	chorioretinopathy and pituitary dysfunction
	chronic peritoneal dialysis
	citrate-phosphate-dextrose
CPDA-1	citrate-phosphate-dextrose-adenine
CPDD	calcium pyrophosphate deposition disease
CPE	cardiogenic pulmonary edema
	chronic pulmonary emphysema
	complete physical examination
CPGN	chronic progressive glomerulonephritis
CPH	chronic persistent hepatitis
CPI	constitutionally psychopathia inferior
CPID	chronic pelvic inflammatory disease
CPIP	chronic pulmonary insufficiency of prematurity
CPK	creatinine phosphokinase (BB, MB, MM are isoenzymes)
CPKD	childhood polycystic kidney disease
CPL	criminal procedure law
CPM	central pontine myelinolysis
	chlorpheniramine maleate
	Clinical Practice Model
	continue present management
	continuous passive motion
	counts per minute
	cyclophosphamide
CPmax	peak serum concentration
CPMDI	computerized pharmacokinetic model-driven drug infusion
CPmin	trough serum concentration
CPMM	constant passive motion machine
CPN	chronic pyelonephritis
CPP	cerebral perfusion pressure
	chronic pelvic pain
CPPB	continuous positive pressure breathing
CPPD	calcium pyrophosphate dihydrate
	cisplatin

CPPV	continuous positive pressure ventilation	CRAO	central retinal artery occlusion
CPR	cardiopulmonary resuscitation	CRBBB	complete right bundle branch block
	tablet (French)	CRC	child-resistant container
CPRAM	controlled partial rebreathing anesthesia method		clinical research center colorectal cancer
		CR & C	closed reduction and cast
CPS	cardiopulmonary support	CrCl	creatinine clearance
	chloroquine-pyremeth-aminesulfadoxine	CRD	childhood rheumatic disease
	clinical pharmacokinetic service		chronic renal disease chronic respiratory disease
	coagulase-positive staphylococci		cone-rod dystrophy congenital rubella deafness
	complex partial seizures		
CPT	chest physio-therapy	CREAT	serum creatinine
	child protection team	CREST	calcinosis, Raynaud's phenomenon, esophageal dysmotility, sclerodactyly, and telangiectasia
CPTH	chronic post-traumatic headache		
CPUE	chest pain of unknown etiology		
CPX	complete physical examination		
		CRF	chronic renal failure corticotropin-releasing factor
CPZ	chlorpromazine Compazine® (this is a dangerous abbreviation)		
		CRI	Cardiac Risk Index
CR	cardiac rehabilitation		catheter-related infection
	cardiorespiratory		chronic renal insufficiency
	case reports		
	chief resident	CRIE	crossed radioimmuno-electrophoresis
	closed reduction		
	colon resection	crit.	hematocrit
	complete remission	CRL	crown rump length
	contact record	CRM +	cross-reacting material positive
	controlled release		
	creamed	CRNA	Certified Registered Nurse Anesthetist
Cr	chromium		
C & R	cystoscopy and retrograde	CRNI	Certified Registered Nurse Intravenous
CR₁	first cranial nerve		
CRA	central retinal artery	CRNP	Certified Registered Nurse Practitioner
	chronic rheumatoid arthritis		
	colorectal anastomosis	CRO	cathode ray oscilloscope
CRAG	cerebral radionuclide angiography	CROS	contralateral routing of signals
CRAMS	Circulation, Respiration, Abdomen, Motor, and Speech	CRP	chronic relapsing pancreatitis coronary rehabilitation program

	C-reactive protein	C/S	cesarean section
CRPD	chronic restrictive pulmonary disease		culture and sensitivity
CRPF	chloroquine-resistant plasmodium falciparum	CSA	controlled substance analogue
CRS	catheter-related sepsis	CsA	cyclosporin
	Chinese restaurant syndrome	CSB	caffeine sodium benzoate
	colon-rectal surgery		Cheyne-Stokes breathing
	congenital rubella syndrome	CSB I & II	Chemistry Screening Batteries I and II
CRST	calcification, Raynaud's phenomenom, scleroderma, and telangiectasia	CSBF	coronary sinus blood flow
		CSC	cornea, sclera, and conjunctiva
CRT	cadaver renal transplant	CSCI	continuous subcutaneous infusion
	cathode ray tube	CSD	cat scratch disease
	central reaction time	C S&D	cleaned, sutured, and dressed
	copper reduction test		
	cranial radiation therapy	CSE	cross-section echocardiography
Cr Tr	crutch training	C sect.	cesarean section
CRTT	Certified Respiratory Therapy Technician	CSF	cerebrospinal fluid
			colony-stimulating factors
CRTX	cast removed take x-ray	CSFP	cerebrospinal fluid pressure
CRU	cardiac rehabilitation unit	C-Sh	chair shower
	clinical research unit	CSH	carotid sinus hypersensitivity
CRV	central retinal vein		
CRVF	congestive right ventricular failure		chronic subdural hematoma
CRVO	central retinal vein occlusion	CSICU	cardiac surgery intensive care unit
CRYST	crystals	CSII	continuous subcutaneous insulin infusion
CS	cat scratch		
	cervical spine	CS IV	clinical stage 4
	cesarean section	CSLU	chronic status leg ulcer
	chest strap	CSM	carotid sinus massage
	cholesterol stone		cerebrospinal meningitis
	cigarette smoker		circulation, sensation, and movement
	clinical stage		
	close supervision	CSME	cotton spot macular edema
	conjunctiva-sclera		
	consciousness	CSNS	carotid sinus nerve stimulation
	Cushing's syndrome		
	cycloserine	CSO	copied standing orders
	consultation	CSOM	chronic serous otitis media
	consultation service		
C&S	conjunctiva and sclera		chronic suppurative otitis media
	culture and sensitivity		

CSP	cellulose sodium phosphate	CT & DB	cough, turn & deep breath
CSR	central supply room	CTD	carpal tunnel decompression
	Cheyne-Strokes respiration		chest tube drainage
	corrective septorhino-plasty		connective tissue disease
CSS	carotid sinus stimulation	CTDW	continues to do well
	chewing, sucking, and swallowing	CTF	Colorado tick fever
		C/TG	cholesterol to triglyceride ratio
CST	cardiac stress test	CTGA	complete transposition of the great arteries
	contraction stress test		
	convulsive shock therapy	CTH	clot to hold
	cosyntropin stimulation test	CTI	certification of terminal illness
	static compliance	CTL	cervical, thoracic, and lumbar
CSU	cardiac surgery unit		
	cardiac surveillance unit		cytotoxic T lymphocytes
	cardiovascular surgery unit	CTM	Chlor-Trimeton®
		CT/MPR	computed tomography with multiplanar reconstructions
	casualty staging unit		
	catheter specimen of urine		
CT	calcitonin	CTN	calcitonin
	cardiothoracic	C & T N, BLE	color and temperature normal, both lower extremities
	carpal tunnel		
	cervical traction		
	chest tube	cTNM	clinical-diagnostic staging of cancer
	circulation time		
	clotting time	CTP	comprehensive treatment plan
	coagulation time		
	coated tablet	CTR	carpal tunnel release
	compressed tablet	CTS	carpal tunnel syndrome
	computed tomography	CTSP	called to see patient
	Coomb's test	CTW	central terminal of Wilson
	corneal thickness	CTX	cyclophosphamide (Cytoxan®)
	corneal transplant		
	corrective therapy	CTXN	contraction
	cytarabine and thioguanine	CTZ	chemoreceptor trigger zone
	cytoxic drug		Co-Trimoxazole (sulfamethoxazole-trimethoprin)
CTA	catamenia (menses)		
	clear to auscultation		
C-TAB	cyanide tablet	Cu	copper
CTAP	computed tomography during arterial portography	CU	cause unknown
		CUC	chronic ulcerative colitis
		CUD	cause undetermined
CTB	ceased to breathe	CUG	cystourethrogram
CTCL	cutaneous T-cell lymphoma	CUP	carcinoma of unknown primary (site)

CUPS	carcinoma of unknown primary site	CVOR	cardiovascular operating room
CUR	curettage	CVP	central venous pressure
CUS	chronic undifferentiated schizophrenia		cyclophosphamide, vincristine and prednisone
	contact urticaria syndrome		
CUSA	Cavitron ultrasonic aspirator	CVPP	lomustine, vinblastine, procarbazine, and prednisone
CUT	chronic undifferentiated type (schizophrenia)	CVR	cerebral vascular resistance
CV	cardiovascular		
	cell volume	CVRI	coronary vascular resistance index
	cisplatin and etoposide		
	color vision	CVS	cardiovascular surgery
	consonant vowel		chorionic villi sampling
CVA	cerebrovascular accident		clean voided specimen
	costovertebral angle	CVSU	cardiovascular specialty unit
CVAH	congenital virilizing adrenal hyperplasia		
		CVUG	cysto-void urethrogram
CVAT	costovertebral angle tenderness	CW	careful watch
			chest wall
CVC	central venous catheter		clockwise
	consonant vowel consonant		compare with
		C/W	consistent with
CVD	collagen vascular disease		crutch walking
CVEB	cisplatin, vinblastine, etoposide, and bleomycin	CWD	cell wall defective
		CWE	cottonwool exudates
		CWMS	color, warmth, movement, and sensation
CVF	cardiovascular failure		
	central visual field		
	cervicovaginal fluid	CWP	childbirth without pain
CVHD	chronic valvular heart disease		coal worker's pneumoconiosis
CVI	carboplatin, etoposide, ifosfamide, and mesna uroprotection	CWS	comfortable walking speed
			cotton wool spots
	cerebrovascular insufficiency	Cx	cancel
			cervix
	continuous venous infusion		culture
			cylinder axis
CVID	common variable immune deficiency	CxMT	cervical motion tenderness
		CXR	chest x-ray
CVN	central venous nutrient	CXTX	cervical traction
CVO	central vein occlusion	CY	cyclophosphamide
	conjugate diameter of pelvic inlet	CyA	cyclosporine
		CyADIC	cyclophosphamide, doxorubicin, and dacarbazine
CvO_2	mixed venous oxygen content		

Cyclo C	cyclocytidine HCl			drug administration
CYL	cylinder			device
CYSTO	cystogram		DAE	diving air embolism
	cystoscopy		DAG	dianhydrogalactitol
CYT	cyclophosphamide		DAH	disordered action of the
CYVA	cyclophosphamide,			heart
DIC	vincristine, adriamycin,		DAI	diffuse axonal injury
	and dacarbazine		DAL	drug analysis laboratory
CZI	crystalline zinc insulin		DAM	diacetylmonoxine
	(regular insulin)		DANA	drug induced antinuclear
CZN	chlorzotocin			antibodies
			DAP	draw a person

D

D	cholecalciferol			diabetes-associated peptide
	daughter		DAR	daily affective rhythm
	day		DARP	drug abuse rehabilitation
	dead			program
	dextrose			drug abuse reporting
	diarrhea			program
	diastole		DAS	developmental apraxia of
	diopter			speech
	distal			died at scene
	divorced		DAT	daunorubicin, cytarabine,
D_1, D_2	dorsal vertebra #1, #2			(ARA-C), and
D50	50% dextrose injection			thioguanine
2/d	twice a day (this is a			dementia of the
	dangerous abbreviation)			Alzheimer type
2 D	two-dimensional			diet as tolerated
3-D	three-dimensional			diphtheria antitoxin
DA	degenerative arthritis			direct agglutination test
	delivery awareness			direct antiglobulin test
	diagnostic arthroscopy		DAW	dispense as written
	direct admission		dB	decibel
	direct agglutination		DB	date of birth
	dopamine			deep breathe
	drug addict			direct bilirubin
	drug aerosol			double blind
D/A	discharge and advise		DB & C	deep breathing and
DA/A	drug/alcohol addiction			coughing
DAB	days after birth		DBD	milolactol (dibromodulici-
DAC	disabled adult child			tol)
	Division of Ambulatory		DBE	deep breathing exercise
	Care		DBED	penicillin G benzathine
DACL	Depression Adjective		DBI®	phenformin HCl
	Checklists		DBIL	direct bilirubin
DACT	dactinomycin		DBP	diastolic blood pressure
DAD	diffuse alveolar damage		DBQ	debrisoquin
	dispense as directed		DBS	diminished breath sounds
			DBZ	dibenzamine

DC	daunorubicin and cytarabine		direct (antiglobulin) Coombs test
	Doctor of Chiropractic	DCTM	delay computer tomographic myelography
D&C	dilation and curettage		
	direct and consensual		
d/c, DC	decrease	DCYS	Department of Children and Youth Services
	diagonal conjugate		
	direct Coombs (test)	DD	dependent drainage
	discharged		dialysis dementia
	discontinue		died of the disease
DC65®	Darvon Compound 65®		differential diagnosis
DCA	sodium dichloroacetate		discharge diagnosis
DCAG	double coronary artery graft		down drain
			dry dressing
DCBE	double contrast barium enema		Duchenne's dystrophy
		D→D	discharge to duty
DCC	day care center	D & D	diarrhea and dehydration
DCCF	dural carotid-cavernous fistula	DDA	dideoxyadenosine
		DDAVP®	desmopressin acetate
DCE	delayed contrast-enhance-ment	DDC	dideoxycytidine
		DDD	defined daily doses
	designated compensable event		degenerative disc disease
			fully automatic pacing
DCFS	Department of Children and Family Services	DDGB	double-dose gallbladder (test)
DCH	delayed cutaneous hypersensitivity	DDHT	double dissociated hypertropia
DCIS	ductal carcinoma *in situ*	DDI	dideoxyinosine
DCMXT	dichloromethotrexate	DDP	cisplatin
DCN	Darvocet N®	DDS	dialysis disequilibrium syndrome
DCNU	chlorozotocin		
DCO	diffusing capacity of carbon monoxide		doctor of dental surgery
			double decidual sac (sign)
DCP®	calcium phosphate, dibasic		4, 4-diaminodiphenyl-sulfone (dapsone)
DCPM	daunorubicin, cytarabine, prednisolone, and mercaptopurine	DDST	Denver Development Screening Test
		DDT	chlorophenothane
DCPN	direction-changing positional nystagmus	DDx	differential diagnosis
		D_5E_{48}	5% Dextrose and Electrolyte 48
DCR	dacryocystorhinostomy		
	delayed cutaneous reaction	D_5E_{75}	5% Dextrose and Electrolyte 75
DCS	decompression sickness	2DE	two dimensional echocardiography
DCSA	double contrast shoulder arthrography		
		D&E	dilation and evacuation
DCT	daunorubicin, cytarabine, and thioguanine	DEA#	Drug Enforcement Administration number
	deep chest therapy		

	(physician's Federal narcotic number)	DFMO	eflornithine (difluoro-methylorithine)
DEC	decrease	DFMR	daily fetal movement record
	diethylcarbamazine		
DECAFS	Department of Children and Family Services	DFO	deferoxamine
		DFOM	deferoxamine
DECEL	deceleration	DFP	diastolic filling period
decub	decubitus		isoflurophate (diisopropyl flurophosphate)
DEET	diethyltoluamide		
DEF	decayed, extracted, or filled	DFR	diabetic floor routine
		DFRC	deglycerolized frozen red cells
	defecation		
	deficiency	DFS	disease-free survival
degen	degenerative	DFU	dead fetus in uterus
del	delivery, delivered	DFW	Dexide face wash
DEP ST SEG	depressed ST segment	DGE	delayed gastric emptying
		DGI	disseminated gonococcal infection
DER	disulfiram-ethanol reaction	DGM	ductal glandular mastectomy
DERM	dermatology		
DES	diethylstilbestrol	DH	delayed hypersensitivity
	diffuse esophageal spasm		dermatitis herpetiformis
	disequilibrium syndrome		developmental history
DESAT	desaturation		diaphragmatic hernia
DET	diethyltryptamine	DHA	dihydroxyacetone
DEV	deviation		docosahexaenoic acid
	duck embryo vaccine	DHAD	mitoxanthrone HCl
DEVR	dominant exudative vitreoretinopathy	DHBV	duck hepatitis B virus
		DHE 45®	dihydroergotamine mesylate
dex.	dexter (right)		
DF	decayed and filled	DHEA	dehydroepiandrosterone
	degree of freedom	DHEAS	dehydroepiandrosterone sulfate
	dengue fever		
	diabetic father	DHF	dengue hemorrhagic fever
	diastolic filling	DHFR	dihydrofolate reductase
	dorsiflexion	DHL	diffuse histocytic lymphoma
	drug free		
	dye free	DHPG	ganciclovir
DFA	diet for age	DHPR	erythrocyte dihydropteri-dine reductase
	difficulty falling asleep		
	direct fluorescent antibody	DHS	Department of Human Services
			duration of hospital stay
DFD	defined formula diets		dynamic hip screw
DFE	distal femoral epiphysis	DHST	delayed hypersensitivity test
DFG	direct forward gaze		
DFI	disease-free interval	DHT	dihydrotachysterol
DFM	decreased fetal movement		dissociated hypertropia
DFMC	daily fetal movement count	DI	(Beck) Depression Inventory

	date of injury	disch.	discharge
	Debrix Index	DISH	diffuse idiopathic skeletal hyperostosis
	detrusor instability		
	diabetes insipidus	D_5ISOM	5% Dextrose and Isolyte M
	diagnostic imaging		
	drug interactions	D_5ISOP	5% Dextrose and Isolyte P
D&I	dry and intact		
diag.	diagnosis	dist.	distal
DIAS BP	diastolic blood pressure		distilled
Diath SW	diathermy short wave	DIT	diiodotyrosine
DIAZ	diazepam		drug-induced thrombocytopenia
DIB	disability insurance benefits		
		DIV	double inlet ventricle
DIC	dacarbazine	DIVA	digital intravenous angiography
	disseminated intravascular coagulation		
		DJD	degenerative joint disease
	drug information center	DK	dark
DID	delayed ischemia deficit		diabetic ketoacidosis
DIE	die in emergency department		diseased kidney
		DKA	diabetic ketoacidosis
DIFF	differential blood count		didn't keep appointment
DIG	digoxin (this is a dangerous abbreviation)	dl	deciliter (100 mL)
		DL	danger list
DIH	died in hospital		deciliter
DIJOA	dominantly inherited juvenile optic atrophy		diagnostic laparoscopy
			direct laryngoscopy
DIL	dilute		drug level
	drug-induced lupus	D_L	maximal diffusing capacity
DILD	diffuse infiltrative lung disease		
		DLB	direct laryngoscopy and bronchoscopy
DILE	drug induced lupus erythematosus		
		DLC	double lumen catheter
DIM	diminish	DLCO sb	diffuse capacity of carbon monoxide, single breath
DIMOAD	diabetes insipidus, diabetes mellitus, optic atrophy, and deafness		
		DLE	discoid lupus erythematosus
DIMS	disorder of initiating and maintaining sleep	DLF	digitalis-like factor
		DLIF	digoxin-like immunoreactive factors
DIP	desquamative interstitial pneumonia		
		DLIS	digoxin-like immunoreactive substance
	distal interphalangeal		
	drip infusion pyelogram	DLMP	date of last menstrual period
	drug-induced parkinsonism		
DIPJ	distal interphalangeal joint	DLNMP	date of last normal menstrual period
DIR	directions		
DIS	Diagnostic Interview Schedule (questionnaire)	D5LR	dextrose 5% in lactated Ringer's injection
		DLS	daily living skills
	dislocation	DM	dermatomyositis

	dextromethorphan	DNKA	did not keep appointment
	diabetes mellitus	DNP	dinitrophenylhydrazine
	diabetic mother		do not publish
	diastolic murmur	DNR	daunorubicin
DMAD	disease-modifying antirheumatic drug		did not respond
			do not report
DMARD	disease modifying antirheumatic drug		do not resuscitate
			dorsal nerve root
DMBA	dimethylbenzantracene	DNS	deviated nasal septum
DMC	dactinomycin, methotrexate, and cyclophosphamide		doctor did not see patient
			do not show
			dysplastic nevus syndrome
DMD	Doctor of Dental Medicine	D_5NSS	5% dextrose in normal saline solution
	Duchenne's muscular dystrophy	DNT	did not test
DME	durable medical equipment	DO	diet order
			distocclusal
DMF	decayed, missing or filled		Doctor of Osteopathy
DMI	desipramine		doctor's order
	diaphragmatic myocardial infarction	D/O	disorder
		DOA	date of admission
DMKA	diabetes mellitus ketoacidosis		dead on arrival
			duration of action
DMO	dimethadone	DOA-DRA	dead on arrival despite resuscitative attempts
DMOOC	diabetes mellitus out of control		
		DOB	dangle out of bed
DMSA	dimercaptosuccinic acid		date of birth
DMSO	dimethyl sulfoxide		dobutamine
DMT	dimethyltryptamine		doctor's order book
DMV	Doctor of Veterinary Medicine	DOC	diabetes out of control
			died of other causes
DMX	diathermy, massage and exercise		drug of choice
		DOCA	desoxycorticosterone acetate
DN	diabetic nephropathy		
	dicrotic notch	DOD	date of death
	down	DOE	dyspnea on exertion
	dysplastic nevus	DOES	disorder of excessive somnolence
D & N	distance and near (vision)		
D_5 1/2NS	dextrose 5% in 0.45% sodium chloride injection	DOH	Department of Health
		DOI	date of injury
		DOL #2	second day of life
DNA	deoxyribonucleic acid	DOLV	double outlet left ventricle
	did not answer	DON	Director of Nursing
	did not attend	DOP	dopamine
	does not apply	DORV	double-outlet right ventricle
DNCB	dinitrochlorobenzene		
DNC	did not come	DORx	date of treatment
DND	died a natural death	DOSS	docusate sodium (dioctyl sodium sulfosuccinate)
DNI	do not intubate		

DOT	date of transcription			diagnostic radiology
	date of transfer			diurnal rhythm
	died on table		DRA	drug-related admissions
	Doppler ophthalmic test		DRE	digital rectal examination
DOX	doxorubicin		DRESS	depth resolved surface
doz	dozen			coil spectroscopy
DP	diastolic pressure		DREZ	dorsal root entry zone
	disability pension		DRG	diagnosis-related groups
	discharge planning		DRGE	drainage
	dorsalis pedis (pulse)		drI	Discharge Readiness
DPA	Department of Public			Index
	Assistance		DRS	Duane's retraction
DPB	days postburn			syndrome
DPC	delayed primary closure		DRSG	dressing
	discharge planning		DRUB	drug screen-blood
	coordinator		DS	deep sleep
DPDL	diffuse poorly			dextrose stick
	differentiated			discharge summary
	lymphocytic lymphoma			disoriented
2,3-DPG	2,3-diphosphoglyceric			double strength
	acid			Down's syndrome
DPH	Department of Public		D/S	5% dextrose and 0.9%
	Health			sodium chloride
	diphenhydramine			injection
	Doctor of Public Health		D&S	diagnostic and surgical
	phenytoin (diphenylhy-			dilation and suction
	dantoin)		D5S	dextrose 5% in 0.9%
DPL	diagnostic peritoneal			sodium chloride
	lavage			(saline)
DPM	distintegrations per		DSA	(angiocardiography)
	minute (dpm)			digital subtraction
	Doctor of Podiatric			angiography
	Medicine		DSD	discharge summary
	drops per minute			dictated
DPT	Demerol®, Phenergan®,			dry sterile dressing
	and Thorazine® (this is		DSDB	direct self-destructive
	a dangerous			behavior
	abbreviation)		dsg	dressing
	diphtheria, pertussis, and		DSI	deep shock insulin
	tetanus (immunization)			Depression Status
	Driver Performance Test			Inventory
DPTPM	diphtheria, pertussis,		DSM	drink skim milk
	tetanus, poliomyelitis,		DSM III	Diagnostic & Statistical
	and measles			Manual, 3rd Edition
DPU	delayed pressure urticaria		DSP	digital signal processor
DPUD	duodenal peptic ulcer		DSRF	drainage subretinal fluid
	disease		DSS	dengue shock syndrome
Dr.	doctor			Disability Status Scale
DR	delivery room			docusate sodium
	diabetic retinopathy		DST	dexamethasone

	suppression test	DV	distance vision
	donor specific transfusion	D&V	diarrhea and vomiting
DSU	day surgery unit	DVA	vindesine
DSV	digital subtraction ventriculography	DVC	direct visualization of vocal cords
DSWI	deep surgical wound infection	DVD	dissociated vertical deviation
DT	delirium tremens	DVI	atrioventricular sequential pacing
	dietetic technician		digital vascular imaging
	diphtheria tetanus	DVIU	direct vision internal urethrotomy
	diphtheria toxoid		
	discharge tomorrow	DVM	Doctor of Veterinary Medicine
D&T	diagnosis and treatment		
DTBC	tubocurarine (d-tubocurarine)	DVP	cyclophosphamide, vincristine, and prednisone
DTC	day treatment center	DVP-Asp	daunorubicin, vincristine, prednisone, and asparaginase
DTD #30	dispense 30 such doses		
DTH	delayed-type hypersensitivity		
DTIC	dacarbazine	DVPA	daunorubicin, vincristine, prednisone, and asparaginase
DTPA	pentetic acid (diethylenetriaminepen- taacetic acid)		
		DVR	Division of Vocational Rehabilitation
DTR	deep tendon reflexes		
DTs	delirium tremens		double valve replacement
DTS	donor specific transfusion	DVSA	digital venous subtraction angiography
DTT	diphtheria tetanus toxoid		
	dithiothreitol	DVT	deep vein thrombosis
DTUS	diathermy, traction, and ultrasound	D$_5$W	5% dextrose (in water) injection
DTV	due to void	DW	deionized water
DTX	detoxification		dextrose in water
DU	diabetic urine		distilled water
	diagnosis undetermined	5 DW	5% dextrose (in water) injection
	duodenal ulcer		
	duroxide uptake	DWDL	diffuse well differentiated lymphocytic lymphoma
DUB	Dubowitz (score)		
	dysfunctional uterine bleeding	DWI	driving while intoxicated
		DWRT	delayed work recall test
DUI	driving under the influence	Dx	diagnosis
		DXM	dexamethasone
DUID	driving under the influence of drugs	DXRT	deep x-ray therapy
		DYF	drag your feet (author's note: see you in court)
DUNHL	diffuse undifferentiated non-Hodgkins lymphoma		
		DZ	diazepam
			disease
DUR	drug use review		dizygotic
	duration		dozen

E

E	edema		extracellular
	engorged		eyes closed
	eosinophil	ECA	ethacrynic acid
	expired		external carotid artery
	eye	ECBD	exploration of common
E2	estradiol		bile duct
E3	estriol	ECC	emergency cardiac care
4E	4 plus edema		endocervical curettage
E →A	say E,E,E, comes out as		external cardiac
	A,A,A upon		compression
	auscultation of lung	ECCE	extracapsular cataract
	showing consolidation		extraction
EA	elbow aspiration	ECD	endocardial cushion
	enteral alimentation		defect
E&A	evaluate and advise	ECEMG	evoked compound
EAA	electrothermal atomic		electromyography
	absorption	ECF	extended care facility
			extracellular fluid
	essential amino acids	ECG	electrocardiogram
EAC	external auditory canal	ECHINO	echinocyte
EACA	aminocaproic acid	ECHO	echocardiogram
EAHF	eczema, allergy, hay, and		enterocytopathogenic
	fever		human orphan (virus)
EAM	external auditory meatus		etoposide, cyclophospha-
EAP	Employment Assistance		mide, Adriamycin®,
	Programs		and vincristine
EAS	external anal sphincter	ECHO/	echocardiography/radionu-
EAST	external rotation,	NV	clide ventriculography
	abduction stress test	ECL	extend of cerebral lesion
EAT	ectopic atrial tachycardia		extracapillary lesions
EAU	experimental autoimmune	ECM	erythema chronicum
	uveitis		migrans
EB	epidermolysis bullosa	ECMO	extracorporeal membrane
	Epstein-Barr		oxygenation
EBA	epidermolysis bullosa		(oxygenator)
	acquisita	ECN	extended care nursery
EBAB	equal breath sounds	ECOG	Eastern Cooperative
	bilaterally		Oncology Group
EBC	esophageal balloon	ECPD	external counterpressure
	catheter		device
EBF	erythroblastosis fetalis	ECR	emergency chemical
EBL	estimated blood loss		restraint
EBM	expressed breast milk	ECRL	extensor carpi radialis
EBS	epidermolysis bullosa		longus
EBV	Epstein-Barr virus	ECS	electrocerebral silence
EC	ejection click	ECT	electroconvulsive therapy
	enteric coated		emission computed
	Escherichia coli		tomography

	enhanced computer tomography		external eye examination
ECU	extensor carpi ulnaris	EEG	electroencephalogram
ECW	extracellular water	EENT	eyes, ears, nose, and throat
ED	elbow disarticulation emergency department epidural	EES®	erythromycin ethylsuccinate
ED$_{50}$	median effective dose	EF	ejection fraction endurance factor extended-field (radiotherapy)
EDAP	Emergency Department Approved for Pediatrics		
EDAX	energy-dispersive analysis of x-rays	EFAD	essential fatty acid deficiency
EDB	ethylene dibromide	EFE	endocardial fibroelastosis
EDC	effective dynamic compliance electrodesiccation and curettage end diastolic counts estimated date of conception estimated date of confinement extensor digitorium communis	EFHBM	eosinophilic fibrohistio-cytic lesion of bone marrow
		EFM	electronic fetal monitor(ing) external fetal monitoring
		EFW	estimated fetal weight
		EF/WM	ejection fraction/wall motion
		e.g.	for example
		EGA	estimated gestational age
EDD	expected date of delivery	EGBUS	external genitalia, Bartholin, urethral, and Skene's glands
EDF	elongation, derotation, and flexion		
EDH	epidural hematoma	EGD	esophagogastroduodenos-copy
EDM	early diastolic murmur		
EDP	emergency department physician end diastolic pressure	EGF	epidermal growth factor
		EGG	electrogastrography
EDR	edrophonium	EGL	eosinophilic granuloma of the lung
EDRF	endothelium derived relaxing factor	EGTA	esophageal gastric tube airway
EDS	Ehlers-Danlos syndrome	EH	educationally handicapped enlarged heart essential hypertension extramedullary hematopoiesis
EDTA	edetic acid (ethylenedini-trilo tetraacetic acid)		
EDV	end-diastolic volume		
EE	end to end equine encephalitis external ear eye and ear	EHDA	etidronate sodium
		EHB	elevate head of bed
		EHE	epithelioid hemangioen-dothelioma
EEA	elemental enteral alimentation end-to-end anastomosis	EHF	epidemic hemorrhagic fever
		EHL	electrohydraulic lithotripsy extensor hallucis longus
EEE	Eastern equine encephalomyelitis edema, erythema, and exudate		
		E & I	endocrine and infertility

EIA	enzyme immunoassay	EMF	erythrocyte maturation
	exercise induced asthma		factor
EIAB	extracranial-intracranial		evaporated milk formula
	arterial bypass	EMG	electromyograph
EIB	exercise induced		emergency
	bronchospasm		essential monoclonal
EID	electroimmunodiffusion		gammopathy
	electronic infusion device	EMIC	emergency maternity and
EIP	end-inspiratory pressure		infant care
EIS	endoscopic injection	E-MICR	electron microscopy
	scleropathy	EMIT	enzyme multiplied
EJ	elbow jerk		immunoassay technique
	external jugular	EMLB	erythromycin lactobionate
EKC	epidemic keratoconjuctivi-	EMMW	extended mandatory
	tis		minute ventilation
EKG	electrocardiogram	EMR	educable mentally
EKO	echoencephalogram		retarded
EKY	electrokymogram		emergency mechanical
E-L	external lids		restraint
ELF	elective low forceps		empty, measure, and
ELH	endolymphatic hydrops		record
ELI	endomyocardial	EMS	early morning stiffness
	lymphocytic infiltrates		emergency medical
ELISA	enzyme-linked		services
	immunosorbent assay		eosinophilia myalgia
Elix	elixir		syndrome
ELLIP	ellipocytosis	EMT	emergency medical
ELOP	estimated length of		technician
	program	EMV	eye, motor, verbal
ELOS	estimated length of stay		(grading for Glasgow
ELP	electrophoresis		coma scale)
ELPS	excessive lateral pressure	EMVC	early mitral valve closure
	syndrome	EMW	electromagnetic waves
ELS	Eaton-Lambert syndrome	EN	enteral nutrition
EM	early memory		erythema nodosum
	ejection murmur	ENA	extractable nuclear
	electron microscope		antigen
	emmetropia	ENC	encourage
	erythema migrans	ENDO	endodontia
	erythema multiforme		endoscopy
	extensive metabolizers		endotracheal
EMA-CO	etoposide, methotrexate,	ENF	Enfamil®
	dactinomycin, and	ENG	electronystagmogram
	leucovorin		engorged
EMB	endometrial biopsy	ENL	erythema nodosum
	endomyocardial biopsy		leprosum
	ethambutol	ENP	extractable nucleoprotein
EMC	encephalomyocarditis	ENT	ears, nose, throat
EMD	electromechanical	EO	elbow orthosis
	dissociation		eosinophilia

	ethylene oxide	EPTS	existed prior to service
	eyes open	ER	emergency room
EOA	esophageal obturator airway		estrogen receptors
			external rotation
	examine, opinion, and advice	E & R	equal and reactive
			examination and report
EOC	enema of choice	ER+	estrogen receptor-positive
EOD	every other day (this is a dangerous abbreviation)	ERA	estrogen receptor assay
			evoked response audiometry
EOG	electro-oculogram	ERCP	endoscopic retrograde cholangiopancreatography
	Ethrane®, oxygen, and gas (nitrous oxide)		
EOM	external otitis media		
	extraocular movement	ERD	early retirement with disability
	extraocular muscles		
EOMI	extraocular muscles intact	ERE	external rotation in extension
EORA	elderly onset rheumatoid arthritis	ERF	external rotation in flexion
eos.	eosinophil		
EP	ectopic pregnancy	ERFC	erythrocyte rosette forming cells
	electrophysiologic		
	elopement precaution	ERG	electroretinogram
	endogenous pyrogen	ERL	effective refractory length
	evoked potentials	ERP	emergency room physician
E&P	estrogen and progesterone		
EPA	eicosapentaenoic acid		endoscopic retrograde pancreatography
EPB	extensor pollicis brevis		
EPC	erosive prepyloric changes		event-related potentials
			estrogen receptor protein
EPF	Enfamil Premature Formula®	ERPF	effective renal plasma flow
EPEG	etoposide	ERT	estrogen replacement therapy
EPI	epinephrine		
	epitheloid cells	ERV	expiratory reserve volume
	exocrine pancreatic insufficiency	ES	emergency service
			end-to-side
EPIS	episiotomy		ex-smoker
epith.	epithelial	ESA	end-to-side anastomosis
EPL	extensor pollicis longus	ESAP	evoked sensory (nerve) action potention
EPM	electronic pacemaker		
EPO	erythropoietin	ESC	end systolic counts
EPP	erythropoietic protoporphyria	ESD	Emergency Services Department
EPR	electrophrenic respiration		esophagus, stomach, and duodenum
	emergency physical restraint	ESF	external skeletal fixation
EPS	electrophysiologic study	ESLD	end-stage liver disease
	extrapyramidal syndrome (symptom)	ESM	ejection systolic murmur
		ESO	esophagus
EPT®	early pregnancy test	ESP	end systolic pressure

	especially	ETP	elective termination of
	extrasensory perception		pregnancy
ESR	erythrocyte sedimentation	ETS	end-to-side
	rate	ETT	endotracheal tube
ESRD	end-stage renal disease		exercise tolerance test
ess.	essential	ETU	emergency and trauma
EST	electroshock therapy		unit
	exercise stress test		emergency treatment unit
ESWL	extracorporeal shockwave	EU	esophageal ulcer
	lithotripsy		etiology unknown
ET	ejection time		excretory urography
	endotracheal	EUA	examine under anesthesia
	enterostomal therapy	EUCD	emotionally unstable
	(therapist)		character disorder
	esotropia	EUG	extrauterine gestation
	essential thrombocythemia	EUM	external urethral meatus
	essential tremor	EUP	extrauterine pregnancy
	eustachian tube	EUS	external urethral sphincter
	exchange transfusion	EV	esophageal varices
	exercise treadmill	EVAC	evacuation
et	and	eval	evaluate
E(T)	intermittent esotropia	EVE	evening
ETA	endotracheal airway	EVS	endoscopic variceal
	ethionamide		sclerosis
et al	and others	ew	elsewhere
ETC	and so forth	EWB	estrogen withdrawal
	estimated time of		bleeding
	conception	EWHO	elbow-wrist-hand orthosis
ETCO₂	end tidal carbon dioxide	EWSCLs	extended-wear soft
ETD	eustachian tube		contact lenses
	dysfunction	EWT	erupted wisdom teeth
ETE	end-to-end	ex	examined
ETF	eustachian tubal function		excision
ETH	elixir terpin hydrate		exercise
	ethanol	exam.	examination
	Ethrane®	EXEF	exercise ejection fraction
ETHc̄C	elixir terpin hydrate with	EXP	experienced
	codeine		exploration
ETI	ejective time index		expose
ETKTM	every test known to man	expect	expectorant
ETO	estimated time of	exp. lap.	exploratory laparotomy
	ovulation	EXT	extension
	ethylene oxide		external
	eustachian tube		extract
	obstruction		extraction
		Ext mon	external monitor
ETOH	alcohol	extrav	extravasation
	alcoholic	ext. rot.	external rotation
ETOP	elective termination of	EXTUB	extubation
	pregnancy	EX U	excretory urogram

F

F	facial
	Fahrenheit
	fair
	fasting
	father
	female
	finger
	firm
	flow
	fluoride
	French
	fundi
F/	full upper denture
/F	full lower denture
(F)	final
F_1	offspring from the first generation
F_2	offspring from the second generation
F II	factor II (two)
F VIII	factor VIII (8)
FA	femoral artery
	folic acid
	forearm
FAAP	family assessment adjustment pass
FAA SOL	formalin, acetic, and alcohol solution
FAAN	Fellow of the American Academy of Nursing
FAAP	Fellow of the American Academy of Pediatrics
FAB	digoxin immune Fab (Digibind®)
	French-American-British Cooperative group
	functional arm brace
FABER	full abduction and external rotation
FABF	femoral artery blood flow
FAC	fluorouracil, Adriamycin®, and cyclophosphamide
	fractional area concentration
FACA	Fellow of the American College of Anaesthetists
FACAG	Fellow of the American College of Angiology
FACAL	Fellow of the American College of Allergists
FACAN	Fellow of the American College of Anesthesiologists
FACAS	Fellow of the American College of Abdominal Surgeons
FACC	Fellow of the American College of Cardiology
FACCP	Fellow of the American College of Chest Physicians
FACCPC	Fellow of the American College of Clinical Pharmacology & Chemotherapy
FACD	Fellow of the American College of Dentists
FACEM	Fellow of the American College of Emergency Medicine
FACEP	Fellow of the American College of Emergency Physicians
FACGE	Fellow of the American College of Gastroenterology
FACH	forceps to after-coming head
FACLM	Fellow of the American College of Legal Medicine
FACN	Fellow of the American College of Nutrition
FACNP	Fellow of the American College of Neuro-psychopharmacology
FACOG	Fellow of the American College of Obstetricians & Gynecologists
FACOS	Fellow of the American College of Orthopedic Surgeons
FACP	Fellow of the American College of Physicians
FACPRM	Fellow of the American

	College of Preventive Medicine	FBH	hydroxybutyric dehydrogenase
FACR	Fellow of the American College of Radiology	FBL	fecal blood loss
		FBRCM	fingerbreadth below right costal margin
FACS	Fellow of the American College of Surgeons	FBS	fasting blood sugar
			fetal bovine serum
FACSM	Fellow of the American College of Sports Medicine	FBU	fingers below umbilicus
		FBW	fasting blood work
FAD	Family Accessment Device	FC	family conference
			febrile convulsions
FAGA	full-term appropriate for gestational age		financial class
			finger clubbing
FAI	functional assessment inventory		finger counting
			flucytosine
FALL	fallopian		foley catheter
FAM	family		foster care
	fluorouracil, Adriamycin, and mitomycin		functional capacity
		5-FC	flucytosine
FAMA	fluorescent antibody to membrane antigen	FC	fever, chills
			finger clubbing
FAME	fluorouracil, doxorubicin, and methyl CCNU		function capacity
			functional class
FANA	fluorescent antinuclear antibody	F + C	flare and cells
		F & C	foam and condom
FAP	familial adenomatous polyposis	F. cath.	foley catheter
		FCC	familial colonic cancer
	familial amyloid polyneuropathy		femoral cerebral catheter
			follicular center cells
	femoral artery pressure		fracture compound comminuted
	fibrillating action potential	FCCL	follicular center cell lymphoma
FAS	fetal alcohol syndrome		
FASHP	Fellow of the American Society of Hospital Pharmacists	FCD	fibrocystic disease
		FCDB	fibrocystic disease of the breast
FAST	fluorescent allergo sorbent technique	FCE	fluorouracil, cisplatin, and etoposide
FAT	fluorescent antibody test	FCH	familial combined hyperlipidemia
FB	fasting blood (sugar)		
	finger breadth	FCHL	familial combined hyperlipemia
	foreign body		
F/B	forward bending	F-CL	fluorouracil and calcium leucovorin
FBC	full blood count		
FBD	fibrocystic breast disease	FCMC	family centered maternity care
	functional bowel disease	FCMD	Fukiyama's congenital muscular dystrophy
FBF	forearm blood flow		
FBG	foreign-body-type granulomata	FCMN	family centered maternity nursing

FCR	flexor carpi radialis	FEM	femoral
FCRB	flexor carpi radialis brevis	Fem-pop	femoral popliteal (bypass)
FCSNVD	fever, chills, sweating, nausea, vomiting, and diarrhea	FEN	fluid, electrolytes, and nutrition
FCU	flexor carpi ulnaris	FENa	fractional extraction of sodium
FD	familial dysautonomia	FEP	free erythrocyte protoporphorin
	fetal demise		
	focal distance	FES	fat embolism syndrome
	forceps delivery		functional electrical stimulation
	full denture		
F & D	fixed and dilated	FeSO$_4$	ferrous sulfate
FDA	Food and Drug Administration	FEUO	for external use only
		FEV$_1$	forced expiratory volume in one second
	fronto-dextra anterior		
FDBL	fecal daily blood loss	FF	fat free
FDG	feeding		fecal frequency
	fluorine-18-labeled deoxyglucose		filtration fraction
			finger to finger
FDGS	feedings		flat feet
FDIU	fetal death in utero		force fluids
FDLMP	first day of last menstrual period		foster father
			fundus firm
FDM	fetus of diabetic mother	F&F	fixes and follows
FDP	fibrin-degradation products	FFA	free fatty acid
		FFB	flexible fiberoptic bronchoscopy
	flexor digitorum profundus		
		FFD	fat-free diet
FDS	flexor digitorum superficialis	FFI	fast food intake
		FFM	fat-free mass
	for duration of stay		five finger movement
Fe	female	FFP	fresh frozen plasma
	iron	FFS	flexible fiberoptic sigmoidoscopy
FEC	fluorouracil, etoposide, and cisplatin		
		FFT	fast-Fourier transforms
	forced expiratory capacity	FFTP	first full-term pregnancy
FECG	fetal electrocardiogram	FG	fibrin glue
FEF	forced expiratory flow rate	FGP	fundic gland polyps
		FH	family history
FEF$_{25\%-75\%}$	forced expiratory flow during the middle half of the forced vital capacity		fetal head
			fetal heart
			fundal height
		FHF	fulminant hepatic failure
FEF$_{x-y}$	forced expiratory flow between two designated volume points in the forced vital capacity	FHH	familial hypocalciuric hypercalcemia
			fetal heart heard
		FHI	Fuch's heterochromic iridocyclitis
FEL	familial erythrophagocytic lymphohistiocytosis		
		FHL	flexor hallucis longus
FeLV	feline leukemia virus	FHNH	fetal heart not heard

FHP	family history positive	F & M	firm and midline (uterus)
FHR	fetal heart rate	FMC	fetal movement count
FHS	fetal heart sounds	FMD	family medical doctor
	fetal hydantoin syndrome		fibromuscular dysplasia
FHT	fetal heart tone		foot and mouth disease
FiCO$_2$	fraction of inspired	FME	full mouth extraction
	carbon dioxide	FMF	familial Mediterranean
FID	father in delivery		fever
FIF	forced inspiratory flow		fetal movement felt
FIGLU	formiminoglutamic acid		forced midexpiratory flow
FIGO	International Federation	FMG	fine mesh gauze
	of Gynecology and		foreign medical graduate
	Obstetrics	FMH	family medical history
FIL	father-in-law		fibromuscular hyperplasia
FIM	functional independence	FML®	fluorometholone
	measure	FMN	first malignant neoplasm
FiO$_2$	fraction of inspired	FMP	fasting metabolic panel
	oxygen		first menstrual period
FIPT	periarteriolar transudate	FMR	fetal movement record
FISP	fast imaging with steady	FMS	fluorouracil, mitomycin,
	state precision		and streptozocin
FITC	fluorescein isothiocynate		full mouth series
FIVC	forced inspiratory vital	FMV	fluorouracil,
	capacity		methyl-CCNU, and
FJROM	full joint range of motion		vincristine
FJS	finger joint size	FMX	full mouth x-ray
FL	fatty liver	FN	false negative
	fetal length		finger-to-nose
	fluid	F to N	finger to nose
	flutamide and leuprolide	FNA	fine-needle aspiration
	acetate	FNAB	fine-needle aspiration
	full liquids		biopsy
FLASH	fast low-angle shot	FNAC	fine-needle aspiratory
FLD	fatty liver disease		cytology
	fluid	FNCJ	fine needle catheter
	flutamide and leuprolide		jejunostomy
	acetate depot	FNF	finger nose finger
FLGA	full-term, large for	FNH	focal nodular hyperplasia
	gestational age	FNR	false negative rate
FLK	funny looking kid (should	FNS	food and nutrition
	never be used: unusual		services
	facial features, is a		functional neuromuscular
	better expression)		stimulation
FLS	flashing lights and/ or	FNT	finger to nose test
	scotoma	FO	foot orthosis
FLU A	influenza A virus		foreign object
FLW	fasting laboratory work		fronto-occipital
FLZ	flurazepam	FOB	father of baby
FM	face mask		fecal occult blood
	fetal movements		feet out of bed

	fiberoptic bronchoscope	FRACTS	fractional urines
	foot of bed	FRC	functional residual capacity
FOBT	fecal occult blood test		
FOC	father of child	FRE	flow-related enhancement
	fluid of choice	FRF	filtration replacement fluid
	fronto-occipital circumference	FRJM	full range of joint movement
FOD	free of disease		
FOEB	feet over edge of bed	FROM	full range of motion
FOG	Fluothane®, oxygen and gas (nitrous oxide)	FS	fingerstick
			flexible sigmoidoscopy
	full-on gain		frozen section
FOI	flight of ideas		full strength
FOM	floor of mouth	F & S	full and soft
FOMi	fluorouracil, Oncovin, (vincristine), and mitomycin	FSALO	Fletcher suite after loading ovoids
		FSALT	Fletcher suite after loading tandem
FOOB	fell out of bed		
FOOSH	fell on outstretched hand	FSB	fetal scalp blood
FOV	field of view	FSBM	full strength breast milk
FP	false positive	FSC	fracture, simple, and complete
	family planning		
	family practice	FSD	fracture, simple, depressed
	flat plate		
	food poisoning	FSE	fetal scalp electrode
	frozen plasma	FSG	focal & segmental glomerulosclerosis
F-P	femoral popliteal		
fpA	fibrinopeptide A	FSGA	full-term, small for gestational age
F.P.A.L.	fullterm, premature, abortion, living		
		FSGS	focal segmental glomerulosclerosis
FPB	flexor pollicis brevis		
FPC	familial polyposis coli	FSH	facioscapulohumeral
	family practice center		follicle stimulating hormone
FPD	feto-pelvic disproportion		
	fixed partial denture	FSHMD	facioscapulohumeral muscular dystrophy
FPG	fasting plasma glucose		
FPHx	family psychiatric history	FSIQ	Full-Scale Intelligence Quotient
FPIA	fluorescence-polarization immunoassay		
		F-SM/C	fungus, smear and culture
FPL	flexor pollicis longus	FSP	fibrin split products
FPM	full passive movements	FSS	French steel sound (dilated to #24FSS)
FPNA	first-pass nuclear angiocardiography		
			full scale score
FPZ	fluphenazine	FSW	field service worker
FPZ-D	fluphenazine decanoate	FT	family therapy
FR	father		filling time
	Father (priest)		finger tip
	flow rate		follow through
	fluid restriction		foot (ft)
F & R	force & rhythm (pulse)		full term

FT$_3$	free triiodorhyroxine		flow volume loop
FT$_4$	free thyroxine	F waves	fibrillatory waves
F$_3$T	trifluridine		flutter waves
FTA	fluorescent titer antibody	FWB	full weight bearing
	fluorescent treponemal antibody	FWW	front wheel walker
		Fx	fractional urine
FTB	fingertip blood		fracture
FTBD	full-term born dead	Fx-dis	fracture-dislocation
FTD	failure to descend	FXN	function
FTE	full-time equivalent	FXR	fracture
FTFTN	finger-to-finger-to-nose	FYI	for your information
FTG	full thickness graft		
FTI	free thyroxine index		

G

G	gallop
	gauge
	good
	grade
	gram (g)
	gravida

FTKA	failed to keep appointment		
FTLB	full-term living birth		
FTLFC	full term living female child		
FTLMC	full term living male child		
FTN	finger-to-nose		
	full term nursery	G +	Gram-positive
FTNB	full-term newborn	G −	Gram-negative
FTND	full-term normal delivery	G1-4	grade 1–4
FTNSD	full-term, normal, spontaneous delivery	G-11	hexachlorophene
		GA	Gamblers Anonymous
FTP	failure to progress		gastric analysis
FTR	for the record		general anesthesia
FTSG	full-thickness skin graft		general appearance
FTT	failure to thrive		gestational age
F & U	flanks and upper quadrants		ginger ale
			glucose/acetone
F/U	follow-up	Ga	gallium
	fundus at umbilicus	GABA	gamma-aminobutyric acid
F ↑U	fingers above umbilicus	GABHS	group A beta hemolytic streptococci
F ↓U	fingers below umbilicus		
5-FU	fluorouracil	GAG	glycosaminoglycan
FUB	function uterine bleeding	Gal	gallon
FUDR®	floxuridine	G'ale	ginger ale
FUN	follow-up note	GALI- PUT	galactose-1-phosphate uridye transferase enzyme
FUNG-C	fungus culture		
FUNG-S	fungus smear		
FUO	fever of undetermined origin	GAS	general adaption syndrome
FUOV	follow-up office visit		Glasgow Assessment Schedule
FUS	fusion		
FV	femoral vein		Global Assessment Scale
FVC	filled voiding flow rate		group *A streptococcus*
	forced vital capacity	Gas Anal F&T	gastric analysis, free and total
FVH	focal vascular headache		
FVL	femoral vein ligation	Ga scan	gallium scan

			gastroenteritis
Gastroc	gastrocnemius		gastroesophageal
GAT	group adjustment therapy	GEN/	general anesthesia with
GATB	General Aptitude Test Battery	ENDO	endotracheal intubation
GAU	geriatric assessment unit	GENT	gentamicin
Gaw	airway conductance	GENTA/P	gentamicin-peak
GB	gallbladder	GENTA/T	gentamicin-trough
G & B	good and bad	GEP	gastroenteropancreatic
GBA	ganglionic-blocking agent	GER	gastroesophageal reflux
GBBS	group B beta hemolytic streptococcus	GERD	gastroesophageal reflux disease
GBE	*Ginkgo biloba* extract	GET	gastric emptying time
GBH	gamma benzene hexachloride (lindane)	GETA	graded exercise test general endotracheal
GBM	glomerular basement membrane	GF	anesthesia gastric fistula
GBMI	guilty but mentally ill		glutenfree
GBP	gastric bypass		grandfather
GBS	gallbladder series	GFAP	glial fibrillary acid protein
	gastric bypass surgery	GFD	gluten-free diet
	group B streptococci	GFM	good fetal movement
	Guillain-Barre syndrome	GFR	glomerular filtration rate
GC	gas chromatography		grunting, flaring, and
	geriatric chair (Gerichair)		retractions
	gonococci (gonorrhea)	GG	gamma globulin
	good condition		guaifenesin
	graham crackers	GGE	generalize glandular
GCI	General Cognitive Index		enlargement
G−C	Gram-negative cocci	GGS	glands, goiter, and
G+C	Gram-positive cocci		stiffness
GCDFP	gross cystic disease fluid protein	GGT	gamma-glutamyl transpeptidase
GCIIS	glucose control insulin infusion system	GGTP	gamma glutamyl transpeptidase
GCM	good central maintained	GH	growth hormone
GCS	Glasgow Coma Scale	GHB	gamma hydroxybutyrate
GCSF	granulocyte colony-stimulating factor	GHb	glycosylated hemoglobin growth hormone
GCT	general care and treatment	GHD	deficiency
	giant cell tumor	GHQ	General Health
GCU	gonococcal urethritis		Questionnaire
GD	Graves' disease	GI	gastrointestinal
Gd	gadolinium		granuloma inguinale
G and D	growth and development	GIB	gastric ileal bypass
GDF	gel diffusion precipitin	GIC	general immunocompetence
GDM	gestational diabetes mellitus	GIDA	Gastrointestinal Diagnostic Area
GE	gainfully employed gastric emptying	GIFT	gamete intrafallopian transfer

GIK	glucose-insulin-potassium	GNR	Gram-negative rods	
ging	gingiva	GnRH	gonadotropin-releasing hormone	
GIP	gastric inhibitory peptide			
	giant cell interstitial pneumonia	GOD	glucose oxidase	
GIS	gas in stomach	GOG	Gynecologic Oncology Group	
	gastrointestinal series	GOK	God only knows	
GIT	gastrointestinal tract	GON	gonococcal ophthalmia neonatorum	
GITS	gastrointestinal therapeutic system	GOO	gastric outlet obstruction	
GITSG	Gastrointestinal Tumor Study Group	GOR	general operating room	
		GOT	glucose oxidase test	
GIWU	gastrointestinal work-up		glutamic-oxaloacetic transaminase (aspartate aminotransferase)	
giv	given			
GJ	gastrojejunostomy			
GL	gastric lavage		goals of treatment	
	greatest length	GP	general practitioner	
GLA	gingivolinguoaxial		Gram-positive	
GLC	gas-liquid chromatography		gutta percha	
		G/P	gravida/para	
GLP	Gambro Liendia Plate	G_4P_{3104}	four pregnancies (gravid), 3 went to term, one premature, no abortion (or miscarriage) and 4 living children (p = para)	
GLU 5	five hour glucose tolerance test			
GLYCOS Hb	glycosylated hemoglobin			
GM	gram			
	grand mal	GPC	giant papillary conjunctivitis	
	grandmother			
GM +	Gram-positive		Gram positive cocci	
GM −	Gram-negative	GPC/TP	glycerylphosphorylcholine to total phosphate	
gm %	grams per 100 milliliters			
GMC	general medical clinic	G6PD	glucose-6-phosphate dehydrogenase	
GM-CSF	granulocyte macrophage colony stimulating factor			
		G-PLT	giant platelets	
GMP	guanosine monophosphate	GPMAL	gravida, para, multiple births, abortions, and live births	
GMS	general medical services			
	Gomori methenamine silver	GPN	graduate practical nurse	
		GPS	Goodpasture's syndrome	
GM&S	general medicine and surgery	GPT	glutamic pyruvic transaminase	
GMTs	geometric mean antibody titers	gr	grain (approximately 60 mg) (this is a dangerous abbreviation)	
GN	glomerulonephritis			
	graduate nurse	G−R	Gram-negative rods	
	Gram negative	G+R	Gram-positive rods	
GNB	Gram-negative bacilli	GRASS	gradient recalled acquisition in a steady state	
GND	Gram-negative diplococci			
GNID	Gram-negative intracellular diplococci	Grav.	gravid (pregnant)	

GRD	gastroesophageal reflux disease	GTT	drop
			glucose tolerance test
GRE	gradient-echo	GTT agar	gelatin-tellurite-tauro-cholate agar
GR-FR	grandfather		
GR-MO	grandmother	GTT3H	glucose tolerence test 3 hours (oral)
GRN	granules		
	green	GTTS	drops
Gr$_1$P$_0$AB$_1$	one pregnancy, no births, and one abortion	GU	genitourinary
		GUS	genitourinary sphincter
GRT	gastric residence time		genitourinary system
	Graduate Respiratory Therapist	GVF	Goldmann visual fields
			good visual fields
GRTT	Graduate Respiratory Therapist Technician	GVHD	graft-versus-host disease
		G/W	glucose water
GS	gallstone	GWA	gunshot wound of the abdomen
	generalized seizure		
	general surgery	GWT	gunshot wound of the throat
	Gram stain		
	grip strength	GXP	graded exercise program
GSD	glucogen storage disease	GZTS	Guilford-Zimmerman Temperament Survey
GSD-1	glycogen storage disease, type 1		
GSE	genital self-examination		
	gluten sensitive enteropathy		

H

	grip strong and equal	H	heart
GSI	genuine stress incontinence		height
			Hemophilis
GSP	general survey panel		heroin
GSPN	greater superficial petrosal neurectomy		hour
			husband
GSR	galvanic skin resistance		hydrogen
GST	gold sodium thiomalate		hyperopia
GSTM	gold sodium thiomalate		hypermetropia
GSW	gunshot wound		hypodermic
GSWA	gunshot wound to abdomen	Ⓗ	hypodermic injection
		H²	hiatal hernia
GT	gait	H₂	hydrogen
	gait training	3H	high, hot, and a helluva lot
	gastrotomy tube		
	group therapy	HA	headache
GTCS	generalized tonic-clonic seizure		hearing aid
			hemadsorption
GTF	gastrostomy tube feedings		hemolytic anemia
GTN	gestational trophoblastic neoplasms		hospital admission
			hyperalimentation
	glomerulo-tubulo-nephritis		hypermetropic astigmatism
GTP	glutamyl transpeptidase		
GTS	Gilles de la Tourette syndrome		hypothalmic amenorrhea
		H/A	head-to-abdomen (ratio)

HAA	hepatitis-associated antigen	HAT	head, arms, and trunk
			hospital arrival time
HACS	hyperactive child syndrome	HAV	hallux abducto valgus
			hepatitis A virus
HAD	human adjuvant disease	HB	heart block
HAE	hearing aid evaluation		heel to buttock
	hepatic artery embolization		hemoglobin (Hb)
			hold breakfast
	hereditary angioedema		housebound
HAGG	hyperimmune antivariola gamma globulin	1 HB	first degree heart block
		HbA₁c	glycosylated hemoglobin
HAI	hemagglutination inhibition assay	HBAC	hyperdynamic beta-adrenergic circulatory
	hepatic arterial infusion		
HAL	hyperalimentation	HBBW	hold breakfast for blood work
HALO	halothane		
HAM	human albumin microspheres	HB core	hepatits B core antigen
		HBD	has been drinking
HAMA	human anti-mouse antibody		hydroxybutyric acid dehydrogenase
HAM-A	Hamilton Anxiety (scale)	HB_e AB	hepatitis B_e antibody
HAM D	Hamilton Depression (scale)	HB_e AG	hepatitis B_e antigen
		HBF	fetal hemoglobin
HAN	heroin associated nephropathy		hepatic blood flow
HANE	hereditary angioneurotic edema	HBGM	home blood glucose monitoring
		HBI	hemibody irradiation
HAP	hospital-acquired pneumonia	HBID	hereditary benign intraepithelial dyskeratosis
HAPC	hospital-acquired penetration contact		
		HBIG	hepatitis B immune globulin
HAPE	high altitude pulmonary edema		
		Hb Kansas	mutant hemoglobin with a low affinity for oxygen
HAPS	hepatic arterial perfusion scintigraphy	HBLV	B-lymphotropic virus human
HAPTO	haptoglobin	HBO	hyperbaric oxygen
HAQ	Headache Assessment Questionnaire	HbO₂	hyperbaric oxygen
			hemoglobin, oxygenated
HAR	high altitude retinopathy	HBOT	hyperbaric oxygen treatment
HARH	high altitude retinal hemorrhage		
		HBP	high blood pressure
HARS	Hamilton Anxiety Rating Scale	HBPM	home blood pressure monitoring
HAS	Hamilton Anxiety (Rating) Scale	HBS	Health Behavior Scale
		HbS	sickle cell hemoglobin
	hyperalimentation solution	HBsAg	hepatitis B surface antigen
HASHD	hypertensive arteriosclerotic heart disease		
		HbSC	sickle cell hemoglobin C

HBSS	Hank's balanced salt solution	HCVD	hypertensive cardiovascular disease
HBV	hepatitis B vaccine	HCWs	health-care workers
	hepatitis B virus	HD	haloperidol decanoate
	honey-bee venom		hearing distance
HBW	high birth weight		heart disease
H/BW	heart-to-body weight (ratio)		heloma durum
			hemodialysis
HC	handicapped		high dose
	head circumference		hip disarticulation
	heel cords		Hodgkin's disease
	Hickman catheter		hospital day
	home care		house dust
	housecall		Huntington's disease
	hydrocortisone	HDAC	high-dose cytarabine
H & C	hot and cold	HDARAC	high dose cytarabine (ARA C)
HCA	health care aide		
H-CAP	hexamethylmelamine, cyclophosphamide, doxorubicin, and cisplatin	HDCV	human diploid cell vaccine
		HDL	high-density lipoprotein
		HDLW	hearing distance for watch in left ear
HCC	hepatocellular carcinoma		
HCD	hydrocolloid dressing	HDMTX	high-dose methotrexate
HCG	human chorionic gonadotropin	HDMTX-CF	high-dose methotrexate and citrovorum factor
HCl	hydrochloric acid	HDMTX /LV	high dose methotrexate and leucovorin
	hydrochloride		
HCL	hairy cell leukemia	HDN	hemolytic disease of the newborn
HCLs	hard contact lenses		
HCM	health care maintenance	HDP	hydroxymethyline diphosphonate
	hypertropic cardiomyopathy		
		HDPAA	heparin-dependent platelet-associated antibody
HCMV	human cytomegalovirus infections		
		HDRS	Hamilton Depression Rating Scale
HCO$_3$	bicarbonate		
HCP	hereditary coporphyria	HDRW	hearing distance for watch in right ear
17-HCS	17-hydroxycorticosteroids		
HCT	hematocrit	HDS	Hamilton Depression (Rating) Scale
	histamine challenge test		
	human chorionic thyrotropin	HDU	hemodialysis unit
		HDV	hepatitis delta virus
	hydrochlorothiazide (this is a dangerous abbreviation)	HE	hard exudate
		H&E	hematoxylin and eosin
	hydrocortisone		hemorrhage and exudate
HCTU	home cervical traction unit		heredity and environment
		HEAT	human erythrocyte agglutination test
HCTZ	hydrochlorothiazide (this is a dangerous abbreviation)		
		HEC	Health Education Center

HEENT	head, eyes, ears, nose, and throat	HFPPV	high-frequency positive pressure ventilation
HEK	human embryonic kidney	HFST	hearing-for-speech test
HEL	human embryonic lung	HFUPR	hourly fetal urine production rate
HELA	Helen Lake (tumor cells)		
HELLP Syndrome	hemolysis, elevated liver enzymes, and low platelet count	HFV	high-frequency ventilation
		HG	hemoglobin
		Hgb	hemoglobin
HEMI	hemiplegia	HGH	human growth hormone
HEMOSID	hemosiderin	HGO	hip guidance orthosis
HEMPAS	hereditary erythrocytic multinuclearity with positive acidified serum test	HGPRT	hypoxanthine-guanine phosphoribosyl-trans-ferase
		HH	hard of hearing
HEMS	helicopter emergency medical services		hiatal hernia
			home health
HEP	heparin		hypogonadotrophic hypogonadism
	hepatic		
	histamine equivalent prick	H&H	hematocrit and hemoglobin
HEPA	hamster egg penetration assay	HHA	hereditary hemolytic anemia
hep cap	heparin cap		home health agency
HERP	human exposure (dose)/rodent potency (dose)	HHC	home health care
		HHD	home hemodialysis
			hypertensive heart disease
HES	hydroxyethyl starch	HHFM	high humidity face mask
	hypereosinophilic syndrome	HHM	humoral hypercalcemia of malignancy
Hex	hexamethylmelamine		
Hexa-CAF	hexamethylmelamine, cyclophosphamide, methotrexate, and fluorouracil	HHN	hand held nebulizer
		HHNC	hyperosmolar hyperglycemic nonketotic coma
HF	hard feces	HHNK	hyperglycemic hyperosmolar nonketotic (coma)
	hay fever		
	head of fetus		
	heart failure	HHS	Health and Human Service (US Department of)
	high frequency		
	house formula		
HFA	health facility administrator	HHT	hereditary hemorrhagic telangiectasis
HFD	high fiber diet	HHTC	high-humidity trach collar
	high forceps delivery	HHTM	high-humidity trach mask
HFHL	high-frequence hearing loss	HI	head injury
			hearing impaired
HFI	hereditary fructose intolerance		hemagglutination inhibition
			hospital insurance
HFJV	high frequency jet ventilation	HIA	hemagglutination inhibition antibody
H flu	Hemophilus influenzae		

5-HIAA	5 hydroxyindoleacetic acid			heparin lock
				Hickman line
HIB	Haemophilus influenzae type b (vaccine)		H&L	heart and lung
hi-cal	high caloric		HLA nega-tive	heart, lungs, and abdomen negative
HID	headache, insomnia, and depression		HLA	human lymphocyte antigen
	herniated intervertebral disc		HLD	haloperidol decanoate
HIDA	hepato-iminodiacetic acid (lidofenin)			herniated lumbar disc
			HLHS	hypoplastic left heart syndrome
HIE	hypoxic-ischemic encephalopathy		HLK	heart, liver, and kidney
HIF	*haemophilus influenzae*		HLT	heart-lung transplantation
	higher integrative functions		HLV	herpes-like virus
				hypoplastic left ventricle
HIHA	high impulsiveness, high anxiety		HM	hand motion
				heart murmur
HIL	hypoxic-ischemic lesion			heavily muscled
HILA	high impulsiveness, low anxiety			hemola molle
				Holter monitor
HIR	head injury routine			human milk
HIS	Hanover Intensive Score			human semisynthetic insulin
	Health Intention Scale		HMA	hemorrhages and microaneurysms
	hospital information system			
HISMS	How I See Myself Scale		HMB	homatropine methylbromide
Histo	histoplasmin skin test		HMBA	hexamethylene bisacetamide
HIT	heparin induced thrombocytopenia			
			HMD	hyaline membrane disease
	histamine inhalation test		HME	heat, massage, and exercise
HIU	head injury unit			
HIV	human immunodeficiency virus		HMDP	hydroxymethyline diphosphonate
			HMETSC	heavy metal screen
HIVD	herniated intervertebral disc		HMG	human menopausal gonadotropin
HJB	Howell-Jolly bodies			
HJR	hepato-jugular reflex		HMG CoA	hepatic hydroxymethyl glutaryl coenzyme A
H-K	hand to knee			
HKAFO	hip-knee-ankle-foot orthosis		HMI	healed myocardial infarction
HKAO	hip-knee-ankle orthosis		HMK	homemaking
HKO	hip-knee orthosis		HMM	hexamethylmelamine
HKS	heel, knee, and shin		HMO	Health Maintenance Organization
HL	hairline			
	half-life		HMP	hexose monophosphate
	hallux limitus			hot moist packs
	haloperidol		HMPAO	hexamethylpropylenamine oxide
	harelip			
	hearing level			

HMR	histocytic medullary reticulosis	HP	hard palate
			hemipelvectomy
HMX	heat massage exercise		hemiplegia
HN	head and neck		hot packs
	head nurse		hydrogen peroxide
	high nitrogen		hydrophilic petrolatum
H&N	head and neck	H&P	history and physical
HNC	hyperosmolar nonketotic coma	HPA	hypothalamic-pituitary-adrenal (axis)
HN₂	mechlorethamine HCl	HPE	history and physical examination
HNKDC	hyperosomolar nonketotic diabetic coma	HPF	high-power field
HNKDS	hyperosomolar nonketotic diabetic state	HPFH	hereditary persistence of fetal hemoglobin
HNLN	hospitalization no longer necessary	HPI	history of present illness
		HPL	human placenta lactogen
HNP	herniated nucleus pulposus	HPLC	high-pressure (performance) liquid chromatography
HNRNA	heterogeneous nuclear ribonucleic acid	HPG	human pituitary gonadotropin
HNS	head and neck surgery head, neck, and shaft	HPL	hyperplexia
HNV	has not voided	HPM	hemiplegic migraine
HO	hand orthosis	HPN	home parenteral nutrition
	Hemotology-Oncology	HPO	hydrophilic ointment
	heterotropic ossification		hypertrophic pulmonary osteoarthropathy
	hip orthosis		
	house officer	HPS	hypertrophic pyloric stenosis
H/O	history of		
H₂O	water	HPT	histamine provocation test
H₂O₂	hydrogen peroxide		hyperparathyroidism
HOA	hip osteoarthritis	hPTH	human parathyroid hormone I₃₄ (teriparatide)
HOB	head of bed		
HOB UPSOB	head of bed up for shortness of breath	HPTM	home prothrombin time monitoring
HOC	Health Officer Certificate	HPV	human papilloma virus
HOCM	high-osmolar contrast media		human parvovirus
		HPZ	high pressure zone
	hypertrophic obstructive cardiomyopathy	HQC	hydroquinone cream
		HR	hallux rigidus
HOG	halothane, oxygen, and gas (nitrous oxide)		Harrington rod
			heart rate
HOH	hard of hearing		hospital record
HOI	hospital onset of infection		hour
HOM	high-osmolar contrast media	H & R	hysterectomy and radiation
HONDA	hypertensive, obese, Negro, diabetic, arthritic	HRA	high right atrium
			histamine releasing activity
HOPI	history of present illness		

HRC	Human Rights Committee	HSSE	high soap suds enema
HRCT	high-resolution computer tomography		histotechnologist
		HSV	herpes simplex virus
HRF	Harris return flow	HSVI	herpes simplex virus type 1
	histamine releasing factor	HT	hammertoe
HRIF	histamine inhibitory releasing factor		hearing test
			heart
HRL	head rotated left		heart transplant
HRLA	human reovirus-like agent		height
HRP	high-risk pregnancy		high temperature
	horseradish peroxidase		hyperthermia
HRR	head rotated right		hubbard tank
HRS	hepatorenal syndrome		hypermetropia
HRT	heart rate		hyperopia
	hormone replacement therapy		hypertension
HS	bedtime	H&T	hospitalization and treatment
	half strength	H(T)	intermittent hypertropia
	hamstrings	5-HT	5-hydroxytryptamine
	Hartman's solution (lactated Ringer's)	ht. aer.	heated aerosol
	heart sounds	HTAT	human tetanus antitoxin
	heavy smoker	HTB	hot tub bath
	heel spur	HTC	hypertensive crisis
	heel stick	HTF	house tube feeding
	hereditary spherocytosis	HTK	heel to knee
	herpes simplex	HTL	hearing threshold level
	high school		human T-cell leukemia
H→S	heel to shin		human thymic leukemia
H&S	hemorrhage and shock	HTLV III	human T cell lymphotrophic virus type III
	hysterectomy and sterilization		
HSA	Health Systems Agency	HTN	hypertension
	human serum albumin	HTP	House-Tree-Person-test
	hypersomnia-sleep apnea	5-HTP	5-hydroxytryptophan
HSBG	heel stick blood gas	HTS	head traumatic syndrome
HSCL	Hopkins Symptom Check List		heel-to-shin
		HTT	hand thrust test
HSE	herpes simplex encephalitis	HTV	herpes-type virus
		HTVD	hypertensive vascular disease
HSG	herpes simplex genitalis	HU	head unit
	histosalpingogram		hydroxyurea
HSL	herpes simplex labialis	HUIFM	human leukocyte interferon meloy
HSM	hepato-splenomegaly		
	holosystolic murmur	HUK	human urinary kallikrein
HSP	Henoch-Schonlein purpura	HUR	hydroxyurea
		HUS	hemolytic uremic syndrome
	hysterosalpingography		
HSR	heated serum reagin		husband

husb	husband	IAC	internal auditory canal
HV	hallux valgus		intra-arterial
	has voided		chemotherapy
	Hemovac®	IAC-CPR	interposed abdominal
	home visit		compressions—cardio-
H&V	hemigastrecomy and		pulmonary resuscitation
	vagotomy	IACP	intra-aortic counterpulsa-
HVA	homovanillic acid		tion
HVGS	high volt galvanic	IADHS	inappropriate antidiuretic
	stimulation		hormone syndrome
HVL	half value layer	IA DSA	intra-arterial subtraction
HW	heparin well		arteriography
	housewife	IAGT	indirect antiglobulin test
hwb	hot water bottle	IAHA	immune adherence
HWFE	housewife		hemagglutination
HWP	hot wet pack	IAI	intra-abdominal infection
Hx	history	IAM	internal auditory meatus
	hospitalization	IAN	intern admission note
HXM	hexamethylmelamine	IAO	immediately after onset
Hy	hypermetropia	IAP	intermittent acute
HYG	hygiene		porphyria
Hyper Al	hyperalimentation	IASD	interatrial septal defect
hypopit	hypopituitarism		immunoaugmentive
Hyst	hysterectomy		therapy
Hz	Hertz	IAT	indirect antiglobulin test
HZ	herpes zoster	IAV	intermittent assist
HZO	herpes zoster		ventilation
	ophthalmicus	IB	ileal bypass
HZV	herpes zoster virus		isolation bed
		IBBB	intra-blood-brain barrier
		IBBBB	incomplete bilateral
			bundle branch block

I

I	impression	IBC	iron binding capacity
	incisal	IBD	inflammatory bowel
	independent		disease
	initial	IBI	intermittent bladder
	inspiration		irrigation
	intact (bag of waters)	*ibid*	at the same place
	intermediate	IBILI	indirect bilirubin
	one	IBNR	incurred but not reported
I_2	iodine	IBOW	intact bag of waters
I^{131}	radioactive iodine	IBRS	Inpatient Behavior Rating
IA	incidental appendectomy		Scale
	intra-amniotic	IBS	irritable bowel syndrome
I & A	irrigation and aspiration	IBU	ibuprofen
IAA	interrupted aortic arch	IBW	ideal body weight
IABC	intra-aortic balloon	IC	between meals
	counterpulsation		immunocompromised
IABP	intra-aortic balloon pump		incomplete
			indirect Coombs (test)

	individual counseling	ICPP	intubated continuous positive pressure
	inspiratory capacity		
	intensive care	ICRF-159	razoxane
	intercostal	ICS	ileocecal sphincter
	intermediate care		intercostal space
	intermittent catheterization	ICSH	interstitial cell-stimulating hormone
	interstitial changes	ICT	icterus
	intracranial		indirect Coombs' test
	irritable colon		inflammation of connective tissue
ICA	intermediate care area		intensive conventional therapy
	internal carotid artery		
	islet-cell antibody		intermittent cervical traction
ICB	intracranial bleeding		
ICBT	intercostobronchial trunk		intracranial tumor
ICC	islet cell carcinoma	ICU	intensive care unit
ICCE	intracapsular cataract extraction		intermediate care unit
		ICV	intracerebroventricular
ICCU	intensive coronary care unit	ICVH	ischemic cerebrovascular headache
	intermediate coronary care unit	ICW	intercellular water
		ID	identification
ICD	instantaneous cardiac death		identify
			ifosfamide, mesna uroprotection, and doxorubicin
	isocitrate dehydrogenase		
ICD 9 CM	International Classification of Diseases, 9th Revision, Clinical Modification		immunodiffusion
			infectious disease (physician or department)
ICDC	implantable cardioverter-defibrillator catheter		initial diagnosis
			initial dose
ICDO	international classification of diseases for oncology		injected dose
			intradermal
ICE	ice, compression, and elevation	id	the same
		I & D	incision and drainage
	individual career exploration	IDA	iron deficiency anemia
ICF	intermediate care facility	IDDM	insulin-dependent diabetes mellitus
	intracellular fluid		
ICG	indocyanine green	IDDS	implantable drug delivery system
ICH	immunocompromised host		
	intracerebral hemorrhage	IDE	Investigational Device Exemption
	intracranial hemorrhage		
ICL	intracorneal lense	IDFC	immature dead female child
ICM	intracostal margin		
ICN	infection control nurse	IDG	interdisciplinary group
	intensive care nursery	IDI	Interpersonal Dependency Inventory
ICP	intracranial pressure		

IDK	internal derangement of knee	IGDE	idiopathic gait disorders of the elderly
IDM	infant of a diabetic mother	IGDM	infant of gestational diabetic mother
IDMC	immature dead male child	IgE	immunoglobulin E
IDR	intradermal reaction	IgG	immunoglobulin G
IDS	infectious disease service	IGIM	immune globulin intramuscular
IDU	idoxuridine		
IDV	intermittent demand ventilation	IGIV	immune globulin intravenous
IDVC	indwelling venous catheter	IgM	immunoglobulin M
		IGR	intrauterine growth retardation
IE	immunoelectrophoresis		
	induced emesis	IGT	impaired glucose tolerance
	inner ear		
	international unit (European abbreviation)	IH	indirect hemagglutination
			infectious hepatitis
i.e.	that is		inguinal hernia
I:E ratio	inspiratory to expiratory time ratio	IHA	immune hemolytic anemia
			indirect hemagglutination
I&E	internal and external	IHC	immobilization hypercalcemia
IEC	inpatient exercise center		
IEF	iso-electric focusing	IHD	intraheptic duct (ule)
IEM	immune electron microscopy		ischemic heart disease
		IHH	idiopathic hypogonadotrophic hypogonadism
IEP	immunoelectrophoresis		
	individualized education program		
		IHS	Indian Health Service
IF	ifosfamide		Iodiopathic Headache Score
	immunofluorescence		
	interferon	IHs	iris hamartomas
	intermaxillary fixation	IHSA	iodinated human serum albumin
	internal fixation		
	intrinsic factor	IHSS	idiopathic hypertrophic subaortic stenosis
	involved field (radiotherapy)		
		IHT	insulin hypoglycemia test
IFA	indirect fluorescent antibody immunofluorescent assay	IHW	inner heel wedge
		IIA	internal iliac artery
		IICP	increased intracranial pressure
IFE	immunofixation electrophoresis		
		IICU	infant intensive care unit
IFM	internal fetal monitoring	IJ	ileojejunal
IFN	interferon		internal jugular
IFOS	ifosfamide	IJD	inflammatory joint disease
IFP	inflammatory fibroid polyps	IJR	idiojunctional rhythm
		IJT	idiojunctional tachycardia
		IJV	internal jugular vein
IgA	immunoglobulin A	IK	immobilized knee
IgD	immunoglobulin D		interstitial keratitis

IL	immature lungs	IMIG	intramuscular
	interleukin (1, 2, and 3)		immunoglobulin
	Intralipid®	IMLC	incomplete mitral leaflet
ILA	indicated low forceps		closure
ILBBB	incomplete left bundle	IMN	internal mammary
	branch block		(lymph) node
ILBW	infant, low birth weight	IMP	impacted
ILD	interstitial lung disease		important
	ischemic leg disease		impression
ILE	infantile lobar emphysema		improved
ILFC	immature living female	IMS	incurred in military
	child		service
ILM	internal limiting	IMT	inspiratory muscle
	membrane		training
ILMC	immature living male	IMV	inferior mesenteric vein
	child		intermittent mandatory
ILMI	inferolateral myocardial		ventilation
	infarct	IMVP-16	ifosfamide, mesna
ILVEN	inflammatory linear		uroprotection,
	verrucal epidermal		methotrexate, and
	nevus		etoposide
IM	infectious mononucleosis	In	inches
	intermetatarsal		indium
	internal medicine	INC	incisal
	intramuscular		incision
IMA	inferior mesenteric artery		incomplete
	internal mammary artery		incontinent
IMAC	ifosfamide, mesna		increase
	uroprotection,		inside-the-needle catheter
	doxorubicin, and	Inc Spir	incentive spirometer
	cisplatin	IND	induced
IMAG	internal mammary artery		Investigational New Drug
	graft		(application)
IMB	intermenstrual bleeding	INDM	infant of nondiabetic
IMC	intramedullary catheter		mother
IMCU	intermediate care unit	INEX	inexperienced
IME	independent medical	INF	infant
	examination		infarction
IMF	ifosfamide, mesna		infected
	uroprotection,		inferior
	methotrexate, and		information
	fluorouracil		infused
	intermaxillary fixation		infusion
IMG	internal medicine group	INFC	infected
	(group practices)		infection
IMH test	indirect microhemaggluti-	ING	inguinal
	nation test	✔ ing	checking
IMI	imipramine	INH	isoniazid
	inferior myocardial	inj	injection
	infarction		injury

INK	injury not known	IPD	immediate pigment darkening
INO	internuclear ophthal-moplegia		inflammatory pelvic disease
INDO	indomethacin		intermittent peritoneal dialysis
inpt	inpatient		interpupillary distance
INS	insurance	IPF	idiopathic pulmonary fibrosis
INST	instrumental delivery		
INT	intermittent needle therapy	IPFD	intrapartum fetal distress
	internal	IPG	impedance plethysmogra-phy
Int mon	internal monitor		individually polymerized grass
INTERP	interpretation		
intol	intolerance	IPH	interphalangeal
int-rot	internal rotation	IPJ	interphalangeal joint
int trx	intermittent traction	IPK	intractable plantar keratosis
intub	intubation		
inver	inversion	IPMI	inferoposterior myocardial infarct
I&O	intake and output		
IO	inferior oblique	IPN	infantile periarteritis nodosa
	initial opening		
	intraocular pressure		intern's progress note
IOC	intern on call	IPOF	immediate postoperative fitting
	intraoperative cholangiogram		
IOCG	intraoperative cholangiogram	IPOP	immediate postoperative prosthesis
IOD	interorbital distance	IPP	inflatable penile prosthesis
IODM	infant of diabetic mother		
IOF	intraocular fluid	IPPA	inspection, palpation, percussion, and auscultation
IOFB	intraocular foreign body		
IOH	idiopathic orthostatic hypotension		
IOI	intraosseous infusion	IPPB	intermittent positive pressure breathing
IOL	intraocular lens		
ION	ischemic optic neuropathy	IPPI	interruption of pregnancy for psychiatric indication
IOP	intraocular pressure		
IORT	intraoperative radiation therapy		
		IPPV	intermittent positive pressure ventilation
IOS	intraoperative sonography	IPS	infundibular pulmonic stenosis
IOV	initial office visit		
IP	incubation period	IPSF	immediate postsurgical fitting
	individualized plan		
	interphalangeal	IPV	inactivated polio vaccine
	intraperitoneal	IPVC	interpolated premature ventricular contraction
IPA	invasive pulmonary aspergillosis		
		IPW	interphalangeal width
	isopropyl alcohol	IQ	intelligence quotient
IPCD	infantile polycystic disease	IR	inferior rectus
			infrared

	internal rotation	ISQ	as before; continue on (*in status quo*)
I&R	insertion and removal		
IRA-EEA	ileorectal anastomoses with end-to-end anastomosis	ISS	Injury Severity Score
		IS10S	10% invert sugar in saline
		IST	insulin sensitivity test
IRB	institutional review board		insulin shock therapy
IRBBB	incomplete right bundle branch block	ISW	interstitial water
		IS10W	10% invert sugar in water
IRBC	immature red blood cell	ISWI	incisional surgical wound infection
IRBP	interphotoreceptor retinoid-binding protein		
		IT	inferior-temporal
IRC	indirect radionuclide cystography		inhalation therapy
			intensive therapy
IRCU	intensive respiratory care unit		intermittent traction
			intertuberous
IRDS	idiopathic respiratory distress syndrome		intrathecal
		ITA	individual treatment assessment
	infant respiratory distress syndrome		
		ITAG	internal thoracic artery graft
IRH	intraretinal hemorrhage		
IRMA	immunoradiometric assay	ITB	iliotibial band
	intraretinal microvascular abnormalities	ITC	Incontinence Treatment Center
IROS	ipsilateral routing of signals	ITCP	idiopathic thrombocytopenia purpura
IRR	intrarenal reflux	ITCU	intensive thoracic cardiovascular unit
irreg	irregular		
IRT	immunoreactive trypsin	ITE	insufficient therapeutic effect
IRV	inspiratory reserve volume		
			in-the-ear (hearing aid)
IS	incentive spirometer	ITGV	intrathoracic gas volume
	induced sputum	ITP	idiopathic thrombocytopenic purpura
	intercostal space		
	inventory of systems		interim treatment plan
	ipecac syrup	ITT	identical twins (raised) together
I/S	instruct/supervise		
ISB	incentive spirometry breathing		insulin tolerance test
		ITVAD	indwelling transcutaneous vascular access device
ISC	isolette servo control		
ISCs	irreversible sickle cells	IU	international unit (this is a dangerous abbreviation as it is read as intravenous)
ISD	inhibited sexual desire		
	initial sleep disturbance		
ISDN	isosorbide dinitrate		
ISG	immune serum globulin	IUC	intrauterine catheter
ISH	isolated systolic hypertension	IUD	intrauterine death
			intrauterine device
ISMA	infantile spinal muscular atrophy	IUDR	idoxuridine
		IUFD	intrauterine fetal death
ISO	isoproterenol		intrauterine fetal distress

IUGR	intrauterine growth retardation	IVLBW	infant of very low birth weight
IUI	intrauterine insemination	IVOX	intravascular oxygenator
IUP	intrauterine pregnancy	IVP	intravenous push
IUPC	intrauterine pressure catheter		intravenous pyelogram
		IVPB	intravenous piggyback
IUPD	intrauterine pregnancy delivered	IVPU	intravenous push
		IVR	idioventricular rhythm
IUP,TBCS	intrauterine pregnancy, term birth, cesarean section	IVS	intraventricular septum irritable voiding syndrome
		IVSD	intraventricular septal defect
IUP,TBLC	intrauterine pregnancy, term birth, living child	IVSE	interventricular septal excursion
IUR	intrauterine retardation	IVSS	intravenous Soluset®
IV	four	IVTTT	intravenous tolbutamide tolerance test
	intravenous (i.v.)		
	symbol for class 4 controlled substances	IVU	intravenous urography
		IWL	insensible water loss
IVA	Intervir-A	IWMI	inferior wall myocardial infarct
IVAP	implantable vascular access device		
		IWML	idiopathic white matter lesion
IVC	inferior vena cava inspiratory vital capacity	IWT	impacted wisdom teeth
	intravenous cholangiogram		
	intraventricular catheter		
IVCD	intraventricular conduction defect		
			J
IVD	intervertebral disk intravenous drip	J	Jewish joint juice
IVDA	intravenous drug abuse		
IVF	*in vitro* fertilization intravenous fluid(s)	JAMG	juvenile autoimmune myasthenia gravis
IVFE	intravenous fat emulsion	JBE	Japanese B encephalitis
IVF-ET	*in vitro* fertilization-embryo transfer	JC	junior clinicians (medical students)
IVFT	intravenous fetal transfusion	JD	jaundice
		JDMS	juvenile dermatomyositis
IVGTT	intravenous glucose tolerance test	JE	Japanese encephalitis
		JER	junctional escape rhythm
IVH	intravenous hyperalimentation	JF	joint fluid
		JFS	Jewish Family Service
	intraventricular hemorrhage	JHR	Jarisch-Herxheimer reaction
IVIG	intravenous immunoglobulin	JI	jejunoileal
		JIB	jejunoileal bypass
IVJC	intervertebral joint complex	JIS	juvenile idiopathic scoliosis
IVL	intravenous lock	JJ	jaw jerk

JLP	juvenile laryngeal papillomatosis	K_3	menadione
JM-9	iproplatin	K_4	menadiol sodium diphosphate
JMS	junior medical student	17K	17-ketosteroids
JND	just noticeable difference	KA	ketoacidosis
jnt	joint	KAB	knowledge, attitude, and behavior
JODM	juvenile onset diabetes mellitus	KABINS	knowledge, attitude, behavior, and improvement in nutritional status
JOMAC	judgment, orientation, memory, affect, and cognition		
JOMACI	judgment, orientation, memory, abstraction, and calculation intact	KAFO	knee-ankle-foot orthosis
		KAO	knee-ankle orthosis
		KAS	Katz Adjustment Scale
JP	Jackson-Pratt (drain) Jobst pump joint protection	KASH	knowledge, abilities, skills, and habits
		K-A units	King-Armstrong units
JPB	junctional premature beats	KC	keratoconjunctivitis knees to chest
JPC	junctional premature contraction	kcal	kilocalorie
JPS	joint position sense	kCi	kilocurie
JPTS	juvenile tropical pancreatitis syndrome	KCl	potassium chloride
		KCS	keratoconjunctivitis sicca
JRA	juvenile rheumatoid arthritis	KD	Kawasaki's disease Keto Diastex® kidney donors knee disarticulation
JRAN	junior resident admission note		
		KDA	known drug allergies
Jr BF	junior baby food	17 Keto	17 ketosteroids
JRC	joint replacement center	KF	kidney function
JT	jejunostomy tube joint	KFAO	knee-foot-ankle orthosis
		KFD	Kyasanur Forrest disease
JTF	jejunostomy tube feeding	KFR	Kayser-Fleischer ring
JTP	joint projection	kg	kilogram
J-Tube	jejunostomy tube	KGC	Keflin®, gentamicin, and carbenicillin
juv.	juvenile		
JVD	jugular venous distention	K24H	potassium, urine 24 hour
JVP	jugular venous pressure jugular venous pulse	KI	karyopyknotic index knee immobilizer potassium iodide
JVPT	jugular venous pulse tracing		
		KID	keratitis, ichthyosis, and deafness (syndrome)
JW	Jehovah's witness		
JXG	juvenile xanthogranuloma	kilo	kilogram
		KISS	saturated solution of potassium iodide
# K		KIT	Kahn intelligence test
K	potassium thousand vitamin K	KJ	kilojoule knee jerk
		KK	knee kick
K_1	phytonadione	KL-BET	Kleihauer-Betke

Kleb	Klebsiella	LA	language age
KLH	keyhole limpet hemocyanin		Latin American
			left atrial
KLS	kidneys, liver, and spleen		left atrium
KM	kanamycin		local anesthesia
$KMnO_4$	potassium permanganate		long acting
KNO	keep needle open	L + A	light and accommodation
KO	keep open		living and active
	knee orthosis	Lab	laboratory
KOH	potassium hydroxide	LAC	laceration
KP	hot pack		long arm cast
	keratoprecipitate	LACT-ART	lactate arterial
Kr	krypton		
KS	Kaposi's sarcoma	LAD	left anterior descending
17-KS	17-ketosteroids		left axis deviation
KSA	knowledge, skills, and abilities	LADCA	left anterior descending coronary artery
KS/OI	Kaposi's sarcoma and opportunistic infections	LADD	left anterior descending diagonal
KT	kidney transplant	LAD-MIN	left axis deviation minimal
KTU	kidney transplant unit		
KUB	kidney, ureter, and bladder	LAE	left atrial enlargement
			long above elbow
KUS	kidney(s), ureter(s), and spleen	LAF	laminar air flow
			Latin-American female
KV	kilovolt		low animal fat
KVO	keep vein open		lymphocyte-activating factor
KVP	kilovolt peak		
KW	Keith-Wagener (ophthalmoscopic finding, graded I-IV)	LAG	lymphangiogram
		LAH	left anterior hemiblock
			left atrial hypertrophy
	Kimmelstiel-Wilson	LAHB	left anterior hemiblock
KWB	Keith, Wagener, Barker	LAK	lymphokine-activated killer
K-wire	Kirschner wire		
		LAL	left axillary line
			limulus amebocyte lysate
	L	LAM	laminectomy
L	fifty		Latin-American male
	left	LANC	long arm navicular cast
	lente insulin	LAN	lymphadenopathy
	lingual	LAO	left anterior oblique
	liter	LAP	laparoscopy
	liver		laparotomy
	lumbar		left arterial pressure
	lung		leucine amino peptidase
Ⓛ	left		leukocyte alkaline phosphatase
$L_1...L_5$	lumbar nerve 1 through 5		
	lumbar vertebra 1 through 5	LAPMS	long arm posterior molded splint

LAPW	left atrial posterior wall	LCA	Leber's congenital amaurosis
LAQ	long arc quad		left coronary artery
LAR	left arm, reclining		left circumflex artery
LAS	laxative abuse syndrome		light contact assist
	leucine acetylsalicylate	LCAT	lecithin cholesterol acyltransferase
	long arm splint	LCB	left costal border
	lymphadenopathy syndrome	LCCA	left common carotid artery
	lymphangioscintigraphy		leukocytoclastic angiitis
L-ASP	asparaginase	LCCS	low cervical cesarean section
LAT	lateral		
	left anterior thigh	LCD	coal tar solution (*liquor carbonis detergens*)
lat.men.	lateral meniscectomy		
LATS	long-acting thyroid stimulator		localized collagen dystrophy
LAV	lymphadenopathy associated virus		low calcium diet
		LCF	left circumflex
LAW	left atrial wall	LCFA	long-chain fatty acid
LB	large bowel	LCFM	left circumflex marginal
	left breast	LCGU	local cerebral glucose utilization
	left buttock		
	live births	LCH	local city hospital
	low back	LCLC	large cell lung carcinoma
	lung biopsy	LCM	left costal margin
	pound		lymphocytic choriomeningitis
L&B	left and below		
LBB	left breast biopsy	LCR	late cortical response
LBBB	left bundle branch block		late cutaneous reaction
LBCD	left border of cardiac dullness	LCS	low constant suction
			low continuous suction
LBD	large bile duct	LCSW	Licensed Clinical Social Worker
	left border dullness		
LBE	long below elbow	LCT	long chain triglyceride
LBH	length, breadth, and height		low cervical transverse
			lymphocytotoxicity
LBM	lean body mass	LCTD	low-calcium test diet
	loose bowel movement	LCV	leucovorin
LBO	large bowel obstruction		low cervical vertical
LBP	low back pain	LCX	left circumflex coronary artery
	low blood pressure		
LBT	low back tenderness	LD	labor and delivery
	low back trouble		lactic dehydrogenase (formerly LDH)
LBV	left brachial vein		
LBW	lean body weight		last dose
	low birth weight		learning disability
LC	leisure counseling		learning disorder
	living children		Legionnaire's disease
	low calorie		lethal dose
	lung cancer		

	levodopa	LEV	levator muscle
	liver disease	LF	Lassa fever
	living donor		left foot
	loading dose		low fat
	longdwell		low forceps
LDB	Legionnaires disease		low frequency
	bacterium	LFA	left femoral artery
LDDS	local dentist		left forearm
LDH	lactic dehydrogenase		left fronto-anterior
LDIH	left direct inguinal hernia		low friction arthroplasty
LDL	low-density lipoprotein	LFC	living female child
L-dopa	levodopa		low fat and cholesterol
LDR	labor, delivery, and	LFD	lactose free diet
	recovery		low fat diet
LDR/P	labor, delivery, recovery,		low fiber diet
	and postpartum		low forceps delivery
LDT	left dorsotransverse	LFL	left frontolateral
LDUB	long double upright brace	LFP	left frontoposterior
LDV	laser Doppler velocimetry	LFS	liver function series
LE	left ear	LFT	latex flocculation test
	left eye		left frontotransverse
	lens extraction		liver function tests
	live embryo	LFU	limit flocculation unit
	lower extremities	LG	large
	lupus erythematosus		laryngectomy
LEA	lumbar epidural		left gluteal
	anesthesia	LGA	large for gestational age
LED	lupus erythematosus		left gastric artery
	disseminatus	LGI	lower gastrointestinal
LEHPZ	lower esophageal high		(series)
	pressure zone	LGL	Lown-Ganong-Levine
LEJ	ligation of the		(syndrome)
	esophagogastric	LGN	lobular glomerulonephritis
	junction	LGV	lymphagranuloma
LEM	lateral eye movements		venerum
	light electron microscope	LH	left hand
LEP	lower esophageal pressure		left hyperphoria
LEP 2	leptospirosis 2		luteinizing hormone
LE prep	lupus erythematosus	LHA	left hepatic artery
	preparation	LHF	left heart failure
L-ERX	leukoerythroblastic	LHG	left hand grip
	reaction	LHH	left homonymous
LES	local excitatory state		hemianopsia
	lower esophageal	LHL	left hemisphere lesions
	sphincter	LHP	left hemiparesis
	lupus erythematosis	LHR	leukocyte histamine
	systemic		release
LESP	lower esophageal	LHRH	luteinizing hormone-
	sphincter pressure		releasing hormone
LET	linear energy transfer		(hypothalamic)

LHS	left hand side		LKKS	liver, kidneys, spleen
LHT	left hypertropia		LKS	liver, kidneys, spleen
LI	lactose intolerance		LKSB	liver, kidneys, spleen, and bladder
	large intestine			
	learning impaired		$\begin{smallmatrix} L & & M \\ K & O & \\ S & & T \end{smallmatrix}$	liver, kidneys, and spleen negative, no masses, or tenderness
Li	lithium			
LIB	left in bottle			
LIC	left iliac crest			
	left internal carotid		LL	large lymphocyte
	leisure interest class			left leg
LICA	left internal carotid artery			left lower
LICD	lower intestinal Crohn's disease			left lung
				lower lid
				lower lip
LICM	left intercostal margin			lower lobe
Li_2CO_3	lithium carbonate			lumbar length
LICS	left intercostal space			lymphocytic leukemia
Lido	lidocaine			lymphoblastic lymphoma
LIF	left iliac fossa		LL2	limb lead two
	liver (migration) inhibitory factor		LLA	limulus lysate assay
			LLB	left lateral border
	left index finger			long leg brace
LIG	ligament		LLC	long leg cast
LIH	left inguinal hernia		LLBCD	left lower border of cardiac dullness
LIHA	low impulsiveness, high anxiety			
			LLD	left lateral decubitus
LILA	low impulsiveness, low anxiety			left length discrepancy
			LLE	left lower extremity
LIMA	left internal mammary artery (graft)		LL-GXT	low-level graded exercise test
LING	lingual		LLL	left lower lid
LIO	left inferior oblique			left lower lobe (lung)
LIP	lithium-induced polydipsia		LLLE	lower lid left eye
			LLLNR	left lower lobe, no rales
	lymphocytic interstitial pneumonia		LLO	Lengionella-like organism
			LLOD	lower lid, right eye
LIQ	liquid		LLOS	lower lid, left eye
	lower inner quadrant		LLQ	left lower quadrant (abdomen)
LIR	left iliac region			
	left inferior rectus		LLR	left lateral rectus
LIS	left intercostal space		LLRE	lower lid, right eye
	low intermittent suction		LLS	lazy leukocyte syndrome
LISS	low ionic strength saline		LLSB	left lower sternal border
LIV	left innominate vein		LLT	left lateral thigh
LIVC	left inferior vena cava		LLWC	long leg walking cast
LIVPRO	liver profile		LLX	left lower extremity
LJM	limited joint mobility		L/M	liters per minute
LK	lamellar keratoplasty		LMA	left mento-anterior
	left kidney			liver membrane autoantibody
LKA	Lazare-Klerman-Armour (Personality Inventory)			

LMB	Laurence-Moon-Biedl syndrome		loss of consciousness
LMC	living male child	LOCM	low-osmolar contrast media
LMCA	left main coronary artery	LOD	line of duty
	left middle cerebral artery	LOIH	left oblique inguinal hernia
LMCAT	left middle cerebral artery thrombosis	LOL	left occipitolateral
LMCL	left midclavicular line		little old lady
LMD	local medical doctor	LOM	left otitis media
	low molecular weight dextran		limitation of motion
			loss of motion
LME	left mediolateral episiotomy		low-osmolar (contrast) media
LMEE	left middle ear exploration	LOMSA	left otitis media, suppurative, acute
LMF	left middle finger	LOMSC	left otitis media, suppurative, chronic
L/min	liters per minute		
LML	left medial lateral	LoNa	low sodium
	left middle lobe	LOP	leave on pass
LMLE	left mediolateral episiotomy		left occiput posterior
		LOQ	lower outer quadrant
LMM	lentigo maligna melanoma	LORS-I	Level of Rehabilitation Scale-I
LMP	last menstrual period	LOS	length of stay
	left mentotoposterior	LOT	left occiput transverse
LMR	left medial rectus		Licensed Occupational Therapist
LMS	lateral medullary syndrome		
LMT	left main trunk	LOV	loss of vision
	left mentotransverse	LOZ	lozenge
LMWD	low molecular weight dextran	LP	light perception
			low protein
LMWH	low molecular weight heparin		lumbar puncture
		L/P	lactate-pyruvate ratio
LN_2	liquid nitrogen	LPA	left pulmonary artery
	lymph nodes	L-PAM	melphalan
LNCs	lymph node cells	LPC	laser photocoagulation
LND	light-near dissociation	LPc̄P	light perception with projection
	lymph node dissection		
LNMP	last normal menstrual period	LPD	low protein diet
			luteal phase defect
LO	lateral oblique (x-ray view)	lpf	low-power field
		LPF	liver plasma flow
	lumber orthosis	LPH	left posterior hemiblock
LOA	leave of absence	LPI	laser peripheral irridectomy
	left occiput anterior		
	lysis of adhesions	LPL	lipoprotein lipase
LOC	laxative of choice	LPM	liters per minute
	level of care	LPN	Licensed Practical Nurse
	level of consciousness	LPO	left posterior oblique
	local		light perception only

LPS	lipopolysaccharide	LSL	left sacrolateral
LR	labor room		left short leg (brace)
	lactated Ringer's (injection)	LSM	late systolic murmur
		LSO	left salpingo-oophorectomy
	lateral rectus		left superior oblique
	left-right		lumbosacral orthosis
	light reflex	LSP	left sacrum posterior
L→R	left to right		liver-specific (membrane) lipoprotein
LR1A	labor room 1A		
LRD	living related donor	L–Spar	Elspar (asparaginase)
	living renal donor	LSR	left superior rectus
LREH	low renin essential hypertension	L/S ratio	lecithin/sphingomyelin ratio
LRF	left rectus femoris	LSS	liver-spleen scan
LRM	left radical mastectomy	LST	left sacrum transverse
LRMP	last regular menstrual period	LSTC	laparoscopic tubal coagulation
LRND	left radical neck dissection	L.S.T.L.	laparoscopic tubal ligation
LRQ	lower right quadrant	L's & T's	lines and tubes
LRS	lactated Ringer's solution	LSV	left subclavian vein
LRT	lower respiratory tract	LSVC	left superior vena cava
LRTI	lower respiratory tract infection	LT	laboratory technician
			left
LRZ	lorazepam		left thigh
LS	left side		leukotrienes
	legally separated		levin tube
	liver scan		light
	liver-spleen		lumbar traction
	low salt	LTA	local tracheal anesthesia
	lumbosacral	LTB	laparoscopic tubal banding
L/S	lecithin-spingomyelin ratio		laryngotracheo-bronchitis
L5-S1	lumbar fifth vertebra to sacral first vertebra	LTB_4	leukotriene B_4
		LTC	left to count
LSA	left sacrum anterior		long-term care
	lipid-bound sialic acid	LTC_4	leukotriene C_4
	lymphosarcoma	LTCF	long-term care facility
LSB	left sternal border	LTCS	low transverse cesarean section
LS BPS	laparoscopic bilateral partial salpingectomy	LTD	largest tumor dimension
LSC	late systolic click	LTG	long-term goal
LSCA	left scapuloanterior	LTGA	left transposition of great artery
LSCP	left scapuloposterior		
LSD	low salt diet	LTL	laparoscopic tubal ligation
	lysergide	LTM	long-term memory
LSE	local side effects	LTOT	long-term oxygen therapy
LSF	low saturated fat	LTS	laparoscopic tubal sterilization
LSKM	liver-spleen-kidney-megalia		
		LTT	lactose tolerance test

	lymphocyte transformation test	LVFP	left ventricular filling pressure
LTV	Luche tumor virus	LVG	left ventrogluteal
LU	living unit	LVH	left ventricular hypertrophy
L & U	lower and upper		
LUA	left upper arm	LVIDd	left ventricle internal dimension diastole
LUE	left upper extremity		
Lues I	primary syphilis	LVIDs	left ventricle internal dimension systole
LUL	left upper lid		
	left upper lobe (lung)	LVL	left vastus lateralis
LUOB	left upper outer buttock	LVMM	left ventricular muscle mass
LUOQ	left upper outer quadrant		
LUQ	left upper quadrant	LVN	Licensed Visiting Nurse
LURD	living unrelated donor		Licensed Vocational Nurse
LUSB	left upper sternal border		
LV	leave	LVOP	left ventricular outflow tract
	left ventricle		
	leucovorin	LVP	large volume parenteral
LVA	left ventricular aneurysm		left ventricular pressure
LVAD	left ventricular assist device	LVPW	left ventricular posterior wall
L-VAM	leuprolide acetate, vinblastine, doxorubicin, and mitomycin	LVR	leucovorin
		LVSEMI	left ventricular subendocardial myocardialischemia
LVAT	left ventricular activation time	LVSP	left ventricular systolic pressure
LVD	left ventricular dysfunction	LVSWI	left ventricular stroke work index
LVDP	left ventricular diastolic pressure	LVV	left ventricular volume
			live varicella vaccine
LVDV	left ventricular diastolic volume	LVW	left ventricular wall
		LVWI	left ventricular work index
LVE	left ventricular enlargement		
LVEDP	left ventricular end diastolic pressure	LVWMA	left ventricular wall motion abnormality
		LVWMI	left ventricular wall motion index
LVEDV	left ventricular end diastolic volume		
		L & W	living and well
LVEF	left ventricular ejection fraction	LWCT	Lee-White clotting time
		LWBS	left without being seen
LVEP	left ventricular end pressure	LWC	leave without consent
		LWP	large whirlpool
LVESVI	left ventricular end-systolic volume index	lx	larynx
			lower extremity
		LXC	laxative of choice
LVET	left ventricular ejection time	LXT	left exotropia
		LYG	lymphmatoid granulomatosis
LVF	left ventricular failure	LYM	lymphocytes

lymphs	lymphocytes		MAB	monoclonal antibody
LYS	lysine		MABP	mean arterial blood pressure
lytes	electrolytes (Na, K, Cl, etc.)		MAAC	no apparent anesthetic complications
			MAC	macrocytic erythrocytes

M

M	male			macula
	marital			maximal allowable concentration
	married			methotrexate, dactinomycin, and cyclophosphamide
	mass			
	medial			
	meta			mid-arm circumference
	meter (m)			minimum alveolar concentration
	million			
	minimum			monitored anesthesia care
	molar		MACC	methotrexate, doxorubicin, cyclophosphamide, and lomustine
	Monday			
	monocytes			
	mother			
	mouth		MACOP-B	methotrexate, doxorubicin, cyclophosphamide, vincristine, prednisone, and bleomycin
	murmur			
	muscle			
	myopia			
	myopic			
	thousand		MACRO	macrocytes
M	murmur		MADRS	Montgomery-Asburg Depression Rating Scale
M_1	first mitral sound			
M1	left mastoid			
M^2	square meters (body surface)		MAE	moves all extremities
			MAEEW	moves all extremities equally well
M2	right mastoid			
M-2	vincristine, carmustine, cyclophosphamide, melphalan, and prednisone		MAEW	moves all extremities well
			MAFAs	movement-associated fetal (heart rate) accelerations
			mag cit	magnesium citrate
MA	machine		mag sulf	magnesium sulfate
	medical assistance		MAHA	macroangiopathic hemolytic anemia
	medical authorization			
	menstrual age		MAI	maximal aggregation index
	mental age			
	Mexican American			minor acute illness
	Miller-Abbott (tube)			*Mycobacterium avium*-intracellulare
	milliamps			
	monoclonal antibodies		MAL	malignant
	motorcycle accident			midaxillary line
M/A	mood and/or affect		malig	malignant
MAA	macroaggregates of albumin		MALT	mucosa-associated lymphoid tissue

MAMC	mid-arm muscle circumference		minimal bacteriocidal concentration
Mammo	mammography	MB-CK	a creatinine kinase isoenzyme
m-AMSA	amsacrine		
Mand	mandibular	MBC	nonbed care
MANOVA	multivariate analysis of variance	MBEST	modulus blipped echo-planar single-pulse technique
MAO	maximum acid output		
MAOI	monoamine oxidase inhibitor	MBD	minimal brain damage minimal brain dysfunction
MAP	mean airway pressure	MBE	medium below elbow
	mean arterial pressure	MBF	meat base formula
	mitomycin, doxorubicin, and cisplatin		myocardial blood flow
		MBFC	medial brachial fascial compartment
MAPS	make a picture story		
	megaloblastic anemia of pregnancy	MBHH	newborn helpful hints
		MBI	methylene blue installation
MAR	medication administration record		
		MBL	menstrual blood loss
MAS	meconium aspiration syndrome	MBM	mothers breast milk
		MBNW	multiple-breath nitrogen washout
	mobile arm support		
MAST	mastectomy	MBO	mesiobuccal occulsion
	military antishock trousers	MC	metatarso - cuneiform
MAT	manual arts therapy		mitoxantrone and cytarabine
	maternal		
	maternity		mixed cellularity
	mature		molluscum contagiosum
	medication administration team		monocomponent highly purified pork insulin
	multifocal atrial tachycardia		mouth care
		m + c	morphine and cocaine
MAVR	mitral and aortic valve replacement	MCA	megestrol, cyclophospha-mide and doxorubicin
max	maxillary		middle cerebral aneurysm
	maximal		middle cerebral artery
MB	buccal margin		monoclonal antibodies
	Mallory body		motorcycle accident
M-BACOD	methotrexate, calcium leucovorin, bleomycin, doxorubicin, cyclophosphamide, vincristine, and dexamethasone		multichannel analyzer
		McB pt	McBurney's point
		MCC	midstream clean-catch
		MCCU	mobile coronary care unit
		MCDT	mast cell degranulation test
MBC	maximum bladder capacity	mcg	microgram (μg)
	maximum breathing capacity	MCGN	minimal-change glomerular nephritis
	methotrexate, bleomycin, and cisplatin	MCH	mean corpuscular hemoglobin

	muscle contraction headache		motor discriminativeacuity
MCHC	mean corpuscular hemoglobin concentration	MDC	medial dorsal cutaneous (nerve)
mCi	millicurie	MDD	major depressive disorder
MCL	medial collateral ligament		manic depressive disorder
	midclavicular line	MDE	major depressive episode
	midcostal line	MDF	myocardial depressant factor
	modified chest lead		
	most comfortable listening level	MDI	manic depressive illness
			metered dose inhaler
MCLNS	mucocutaneous lymph node syndrome		methylenedioxyindenes
			multiple daily injection
			multiple dosage insulin
MCMI	Million Clinical Multiaxial Inventory	MDIA	Mental Development Index, Adjusted
mcmol	micromoles	MDII	multiple daily insulin injection
MCP	metacarpophalangeal joint		
	metoclopramide	MDM	middiastolic murmur
MCS	microculture and sensitivity		minor determinant mix (of penicillin)
MCSA	minimal crosssectional area	MDP	methylene diphosphonate
		MDPI	maximum daily permissible intake
MCT	manual cervical traction		
	mean circulation time	MDR	minimum daily requirement
	medium chain triglyceride		
	medullary carcinoma of the thyroid	MDS	maternal deprivation syndrome
			myelodysplastic syndromes
MCTC	metrizamide computer tomography cisternogram		
		MDT	multidisciplinary team
MCTD	mixed connective tissue disease	MDTM	multidisciplinary team meeting
MCU	micturating cystourethrogram	MDTP	multidisciplinary treatment plan
MCV	mean corpuscular volume	MDUO	myocardial disease of unknown origin
MD	maintenance dialysis		
	major depression	MDV	Marek's disease virus
	mammary dysplasia		multiple dose vial
	manic depression	MDY	month, date, and year
	medical doctor	ME	macula edema
	mediodorsal		manic episode
	mental deficiency		medical examiner
	movement disorder		middle ear
	muscular dystrophy	M/E	myeloid-erythroid (ratio)
MDA	malondialdehyde	MEA-I	multiple endocrine adenomatosis type I
	manual dilation of the anus		
		MEB	methylene blue
	methylenedioxyamphetamine	MEC	meconium
			middle ear canals

MeCCNU	semustine			metabolic
MECG	maternal electrocardio-gram			metastasis
		META		metamyelocytes
MeCP	methyl-CCNU, cyclophosphamide, and prednisone	METHb		methemoglobin
		methyl CCNU		semustine
MED	medial	methyl G		mitroguazone dihydrochloride
	median erythrocyte diameter	methyl GAG		mitroguazone dihydrochloride
	medical	MET		metamyelocytes
	medication	METS		metabolic equivalents (multiples of resting oxygen uptake)
	medicine			
	medium			
	minimum effective dose			metastasis
MEDAC	multiple endocrine deficiency-autoimmune-candidiasis	METT		maximum exercise tolerance test
		MEV		million electron volts
MED-LARS	Medical Literature Analysis and Retrieval System	MEX		Mexican
		MF		Malassezia furfur
				masculinity/femininity
MEE	measured energy expenditure			meat free
	middle ear effusion			methotrexate, fluorouracil and calcium leucovorin
MEF	maximum expired flow rate			midcavity forceps
	middle ear fluid			mycosis fungoides
MEFR	mid expiratory flow rate			myocardial fibrosis
MEFV	maximum expiratory flow-volume	M & F		male and female
				mother and father
MEG	magnetoenephalogram	MFAT		multifocal atrial tachycardia
	magnetoencephalogram			
MEL B	melarsoprol	MFB		metallic foreign body
men	meningeal	MFD		midforceps delivery
	meninges			milk-free diet
	meningitis	MFEM		maximal forced expiratory maneuver
MEN (II)	memory			
	multiple endocrine neoplasia (type II)	MFH		malignant fibrous histiocytoma
MEO	malignant external otitis	MFR		mid-forceps rotation
MEOS	microsomal ethanol oxidizing system	MFT		muscle function test
		MFVNS		middle fossa vestibular nerve section
mEq	milliequivalent			
mEq/24 H	millequivalents per 24 hours	MFVPT		Motor Free Visual Perception Test
mEq/L	milliequivalents per liter	MG		Marcus Gunn
M/E ratio	myeloid/erythroid ratio			milligram (mg)
MEP	meperidine			myasthenia gravis
MES	mesial	Mg		magnesium
MET	medical emergency treatment	mg%		milligrams per 100 milliliters

mg/dl	milligrams per 100 milliliters		malignant hyperthermia susceptible
MGF	maternal grandfather	MHW	medial heel wedge
mg/kg	milligram per kilogram		mental health worker
mg/kg/d	milligram per kilogram per day	MHz	megahertz
		MI	membrane intact
mg/kg/hr	milligram per kilogram per hour		mental illness
			mental institution
MGM	maternal grandmother		mitral insufficiency
	milligram (mg is correct)		myocardial infarction
MGN	membranous glomerulonephritis	MIA	medically indigent adult
			missing in action
MgO	magnesium oxide	MIC	maternal and infant care
MGP	Marcus-Gunn's pupil		medical intensive care
MgSO₄	magnesium sulfate (Epsom salt)		microscope
			microcytic erythrocytes
MGUS	monoclonal gammapathies of undetermined significance		minimum inhibitory concentration
		MICN	mobile intensive care nurse
M-GXT	multi-stage graded exercise test	MICR	methacholine inhalation challenge response
MH	malignant hyperthermia	MICRO	microcytes
	marital history	MICU	medical intensive care unit
	menstrual history		
	mental health		mobile intensive care unit
	moist heat	MID	multi-infarct dementia
MHA	mental health assistant	Mid I	middle insomnia
	microangiopathic hemolytic anemia	MIE	medical improvement expected
	microhemagglutination	MIF	merthiolateiodine-formalin
MHB	maximum hospital benefit		migration inhibitory factor
	methemoglobin	MIFR	mid-inspiratory flow rate
MHBSS	modified Hank's balanced salt solution	MIH	migraine with interparoxysmal headache
MHC	major histocompatibility complex		
		MIL	military
	mental health center		mother-in-law
	mental health counselor	MIN	mineral
M/hct	microhematocrit		minimum
mHg	millimeters of mercury		minor
MHI	Mental Health Index (information)		minute (min)
		MINE	mesna uroprotection, ifosfamide, mitoxantrone, and etoposide
MH/MR	mental health & mental retardation		
MHN	massive hepatic necrosis	MINE	medical improvement not expected
MHRI	Mental Health Research Institute		
		MIO	minimum identifiable odor
MHS	major histocompatibility system		

MIP	maximum inspiratory pressure	MLU	mean length of utterance
	medical improvement possible	MM	malignant melanoma
			Marshall-Marchetti
	metacarpointerphalangeal		medial malleolus
MIRD	Medical Internal Radiation Dose		meningococcic meningitis
			mercaptopurine and methotrexate
MIRP	myocardial infarction rehabilitation program		methadone maintenance
			millimeter (mm)
MIS	mitral insufficiency		morbidity and mortality
MISC	miscarriage		motor meal
	miscellaneous		mucous membrane
MISO	misonidazole		multiple myeloma
MISS	Modified Injury Severity Score (scale)	mM.	millimole
		M&M	milk and molasses
MIT	meconium in trachea		morbidity and mortality
MITO-C	mitomycin	MMA	methylmalonic acid
mix mon	mixed monitor	MMC	mitomycin (mitomycin C)
MJ	marijuana	MMECT	multiple monitor electroconvulsive therapy
	mega joule		
MJT	Mead Johnson tube		
MK-CSF	megakrayocyte colony stimulating-factor	MMEFR	maximal midexpiratory flow rate
MKAB	may keep at bedside	MMF	mean maximum flow
ML	middle lobe	MMFR	maximal mid-expiratory flow rate
	midline		
mL	milliliter	mmHg	millimeters of mercury
M/L	monocyte to lymphocyte (ratio)	MMI	methimazole
		MMK	Marshall-Marchetti-Krantz (cystourethroplexy)
	mother-in-law		
MLA	mentolaeva anterior	MMM	myelofibrosis with mycloid metaplasia
MLC	minimal lethal concentration		
		MMMT	metastatic mixed Müllerian tumor
	mixed lymphocyte culture		
	multi-level care	MMOA	maxillary mandibular odentectomy alveolectomy
	multilumen catheter		
MLD	masking level difference		
	metachromatic leukodystrophy	mmol	millimole
		MMPI	Minnesota Multiphasic Personality Inventory
	minimal lethal dose		
MLE	midline episiotomy	MMPI-D	Minnesota Multiphasic Personality Inventory-Depression Scale
MLF	median longitudinal fasciculus		
MLNS	mucocutaneous lymph node syndrome		
		6-MMPR	6 methylmercaptopurine riboside
MLR	middle latency response		
	mixed lymphocyte reaction	MMR	measles, mumps, and rubella
	multiple logistic regression		midline malignant reticulosis

MMS	Mini-Mental State (examination)	MOFS	multiple-organ failure syndrome
MMT	manual muscle test Mini Mental Test	MOJAC	mood orientation, judgement, affect, and content
MMTP	Methadone Maintenance Treatment Program	MOM	milk of magnesia
MMV	mandatory minute volume		mucoid otitis media
MMWR	Morbidity & Mortality Weekly Report	MON	monitor
MN	midnight	mono.	infectious mononucleosis monocyte
Mn	manganese		monospot
M&N	morning and night	MOP	medical outpatient
MNC	mononuclear leukocytes	MOPP	mechlorethamine, vincristine, procarbazine, and prednisone
M/NCV	motor nerve conduction velocity		
MND	modified neck dissection motoneuron disease	MOPV	monovalent oral poliovirus vaccine
MNG	multinodular goiter	MOR	morphine
MNR	marrow neutrophil reserve	MOS	mirrow optical system
Mn SSEPS	median nerve somato-sensory evoked potentials		months
		mOsm	milliosmole
		mOsmol	milliosmole
MNTB	medial nucleus of the trapezoid body	MOT	motility examination
MO	medial oblique (x-ray view)	MOTT	mycobacteria other than tubercle
	mesio-occlusal	MOUS	multiple occurrences of unexplained symptoms
	mineral oil		
	month (mo)	MOV	multiple oral vitamin
	months old	MP	melphalan and prednisone
	morbidly obese		menstrual period
	mother		mercaptopurine
Mo	molybdenum		metacarpal phalangeal joint
MOA	mechanism of action		
MoAb	monoclonal antibody		moist park
MOB	medical office building		mouthpiece
MOB-PT	mitomycin, vincristine, bleomycin, and cisplatin	4MP4	methylpyrazole
		6-MP	mercaptopurine
MOC	mother of child	MPA	main pulmonary artery medroxyprogesterone acetate
MOD	maturity onset diabetes medical officer of the day mesio-occlusodistal moderate		
		MPAG	McGill Pain Assessment Questionnaire
MODM	mature-onset diabetes mellitus	MPAP	mean pulmonary artery pressure
MODY	maturity onset diabetes of the youth	MPB	male pattern baldness
		MPC	mucopurulent cervicitis
MOF	methotrexate, vincristine, and fluorouracil	MPCN	microscopically positive, and culturally negative

MPD	maximum permissable dose	MRD	margin reflex distance
	multiple personality disorder		Medical Records Department
MPGN	membranoproliferative glomerulonephritis	MRDD	Mental Retardation and Development Disabilities
MPH	Master of Public Health methylphenidate	MRDM	malnutrition-related diabetes mellitus
MPJ	metacarpophalangeal joint	MRE	manual resistance exercise
mpk	milligram per kilogram	MRG	murmurs, rubs, and gallops
MPL	maximum permissable level	MRH	Maddox rod hyperphoria
MPM	Mortality Prediction Model	MRI	magnetic resonance imaging
MPOA	medial preoptic area	MRM	modified radical mastectomy
MPP	massive periretinal proliferation	mRNA	messenger ribonucleic acid
MPQ	McGill Pain Questionnaire	MRS	magnetic resonance spectroscopy
MPPT	methylprednisolone pulse therapy		methicillin resistant *Staphylococcus aureus*
MPS	mucopolysaccharidosis multiphasic screening	MRSA	methicillin-resistant *Staphylococcus aureus*
MPSS	methylprednisolone sodium succinate	MRSE	methicillin-resistant *staphylococcus epidermitis*
MPTR	motor, pain, touch, reflex, and deficit	MS	mass spectroscopy
MPV	mean platelet volume		medical student
MQ	memory quotient		mental status
MR	magnetic resonance		milk shake
	Maddox rod		minimal support
	may repeat		mitral sounds
	measles-rubella		mitral stenosis
	medial rectus		morning stiffness
	medical record		morphine sulfate
	mental retardation		multiple sclerosis
	milliroentgen		muscle strength
	mitral regurgitation		musculoskeletal
	moderate resistance		
M&R	measure and record	M & S	microculture and sensitivity
MR × 1	may repeat times one (once)	MS III	third-year medical student
MRA	main renal artery	MSAF	meconium stained amniotic fluid
	medical record administrator	MSAFP	maternal serum alpha fetoprotein
	mid-right atrium	MSAP	mean systemic arterial pressure
MRAN	medical resident admitting note		
MRAP	mean right atrial pressure	MSBOS	maximum surgical blood order schedule
MRAS	main renal artery stenosis		

MSCA	McCarthy Scales of Children's Abilities	MT		empty
				malaria therapy
MSCU	medical special care unit			malignant teratoma
MSCWP	musculoskeletal chest wall pain			medical technologist
				metatarsal
MSD	microsurgical discectomy			muscles and tendons
	mid-sleep disturbance			music therapy
MSE	Mental Status Examination	M/T		masses of tenderness
				myringotomy with tubes
Msec	milliseconds	M & T		Monilia and Trichomonas
MSEL	myasthenic syndrome of Eaton-Lambert			myringotomy and tubes
		MTAD		tympanic membrane of the left ear
MSER	mean systolic ejection rate	MTAS		tympanic membrane of the left ear
	Mental Status Examination Record	MTAU		tympanic membranes of both ears
MSF	meconium-stained fluid			
	megakaryocyte stimulating factor	MTB		*Mycobacterium tuberculosis*
MSG	methysergide	MTBE		methyl tert-butyl ether
	monosodium glutamate	MTD		Monroe Tidal drainage
MSH	melanocyte-stimulating hormone	MTDI		maximum tolerable daily intake
MSIR®	morphine sulfate immediate release tablets	MTET		modified treadmill exercise testing
		MTG		mid-thigh girth
MSK	medullary sponge kidney	MTI		malignant teratoma intermiate
MSL	midsternal line			
MSLT	multiple sleep latency test	MTM		modified Thayer-Martin medium
MSO₄	morphine sulfate (this is a dangerous abbreviation)	MTP		master treatment plan
				medical termination of pregnancy
MSPN	medical student progress notes			metatarsal phalangeal
MSPU	medical short procedure unit	MTR-O		no masses, tenderness, or rebound
MSR	muscle stretch reflexes	MTRS		Licensed Master Therapeutic Recreation Specialist
MSS	Marital Satisfaction Scale			
	minor surgery suite			
	muscular subaortic stenosis	MTST		maximal treadmill stress test
MST	mean survival time	MTU		malignant teratoma undifferentiated
MSTA®	mumps skin test antigen			methylthiouracil
MSTI	multiple soft tissue injuries	MTX		methotrexate
		MTZ		mitoxantrone
MSU	maple syrup urine	MU		million units
	midstream urine	mU		milliunits
MSUD	maple-syrup urine disease	MUAC		middle upper arm circumference
MSW	Master of Social Work			
	multiple stab wounds			

MUGA	multiple gated acquisition		motor, vascular, and
MUGX	multiple gated acquisition		sensory
	exercise	MVV	maximum voluntary
mus-lig	musculoligamentous		ventilation
MUU	mouse uterine units		mixed vespid venom
MV	mechanical ventilation	MWD	microwave diathermy
	millivolts	MWI	Medical Walk-In (Clinic)
	minute volume	MWS	Mickety-Wilson syndrome
	mitoxantrone and	MWT	malpositioned wisdom
	etoposide		teeth
	mitral valve	Mx	myringotomy
	mixed venous	My	myopia
	multivesicular	myelo	myelocytes
MVA	malignant vertricular		myelogram
	arrhythmias	MYD	mydriatic
	mitral valve area	MyG	myasthenia gravis
	motor vehicle accident	MZ	monozygotic
M-VAC	methotrexate, vinblastine,	MZL	marginal zone lymphocyte
	doxorubicin, and		
	cisplatin		
MVAC	methotrexate, vinblastine,		**N**
	doxorubicin, and		
	cisplatin	N	negative
MVB	mixed venous blood		Negro
MVC	maximal voluntary		nerve
	contraction		never
MVD	microvascular		no
	decompression		nodes
	mitral valve disease		normal
	multivessel disease		not
MVE	mitral valve (leaflet)		noun
	excursion		NPH insulin
MVI	multiple vitamin injection		size of sample
MVI®	trade name for parenteral	N_2	nitrogen
	multivitamins	5'-N	5'-Nucleotidase
MVI 12®	trade name for parenteral	Na	sodium
	multivitamins	NA	Native American
MVO_2	myocardial oxygen		Narcotics Anonymous
	consumption		Negro adult
MVP	mean venous pressure		nicotinic acid
	mitral valve prolapse		not admitted
MVPP	mechlorethamine,		not applicable
	vinblastine,		not available
	procarbazine, and		nurse aide
	prednisone		Nurse Anesthetist
MVR	massive vitreous		nursing assistant
	retraction	N & A	normal and active
	mitral valve regurgitation	NAA	neutron activation
	mitral valve replacement		analysis
MVS	mitral valve stenosis		no apparent abnormalities

NABS	normoactive bowel sounds		normal bowel movement
			nothing by mouth
NaClO	sodium hypochlorite	NBN	newborn nursery
NaCl	sodium chloride (salt)	NBP	needle biopsy of prostate
NAD	no active disease	NBQC	narrow base quad cane
	no acute distress	NBS	newborn screen (serum thyroxine and phenylketonuria)
	no apparent distress		
	no appreciable disease		
	normal axis deviation		no bacteria seen
	nothing abnormal detected		normal bowel sound
NADPH	nicotinamide adenine dinucleotide phosphate	NBT	nitroblue tetrazolium reduction (tests)
NADSIC	no apparent disease seen in chest	NBTE	nonbacterial thrombotic endocarditis
NaF	sodium fluoride	NBTNF	newborn, term, normal female
NAF	nafcillin		
	Negro adult female	NBTNM	newborn, term, normal, male
NAG	narrow angle glaucoma		
NaHCO₃	sodium bicarbonate	NC	nasal cannula
NAI	no acute inflammation		Negro child
	non-accidental injury		neurologic check
NaI	sodium iodide		no change
NANB	non-A, non-B (hepatitis)		no charge
NAP	narrative, assessment, and plan		no complaints
			noncontributory
NAPA	N-acetyl procainamide		nose clips
NAPD	no active pulmonary disease		not completed
			not cultured
Na Pent	Pentothal Sodium®	NCA	neurocirculatory asthenia
NAR	not at risk		no congenital abnormalities
NARC	narcotic(s)		
NAS	nasal	NCAS	neocarzinostatin
	neonatal abstinence syndrome	NC/AT	normal cephalic atraumatic
	no added salt	NCB	no code blue
NAT	no action taken	NCC	no concentrated carbohydrates
NB	nail bed		
	needle biopsy	NCD	normal childhood diseases
	newborn		not considered disabling
	nitrogen balance	NCF	neutrophilic chemotactic factor
	note well		
NBD	neurologic bladder dysfunction	NCI	National Cancer Institute
		NCJ	needle catheter jejunostomy
	no brain damage		
NBF	not breast fed	NCL	neuronal ceroid lipofuscinosis
NBI	no bone injury		
NBICU	newborn intensive care unit		nuclear cardiology laboratory
NBM	no bowel movement	NCM	nailfold capillary microscope
	normal bone marrow		

NCNC	normochromic, normocytic		norepinephrine
NCO	no complaints offered		not elevated
	non-commissioned officer	NEC	not examined
NCP	nursing care plan		necrotizing entercolitis
NCPAP	nasal continuous positive airway pressure	NED	not elsewhere classified
		NEEP	no evidence of disease
NCPR	no cardiopulmonary resuscitation		negative end-expiratory pressure
NCRC	non-child resistant container	NEF	negative expiratory force
		NEFA	non-esterified fatty acids
NCS	nerve conduction studies	NEG	negative
	no concentrated sweets		neglect
	zinostatis (neocarzinosta-tin)	NEPHRO	nephrogram
		NEM	no evidence of malignancy
NCT	neutron capture therapy	NEMD	nonspecific esophageal motility disorder
	noncontact tonometry		
NCV	nerve conduction velocity	NEOH	neonatal high risk
ND	nasal deformity	NEOM	neonatal medium risk
	natural death	NEP	no evidence of pathology
	neurological development	NER	no evidence of recurrence
	no disease	NERD	no evidence of recurrent disease
	nondisabling		
	none detectable	NES	not elsewhere specified
	normal delivery	NET	naso-endotracheal tube
	normal development	NETT	nasal endotracheal tube
	nose drops	NEX	nose to ear to xiphoid
	not diagnosed	NF	Negro female
	not done		neurofibromatosis
	nothing done		none found
N&D	nodular and diffuse		not found
Nd	neodymium		nursed fair
NDA	New Drug Application	NFD	no family doctor
	no data available	NFL	nerve fiber layer
	no detectable activity	NFP	no family physician
NDD	no dialysis days	NFTD	normal full term delivery
NDI	neurogenic diabetes insipidus	NFTSD	normal full-term spontaneous delivery
Nd/NT	nondistended, nontender	NFTT	nonorganic failure to thrive
NDP	net dietary protein		
NDR	neurotic depressive reaction	NFW	nursed fairly well
		NG	nanogram
	normal detrusor reflex		nasogastric
NDT	neurodevelopmental treatment		nitroglycerin
			no growth
	noise detection threshold	NGB	neurogenic bladder
NDV	Newcastle disease virus	NGF	nerve growth factor
NE	never exposed	n giv	not given
	no effect	NGR	nasogastric replacement
	no enlargement		

NGRI	not guilty by reason of insanity	NINU	neuro intermediate nursing unit
NGT	nasogastric tube	NINVS	non-invasive
	normal glucose tolerance		neurovascular studies
NGU	nongonococcal urethritis	NIP	no infection present
NH	nursing home		no inflammation present
NHC	neighborhood health center	Nitro	nitroglycerin (this is a dangerous abbreviation)
	neonatal hypocalcemia		sodium nitroprusside
	nursing home care	NJ	nasojejunal
NH_3	ammonia	NK	natural killer (cells)
NH_4Cl	ammonium chloride		not known
NHCU	nursing home care unit	NKA	no known allergies
NHD	normal hair distribution	NKC	nonketotic coma
NHL	nodular histiocytic lymphoma	NKDA	no known drug allergies
		NKFA	no known food allergies
	non-Hodgkin's lymphomas	NKHA	nonketotic hyperosmolar acidosis
nHL	normalized hearing level	NKHS	nonketotic hyperosmolar syndrome
NHP	nursing home placement		
NI	neurological improvement	NKMA	no known medication allergies
	no information		
	not identified	NL	nasolacrimal
	not isolated		normal
NIA	no information available	NLB	needle liver biopsy
NIAL	not in active labor	NLC & C	normal libido, coitus, and climax
NICC	neonatal intensive care center		
		NLD	nasolacrimal duct
NICU	neonatal intensive care unit		necrobiosis lipoidica diabeticorum
	neurosurgical intensive care unit	NLE	nursing late entry
		NLF	nasolabial fold
NIDD	non-insulin-dependent diabetes	NLP	no light perception
			nodular liquifying panniculitis
NIDDM	non-insulin-dependent diabetes mellitus	NLS	neonatal lupus syndrome
NIF	negative inspiratory force	NLT	not later than
	not in file		not less than
NIG	NSAIA (non-steroidal anti-inflamatory agent) induced gastropathy	NM	neuromuscular
			Negro male
			nodular melanoma
NIH	National Institutes of Health		nonmalignant
			not measurable
NIHL	noise-induced hearing loss		not measured
			not mentioned
NIL	not in labor		nuclear medicine
NIMHDIS	National Institute for Mental Health Diagnostic Interview Schedule	N & M	nerves and muscles
			night and morning
		NMD	normal muscle development

NMI	no mental illness	NOD	nonobese diabetic
	no middle initial		notify of death
	normal male infant	NOK	next of kin
NMN	no middle name	NOM	nonsuppurative otitis
nmol	nanomole		media
NMP	normal menstrual period	NOMI	nonocclusive mesenteric
NMR	nuclear magnetic		infarction
	resonance (same as	non pal	not palpable
	magnetic resonance	NOOB	not out of bed
	imaging)	NOR	normal
NMS	neuroleptic malignant		nortriptyline
	syndrome	NOR-EPI	norepinephrine
NMSE	normalized mean square	norm	normal
	root	NOS	not on staff
NMSIDS	near-miss sudden infant		not otherwise specified
	death syndrome	NOSIE	Nurse's Observation
NMT	nebulized mist treatment		Scale for Inpatient
	no more than		Evaluation
NMTB	neuromuscular	NOT	nocturnal oxygen therapy
	transmission blockade	NP	nasal prongs
NN	neonatal		nasopharyngeal
	normal nursery		near point
	nurses' notes		neurophysin
N/N	negative/negative		neuropsychiatric
NND	neonatal death		newly presented
NNE	neonatal necrotizing		nonpalpable
	enterocolitis		no pain
NNM	Nicolle-Novy-MacNeal		not performed
	(media)		not pregnant
NNL	no new laboratory (test		not present
	orders)		nursed poorly
NNO	no new orders		nuclear pharmacist
NNP	Neonatal Nurse		nuclear pharmacy
	Practitioner		nurse practitioner
NNS	neonatal screen	NPA	nasal pharyngeal airway
	(hematocrit, total		near point of
	bilirubin, and total		accommodation
	protein)	NPAT	nonparoxysmal atrial
NNU	net nitrogen utilization		tachycardia
NO	nasal oxygen	NPC	near point convergences
	nitrous oxide		nodal premature
	none obtained		contractions
	nonobese		nonpatient contact
	number (no.)		nonpro ductive cough
	nursing office		nonprotein calorie
N_2O	nitrous oxide	NPDL	nodular poorly
$N_2O:O_2$	nitrous oxide to oxygen		differentiated
	ratio		lymphocytic
noc.	night	NPDR	nonproliferative diabetic
noct	nocturnal		retinopathy

NPE	neuropsychologic examination	NRC	National Research Council
	no palpable enlargement		normal retinal correspondence
	normal pelvic examination		Nuclear Regulatory Commission
NPF	nasopharyngeal fiberscope	NREM	nonrapid eye movement
	no predisposing factor	NREMS	nonrapid eye movement sleep
NPH	a type of insulin (Isophane)	NRF	normal renal function
	no previous history	NRI	nerve root involvement
	normal pressure hydrocephalus		nerve root irritation
NPG	nonpregnant	NRM	normal range of motion
NPhx	nasopharynx		normal retinal movement
NPI	no present illness	NRN	no return necessary
NPJT	nonparoxysmal junctional tachycardia	NROM	normal range of motion
		NRT	neuromuscular reeducation techniques
NPN	nonprotein nitrogen		
NPO	nothing by mouth	NS	nephrotic syndrome
NPP	normal postpartum		neurological signs
NPPNG	nonpenicillinase-producing *Neisseria gonorrhoeae*		neurosurgery
			nipple stimulation
			nonsmoker
NPR	normal pulse rate		normal saline solution (0.9% sodium chloride solution)
	nothing per rectum		
NPSA	nonphysician surgical assistant		no sample
			not seen
NPT	nocturnal penile tumescence		not significant
			nuclear sclerosis
	normal pressure and temperature		nylon suture
		N s̄ E	nausea without emesis
NPU	net protein utilization	NSA	no salt added
NQMI	non-Q wave myocardial infarction		no significant abnormality
			normal serum albumin
NR	do not repeat	NSABP	National Surgical Adjuvant Breast Project
	no refills		
	no report	NSAD	no signs of acute disease
	no response	NSAIA	non-steroidal antiinflammatory agent
	no return		
	nonreactive	NSAID	non-steroidal antiinflammatory drug
	nonrebreathing		
	normal range	NSC	no significant change
	normal reaction		not service-connected
	not reached	NSCD	nonservice-connected disability
NRAF	non-rheumatic atrial fibrillation		
		NSCLC	non-small-cell lung cancer
NRBC	normal red blood cell	NSD	no significant disease (difference, defect, deviation)
	nucleated red blood cell		
NRBS	non-rebreathing system		

	nominal standard dose	NSVD	normal spontaneous vaginal delivery	
	normal spontaneous delivery	NSX	neurosurgical examination	
NSDA	non-steroid dependent asthmatic	NSY	nursery	
NSE	neuron-specific enolase	NT	nasotracheal	
	normal saline enema (0.9% sodium chloride)		normal temperature nortriptyline	
NSFTD	normal spontaneous full-term delivery		not tender not tested nourishment taken	
NSG	nursing	N&T	nose and throat	
NSI	negative self-image	NTBR	not to be resuscitated	
	no signs of infection	NTC	neurotrauma center	
	no signs of inflammation	NTD	neural tube defects	
NSILA	nonsuppressible insulin-like activity	NTE	not to exceed	
NSN	nephrotoxic serum nephritis	NTF	normal throat flora	
		NTG	nitroglycerin nontoxic goiter	
NSO	Neosporin® ointment		nontreatment group	
NSP	neck and shoulder pain	NTGO	nitroglycerin ointment	
NSPVT	nonsustained polymorphic ventricular tachycardia	NTM	nocturnal tumescence monitor	
NSR	nasoseptal repair	NTMB	nontuberculous myobacteria	
	nonspecific reaction	NTMI	non-transmural myocardial infarction	
	normal sinus rhythm not seen regularly			
NSS	normal size and shape	NTND	not tender, not distended	
	not statistically significant	NTP	Nitropaste® (nitroglycerin ointment)	
	nutritional support service			
	sodium chloride 0.9% (normal saline solution)		normal temperature and pressure	
1/2 NSS	sodium chloride 0.45% (1/2 normal saline solution)		sodium nitroprusside	
		NTS	nasotracheal suction nucleus tractus solitarii	
NSSL	normal size, shape, and location	NTT	nasotracheal tube	
NSSP	normal size, shape, and position	NU	name unknown	
		NUD	nonulcer dyspepsia	
NSSTT	nonspecific ST and T (wave)	NUG	necrotizing ulcerative gingivitis	
NSST-TWCS	nonspecific ST-T wave changes	nullip	nullipara	
NST	non-stress test	NV	nausea and vomiting	
	not sooner than		near vision	
	nutritional support team		neurovascular	
NSTT	nonseminomatous testicular tumors		next visit nonvaccinated	
NSU	neurosurgical unit		nonvenereal	
	nonspecific urethritis		nonveteran	
			normal value	
			not verified	
NSV	nonspecific vaginitis	N&V	nausea and vomiting	

NVA	near visual acuity		pint
NVAF	nonvalvular atrial fibrillation		without
		$_1O_2$	singlet oxygen
NVD	nausea, vomiting, and diarrhea	O_2	both eyes
			oxygen
	neck vein distention	O_{2v}	superoxide
	neovascularization of the disc	OA	occiput anterior
			oral airway
	neurovesicle dysfunction		oral alimentation
	no venereal disease		osteoarthritis
	nonvalvular disease		Overeaters Anonymous
NVE	neovascularization elsewhere	O & A	observation & assessment
			odontectomy and alveoloplasty
NVG	neovascular glaucoma	OAC	oral anticoagulant(s)
	neoviridogrisein		overaction
NVL	neurovascular laboratory	OAD	obstructive airway disease
NVS	neurological vital signs		occlusive arterial disease
NVSS	normal variant short stature	OAE	otoacoustic emissions
NW	naked weight	OAF	osteoclast activating factor
	nasal wash		
	not weighed	OAG	open angle glaucoma
NWB	non-weight bearing	OASDHI	Old Age, Survivors, Disability, and Health Insurance
NWC	number of words chosen		
NWD	neuroleptic withdrawal		
Nx	nephrectomy	OASO	overactive superior oblique
NYD	not yet diagnosed		
NYHA	New York Heart Association (classification of heart disease)	OASR	overactive superior rectus
		OAW	oral airway
		OB	obese
			obstetrics
nyst	nystagmus		occult blood
NZ	enzyme	OBE-CALP	placebo capsule or tablet
		OBG	obstetrics and gynecology
	O	Ob-Gyn	obstetrics and gynecology
O	eye	Obj	objective
	objective findings	obl	oblique
	obvious	OBRR	obstetric recovery room
	occlusal	OBS	obstetrical service
	often		organic brain syndrome
	open	OBT	obtained
	oral	OC	obstetrical conjugate
	ortho		office call
	other		on call
	oxygen		only child
	pint		oral care
	zero		oral contraceptive
ō	negative	O & C	onset and course
	none	OCA	oculocutaneous albinism

	open care area	ODN	optokinetic nystagmus
	oral contraceptive agent	ODP	occipitodextra transerve
OCAD	occlusive carotid artery disease		offspring of diabetic parents
OCC	occlusal	OE	on examination
OCCC	open chest cardiac compression		orthopedic examination
			otitis externa
occl	occlusion	O&E	observation and
OCCM	open chest cardiac massage		examination
		OEC	outer ear canal
OCC PR	open-chest cardiopulmo-nary resuscitation	OER	oxygen enhancement ratios
OCC Th	occupational therapy	OET	oral esophageal tube
Occup Rx	occupational therapy	OETT	oral endotracheal tube
OCD	obsessive-compulsive disorder	OF	occipital-frontal
			optic fundi
	osteochondritis dissecans	OFC	occipital-frontal circumference
OCG	oral cholecystogram		
OCL®	oral colonic lavage		orbitofacial cleft
OCP	oral contraceptive pills	OG	Obstetrics-Gynecology
	ova, cysts, parasites		orogastric (feeding)
11-OCS	11-oxycorticosteroid	OGTT	oral glucose tolerance test
OCT	ornithine carbamyl transferase	OH	occupational history
			on hand
	oxytocin challenge test		open heart
OCU	observation care unit		oral hygiene
OD	doctor of optometry		orthostatic hypotension
	Officer-of-the-Day		outside hospital
	once daily (this is a dangerous abbreviation as it is read as right eye)	17 OH	17-hydroxycorticosteroids
		OHA	oral hypoglycemic agents
		OH Cbl	hydroxycobalamine
		17-OHCS	17-hydroxycorticosteroids
	on duty	OHD	hydroxy vitamin D
	optic disc		organic heart disease
	outdoor	OHF	omsk hemorrhagic fever
	overdose		overhead frame
	right eye	OHG	oral hypoglycemic
Δ OD 450	deviation of optical density at 450	OHI	oral hygiene instructions
		OHIAA	hydroxyindolacetic acid
ODA	occipitodextra anterior	OHL	oral hairy leukoplakia
	osmotic driving agent	OHP	oxygen under hyperbaric pressure
ODAC	on demand analgesia computer		
		OHRR	open heart recovery room
ODAT	one day at a time	OHS	occupational health service
ODC	ornithine decarboxylase		
	outpatient diagnostic center		ocular hypoperfusion syndrome
			open heart surgery
ODCH	ordinary diseases of childhood	OI	opportunistic infection
ODM	ophthalmodynamometry		osteogenesis imperfecta

	otitis interna	OMSC	otitis media secretory (or suppurative) chronic
OIF	oil-immersion field		
OIH	orthoiodohippurate	OMVC	open mitral valve commissurotomy
OIHA	orthoiodohippuric acid		
OJ	orange juice (this is a dangerous abbreviation)	OMVI	operating motor vehicle intoxicated
	orthoplast jacket	ON	every night (this is a dangerous abbreviation)
OK	all right		
	approved		optic neuropathy
	correct		oronasal
OKAN	optokinetic after nystagmus		Ortho-Novum®
			otic nerve
OKN	optokinetic nystagmus		overnight
OL	left eye	ONC	over-the-needle catheter
OLA	occiput left anterior	ONH	optic nerve head
OLP	occipitolaevoanterior		optic nerve hypoplasia
OLR	otology, laryngology, and rhinology	ONTR	orders not to resuscitate
		OO	oral order
OLT	occipitolaevoposterior	o/o	on account of
	orthotopic liver transplantation	OOB	out of bed
		OOBBRP	out of bed with bathroom privileges
OLTx	orthotopic liver transplantation		
		OOC	onset of contractions
OM	every morning (this is a dangerous abbreviation)		out of cast
			out of control
	obtuse marginal	OOH&NS	ophthalmology, otorhinolaryngology, and head and neck surgery
	osteomalacia		
	osteomyelitis		
	otitis media		
OMAS	otitis media, acute, suppurating	OOL	onset of labor
		OOLR	ophthalmology, otology, laryngology, and rhinology
OMCA	otitis media, catarrhalis, acute		
		OOP	out of pelvis
OMCC	otitis media, catarrhalis, chronic		out of plaster
			out on pass
OME	office of Medical Examiner	OOR	out of room
		OOS	out of stock
	otitis media with effusion	OOT	out of town
7-OMEN	menogaril	OOW	out of wedlock
OMH	organic marine hydrocolloid	OP	oblique presentation
			occiput posterior
OMI	old myocardial infarct		open
OMPA	otitis media, purulent, acute		operation
			oropharynx
OMPC	otitis media, purulent, chronic		oscillatory potentials
			osteoporosis
OMR	operative mortality rate		outpatient
OMSA	otitis media secretory (or suppurative) acute	O&P	ova and parasites

OPA	outpatient anesthesia		opening snap
	oral pharyngeal airway		oral surgery
OPB	outpatient basis		osmium
OPC	outpatient clinic	OSA	obstructive sleep apnea
OPCA	olivopontocerebellar atrophy	OSAS	obstructive sleep apnea syndrome
op cit	in the work cited	OSD	overside drainage
OPD	outpatient department	OSFT	outstretched fingertips
O'p'-DDD	mitotane	OSHA	Occupational Safety & Health Administration
OPE	outpatient evaluation		
OPG	ocular plethysmography	OSM S	osmolarity serum
OPM	occult primary malignancy	OSM U	osmolarity urine
		OSN	off service note
OPP	opposite	OSS	osseous
OPPG	oculopneumoplethysmography		over-shoulder strap
OPS	operations	OT	occiput transverse
	outpatient surgery		occupational therapy
OPT	optimum		old tuberculin
	outpatient treatment	OTA	open to air
OPT c O$_2$	Ohio pediatric tent with oxygen	OTC	ornithonetranscarbamoylase
OPT c CA	Ohio pediatric tent with compressed air		over the counter (sold without prescription)
OPV	oral polio vaccine	OTD	out the door
OR	oil retention	OTH	other
	open reduction	OTO	otology
	operating room	OTR	Occupational Therapist, Registered
ORCH	orchiectomy		
ORIF	open reduction internal fixation	OT/RT	occupational therapy/recreational therapy
ORL	otorhinolaryngology	OTS	orotracheal suction
ORN	operating room nurse	OTT	orotracheal tube
OROS	ostomotic release oral system	OU	both eyes
		OURQ	outer upper right quadrant
ORP	occiput right posterior		
ORS	oral rehydration salts	OV	office visit
ORT	operating room technician Registered Occupational Therapist		ovary
			ovum
		OVAL	ovalocytes
OR XI	oriented to time	OW	once weekly (this is a dangerous abbreviation)
OR X2	oriented to time and place		
OR X3	oriented to time, place, and person		outer wall
			out of wedlock
OS	left eye	OWNK	out of wedlock not keeping
	mouth (this is a dangerous abbreviation as it is read as left eye)		
		Oxi	oximeter (oximetry)
		OXZ	oxazepam
	occipitosacral	oz	ounce

P

P	para
	peripheral
	phosphorus
	pint
	plan
	protein
	pulse
	pupil
$\bar{p}$	after
/P	partial lower denture
P/	partial upper denture
P_2	pulmonic second heart sound
^{32}P	radioactive phosphorus
PA	paranoid
	pernicious anemia
	phenol alcohol
	physician assistant
	pineapple
	posterior-anterior (x-ray)
	presents again
	professional association
	psychiatric aide
	pulmonary artery
P&A	percussion and auscultation
	position and alignment
$P_2 > A_2$	pulmonic second heart sound greater than aortic secondheart sound
PAB	premature atrial beat
PAC	premature atrial contraction
PACH	pipers to after coming head
$PaCO_2$	arterial carbon dioxide tension
PAC-V	cisplatin, doxorubicin, and cyclophosphamide
PACU	post anesthesia care unit
PAD	primary affective disorder
PADP	pulmonary artery diastolic pressure
PAE	postanoxic encephalopathy
	postantibiotic effect

	progressive assistive exercise
PAEDP	pulmonary artery and end-diastole pressure
PAF	paroxysmal atrial fibrillation
	platelet activating factor
PA&F	percussion, auscultation, and fremitus
PAGA	premature appropriate for gestational age
PAGE	polyacrylamide gel electrophoresis
PAH	para-aminohippurate
	pulmonary arterial hypertension
PAI	plasminogen activator inhibitor
	platelet accumulation index
PAIVS	pulmonary atresia with intact ventricle septum
PAL	posterior axillary line
Pa Line	pulmonary artery line
PALN	para-aortic lymph node
PALS	pediatric advanced life support
PAM	penicillin aluminum monostearate
2-PAM	pralidoxime
PAMP	pulmonary arterial (artery) mean pressure
PAN	periodic alternating nystagmus
	polyarteritis nodosa
PANESS	physical and neurological examination for soft signs
PAO_2	arterial oxygen tension
PAO	peak acid output
PAOP	pulmonary artery occlusion pressure
PAP	passive aggressive personality
	peroxidase-anti-peroxidase
	prostatic acid phosphatase
	pulmonary artery pressure
Pap smear	Papanicolaou smear
PA/PS	pulmonary atresia/ pulmonary stenosis

PAR	parafin			phenobarbital
	parallel		P&B	pain and burning
	platelet aggregate ratio			phenobarbital &
	postanesthetic recovery			belladonna
	pulmonary arteriolar		PBA	percutaneous bladder
	resistance			aspiration
PARA	number of pregnancies		PBC	point of basal
para	paraplegic			convergence
PAROM	passive assistance range			primary biliary cirrhosis
	of motion		PBD	percutaneous biliary
PARR	postanesthesia recovery			drainage
	room		PBE	partial breech extraction
PARU	postanesthetic recovery		PBF	placental blood flow
	unit			pulmonary blood flow
PAS	periodic acid-Schiff		PBG	porphobilinogen
	(reagent)		PBI	protein-bound iodine
	peripheral anterior		PBK	pseudophakic bullous
	synechia			keratopathy
	pneumatic antiembolic		PBL	peripheral blood
	stocking			lymphocyte
	postanesthesia score		PBMC	peripheral blood
	premature auricular			mononuclear cell
	systole		PBMNC	peripheral blood
	Professional Activities			mononuclear cell
	Study		PBN	polymyxin B sulfate,
	pulmonary artery stenosis			bacitracin, and
PAS or	para-aminosalicyclic acid			neomycin
PASA			PBO	placebo
Pas Ex	passive exercise		PBPI	penile-brachial pulse
PASG	pneumatic antishock			index
	garment		PBS	phosphate-buffered
PASP	pulmonary artery systolic			saline
	pressure		PBT$_4$	protein-bound thyroxine
PAT	paroxysmal atrial		PBV	percutaneous balloon
	tachycardia			valvuloplasty
	patella		PBZ	phenoxybenzamine
	patient			phenylbutazone
	percent acceleration time			pyribenzamine
	preadmission testing		ΦBZ	phenylbutazone
	pregnancy at term		PC	after meals
Path.	pathology			packed cells
PAV	Pavulon®			platelet concentrate
PAWP	pulmonary artery wedge			poor condition
	pressure			popliteal cyst
PB	parafin bath			posterior chamber
	power building			present complaint
	powder board			productive cough
	premature beat			professional corporation
	protein-bound		PCA	passive cutaneous
Pb	lead			anaphylaxis

	patient care assistant (aide)	PCO$_2$	carbon dioxide pressure (or tension)
	patient controlled analgesia	PCOD	polycystic ovarian disease
	postconceptional age	PCP	patient care plan
	posterior cerebral artery		phencyclidine
	posterior communicating artery		*pneumonocystis carinii* pneumonia
	procainamide		primary care person
	procoagulation activity		primary care physician
PCB	pancuronium bromide		pulmonary capillary pressure
	para cervical block	PCR	polymerase chain reaction
	prepared childbirth		protein catabolic rate
PCBs	polychlorinated biphensyls	PCS	patient care system
PCC	pheochromocytoma		portable cervical spine
	poison control center		portacaval shunt
PCCC	pediatric critical care center		postconcussion syndrome
PCCU	post coronary care unit	P c/s	primary cesarean section
PCD	postmortem cesarean delivery	PCT	post coital test
PCE	physical capacities evaluation		progestin challenge test
PCE®	erythromycin particles in tablets	PCU	palliative care unit
			primary care unit
PCFT	platelet complement fixation test		progressive care unit
			protective care unit
PCG	phonocardiogram	PCV	packed cell volume
PCGG	percutaneous coagulation of gasserian ganglion	PCWP	pulmonary capillary wedge pressure
PCH	paroxysmal cold hemoglobinuria	PCX	paracervical
PC&HS	after meals and at bedtime	PCXR	portable chest radiograph
PCI	prophylactic cranial irradiation	PCZ	procarbazine
			prochlorperazine
PCIOL	posterior chamber intraocular lens	PD	interpupillary distance
			Parkinson's disease
PCKD	polycystic kidney disease		percutaneous drain
PCL	posterior chamber lens		peritoneal dialysis
	posterior cruciate ligament		personality disorder
			poorly differentiated
PCM	protein-calorie malnutrition		postural drainage
			prism diopter
PCMX	chloroxylenol	P/D	packs per day (cigarettes)
PCN	penicillin	PDA	parenteral drug abuser
	percutaneous nephrostomy		patent ductus arteriosus
PCO	polycystic ovary	PDD	cisplatin
		PDE	paroxysmal dyspnea on exertion
			pulsed Doppler echocardiography
		PDFC	premature dead female child

PDGF	platelet derived growth factor	PECHO	prostatic echogram
PDGXT	predischarge graded exercise test	$PECO_2$	mixed expired carbon dioxide tension
PDL	poorly differentiated lymphocytic	Peds.	pediatrics
		PEEP	positive end-expiratory pressure
	progressively diffused leukoencephalopathy	PEFR	peak expiratory flow rate
PDL-D	poorly differentiated lymphocytic-diffuse	PEG	percutaneous endoscopic gastrostomy
PDL-N	poorly differentiated lymphocytic-nodular		pneumoencephalogram
			polyethylene glycol
PDMC	premature dead male child	PEG-ELS	polyethylene glycol and iso-osmolar electrolyte solution
PDN	prednisone		
	private duty nurse	PEGG	Parent Education and Guidance Group
PD & P	postural drainage and percussion	PEJ	percutaneous endoscopic jejunostomy
PDR	Physician's Desk Reference	PEM	protein-energy malnutrition
	postdelivery room	PEMA	phenylethylmalonamide
	proliferative diabetic retinopathy	PEMS	physical, emotional, mental, and safety
PDRcVH	proliferative diabetic retinopathy with vitreous hemorrhage	PEN	parenteral and enteral nutrition
PDS	pain dysfunction syndrome	PENS	percutaneous epidural nerve stimulator
PDT	photodynamic therapy	PEP	pre-ejection period
PDU	pulsed Doppler ultrasonography		protein electrophoresis
PE	cisplatin and etoposide	PER	by pediatric emergency room
	physical examination		protein efficiency ratio
	physical exercise	PERC	perceptual
	plasma exchange		percutaneous
	plural effusion	perf.	perfect
	polyethylene		perforation
	pressure equalization	Peri Care	perineum care
	pulmonary edema	PERL	pupils equal, reactive to light
	pulmonary embolism		
P_1E_1®	epinephrine 1%, pilocarpine 1% ophthalmic solution	per os	by mouth (this is a dangerous abbreviation as it is read as left eye)
PEA	pelvic examination under anesthesia	PERR	pattern evoked retinal response
PEARLA	pupils equal and react to light and accommodation	PERRLA	pupils, equal, round, reactive to light and accommodation
PEB	cisplatin, etoposide, and bleomycin	PERRRLA	pupils equal, round, regular, react to light and accommodation

PES	pre-excitation syndrome	PGL	persistent generalized lymphadenopathy
	pseudoexpoliation syndrome	PGM	paternal grandmother
peSPL	peak equivalent sound pressure level	PGP	paternal grandparent
		PgR	progesterone receptor
PET	poor exercise tolerance	PGU	postgonococcal urethritis
	positron-emission tomography	PGY-1	post-graduate year one
		pH	hydrogen ion concentration
	pre-eclamptic toxemia		
	pressure equalizing tubes	PH	past history
PETN	pentaerythritol tetranitrate		personal history
PEx	physical examination		pinhole
PF	peripheral fields		poor health
	plantar flexion		pubic hair
	power factor		public health
	preservative free	Ph[1]	Philadelphia chromosome
	prostatic fluid	PHA	arterial pH
PF3	platelet factor 3		passive hemagglutinating
PFA	foscarnet (phosphonoformatic acid)		peripheral hyperalimentation
PFC	persistent fetal circulation		phytohemagglutinin
PFFFP	Pall filtered fresh frozen plasma		phytohemagglutinin antigen
PFJS	patellofemoral joint syndrome	PHAR	pharmacist
			pharmacy
PFM	porcelain fused to metal		pharynx
PFO	patent foramen ovule	Pharm	Pharmacy
PFPC	Pall filtered packed cells	PharmD	Doctor of Pharmacy
PFR	parotid flow rate	PHC	primary hepatocellular carcinoma
	peak flow rate		
PFRC	plasma-free red cells	PhD	Doctor of Philosophy
PFT	pulmonary function test	PHH	posthemorrhagic hydrocephalus
PFU	plaque-forming unit		
PFW	pHisoHex® face wash	PHI	prehospital index
PFWB	Pall filtered whole blood	PHIS	posthead injury syndrome
PG	paged in hospital	PHL	Philadelphia (chromosome)
	paregoric		
	phosphatidyl glycerol	PHN	post herpetic neuralgia
	polygalacturonate		public health nurse
	pregnant	PHPT	primary hyperparathyroidism
PGA	prostaglandin A		
PGE	posterior gastroenterostomy	PHPV	persistent hyperplastic primary vitreous
PGE2	prostaglandin E2	PHS	partial hospitalization program
PGF	paternal grandfather		
PGF2 α	prostaglandin F2 α		US Public Health Service
PGH	pituitary growth hormones	PHT	phenytoin
PGI	potassium, glucose, and insulin		portal hypertension
			primary hyperthyroidism
PGI$_2$	epoprostenol		pulmonary hypertension

PHx	past history		proximal interphalangeal (joint)
Phx	pharynx		
PI	package insert	PISA	phase invariant signature algorithm
	pancreatic insufficiency		
	peripheral iridectomy	Pit	patellar inhibition test
	poison ivy		Pitocin®
	postinjury		Pitressin® (this is a dangerous abbreviation)
	premature infant		
	present illness		pituitary
	pulmonary infarction	PITP	pseudo-idiopathic thrombocytopenic purpura
PIAT	Peabody Individual Achievement Test		
PIC	peripherally inserted catheter	PITR	plasma iron turnover rate
		PIV	peripheral intravenous
PICA	Porch Index of Communicative Ability	PIVD	protruded intervertebral disc
	posterior inferior cerebellar artery	PIWT	partially impacted wisdom teeth
	posterior inferior communicating artery	PJB	premature junctional beat
		PJC	premature junctional contractions
PICC	peripherally inserted central catheter	PJS	peritoneojugular shunt
			Peutz-Jeghers syndrome
PICU	pediatric intensive care unit	PK	penetrating keratoplasty
		PKB	prone knee bend
PID	pelvic inflammatory disease	PKD	polycystic kidney disease
		PKP	penetrating keratoplasty
	prolapsed intervertebral disc	PK Test	Prausnitz-Kunstner transfer test
PIE	pulmonary infiltration with eosinophilia	PKU	phenylketonuria
	pulmonary interstitial emphysema	PL	light perception
			place
PIF	peak inspiratory flow		plantar
PIFG	poor intrauterine fetal growth		transpulmonary pressure
		PLAP	placental alkaline phosphatase
PIG	pertussis immune globulin		
PIGI	pregnancy-induced glucose intolerance	PLBO	placebo
		PLED	periodic lateralizing epileptiform discharge
PIH	pregnancy induced hypertension	PLFC	premature living female child
PIMS	programmable implantable medication system		
		PLH	paroxysmal localized hyperhidrosis
		PLL	prolymphocytic leukemia
PIO	pemoline	PLMC	premature living male child
PIOK	poikilocytosis		
PI-PB	performance intensity-phonemically balanced	PLN	pelvic lymph node
			popliteal lymph node
PIP	peak inspiratory pressure	PLR	pupillary light reflex
	postinfusion phlebitis	PLS	plastic surgery

	Preschool Language Scale		posterior myocardial
	primary lateral sclerosis		infarction
PLSO	posterior leafspring orthosis	PML	polymorphonuclear leukocytes
PLSURG	plastic surgery		progressive multifocal leukoencephalopathy
PLT	platelet		
PLT EST	platelet estimate	PMMF	pectoralis major mycutaneous flat
plts	platelets		
PLV	posterior left ventricular	PMN	polymorphonuclear leukocyte
PM	afternoon		
	evening	PMNN	polymorphonuclear neutrophil
	pacemaker		
	petit mal	PMO	postmenopausal osteoporosis
	physical medicine		
	polymyositis	PMP	pain management program
	poor metabolizers		
	post mortem		previous menstrual period
	presents mainly		psychotropic medication plan
	pretibial myxedema		
	primary motivation	PMPO	postmenopausal palpable ovary
	prostatic massage		
PMA	premenstrual asthma	PMR	polymorphic reticulosis
	Prinzmetal's angina		polymyalgia rheumatica
PMB	polymorphonuclear basophil (leukocytes)	PM&R	physical medicine and rehabilitation
	polymyxin B	PMS	postmenopausal syndrome
	postmenopausal bleeding		post-marketing surveillance
PMC	premature mitral closure		
	pseudomembranous colitis		premenstrual syndrome,
PMCP	para-monochlorophenol	PMT	premenstrual tension
PMD	perceptual motor development	PMTS	premenstrual tension syndrome
	primary myocardial disease	PMV	prolapse of mitral valve
		PMW	pacemaker wires
	private medical doctor	PN	parenteral nutrition
PME	polymorphonuclear esosinophil (leukocytes)		percussion note
			percutaneous nephrostogram
	post menopausal estrogen		
PMEC	pseudomembranous enterocolitis		periarteritis nodosa
			pneumonia
PMF	progressive massive fibrosis		polynephritis
			poorly nourished
PMH	past medical history		postnasal
PMI	past medical illness		postnatal
	patient medication instructions		practical nurse
			premie nipple
	plea of mental incompetence		primary nurse
			progress note
	point of maximal impulse	P & N	psychiatry and neurology

PNAB	percutaneous needle aspiration biopsy	PNV	prenatal vitamins
PNAS	prudent no salt added	Pnx	pneumonectomy pneumothorax
PNB	percutaneous needle biopsy	PO	by mouth (*per os*) phone order
	premature newborn		postoperative
	premature nodal beat	PO$_2$	partial pressure of oxygen
PNC	penicillin	PO$_4$	phosphate
	peripheral nerve conduction	POA	pancreatic oncofetal antigen
	premature nodal contraction	POAG	primary open-angle glaucoma
	prenatal care	POB	phenoxybenzamine
	prenatal course		place of birth
	Psychiatric Nurse Clinician	POC	postoperative care product of conception
PND	paroxysmal nocturnal dyspnea	POD	pacing on demand polycystic ovarian disease
	pelvic node dissection	POD 1	postoperative day one
	postnasal drip	POE	position of ease
	pregnancy, not delivered	POEMS	plasma cell dyscasia with polyneuropathy,
PNET-MB	primitive neuroectodermal tumors-medulloblastoma		organomegaly, endocrinopathy, monoclonal
PNF	proprioceptive neuromuscular fasciculation reaction		(M)-protein, and skin changes
PNH	paroxysmal nocturnal hemoglobinuria	POF	position of function
		P of I	proof of illness
PNI	peripheral nerve injury prognostic nutrition index	POG	Pediatric Oncology Group Penthrane®-oxygen gas (nitrous oxide)
PNL	percutaneous nephrostolithotomy		products of gestation
PNMG	persistent neonatal myasthenia gravis	POHA	preoperative holding area
		POHI	physically or otherwise health impaired
PNP	peak negative pressure Pediatric Nurse Practitioner	POI	Personal Orientation Inventory
	progressive nuclear palsey	POIK	poikilocytosis
	purine nucleoside phosphorylase	POL	premature onset of labor
PNS	partial nonprogressing stroke	POLY	polychromic erythrocytes polymorphonuclear leukocyte
	peripheral nervous system practical nursing student	POLY-CHR	polychromatophilia
PNT	percutaneous nephrostomy tube	POM	pain on motion polyoximethylene
pnthx	pneumothorax		prescription-only
PNU	protein nitrogen units		medication

POMP	prednisone, vincristine, methotrexate, and mercaptopurine
POMR	problem-oriented medical record
POMS	Profile of Mood States
PONI	postoperative narcotic infusion
POP	pain on palpation
	persistent occipitoposterior
	plaster of paris
	popiliteal
POp	postoperative
poplit	popliteal
POR	problem-oriented record
PORK	porkilocytosis
PORP	partial ossicular replacement prosthesis
PORT	perioperative respiratory therapy
	postoperative respiratory therapy
POS	parosteal osteosarcoma
	positive
poss	possible
post	post mortem examination (autopsy)
post op	postoperative
Post Sag D	posterior sagittal diameter
post tib	posterial tibial
POU	placenta, ovaries, and uterus
POW	prisoner of war
PP	near point of accommodation
	paradoxical pulse
	partial upper and lower dentures
	pedal pulse
	peripheral pulses
	pin prick
	plasmapheresis
	plaster of paris
	poor person
	posterior pituitary
	postpartum
	postprandial
	presenting part

	private patient
	protoporphyria
	proximal phalanx
	pulse pressure
	push pills
P&P	pins and plaster
	policy and procedure
PPA	palpitation, percussion, and auscultation
	phenylpropanolamine
	phenylpyruvic acid
	postpartum amenorrhea
PP&A	palpation, percussion, and auscultation
PPAS	post-polio atrophy syndrome
PPB	parts per billion
	positive pressure breathing
PPBE	postpartum breast engorgment
PPBS	post prandial blood sugar
PPC	progressive patient care
PPD	packs per day
	posterior polymorphous dystrophy
	postpartum day
	purified protein derivative (of tuberculin)
P & PD	percussion & postural drainage
PPD-B	purified protein derivative, Battey
PPD-S	purified protein derivative, standard
PPF	plasma protein fraction
PPG	photoplethysmography
	postprandial glucose
PPGI	psychophysiologic gastrointestinal (reaction)
PPH	postpartum hemorrhage
	primary pulmonary hypertension
PPHN	persistent pulmonary hypertension of the newborn
PPI	benzylpenicilloylpolysine
	patient package insert
	Present Pain Intensity

PPL	pars plana lensectomy		prolonged remission
PPLO	pleuro-pneumonia-like organisms		Puerto Rican pulse rate
PPM	parts per million permanent pacemaker	P & R	pelvic and rectal pulse and respiration
PPMA	post-poliomyelitis muscular atrophy	PRA PRAT	plasma renin activity platelet radioactive antiglobulin test
PPMS	psychophysiologic musculoskeletal (reaction)	PRBC PRC	packed red blood cells packed red cells
PPN	peripheral parenteral nutrition	PRCA	peer review committee pure red cell aplasia
PPNAD	primary pigmented nodular adrenocortical disease	PRD PRE	polycystic renal disease passive resistance exercises
PPNG	penicillinase producing *Neisseria gonorrhoeae*		progressive resistive exercise
PPO	prefered provider organization	Pred preg	prednisone Pregestimil®
PPP	pedal pulse present	PREMIE	premature infant
	peripheral pulses palpable	pre-op	before surgery
	postpartum psychosis	prep	prepare for surgery
	protamine paracoagulation phenomenon		preposition
PPPBL	peripheral pulses palpable both legs	PRERLA	pupils round, equal, react to light and accommodation
PPPG	post prandial plasma glucose	prev	prevent previous
PPR	patient progress record	PRFN	percutaneous radio frequency
PPRC	Physician Payment Review Commission	PRG	phleborheogram
PPROM	prolonged premature rupture of membranes	PRH	past relevant history preretinal hemorrhage
PPS	peripheral pulmonary stenosis	PRI prim	Pain Rating Index primary
	postpartum sterilization	PRIMIP	primipara (1st pregnancy)
PPTL	postpartum tubal ligation	PRISM	Pediatric Risk of Mortality Score
PPU	perforated peptic ulcer		
PPV	positive predictive value	PRL	prolactin
PPVT	Peabody Picture Vocabulary Test	PRLA	pupils react to light and accommodation
PQ	pronator quadratus	PRM	phosphoribomutase
PR	far point of accommoda- tion		photoreceptor membrane prematurely ruptured membrane
	partial remission	PRM-SDX	pyrimethamine sulfadoxine
	patient relations		
	per rectum	PRN	as occasion requires
	premature	PRO	pronation
	profile		protein
	progressive resistance		

	prothrombin		peripheral smear
prob	probable		plastic surgery (surgeon)
PROCTO	procotoscopic		pressure support
	proctology		protective services
prog.	prognathism		pulmonary stenosis
	prognosis		pyloricstenosis
	program		serum from pregnant
	progressive		women
PROM	passive range of motion	P/S	polyunsaturated to
	premature rupture of		saturated fatty acids
	membranes		ratio
ProMACE	prednisone, methotrexate,	P & S	pain and suffering
	calcium leucovorin,		paracentesis and suction
	doxorubicin,	PsA	psoriatic arthritis
	cyclophosphamide, and	PS I	healthy patient with
	etoposide		localized pathological
Promy	promyelocyte		process
PRO MYELO	promyelocytes	PS II	a patient with mild to moderate systemic
PRON	pronation		disease
pros	prostate	PS III	a patient with severe
	prosthesis		systemic disease
prov	provisional		limiting activity but not
PROVIMI	proteins, vitamins, and		incapacitating
	minerals	PS IV	a patient with
PROX	proximal		incapacitating systemic
PRP	panretinal photocoagula-		disease
	tion	PS V	Moribund patient not
	penicllinase-resistant		expected to live.
	penicllin		(These are American
	polyribose ribitol		Society of
	phosphate		Anesthesiologists'
	progressive rubella		physical status patient
	panencephalitis		classifications.
PRPP	5-phosphoribosyl-		Emergency operations
	1-pyrophosphate		are designated by "E"
PRRE	pupils round regular, and		after the classification).
	equal	PSA	product selection allowed
PRSs	positive rolandic spikes		prostate-specific antigen
PRTH-C	prothrombin time control	PsA	psoriatic arthritis
PRV	polycythemia rubra vera	PSC	Pediatric Symptom
PRVEP	pattern reversal visual		Checklist
	evoked potentials		posterior subcapsular
PRW	polymerized ragweed		cataract
PRZ	prazepam		primary sclerosing
PRZF	pyrazofurin		cholangitis
PS	paradoxic sleep	PSCT	peripheral stem cell
	paranoid schizophrenia		transplant
	pathologic stage	PSE	portal systemic
	performance status		encephalopathy

PSF	posterior spinal fusion		peak and trough
PSGN	post streptococcal		permanent and total
	glomerulonephritis	PTA	percutaneous transluminal
PSH	past surgical history		angioplasty
	post spinal headache		Physical Therapy
PSI	Physiologic Stability		Assistant
	Index		plasma thromboplastin
	pounds per square inch		antecedent
PSIS	posterior superior iliac		post-traumatic amnesia
	spine		pretreatment anxiety
PSM	presystolic murmur		prior to admission
P/sore	pressure sore		pure-tone average
PSP	pancreatic spasmolytic	PTB	patellar tendon bearing
	peptide		prior to birth
	phenolsulphthalein		pulmonary tuberculosis
	progressive supranuclear	PTBA	percutaneous transluminal
	palsy		balloon angioplasty
PSRBOW	premature spontaneous	PTBD-EF	percutaneous transhepatic
	rupture of bag of		biliary drainage—en-
	waters		teric feeding
PSS	painful shoulder	PTBS	posttraumatic brain
	syndrome		syndrome
	physiologic saline	PTB-	patellar tendon
	solution (0.9% sodium	SC-SP	bearing-supracondylar-
	chloride)		suprapatellar
	progressive systemic	PTC	patient to call
	sclerosis		percutaneous transhepatic
PST	paroxysmal supraventricu-		cholangiography
	lar tachycardia		plasma thromboplastin
	platelet survival time		components
PSV	pressure supported		prior to conception
	ventilation	PT-C	prothrombin time control
PSVT	paroxysmal supraventricu-	PTCA	percutaneous transluminal
	lar tachycardia		coronary angioplasty
PSW	psychiatric social worker	PTCL	peripheral T-cell
PT	cisplatin		lymphoma
	parathormone	PTCR	percutaneous transluminal
	parathyroid		coronary recanalization
	paroxysmal tachycardia	PTD	period to discharge
	patient		permanent and total
	phenytoin		disability
	phototoxicity		prior to delivery
	physical therapy	PTDP	permanent transvenous
	pine tar		demand pacemaker
	pint	PTE	pretibial edema
	posteriortibial		proximal tibial epiphysis
	preterm		pulmonary thromboembo-
	prothrombin time		lism
P&T	paracentesis and tubing	PTED	pulmonary thromboem-
	(of ears)		bolic disease

PTFE	polytetrafluorethylene		pregnancy urine
PTG	parathyroid gland	PUBS	percutaneous umbilical
	teniposide		blood sampling
PTH	parathyroid hormone	PUD	peptic ulcer disease
	post transfusion hepatitis	PUE	pyrexia of unknown
	prior to hospitalization		etiology
PTHC	percutaneous transhepatic	PUFA	polyunsaturated fatty
	cholangiography		acids
PTJV	percutaneous transtracheal	pul.	pulmonary
	jet ventilation	PUN	plasma urea nitrogen
PTL	pre-term labor	PUO	pyrexia of unknown
	Sodium Pentothal®		origin
PTMDF	pupils, tension, media,	PUP	percutaneous ultrasonic
	disc, and fundus		pyelolithotomy
PTNM	postsurgical resection-	PUPP	pruritic urticarial papules
	pathologic staging of		and plaque of
	cancer		pregnancy
PTO	please turn over	PUVA	psoralen-ultraviolet-light
PTP	posterior tibial pulse		(treatment)
PTPM	posttraumatic progressive	PV	papillomavirus
	myelopathy		per vagina
PTPN	peripheral (vein) total		polio vaccine
	parenteral nutrition		polycythemia vera
PTR	patella tendon reflex		popliteal vein
	patient to return		portal vein
	prothrombin time ratio		postvoiding
PT-R	prothrombin time ratio		pulmonary vein
PTS	patellar tendon suspension	P&V	peak and valley (this is a
	permanent threshold shift		dangerous abbreviation)
	prior to surgery		use peak and trough
PTSD	post-traumatic stress		pyloroplasty and
	disorder		vagotomy
PTT	partial thromboplastin	PVA	polyvinyl alcohol
	time		Prinzmental's variant
	platelet transfusion		angina
	therapy	PVB	cisplatin, vinblastine, and
PTT-C	partial thromboplastin		bleomycin
	time control		premature ventricular
PTU	pain treatment unit		beat
	propylthiouracil	PVC	polyvinyl chloride
PTV	posterior tibial vein		postvoiding cystogram
PTWTKG	patient's weight in		premature ventricular
	kilograms		contraction
PTX	parathyroidectomy		pulmonary venous
	pelvic traction		congestion
	pneumothorax	PVD	patient very disturbed
PTZ	pentylenetetrazol		peripheral vascular
	phenothiazine		disease
PU	pelvic-ureteric		posterior vitreous
	peptic ulcer		detachment

	premature ventricular depolarization	PVT	pulmonic valve stenosis
PVE	perivenous encephalomyelitis		paroxysmal ventricular tachycardia
	premature ventricular extrasystole	PW	private
	prosthetic value endocarditis		pacing wires
			patient waiting
			puncture wound
PVF	peripheral visual field	P&W	pressures and waves
PVFS	postviral fatigue syndrome	PWB	partial weight bearing
			psychological well-being
PVH	periventricular hemorrhage	PWI	pediatric walk-in clinic
			posterior wall infarct
	pulmonary vascular hypertension	PWLV	posterior wall of left ventricle
PVI	peripheral vascular insufficiency	PWM	pokeweed mitogens
PVK	penicillin V potassium	PWP	pulmonary wedge pressure
PVM	proteins, vitamins, and minerals	PWS	port-wine stain
		PWV	polistes wasp venom
PVNS	pigmented villonodular synovitis	Px	physical exam
			pneumothorax
PVO	peripheral vascular occlusion		prognosis
		PXE	pseudoxanthoma elasticum
	pulmonary venous occlusion	PY	pack years
PVO_2	mixed venous pressure of oxygen	PYP	pyrophosphate
		PZ	peripheral zone
		PZA	pyrazinamide
PVOD	pulmonary vascular obstructive disease	PZI	protamine zinc insulin
PVP	cisplatin and etoposide		

Q

PVP	peripheral venous pressure	q	every
	polyvinylpyrrolidone	QA	quality assurance
P-VP-B	cisplatin, etoposide, and bleomycin	QAM	every morning (this is a dangerous abbreviation)
PVR	peripheral vascular resistance	QC	quality control
			quick catheter
	postvoiding residual	QCA	quantitative coronary angiography
	proliferative vitreoretinopathy	qd	every day (this is a dangerous abbreviation as it is read as four times daily)
	pulmonary vascular resistance		
	pulse-volume recording		
PVS	percussion, vibration and suction	q4h	every four hours
		qh	every hour
	peritoneovenous shunt	qhs	every night (this is a dangerous abbreviation as it is read as every hour)
	persistent vegetative state		
	Plummer-Vinson syndrome		

qid	four times daily	
QIG	quantitative immunoglob-ulins	
QMI	Q wave myocardial infarction	
QMRP	qualified mental retardation professional	
QMT	quantitative muscle testing	
q.n.	every night (this is a dangerous abbreviation as it is read as every hour)	
q.n.s.	quantity not sufficient	
qod	every other day (this is a dangerous abbreviation as it is read as every day or four times a day)	
qoh	every other hour (this is a dangerous abbreviation as it is read as every day or four times a day)	
QON	every other night (this is a dangerous abbreviation)	
qpm	every evening (this is a dangerous abbreviation)	
QR	quiet room	
QRS	principal deflection in an electrocardiogram	
Q.S.	every shift sufficient quantity	
Qs/Qt	intrapulmonary shunt fraction	
QSP	physiological shunt fraction	
qt	quart	
QTC	quantitative tip cultures	
QUAD	quadrant quadriceps quadriplegic	
QU	quiet	
QUART	quadrantectomy, axillary dissection, and radiotherapy	
qwk	once a week (this is a dangerous abbreviation)	

R

R	rate
	rectal
	rectum
	regular
	regular insulin
	resistant
	respiration
	right
	roentgen
Ⓡ	right
RA	rales
	repeat action
	retinoic acid
	rheumatoid arthritis
	right arm
	right atrium
	right auricle
	room air
RAA	renin-angiotensin-aldoste-rone
RAAS	renin-angiotensin-aldoste-rone system
RABG	room air blood gas
RAC	right atrial catheter
RACCO	right anterior caudocranial oblique
RACT	recalcified whole-blood activated clotting time
RAD	ionizing radiation unit radical radiology reactive airway disease right axis deviation
RAE	right atrial enlargement
RAEB	refractory anemia, erythroblastic
RAG	room air gas
RAH	right atrial hypertrophy
RAIU	radioactive iodine uptake
RALT	routine admission laboratory tests
RAM	radioactive material rapid alternating movements
RAN	resident's admission notes
R_2AN	second year resident's admission notes

RAO	right anterior oblique	RCD	relative cardiac dullness
RAP	right atrial pressure	RCF	Reiter complement
RAQ	right anterior quadrant		fixation
RAPD	relative afferent pupillary defect	RCHF	right-sided congestive heart failure
RAS	renal artery stenosis	RCM	radiographic contrast
RAST	radioallergosorbent test		media
RAT	right anterior thigh		retinal capillary
RA test	test for rheumatoid factor		microaneurysm
RATx	radiation therapy		right costal margin
R(AW)	airway resistance	RCPM	raven coloured
RB	retinoblastoma		progressive matrices
	retrobulbar	RCPT	Registered Cardiopulmo-
	right buttock		nary Technician
R & B	right and below	RCS	repeat cesarean section
RBA	right basilar artery		reticulum cell sarcoma
	right brachial artery	RCT	randomized clinical trial
RBB	right breast biopsy		Registered Care
RBBB	right bundle branch block		Technologist
RBBX	right breast biopsy examination		root canal therapy
			Rorschach Content Test
RBC	red blood cell (count)	RCV	red cell volume
RBCD	right border cardiac dullness	R.D.	Registered Dietitian
		RD	Raynaud's disease
RBCM	red blood cell mass		reflex decay
RBC s/f	red blood cells spun filtration		renal disease
			respiratory disease
RBCV	red blood cell volume		retinal detachment
RBD	right border of dullness		Reye's disease
RBE	relative biologic effectiveness		right deltoid
			ruptured disc
RBF	renal blood flow	RDA	recommended daily
RBG	random blood glucose		allowance
RBOW	rupture bag of water	RDG	right dorsogluteal
RBP	retinol-binding protein	RDH	Registered Dental
RBS	random blood sugar		Hygienist
RBV	right brachial vein	RDIH	right direct inguinal
RC	Red Cross		hernia
	Roman Catholic	RDOD	retinal detachment, right
	rotator cuff		eye
R/C	reclining chair	RDOS	retinal detachment, left
RCA	radionuclide cerebral angiogram		eye
		RDP	right dorsoposterior
	right coronary artery	RDPE	reticular degeneration of
RCBF	regional cerebral blood flow		the pigment epithelium
		RDS	research diagnostic
RCC	renal cell carcinoma		criteria
RCCT	randomized controlled clinical trial		respiratory distress syndrome

RDT	regular dialysis (hemodialysis) treatment	REPS	repetitions
		RER	renal excretion rate
		RES	resection
RDTD	referral, diagnosis, treatment, and discharge		resident
			reticuloendothelial system
		RESC	resuscitation
RDVT	recurrent deep vein thrombosis	resp.	respirations
			respiratory
		REST	restoration
RDW	red (cell) distribution width	RET	retention
			reticulocyte
RE	concerning		retina
	rectal examination		retired
	reflux esophagitis		return
	regional enteritis		right esotropia
	reticuloendothelial	retic	reticulocyte
	retinol equivalents	REV	reverse
	right ear		review
	right eye		revolutions
R & E	rest and exercise	RF	renal failure
	round and equal		rheumatic fever
R↑E	right upper extremity		rheumatoid factor
RE✔	recheck		risk factor
REC	rear end collision	R&F	radiographic and fluoroscopic
	recommend		
	record	RFA	right femoral artery
	recovery		right fronto-anterior
	recreation	RFL	right frontolateral
	recur	RFLP	restriction fragment length polymorphism
RECT	rectum		
RED SUBS	reducing substances	RFM	rifampin
REE	resting energy expenditure	RFP	request for payment
R-EEG	resting electroencephalo-gram		right frontoposterior
		RFS	rapid frozen section
REF	referred	RFT	right frontotransverse
	refused		routine fever therapy
	renal erythropoietic factor	RG	right gluteal
ref →	refer to	RGM	right gluteus medius
Reg block	regional block anesthesia	RGO	reciprocating gait orthosis
regurg	regurgitation	Rh	Rhesus factor in blood
rehab	rehabilitation	RH	reduced haloperidol
REL	relative		rest home
	religion		retinal hemorrhage
REM	rapid eye movement		right hand
	recent event memory		right hyperphoria
REMS	rapid eye movement sleep		room humidifier
REP	repair	RHB	raise head of bed
	repeat	RHC	respiration has ceased
	report	RHD	relative hepatic dullness
repol	repolarization		rheumatic heart disease

RHF	right heart failure		right lung
RHG	right hand grip		Ringer's lactate
RHH	right homonymous hemianopsia	R→L	right to left
		RLBCD	right lower border of cardiac dullness
RHL	right hemisphere lesions		
rHmEPO	recombinant human erythropoietin	RLC	residual lung capacity
		RLD	related living donor
RHS	right hand side		right later decubitus
RHT	right hypertropia	RLE	right lower extremity
RHW	radiant heat warmer	RLF	retrolental fibroplasia
RI	regular insulin	RLL	right lower lobe
	rooming in	RLN	recurrent laryngeal nerve
RIA	radioimmunoassay	RLQ	right lower quadrant
RIAT	radioimmune antiglobulin test	RLR	right lateral rectus
		RLS	Ringer's lactate solution
RIC	right iliac crest	RLT	right lateral thigh
	right internal carotid (artery)	RLTCS	repeat low transverse cesarean section
RICE	rest, ice, compression, and elevation	RM	radical mastectomy
			repetitions maximum
RICM	right intercostal margin		respiratory movement
RICS	right intercostal space		room
RICU	respiratory intensive care unit	R&M	routine and microscopic
		RMA	right mento-anterior
RID	radial immunodiffusion	RMCA	right main coronary artery
	ruptured intervertebral disc		right middle cerebral artery
RIE	rocket immunoelectro-phoresis	RMCL	right midclavicular line
		RMD	rapid movement disorder
RIF	rifampin	RME	resting metabolic expenditure
	right iliac fossa		
	right index finger		right mediolateral episiotomy
	rigid internal fixation		
RIG	rabies immune globulin	RMEE	right middle ear exploration
RIH	right inguinal hernia		
RIMA	right internal mammary anastamosis	RMK #1	remark number 1
		RML	right mediolateral
RIND	reversible ischemic neurologic defect		right middle lobe
		RMLE	right mediolateral episiotomy
RIP	radioimmunoprecipitin test		
		RMP	right mentoposterior
	rapid infusion pump	RMR	resting metabolic rate
RIR	right inferior rectus		right medial rectus
RISA	radioactive iodinated serum albumin	RMS	repetitive motion syndrome
RIST	radioimmunosorbent test	RMS®	Rectal Morphine Sulfate (suppository)
RK	radial keratotomy		
	right kidney	RMSE	root mean square error
RL	right lateral	RMSF	Rocky Mountain spotted fever
	right leg		

RMT	Registered Music Therapist			Registered Physician's Assistant
	right mentotransverse			right pulmonary artery
RN	Registered Nurse	RPCF		Reiter protein
RNA	radionuclide angiography			complement fixation
	ribonucleic acid	RPD		removable partial denture
RND	radical neck dissection	RPE		rating of perceived
RNEF	resting (radio-) nuclide			exertion
	ejection fraction			retinal pigment
RO	routine order			epithelium
R/O	rule out	RPF		relaxed pelvic floor
ROA	right occiput anterior			renal plasma flow
ROAC	repeated oral doses of	RPG		retrograde pyelogram
	activated charcoal	RPGN		rapidly progressive
ROC	receiver operating			glomerulonephritis
	characteristic	RPH		retroperitoneal
	resident on call			hemorrhage
	residual organic carbon	R.Ph.		Registered Pharmacist
ROI	region of interest	RPHA		reverse passive
ROIDS	hemorrhoids			hemagglutination
ROIH	right oblique inguinal	RPICCE		round pupil intracapsular
	hernia			cataract extraction
ROL	right occipitolateral	RPL		retroperitoneal
ROM	range of motion			lymphadenectomy
	right otitis media	RPN		renal papillary necrosis
	rupture of membranes			resident's progress notes
Romb	Romberg	R_2PN		second year resident's
ROMSA	right otitis media,			progress notes
	suppurative, acute	RPO		right posterior oblique
ROMSC	right otitis media,	RPP		rate-pressure product
	suppurative, chronic	RPR		rapid plasma reagin (test
ROP	retinopathy of prematurity			for syphilis)
	right occiput posterior			Reiter protein reagin
RoRx	radiation therapy	RPT		Registered Physical
ROS	review of systems			Therapist
	rod outer segments	RPTA		Registered Physical
ROSC	restoration of spontaneous			Therapist Assistant
	circulation	RQ		respiratory quotient
ROT	remedial occupational	RR		recovery room
	therapy			regular respirations
	right occipital transverse			respiratory rate
	rotator			retinal reflex
ROUL	rouleaux	R/R		rales-rhonchi
RP	radial pulse	R&R		rate and rhythm
	radiopharmaceutical			recent and remote
	Raynaud's phenomenon			recession and resection
	retinitis pigmentosa			rest and recuperation
	retrograde pyelogram	RRA		radioreceptor assay
RPA	radial photon			Registered Record
	absorptiometry			Administrator

RRAM	rapid rhythmic alternating movements	RSW	right-sided weakness
RRCT, no(m)	regular rate, clear tones, no murmurs	RT	radiation therapy
			recreational therapy
			rectal temperature
RRE	round, regular, and equal (pupils)		renal transplant
			repetition time
RREF	resting radionuclide ejection fraction		respiratory therapist
			right
rRNA	ribosomal ribonucleic acid		right thigh
RRND	right radical neck dissection		running total
		R/t	related to
RROM	resistive range of motion	RTA	renal tubular acidosis
RRR	regular rhythm and rate	RTC	return to clinic
RRRN	round, regular, and react normally		round the clock
		RTER	return to emergency room
RRT	Registered Respiratory Therapist	rt. ↑ ext.	right upper extremity
		RTF	return to flow
RS	Raynaud's syndrome	RTL	reactive to light
	Reiter's syndrome	RTM	routine medical care
	Reye's syndrome	RTN	renal tubular necrosis
	rhythm strip	RTNM	retreatment staging of cancer
	right side		
	Ringer's solution	RTO	return to office
R/S	rest stress	RTOG	Radiation Therapy Oncology Group
	rupture spontaneous		
RSA	right sacrum anterior	rtPA	recombinant tissue-type plasminogen
	right subclavian artery		
RScA	right scapuloanterior	RTRR	return to recovery room
RScP	right scapuloposterior	RTS	real time scan
rscu-PA	recombinant, single-chain, urokinase-type plasminogen activator		return to sender
		RT₃U	resin triiodothyronine uptake
		RTUS	realtime ultrasound
RSDS	reflex-sympathetic dystrophy syndrome	RTW	return to work
		RTWD	return to work determination
R-SICU	respiratory-surgical intensive care unit		
		RTx	radiation therapy
RSO	right salpingo-oophorectomy	RU	routine urinalysis
		RUA	routine urine analysis
	right superior oblique	RUE	right upper extremity
RSP	right sacroposterior	RUG	retrograde urethrogram
RSR	regular sinus rhythm	RUL	right upper lobe
	relative survival rate	RUOQ	right upper outer quadrant
	right superior rectus	rupt.	ruptured
RSS	Russian spring-summer (encephalitis)	RUQ	right upper quadrant
		RURTI	recurrent upper respiratory tract infection
RST	right sacrum transverse		
RSTs	Rodney Smith tubes		
RSV	respiratory syncytial virus	RUSB	right upper sternal border
	right subclavian vein	RV	rectovaginal

	residual volume		take
	respiratory volume		therapy
	return visit		treatment
	right ventricle	RXN	reaction
	rubella vaccine	RXT	radiation therapy
RVAD	right ventricular assist device		right exotropia
RVD	relative vertebral density		
RVE	right ventricular enlargement		**S**
RVEDP	right ventricular end-diastolic pressure	S	sacral
			second (s)
RVET	right ventricular ejection time		semilente insulin
			sensitive
RVF	Rift-Valley fever		serum
	right ventricular function		single
RVG	radionuclide ventriculography		sister
			son
	right ventrogluteal		subjective findings
RVH	right ventricular hypertrophy		suction
			sulfur
RVIDd	right ventricle internal dimension diastole		supervision
		$\bar{s}$	without (this is a dangerous abbreviation)
RVL	right vastus lateralis		
RVO	relaxed vaginal outlet	S_1	first heart sound
	retinal vein occlusion	S_2	second heart sound
	right ventricular outflow	S_3	third heart sound (ventricular gallop)
	right ventricular overactivity	S_4	fourth hear sound (atrial gallop)
RVOT	right ventricular outflow tract	$S_1...S_5$	sacral vertebra 1 through 5
RVR	rapid ventricular response		
RVP	right ventricular pressure	SA	salicylic acid
RVS	rabies vaccine, adsorbed		sleep apnea
RVSWI	right ventricular stroke work index		sinoatrial
			sinoatrial
RVT	renal vein thrombosis		Spanish American
RV/TLC	residual volume to total lung capacity ratio		suicide alert
			suicide attempt
RVV	rubella vaccine virus		surface area
RVVT	Russell's viper venom time		surgical assistant
			sustained action
RW	ragweed	S/A	same as
R/W	return to work		sugar and acetone
RWM	regional wall motion	S&A	sugar and acetone
Rx	drug	SAA	same as above
	medication	SAB	serum albumin
	pharmacy		spontaneous abortion
	prescription		subarachnoid bleed
	radiotherapy		subarachnoid block

SAC	short arm cast	SARA	sexually acquired reactive arthritis
	substance abuse counselor		system for anesthetic and respiratory administration
SACC	short arm cylinder cast		
SACH	solid ankle cushion heel		
SAD	seasonal affective disorder	SAS	saline, agent, and saline
	Self-Assessment Depression (scale)		self-rating anxiety scale
			short arm splint
	subacute dialysis		sleep apnea syndrome
	sugar and acetone determination		subarachnoid space
			sulfasalazine
SADL	simulated activities of daily living	SASH	saline, agent, saline, and heparin
SADR	suspected adverse drug reaction	SAT	saturated
			saturation
SADS	Schedule for Affective Disorders and Schizophrenia		Saturday
			speech awareness threshold
			subacute thyroiditis
SAE	short above elbow (cast)		
SAF	self-articulating femoral	SATL	surgical Achilles tendon lengthening
Sag D	sagittal diameter		
SAH	subarachnoid hemorrhage	SAVD	spontaneous assisted vaginal delivery
	systemic arterial hypertension		
		SB	safety belt
SAI	Sodium Amytal interview		sandbag
SAL	salicylate		Sengstaken-Blakemore (tube)
	Salmonella		
SAL 12	sequential analysis of 12 chemistry constituents		sinus bradycardia
			small bowel
SAM	self-administered medication		spina bifida
			stand-by
	systolic anterior motion		Stanford-Binet
SAN	side-arm nebulizer		sternal border
	sinoatrial node		stillbirth
	slept all night		stillborn
SANC	short arm navicular cast	Sb	antimony
sang	sanguinous	S/B	side bending
SAO	small airway obstruction	SBA	serum bactericidal activity
SaO$_2$	arterial oxygen percent saturation		standby assistant (assistance)
SAPD	self-administration of psychotropic drugs	SBC	standard bicarbonate
			strict bed confinement
SAPH	saphenous	SBE	short below elbow (cast)
SAPS	short arm plaster splint		shortness of breath on exertion
	Simplified Acute Physiology Score		subacute bacterial endocarditis
SAQ	short arc quad		
SAR	seasonal allergic rhinitis	SBFT	small bowel follow through
	sexual attitudes reassessment		
		SBG	stand-by guard

SBGM	self blood glucose monitoring	SCC	sickle cell crisis squamous cell carcinoma
SBI	systemic bacterial infection	SCCa	squamous cell carcinoma
SB-LM	Stanford Binet Intelligence Test-Form LM	SCCA	semi-closed circle absorber
		SCD	sequential compression device
SBO	small bowel obstruction		service connected disability
SBOD	scleral buckle, right eye		sickle cell disease
SBOH	State Board of Health		spinal cord disease
SBOM	soybean oil meal		subacute combined degeneration
SBOS	scleral buckle, left eye		
SBP	school breakfast program		sudden cardiac death
	scleral buckling procedure	ScDA	scapulodextra anterior
	small bowel phytobezoars	ScDP	scapulodextra posterior
	spontaneous bacterial peritonitis	SCE	sister chromatid exchange
	systolic blood pressure	SCEMIA	self-contained enzymic membrane immunoassay
SBQC	small based quad cane		
SBR	strict bed rest	SCEP	somatosensory cortical evoked potential
SBS	shaken baby syndrome short bowel syndrome	SCFE	slipped capitol femoral epiphysis
SBT	serum bactericidal titers	SCG	sodium cromoglycate
SBTT	small bowel transit time	SCh	succinylcholine chloride
SC	schizophrenia	SCHISTO	schistocytes
	self-care	SCHIZ	schizocytes
	serum creatinine		schizophrenia
	service connected	SCHLP	supracricord hemilaryngopharyngec- tomy
	sickle-cell		
	Snellen's chart		
	spinal cord	SCI	spinal cord injury
	sternoclavicular	SCID	severe combined immunodeficiency disorders
	subclavian		
	subclavian		
	subcutaneous	SCIPP	sacrococcygeal to inferior pubic point
	sulfur colloid		
	without correction (without glasses)	SCIU	spinal cord injury unit
SCA	subcutaneous abdominal (block)	SCIV	subclavian intravenous
		SCL	skin conductance level symptom checklist
SCAN	suspected child abuse and neglect	SCL-90	symptoms checklist—90 items
SCAT	sheep cell agglutination titer	ScLA	scapulolaeva anterior
	sickle cell anemia test	SCLC	small-cell lung cancer
SCB	strictly confined to bed	SCLE	subcutaneous lupus erythematosis
SCBC	small cell bronchogenic carcinoma		
SCBF	spinal cord blood flow	ScLP	scapulolaeva posterior

SCLs	soft contact lenses	SDB	sleep disordered breathing
SCM	sensation, circulation, and motion	SDC	serum digoxin concentration
	spondylitic caudal myelopathy		sodium deoxycholate
	sternocleidomastoid	SD&C	suction, dilation, and curettage
SCMD	senile choroidal macular degeneration	SDB	self-destructive behavior
SCN	special care nursery	SDC	sleep disorders center
SCOP	scopolamine	SDD	selective digestive (tract) decontamination
SCP	sodium cellulose phosphate	SDH	subdural hematoma
SCR	special care room (seclusion room)	SDL	serum digoxin level
			serum drug level
	spondylitic caudal radioculopathy		speech discrimination loss
SCr	serum creatinine	SDP	sacrodextra posterior
SCT	sickel cell trait		stomach, duodenum, and pancreas
	sugar coated tablet	SDS	same day surgery
SCU	self-care unit		Self-Rating Depression Scale
	special care unit	SDT	sacrodextra transversa
SCUF	slow and continuous ultrafiltration		speech detection threshold
		SDU	step-down unit
SCUT	schizophrenia chronic undifferentiated type	SE	saline enema
SCV	subclavian vein		side effect
	subcutaneous vaginal (block)		soft exudates
			spin echo
SD	scleroderma		standard error
	senile dementia		Starr-Edwards
	septal defect	Se	selenium
	severely disabled	sec	second
	shoulder disarticulation		secondary
	spontaneous delivery		secretary
	standard deviation	SECPR	standard external cardiopulmonary resuscitation
	standard diet		
	sterile dressing	SED	sedimentation
	straight drainage		spondyloepiphyseal dysplasia
	streptozocin and doxorubicin	sed rt	sedimentation rate
	sudden death	SEER	Surveillance, Epidemiology, and End Results (program)
	surgical drain		
S & D	stomach and duodenum		
SDA	sacrodextra anterior	SEG	segment
	Seventh-Day Adventist	segs	segmented neutrophils
	steroid-dependent asthmatic	SEH	subependymal hemorrhage
SDAT	senile dementia of Alzheimer's type	SEI	subepithelial (comeal) infiltrate

SELFVD	sterile elective low forceps vaginal delivery		specific gravity
			Swan-Ganz
SEM	scanning electron microscopy	SGA	small for gestational age
		SGC	Swan-Ganz catheter
	semen	SGD	straight gravity drainage
	standard error of mean	SGE	significant glandular enlargement
	systolic ejection murmur		
SEMI	subendocardial myocardial infarction	$\bar{s}$ gl	without correction/ without glasses
SENS	sensitivity	SGOT	serum glutamic oxaloacetic transaminase (same as AST)
	sensorium		
SEP	separate		
	somatosensory evoked potential	SGPT	serum glutamic pyruvic transaminase (same as ALT)
	systolic ejection period		
SEQ	sequella	SGS	second generation sulfonylurea
SER	scanning equalization radiography		
			subglottic stenosis
SER-IV	supination external rotation, type 4 fracture	SH	serum hepatitis
			short
SERs	somatosensory evoked responses		shoulder
			shower
SES	socioeconomic status		social history
SEWHO	shoulder-elbow-wrist-hand orthosis		surgical history
		S&H	speech and hearing
SF	salt free	S/H	suicidal/homicidal ideation
	saturated fat		
	scarlet fever	SHA	super heated aerosol
	seizure frequency	S Hb	sickle hemoglobin screen
	seminal fluid	SHEENT	skin, head, eyes, ears, nose, and throat
	soft feces		
	spinal fluid	Shig	*Shigella*
	sugar free	SHL	supraglottic horizontal laryngectomy
	symptom-free		
	synovial fluid	SHS	student health service
S&F	soft and flat	SI	International System of Units
SFA	saturated fatty acids		
	superficial femoral artery		sacroiliac
SFC	spinal fluid count		self-inflicted
SFEMG	single-fiber electromyography		seriously ill
			small intestine
SFP	spinal fluid pressure		strict isolation
SFPT	standard fixation preference test		stress incontinence
			stroke index
SFTR	sagittal, frontal, transverse, rotation	SIADH	syndrome of inappropriate antidiuretic hormone secretion
SFV	superficial femoral vein		
SG	salivary gland	S & I	suction and irrigation
	serum glucose		
	skin graft	SIB	self-injurious behavior

sibs	siblings	SLE	slit lamp examination
SICT	selective intracoronary thrombolysis		systemic lupus erythematosus
SICU	surgical intensive care unit	SLFVD	sterile low forceps vaginal delivery
SIDS	sudden infant death syndrome	SLGXT	symptom limited graded exercise test
Sig.	let it be marked (appears on prescription before directions for patient)	SLK	superior limbic keratoconjunctivitis
SIJ	sacroiliac joint	SLMFVD	sterile low mid-forceps vaginal delivery
SILFVD	sterile indicated low forceps vaginal delivery	SLMP	since last menstrual period
SIM	selective ion monitoring Similac®	SLN	superior laryngeal nerve
Sim c̄ Fe	Similac with iron®	SLNTG	sublingual nitroglycerin
SIMV	synchronized intermittent mandatory ventilation	SLNWBC	short leg nonweight-bearing cast
SIS	sister	SLNWC	short leg non-walking cast
SISI	short increment sensitivity index	SLO	streptolysin O
		SLR	straight leg raising
SIT	Slossen Intelligence Test sperm immobilization test	SLRT	straight leg raising test
		SLS	short leg splint single limb support
SIT BAL	sitting balance	SLT	swing light test
SIT TOL	sitting tolerance	SLT	sacrolaeva transversa
SIV	Simian immunodeficiency virus	sl. tr.	slight trace
SIW	self-inflicted wound	SLUD	salivation, lacrimation, urination, and defecation
SJS	Stevens-Johnson syndrome		
	Swyer-James syndrome	SLWC	short leg walking cast
SK	senile keratosis SmithKline® solar keratosis streptokinase	SM	sadomasochism skim milk small streptomycin systolic murmur
SK 65®	propoxyphene HCl 65 mg	SMA	sequential multiple analyzer simultaneous multichannel auto-analyzer spinal muscular atrophy superior mesenteric artery
SKAO	supracondylar knee-ankle orthosis		
SK-SD	streptokinase streptodornase		
SL	sensation level shortleg slight sublingual	SMA-6	sequential multipler analyzer for sodium, potassium, CO_2, chloride, glucose, and BUN
S/L	slit lamp (examination)		
SLA	sacrolaeva anterior slide latex agglutination		
SLB	short leg brace	SMA-7	sodium, potassium, CO_2, chloride, glucose, BUN, and creatinine
SLC	short leg cast		
SLCC	short leg cylinder cast		

SMA-12	glucose, BUN, uric acid, calcium, phosphorus, total protein, albumin, cholesterol, total bilirubin, alkaline phosphatase, SGOT, and LDH			standardized mortality ratio
				submucosal resection
			SMRR	submucous resection and rhinoplasty
			SMS	senior medical student
				somatostatin
SMA-23	includes the entire SMA-12 plus sodium, potassium, CO_2, chloride, direct bilirubin, triglyceride, SGPT, indirect bilirubin, R fraction, and BUN/creatinine ratio		SMV	submentovertical
				superior mesenteric vein
			SMVT	sustained monomorphic ventricular tachycardia
			SN	sciatic notch
				student nurse
			Sn	tin
			S/N	signal to noise ratio
			SNA	specimen not available
SMAS	superficial musculoapo-neurotic system		SNAP	sensory nerve action potential
SMBG	self-monitoring blood glucose		SNB	scalene node biopsy
			SNC	skilled nursing care
SMC	special mouth care		SNCV	sensory nerve conduction velocity
SMCD	senile macular chorioretinal degeneration		SND	single needle device
				sinus node dysfunction
SMD	senile macular degeneration		SNE	subacute necrotizing encephalomyelopathy
SMF	streptozocin, mitomycin, and fluorouracil		SNF	skilled nursing facility
			SNGFR	single nephron glomerular filtration rate
SMFVD	sterile mid-forceps vaginal delivery		SNHL	sensorineural hearing loss
SMI	sensory motor integration (group)		SNOOP	Systematic Nursing Observation of Psychopathology
	severely mentally impaired		SNP	sodium nitroprusside
	small volume infusion		SNS	sterile normal saline (0.9% sodium chloride)
	sustained maximal inspiration			
	safety, monitoring, intervention, length of stay and evaluation		SNT	sinuses, nose, and throat
				suppan nail technique
			SO	second opinion
SMILE	sustained maximal inspiratory lung exercises			shoulder orthosis
				significant other
				sphincter of Oddi
SMO	Senior Medical Officer			standing orders
	slip made out			suboccipital
SMON	subacute myeloopticoneu-ropathy			superior oblique
				supraoptic
				supraorbital
SMP	self-management program			sutures out
SMR	senior medical resident		S-O	salpingo-oophorectomy
	skeletal muscle relaxant		S&O	salpingo-oophorectomy

SO₃	sulfite		speech
SO₄	sulfate		spouse
SOA	serum opsonic activity		stand pivot
	spinal opioid analgesia		suicide precautions
	supraorbital artery		suprapubic
	swelling of ankles	sp	species
SOAA	signed out against advice	S/P	semiprivate
SOAM	sutures out in the morning		serum protein
SOAMA	signed out against medical advice		spinal
			stand and pivot
SOAP	subjective, objective, assessment, and plans		status post
			suicide precautions
SOAPIE	subjective, objective, assessment, plan, intervention, and evaluation		suprapubic
			systolic pressure
		SPA	albumin human (formerly known as salt-poor albumin)
SOB	shortness of breath (this abbreviation has caused problems)		serum prothrombin activity
	see order book		stimulation produced analgesia
	side of bed		
SOC	socialization	SPAG	small particle aerosol generator
	standard of care		
S & OC	signed and on chart (e.g. permit)	SPAMM	spatial modulation of magnetization
SOD	sinovenous occlusive disease	SPBI	serum protein bound iodine
	superoxide dysmutase	SPBT	suprapubic bladder tap
	surgical officer of the day	SPD	subcorneal pustular dermatosis
SOG	suggestive of good		
SOL	solution	SPET	single-photon emission tomography
	space occupying lesion		
SOM	serous otitis media	SPE	serum protein electrophoresis
SOMI	sterno-occipital mandibular immobilizer	SPEC	specimen
Sono	sonogram	SPECT	single photon emission computer tomography
SONP	solid organs not palpable		
SOP	standard operating procedure	Spec Ed	special education
		SPEP	serum protein electrophoresis
SOPM	stitches out in afternoon		
SOR	sign own release	SPET	single-photon emission tomography
SOS	may be repeated once if urgently required (Latin: si opus sit)	SPF	split products of fibrin
			sun protective factor
	self-obtained smear	sp fl	spinal fluid
SOT	something other than	SPG	sphenopalatine ganglion
	stream of thought	Sp.G.	specific gravity
SP	sacrum to pubis	SPH	spherocytes
	semiprivate	SPHERO	spherocytes
	sequential pulse	SPI	speech processor interface

SPIA	solid phase immunoabsorbent assay	SRH	signs of recent hemorrhage
SPIF	spontaneous peak inspiratory force	SRIF	somatotropin-releaseinhibiting factor (Somatostin)
SPL	sound pressure level		
SPK	superficial punctate keratitis	SRMD	stress-related mucosal damage
SPMA	spinal progressive muscle atrophy	SR/NE	sinus rhythm, no ectopy
		SRNVM	senile retinal neovascular membrane
SPN	solitary pulmonary nodule		subretinal neovascular membrane
	student practical nurse		
spont	spontaneous	SRO	single room occupancy
SPP	species (specus)	SROM	spontaneous rupture of membrane
	suprapubic prostatectomy		
SPROM	spontaneous premature rupture of membrane	SRP	stapes replacement prosthesis
SPS	simple partial seizure	SRS-A	slow-reacting substance of anaphylaxis
	sodium polyethanol sulfanate	SRT	sedimentation rate test
	systemic progressive sclerosis		speech reception threshold
			sustained release theophylline
SPT	skin prick test		
SP TAP	spinal tap	SRU	side rails up
SPU	short procedure unit	SRUS	solitary rectal ulcer syndrome
SPVR	systemic peripheral vascular resistance		
		SS	half
SQ	status quo		sacrosciatic
	subcutaneous (this is a dangerous abbreviation)		saline solution
			saliva sample
Sq CCa	squamous cell carcinoma		salt substitute
SR	screen		sickle cell
	sedimentation rate		Sjögren's syndrome
	side rails		sliding scale
	sinus rhythm		slip sent
	smooth-rough		Social Security
	sustained release		social service
	system review		somatostatin
S&R	seclusion and restraint		susceptible
SRBC	sheep red blood cells		symmetrical strength
	sickle red blood cells	S&S	shower and shampoo
SRBOW	spontaneous rupture of bag of waters		signs and symptoms
			support & stimulation
SRD	service-related disability	SSA	sagittal split advancement
	sodium-restricted diet		salicylsalicylic acid (salsalate)
SRF	somatotropin releasing factor		Sjögren's syndrome antigen A
	subretinal fluid		
SRF-A	slow releasing factor of anaphylaxis		Social Security Administration

	sulfasalicylic acid (test)	ST	esotropic
SSc	systemic sclerosis		sacrum transverse
SSCA	single shoulder contrast arthrography		shock therapy
			sinus tachycardia
SSCP	substernal chest pain		skin test
SSCr	stainless steel crown		slight trace
SSCVD	sterile spontaneous controlled vaginal delivery		speech therapist
			split thickness
			stomach
SSD	sickle cell disease		straight
	silver sulfadiazine		stress testing
	Social Security disability		stretcher
	source to skin distance		subtotal
SSDI	Social Security disability income	STA	second trimester abortion
			superficial temporal artery
SSE	saline solution enema	stab.	polymorphonuclear leukocytes (white blood cells, in nonmature form)
	soapsuds enema		
	systemic side effects		
SSEPs	somatosensory evoked potentials	STAI	State-Trait Anxiety Inventory
SSF	subscapular skinfold (thickness)	STAI-I	State-Trait-Anxiety Index—I
SSG	sublabial salivary gland	staph	*Staphylococcus aureus*
SSI	sub-shock insulin	stat	immediately
	Supplemental Security Income	STB	stillborn
		STBAL	standing balance
SSKI	saturated solution of potassium iodide	ST BY	stand by
		STC	serum theophylline concentration
SSM	superficial spreading melanoma		stimulate to cry
SSN	Social Security number		subtotal colectomy
SSO	Spanish speaking only		sugar tongue cast
SSOP	Second Surgical Opinion Program	STD	sexually transmitted diseases
			skin test dose
SSPE	subacute sclerosing panencephalitis		skin to tumor distance
			sodium tetradecylsulfate
SSPL	saturation sound pressure level	STD TF	standard tube feeding
SSPU	surgical short procedure unit	STEAM	stimulated-echo acquisition mode
SSS	layer upon layer	STET	single photon emission tomography
	scalded skin syndrome		
	sick sinus syndrome		submaximal treadmill exercise test
	sterile saline soak		
SSSB	sagittal split setback	STETH	stethoscope
SSSS	staphylococcal scalded skin syndrome	STF	special tube feeding
			standard tube feeding
SST	sagittal sinus thrombosis	STG	short-term goals
SSX	sulfisoxazole acetyl		split-thickness graft
S/SX	signs/symptoms		

STH	soft tissue hemorrhage	sub q	subcutaneous (this is a
	somatotrophic hormone		dangerous abbreviation
	subtotal hysterectomy		since the q is mistaken
	supplemental thyroid		for every, when a
	hormone		number follows)
STI	soft tissue injury	SUD	sudden unexpected death
STJ	subtalar joint	SUDS	Subjective Unit of
STK	streptokinase		Distress Scale
STL	serum theophylline level	SUI	stress urinary
STLE	St. Louis encephalitis		incontinence
STLOM	swelling, tenderness, and		suicide
	limitation of motion	SUID	sudden unexplained infant
STM	short-term memory		death
	streptomycin	SULF-	trimethoprim and
STNM	surgical-evaluative staging	PRIM	sulfamethoxazole
	of cancer	SUN	serum urea nitrogen
STNR	symmetrical tonic neck	SUP	superior
	reflex		supination
STORCH	syphilis, toxoplasmosis,		supinator
	other agents, rubella,		symptomatic uterine
	cytomegalovirus, and		prolapse
	herpes (maternal	supp	suppository
	infections)	SUR	surgery, surgical
STP	sodium thiopental	Surgi	surgigator
STPD	standard temperature and	SUUD	sudden unexpected,
	pressure-dry		unexplained death
STR	stretcher	SUX	succinylcholine
strep	*streptococcus*		suction
	streptomycin	SV	seminal vesical
STS	serologic test for syphilis		sigmoid volvulus
	sodium tetradecyl sulfate		single ventricle
	soft tissue swelling		stock volume
STSG	split thickness skin graft	SVB	saphenous vein bypass
STT	scaphoid, trapezium	SVC	slow vital capacity
	trapezoid		superior vena cava
	skin temperature test	SVCO	superior vena cava
STTOL	standing tolerance		obstruction
STU	shock trauma unit	SVCS	superior vena cava
STV	short term variability		syndrome
STZ	streptozocin	SVD	single vessel disease
S&U	supine and upright		spontaneous vaginal
SU	sensory urgency		delivery
	Somogyi units	SVE	sterile vaginal
SUA	serum uric acid		examination
	single umbilical artery		*Streptococcus viridans*
SUB	Skene's urethra and		endocarditis
	Bartholins glands	SVG	saphenous vein graft
SUBL	sublingual	SVL	severe visual loss
Subcu	subcutaneous	SVN	small volume nebulizer

SVO$_2$	mixed venous oxygen saturation			tension
				testicles
SVP	spontaneous venous pulse			thoracic
SVPB	supraventricular			trace
	premature beat	t		teaspoon (5 mL) (this is a dangerous abbreviation)
SVPC	supraventricular			
	premature contraction	T+		increase tension
SVR	supraventricular rhythm	T$_{1/2}$		half-life
	systemic vascular	T$_1$		tricuspid first sound
	resistance	T$_3$		triiodithyronine
		T-		decreased tension
SVRI	systemic vascular	T-2		dactinomycin,
	resistance index			doxorubicin,
SVT	supraventricular			vincristine, and
	tachycardia			cyclophosphamide
SW	sandwich	T3		Tylenol® with codeine 30
	Social Worker			mg (this is a dangerous
	stab wound			abbreviation)
SWD	short wave diathermy			
SWFI	sterile water for injection	T$_4$		levothyroxine
SWG	standard wire gauge			thyroxine
SWI	sterile water for injection	T$_{3/4}$ind		triiodoithyronine to
S&WI	surgical wound infection			thyroxine index
	skin and wound isolation	T-7		free thyroxine factor
SWOG	Southwest Oncology	T$_1$...T$_{12}$		thoracic nerve 1 through
	Group			12
SWP	small whirlpool			thoracic vertebra 1
SWS	slow wave sleep			through 12
	student ward secretary	TA		Takayasu's arteritis
	Sturge-Weber syndrome			temperature axillary
SWT	stab wound of the throat			temporal arteritis
SWU	septic work-up			therapeutic abortion
Sx	signs			tracheal aspirate
	surgery			traffic accident
	symptom			tricuspid atresia
SXR	skull X-ray	Ta		tonometry applanation
syr	syrup	T&A		tonsillectomy and
SYS BP	systolic blood pressure			adenoidectomy
SZ	schizophrenic	T(A)		axillary temperature
	seizure	TAA		thoracic aortic aneurysm
	suction			total ankle arthroplasty
SZN	streptozocin			transverse aortic arch
				triamcinolone acetonide
				tumor associated antigen
	T			(antibodies)
T	tablespoon (15 mL) (this	TAB		tablet
	is a dangerous			therapeutic abortion
	abbreviation)			triple antibiotic
	temperature			(bacitracin, neomycin,
	tender			and polymyxin—this is

		TAT	tetanus antitoxin
	a dangerous abbreviation)		till all taken
TAC	tetracaine, Adrenalin® and cocaine		Thematic Apperception Test
	triamcinolone cream	TB	total base
TAD	transverse abdominal diameter		total bilirubin
			total body
TADAC	therapeutic abortion, dilation, aspiration, and curettage		tuberculosis
		TBA	to be absorbed
			to be added
TAE	transcatheter arterial embolization		to be admitted
			total body (surface) area
TAF	tissue angiogenesis factor	TBB	transbronchial biopsy
TAH	total abdominal hysterectomy	tbc	tuberculosis
		TBE	tick-born encephalitis
	total artificial heart	TBF	total body fat
TAHBSO	total abdominal hysterectomy, bilateral salpingo-oophorectomy	TBG	thyroxine-binding globulin
		TBI	toothbrushing instruction
TAL	tendon Achilles lengthening		total body irradiation
		T bili	total bilirubin
	total arm length	TBK	total body potassium
TAML	therapy-related acute myelogenous leukemia	tbl.	tablespoon (15 mL)
		TBLB	transbronchial lung biopsy
TAM	tamoxifen	TBLC	term birth, living child
	teenage mother	TBLF	term birth, living female
TANI	total axial (lymph) node irradiation	TBLM	term birth, living male
		TBM	tracheobronchomalacia
TAO	thromboangitis obliterans		tubule basement membrane
	troleandomycin		
TAP	tonometry by applanation	TBNA	total body sodium
TAPVC	total anomalous pulmonary venous connection		transbronchial needle aspiration
			treated but not admitted
TAPVD	total anomalous pulmonary venous drainage	TBP	total-body photographs
		TBPA	thyroxine-binding prealbumin
TAPVR	total anomalous pulmonary venous return	TBR	total bed rest
		TBSA	total burn surface area
		tbsp	tablespoon (15 mL)
TAR	thrombocytopenia with absent radius	TBT	tolbutamide test
			tracheal bronchial toilet
	total ankle replacement	TBV	total blood volume
	treatment authorization request		transluminal balloon valvuloplasty
TARA	total articular replacement arthroplasty	TBW	total body water
		TBX_2	thromboxane B2
TAS	therapeutic activities specialist	TBX®	thiabendazole
		TC	throat culture
	typical absence seizures		tissue culture

	transcobalamin	TCOM	transcutaneous oxygen monitor
	trauma center		
	true conjugate	TcPCO$_2$	transcutaneous carbon dioxide
	tubocurarine		
Tc	technetium	TcPO$_2$	transcutaneous oxygen
T/C	telephone call	TCT	thyrocalcitonin
	to consider	TCVA	thromboembolic cerebral vascular accident
T&C	turn and cough		
	type and crossmatch	TD	Takayasu's disease
T&C#3	Tylenol® with 30 mg codeine		tardive dyskinesia
			tetanus-diphtheria toxoid (pediatric use)
TCA	team conference		
	terminal cancer		tidal volume
	thioguianine and cytarabine		tone decay
			transverse diameter
	trichloroacetic acid		travelers diarrhea
	tricuspid atresia		treatment discontinued
	tricyclic antidepressant	Td	tetanus-diphtheria toxoid (adult type)
TCABG	triple coronary artery bypass graft		
		TDD	thoracic duct drainage
TCAD	tricyclic antidepressant	TDE	total daily energy (requirement)
TCBS agar	thiosulfate-citrate-bile salt-sucrose agar		
		TDF	tumor dose fractionation
TCC	transitional cell carcinoma		
TCD	transverse cardiac diameter	TDI	toluene diisocyanate
		TDK	tardive diskinesia
TCCB	transitional cell carcinoma of bladder	TDL	thoracic duct lymph
		TDM	therapeutic drug monitoring
TCDB	turn, cough, and deep breath		
		TDN	transdermal nitroglycerin
TCDD	tetrachlorodibenzo-p-dioxin	TDNTG	transdermal nitroglycerin
		TdP	torsade de pointes
TCE	tetrachloroethylene	TdR	Thymidine
T cell	small lymphocyte	TDT	tentative discharge tomorrow
TCH	turn, cough, hyperventilate		
		TDWB	touch down weight bearing
TCID	tissue culture infective dose		
		TDx®	fluorescence polarization immunoassay
TCM	tissue culture media		
	traditional Chinese medicine	TE	echo time
			tennis elbow
	transcutaneous monitor		trace elements
TCMH	tumor-direct cell-mediated hypersensitivity		tracheoesophageal
		T&E	trial and error
TCMZ	trichloromethiazide	TEA	thromboendarterectomy
TCN	tetracycline		total elbow arthroplasty
TCNS	transcutaneous nerve stimulator	TEC	total eosinophil count
		T&EC	trauma and emergency center
TCNU	tauromustine		
TcO$_4$	pertechnetate	TEDS®	Anti-embolism Stockings

TEE	transesophageal echocardiography			total hysterectomy
		T&H		type and hold
TEF	tracheoesophageal fistula	THA		tacrine (tetrahydroacridine)
TEG	thromboelastogram			
TEI	transesophageal imaging			total hip arthroplasty
TEL	telemetry			transient hemispheric attack
tele	telemetry			
TEM	transmission electron microscopy	THAM®		tromethamine
		THC		tetrahydrocannibinol (dronabinol)
TEN	tension (intraocular pressure)			
				transhepatic cholangiogram
	toxic epidermal necrolysis			
TEN®	Total Enteral Nutrition	TH-CULT		throat culture
TENS	transcutaneous electrical nerve stimulation	THE		transhepatic embolization
		Ther Ex		therapeutic exercise
TEP	tracheoesophageal puncture	THI		transient hypogammaglobinemia of infancy
	tubal ectopic pregnancy	THKAFO		trunk-hip-knee-ankle-foot orthosis
TER	total elbow replacement			
TERB	terbutaline	THP		take home packs
tert.	tertiary			trihexphenidyl
TES	Treatment Emergent Symptoms	THR		total hip replacement
				training heart rate
TESPA	thiotepa	TI		tricuspid insufficiency
TET	transcranial electrostimulation therapy	TIA		transient ischemic attack
		tib.		tibia
	treadmill exercise test	TIBC		total iron-binding capacity
TF	tactile fremitus	TIC		trypsin-inhibitor capacity
	tetralogy of Fallot	TID		three times a day
	to follow	TIE		transient ischemic episode
	tube feeding	TIG		tetanus immune globulin
TFB	trifascicular block	TIL		tumor-infiltrating lymphocytes
TFL	tensor fascia lata			
TFT	trifluridine (trifluorothymidine)	TIN		three times a night (this is a dangerous abbreviation)
TFTs	thyroid function tests			
TG	triglycerides	tinct		tincture
6-TG	thioguanine	TIS		tumor *in situ*
TGA	transient global amnesia	TISS		Therapeutic Intervention Scoring System
	transposition of the great arteries	TIT		Treponema (pallidum) immobilization test
TGFA	triglyceride fatty acid			
TGS	tincture of green soap			triiodothyronine
TGT	thromboplastin generation test	TIVC		thoracic inferior vena cava
TGV	thoracic gas volume	+tive		positive
TGXT	thallium-graded exercise test	TIW		three times a week (this is a dangerous abbreviation)
TH	thrill			
	thyroid hormone	TJ		triceps jerk

TJA	total joint arthroplasty		trimethoxybenzoates
TJN	twin jet nebulizer	TMC	transmural colitis
TK	thymidine kinase		triamicinolone
TKA	total knee arthroplasty	TME	thermolysin-like
TKD	tokodynamometer		metalleondopeptidase
TKE	terminal knee extension	TMET	tread mill exercise test
TKNO	to keep needle open	TMI	threatened myocardial
TKP	thermokeratoplasty		infarction
TKO	to keep open	TMJ	temporomandibular joint
TKR	total knee replacement	TMM	torn medial meniscus
TKVO	to keep vein open	Tmm	McKay-Marg tension
TL	team leader	TMP	thallium myocardial
	trial leave		perfusion
	tubal ligation		transmembrane pressure
Tl	thallium		trimethoprim
TLA	translumbar arteriogram	TMP/SMX	trimethoprimsulfamethox-
	(aortogram)		azole
T/L	terminal latency	TMR	trainable mentally
TLC	tender loving care		retarded
	thin layer chromatography	TMST	treadmill stress test
	total lung capacity	TMT	treadmill test
	total lymphocyte count	TMTC	too many to count
	triple lumen catheter	TMTX	trimethexate
TLD	thermoluminescent	TMX	tamoxifen
	dosimeter	TMZ	temazepam
TLI	total lymphoid irradiation	TN	normal intraocular tension
	translaryngeal intubation		team nursing
TLNB	term living newborn		temperature normal
TLP	transitional living	T&N	tension and nervousness
	program	TNA	total nutrient admixture
TLR	tonic labyrinthine reflex	TNB	term newborn
TLS	tumor lysis syndrome		Tru-Cut® needle biopsy
TLSO	thoracic lumbar sacral	TNF	tumor necrosis factor
	orthosis	TNG	nitroglycerin
TLSSO	thoracolumbosacral spinal	TNI	total nodal irradiation
	orthosis	TNM	primary tumor, regional
TLV	total lung volume		lymph nodes, and
TM	temperature by mouth		distant metastasis (used
	Thayer Martin (culture)		with subscripts for the
	trabecular meshwork		staging of cancer)
	transcendental meditation	TNS	transcutaneous nerve
	tumor		stimulation (stimulator)
	tympanic membrane	TNT	tramcinolone and nystatin
T & M	type and crossmatch	TNTC	too numerous to count
TMA	thrombotic microangiopa-	TO	old tuberculin
	thy		telephone order
	transmetatarsal		total obstruction
	amputation		transfer out
TMB	transient monocular	T(O)	oral temperature
	blindness	T&O	tubes and ovaries

TOA	time of arrival	TPC	total patient care
	tubo-ovarian abscess	TPD	tropical pancreatic
TOB	tobramycin		diabetes
TOCE	transcatheter oily	TPE	therapeutic plasma
	chemoembolization		exchange
TOCO	tocodynamometer		total protective
TOD	intraocular pressure of the		environment
	right eye	TPF	trained participating father
TOF	tetralogy of Fallot	TPH	thromboembolic
	total of four		pulmonary hypertension
TOGV	transposition of the great		trained participating
	vessels		husband
TOH	throughout hospitalization	T PHOS	triple phosphate crystals
TOL	trial of labor	TPI	*Treponema pallidium*
TOM	tomorrow		immobilization
	transcutaneous oxygen	T plasty	tympanoplasty
	monitor	TPM	temporary pacemaker
Tomo	tomography	TPN	total parenteral nutrition
TON	tonight	TP & P	time, place, and person
TOP	termination of pregnancy	TPO	thrombopoietin
TOPV	trivalent oral polio		trial prescription order
	vaccine	TPPN	total peripheral parenteral
TORCH	toxoplasmosis, other		nutrition
	(syphillis, hepatitis,		trans pars plana
	Zoster), rubella,cy-		vitrectomy
	tomegalovirus, and	TPR	temperature
	herpes simplex		temperature, pulse, and
	(maternal infections)		respiration
TORP	total ossicular		total peripheral resistance
	replacement prosthesis	T PROT	total protein
TOS	intraocular pressure of the	TPT	time to peak tension
	left eye		treadmill performance test
	thoracic outlet syndrome	TPVR	total peripheral vascular
TOT BILI	total bilirubin		resistance
TP	temperature and pressure	TR	therapeutic recreation
	temporoparietal		tincture
	therapeutic pass		to return
	thrombophlebitis		trace
	Todd's paralysis		transfusion reaction
	total protein		transplant recipients
	treating physician		treatment
T & P	temperature and pulse		tricuspid regurgitation
	turn and position		tremor
TPA	alteplase, recombinant		tumor registry
	(tissue plasminogen	T(R)	rectal temperature
	activator)	T & R	tenderness and rebound
	tissue polypeptide antigen	TRA	therapeutic recreation
	total parenteral		associate
	alimentation		to run at

trach.	tracheal		Tay-Sachs disease
	tracheostomy	T set	tracheotomy set
Trans D	transverse diameter	TSE	testicular self-examination
TRAS	transplant renal artery stenosis	TSF	tricep skin fold
		TSH	thyroid-stimulating hormone
TRC	tanned red cells		
TRD	tongue-retaining device	tsp	teaspoon (5 mL)
	traction retinal detachment	TSP	total serum protein
		TSPA	thiotepa
Tren	Trendelenberg	TSR	total shoulder replacement
TRH	protirelin (thyrotropin-releasing hormone)	TSS	toxic shock syndrome
		TST	titmus stereocuity test
TRI	trimester		trans-scrotal testosterone
TRIG	triglycerides		treadmill stress test
TRISS	Trauma Score and Injury Severity Score	T&T	tobramycin and ticarcillin
			touch and tone
TRM-SMX	trimethoprimsulfamethoxazole	TT	tetanus toxoid
			thrombin time
tRNA	transfer ribonucleic acid		thymol turbidity
TRND	Trendelenburg		tilt table
TRO	to return to office		tonometry
TRP	tubular reabsorption of phosphate		transtracheal
			twitch tension
TRS	Therapeutic Recreation Specialist	T/T	trace of ___ /trace of___
		TT4	total thyroxine
TRT	thermoradiotherapy	TTA	total toe arthroplasty
T3RU	triiodothyroxine resin uptake	TTD	temporary total disability
			transverse thoracic diameter
TRUS	transrectal ultrasound		
TRUSP	transrectal ultrasound of the prostate	TTN	transient tachypnea of the newborn
TRZ	triazolam	TTNA	transthoracic needle aspiration
TS	temperature sensitive		
	test solution	TTNB	transient tachypnea of the newborn
	toe signs		
	Tourette's syndrome	TTO	to take out
	transsexual		transtracheal oxygen
	Trauma Score	TTOD	tetanus toxoid outdated
	tricuspid stenosis	TTOT	transtracheal oxygen therapy
TSA	toluenesulfonic acid		
	total shoulder arthroplasty	TTP	thrombotic thrombocytopenic purpura
TSAR®	tape surrounded Appli-rulers		
		TTR	triceps tendon reflex
TSBB	transtracheal selective bronchial brushing	TTS	tarsal tunnel syndrome
			temporary threshold shift
TSC	technetium sulfur colloid		through the skin
	theophylline serum concentration		transdermal therapeutic system
TSD	target to skin distance	TTT	tolbutamide tolerance test

TTUTD	tetanus toxoid up-to-date		TWG	total weight gain
TTVP	temporary transvenous pacemaker		TWHW ok	toe walking and heel walking all right
TTWB	touch toe weight bearing		TWR	total wrist replacement
TU	Todd units		TWWD	tap water wet dressing
	transrectal ultrasound		Tx	therapy
	tuberculin units			traction
TUF	total ultrafiltration			transfuse
TUN	total urinary nitrogen			transplant
TUPR	transurethral prostatic resection			treatment
				tympanostomy
TUR	transurethral resection		T & X	type and crossmatch
T_3UR	triiodothyronine uptake ratio		TxA_2	thromboxane A_2
			TXM	type and crossmatch
TURB	turbidity			T cell crossmatch
TURBN	transurethral resection bladder neck		TYCO #3	Tylenol® with 30 mg of codeine (#1=7.5 mg,
TURBT	transurethral resection bladder tumor			#2=15 mg and#4=60 mg of codeine present
TURP	transurethral resection of prostate		Tyl	Tylenol® tyloma (callus)
TURV	transurethral resection valves		TYMP	tympanogram
TUU	transureteroureterostomy		TZ	transition zone
TV	television			
	temporary visit			

U

	tidal volume		U	ultralente insulin
	transvenous			units (this is the most dangerous abbreviation
	trial visit			—spell out "unit")
	Trichomonas vaginalis			urine
T/V	touch-verbal		U/1	1 finger breadth below umbilicus
TVC	triple voiding cystogram			
	true vocal cord		1/U	1 finger over umbilicus
TVDALV	triple vessel disease with an abnormal left ventricle		U/	at umbilicus
			UA	umbilical artery
				unauthorized absence
TVF	tactile vocal fremitus			uncertain about
TVH	total vaginal hysterectomy			upper arm
TVN	tonic vibration response			upper airway
TVP	transvenous pacemaker			uric acid
	transvesicle prostatectomy			urinalysis
TVSC	transvaginal sector scan		UAC	umbilical artery catheter
TVU	total volume of urine			under active
TVUS	transvaginal ultrasound			upper airway congestion
TW	tapwater		UAL	umbilical artery line
	test weight			up *ad lib*
TWD	total white and differential count		UAO	upper airway obstruction
TWE	tapwater enema		UAPF	upon arrival patient found
TWETC	tapwater enema till clear		UAT	up as tolerated

UAVC	univentricular atrioventricular connection	UESP	upper esophageal sphincter pressure
UBF	unknown black female	UF	ultrafiltration until finished
UBI	ultraviolet blood irradiation	UFC	urine-free cortisol
		UFF	unusual facial features
UBM	unknown black male	UFFI	urea formaldehyde foam insulation
UBW	usual body weight		
UC	ulcerative colitis	UFN	until further notice
	umbilical cord	UFO	unflagged order
	unconscious	UFR	ultrafiltration rate
	urea clearance	UG	until gone
	urine culture		urinary glucose
	uterine contraction		urogenital
U&C	urethral & cervical	UGDP	University Group Diabetes Project
	usual and customary		
UCD	urine collection device	UGH	uveitis, glaucoma, and hyphema
	usual childhood diseases		
UCE	urea cycle enzymopathy	UGI	upper gastrointestinal series
UCG	urinary chorionicgonado-tropins		
		UGIH	upper gastrointestinal (tract) hemorrhage
UCHD	usual childhood diseases		
UCHS	uncontrolled hemorrhagic shock	UGK	urine glucose ketones
		UH	umbilical hernia
UCI	urethral catheter in		University Hospital
	usual childhood illnesses	UHBI	upper hemibody irradiation
UCL	uncomfortable loudness level		
		UHDDS	Uniform Hospital Discharge Data Set
UCO	urethral catheter out		
UCP	urethral closure pressure	UHP	University Health Plan
UCR	unconditioned response	UI	urinary incontinence
	usual, customary, and reasonable	UIBC	unsaturated iron binding capacity
UCRE	urine creatinine	UID	once daily (this is a dangerous abbreviation, spell out "once daily")
UCS	unconscious		
UCX	urine culture		
UD	as directed	UIQ	upper inner quadrant
	urethral discharge	UK	unknown
	uterine distension		urine potassium
UDC	usual diseases of childhood		urokinase
		U/L	upper and lower
UDCA	ursodeoxycholic acid	U & L	upper and lower
UDN	updraft nebulizer	ULLE	upper lid, left eye
UDO	undetermined origin	ULN	upper limits of normal
UDS	unconditioned stimulus	ULQ	upper left quadrant
UE	under elbow	ULRE	upper lid, right eye
	undetermined etiology	ULYTES	electrolytes, urine
	upper extremity	UM	unmarried
UES	upper esophageal sphincter	umb ven	umbilical vein
		UN	undernourished

	urinary nitrogen	USI	urinary stress incontinence
UNA	urinary nitrogen appearance	USMC	United States Marine Corp
UNa	urine sodium		
unacc	unaccompanied	USN	ultrasonic nebulizer
ung	ointment		United States Navy
UNK	unknown	USP	United States Pharmacopeia
UNOS	United Network of Organ Sharing		
		USPHS	United States Public Health Service
UO	under observation		
	undetermined origin	USUCVD	unsterile uncontrolled vaginal delivery
	urinary output		
UOP	urinary output	USVMD	urine specimen volume measuring device
UOQ	upper outer quadrant		
Uosm	urinary osmolality	UTD	up to date
✔ up	check up	ut dict	as directed
UP	unipolar	UTF	usual throat flora
UPJ	ureteropelvic junction	UTI	urinary tract infection
UPOR	usual place of residence	UTO	unable to obtain
UPPP	uvulopalatopharyngo-plasty		upper tibial osteotomy
		UTS	ulnar tunnel syndrome
U/P ratio	urine to plasma ratio		ultrasound
UPT	uptake	UUN	urinary urea nitrogen
	urine pregnancy test	UV	ultraviolet
UR	utilization review		ureterovesical
URD	undifferentiated respiratory disease		urine volume
		UVA	ultraviolet A light
URI	upper respiratory infection		ureterovesical angle
URIC A	uric acid	UVB	ultraviolet B light
url	unrelated	UVC	umbilical vein catheter
UROB	urobilinogen	UVJ	ureterovesical junction
urol	urology	UVL	ultraviolet light
URQ	upper right quadrant		umbilical venous line
URTI	upper respiratory tract infection	UVR	ultraviolet radiation
		U/WB	unit of whole blood
US	ultrasonography	UW	unilateral weakness
	unit secretary	UWF	unknown white female
USA	unit services assistant	UWM	unknown white male
	United States Army		unwed mother
USAF	United States Air Force		
USAN	United States Adopted Names		

V

USAP	unstable angina pectoris	V	five
USB	upper sternal border		gas volume
USCVD	unsterile controlled vaginal delivery		minute volume
			vagina
USDA	United States Department of Agriculture		vein
			verb
USG	ultrasonography		vomiting
USH	usual state of health	v̇	Ventilation (L/min)

+V	positive vertical divergence	VATER	vertebral, anal, tracheal, esophageal and renal anomalies
V&C	vertical and centric (a bite)	VATH	vinblastine, doxorubicin, thiotepa, and fluoxymesterone
V_1 to V_6	precordial chest leads		
VA	vacuum aspiration	VB	Van Buren (catheter)
	valproic acid		venous blood
	Veterans Administration		vinblastine and methotrexate
	visual acuity		
V_A	minute alveolar ventilation	VB_1	first voided bladder specimen
VAB	vinblastine, dactinomycin, bleomycin, cisplatin, and cyclophosphamide	VB_2	second midstream bladder specimen
VAC	ventriculo-arterial connections	VBAC	vaginal birth after cesarean
	vincristine, dactinomycin, and cyclophosphamide	VBAP	vincristine, carmustine, doxorubicin, and prednisone
	vincristine, doxorubicin, and cyclophosphamide	VBC	vinblastine, bleomycin, and cisplatin
VAD	vascular (venous) access device	VBD	vinblastine, bleomycin, and cisplatin
	vincristine, doxorubicin, and dexamethasone	VBG	venous blood gas
VADRIAC	vincristine, doxorubicin, and cyclophosphamide		vertical banded gastroplasty
vag.	vagina	VBI	vertebrobasilar insufficiency
VAG HYST	vaginal hysterectomy	VBL	vinblastine
VAH	Veterans Administration Hospital	VBP	vinblastine, bleomycin, and cisplatin
VAIN	vaginal intrapiethelial neoplasia	VBS	vertebral-basilar system
VALE	visual acuity, left eye	VC	color vision
VAMC	Veterans Administration Medical Center		etoposide and carboplatin
			pulmonary capillary blood volume
VAMS	Visual Analogue Mood Scale		vena cava
VANCO/P	vancomycin-peak		vital capacity
VANCO/T	vancomycin-trough		vocal cords
VAP	venous access port	VCAP	vincristine, cyclophosphamide, doxorubicin, and prednisone
	vincristine, asparaginase, and prednisone		
VAR	variant	VCCA	velocity common carotid artery
VARE	visual acuity, right eye	VCG	vectocardiography
VAS	vascular	VCO	centilator CPAP oxyhood
	visual analogue scale		
VASC	Visual-Auditory Screen Test for Children	VCR	vincristine sulfate
		VCT	venous clotting time
VAS RAD	vascular radiology	VCU	voiding cystourethrogram

VCUG	vesicoureterogram	VEP	visual evoked potential
	voiding cystourethrogram	VER	ventricular escape rhythm
VD	venereal disease		visual evoked responses
	voided	VET	veteran
	volume of distribution	VF	left leg (electrode)
V_D	deadspace volume		ventricular fibrillation
V&D	vomiting and diarrhea		vision field
VDA	venous digital angiogram		vocal fremitus
	visual discriminatory	VFI	visual fields intact
	acuity	V. Fib	ventricular fibrillation
VDAC	vaginal delivery after	VFP	vitreous fluorophotometry
	cesarean	VFPN	Volu-feed premie nipple
VDD	atrial synchronous	VFRN	Volu-feed regular nipple
	ventricular inhibited	VG	vein graft
	pacing		ventricular gallop
VDG	venereal disease—gon-		very good
	orrhea	VGH	very good health
Vdg	voiding	VH	vaginal hysterectomy
VDH	valvular disease of the		Veterans Hospital
	heart		viral hepatitis
VDL	vasodepressor lipid		vitreous hemorrhage
	visual detection level	VHD	valvular heart disease
VD or M	venous distention or	VI	six
	masses		volume index
VDP	vinblastine, decarbazine,	vib	vibration
	and cisplatin	VICA	velocity internal carotid
VDRL	Venereal Disease		artery
	Research Laboratory	VID	videodensitometry
	(test for syphilis)	VIG	vaccinia immune globulin
VDRR	vitamin D-resistant rickets	VIN	vaginal intra-epiheal
VDS	venereal disease—syphilis		neoplasia
	vindesine	VIP	etopside, ifosfamide, and
VDT	video display terminal		cisplatin
VD/VT	dead space to tidal		vasoactive intestinal
	volume ratio		peptide
VE	vaginal examination		vasoactive intracorpeal
	vertex		pharmacotherapy
	vocational evaluation		very important patient
V_E	minute volume (expired)		vinblastine, ifosfamide,
VEA	ventricular ectopic		and cisplatin
	activity		voluntary interruption of
VEB	ventricular ectopic beat		pregnancy
VED	ventricular ectopic	VISC	vitreous infusion suction
	depolarization		cutter
VEE	Venezuelan equine	VIT	venom immunotherapy
	encephalitis		vital
VENT	ventilation		vitamin
	ventilator	vit. cap.	vital capacity
	ventral	VIZ	namely
	ventricular	VKC	vernal keratoconjunctivitis

VL	left arm (electrode)	VPDF	vegetable protein diet plus fiber
VLBW	very low birth weight		
VLCD	very low calorie diet	VPDs	ventricular premature depolarizations
VLCFA	very long chain fatty acids		
		VPI	velopharyngeal insufficiency
VLDL	very low density lipoprotein		
		VPL	vento-posterolateral
VLH	ventrolateral nucleus of the hypothalamus	VPR	volume pressure response
		VQ	ventilation perfusion
VM 26	teniposide	VR	valve replacement
VMA	vanillylmandelic acid		right arm (electrode)
VMCP	vincristine, melphalan, cyclophosphamide, and prednisone		ventricular rhythm
			verbal reprimand
			vocational rehabilitation
VMH	ventromedial hypothalamus	VRA	visual reinforcement audiometry
VMO	vastic medalis oblique	VRC	vocational rehabilitation counselor
VMR	vasomotor rhinitis		
VN	visiting nurse	VRI	viral respiratory infection
VNA	Visiting Nurses' Association		
		VRL	ventral root, lumbar
VNC	vesicle neck contracture	VRT	variance of resident time
VO	verbal order		ventral root, thoracic
VOCAB	vocabulary		Visual Retention Test
VOCTOR	void on call to operating room	VS	versus
			very sensitive
VOD	venocclusive disease		vital signs
	vision right eye	VSBE	very short below elbow (cast)
VOL	volume		
	voluntary	VSD	ventricular septal defect
VOO	continuous ventricular asynchronous pacing	VSI	visual motor integration
		VSO	vertical subcondylar oblique
VOR	vestibular ocular reflex		
VOS	vision left eye	VSOK	vital signs normal
VOT	Visual Organization Test	VSR	venous stasis retinopathy
VOU	vision both eyes	VSS	vital signs stable
VP	etoposide	VT	ventricular tachycardia
	variegate porphyria	v. tach.	ventricular tachycardia
	venous pressure	VTE	venous thromboembolism
	ventricularoperitoneal	VTEC	verotoxin-producing *Escherichia coli*
	ventricul-peritoneal		
V & P	vagotomy and pyloroplasty	VTX	vertex
		VV	varicose veins
	ventilation and perfusion	V&V	vulva and vagina
VP-16	etoposide	V/V	volume to volume ratio
VPA	valproic acid	VVD	vaginal vertex delivery
VPB	ventricular premature beat	VVFR	vesicovaginal fistula repair
VPC	ventricular premature contractions	V/VI	grade 5 on a 6 grade basis

VVOR	visual-vestibulo-ocular-reflex	W Bld	whole blood
		WBN	wellborn nursery
VVT	ventricular synchronous pacing	WBQC	wide base quad cane
		WBR	whole body radiation
VW	vessel wall	WBS	whole body scan
VWD	von Willebrand's disease	WBTF	Waring Blender tube feeding
VWM	ventricular wall motion		
V_x	vitrectomy	WBTT	weight bearing to tolerance
VZ	varicella zoster		
VZIG	varicella zoster immune globulin	WBUS	weeks by ultrasound
		WC	ward clerk
VZV	varicella zoster virus		ward confinement
			wet compresses
			wheelchair
W			white count
			whooping cough
w	week		will call
	weight	WCC	well child care
	white		white cell count
	widowed	WD	ward
	wife		well developed
	with		well differentiated
WA	when awake		wet dressing
	while awake		Wilson's disease
	wide awake		word
W or A	weakness or atrophy		wound
WAF	weakness, atrophy, and fasciculation	W/D	warm and dry
			withdrawal
	white adult female	W→D	wet to dry
WAIS	Wechsler Adult Intelligence Scale	W4D	Worth four-dot (test)
		WDCC	well-developed collateral circulation
WAIS-R	Wechsler Adult Intelligence Scale-Revised		
		WDF	white divorced female
		WDHA	watery diarrhea, hypokalemia, and achlorhydria
WAM	white adult male		
WAP	wandering atrial pacemaker		
		WDLL	well-differentiated lymphocytic lymphoma
WAS	Wishott-Aldrich syndrome		
WASS	Wasserman test	WDM	white divorced male
WAT	word association test	WDWN-BM	well-developed, well-nourished black male
WB	waist belt		
	weight bearing		
	well baby	WDWN-WF	well-developed, well-nourished white female
	Western blot		
	whole blood		
WBAT	weight bearing as tolerated	WE	weekend
		W/E	weekend
WBC	well baby clinic	WEE	Western equine encephalitis
	white blood cell (count)		
WBCT	whole blood clotting time		
WBH	whole-body hyperthermia	WEP	weekend pass

WF	white female			written order
WFI	water for injection	W/O	water in oil
WFL	within functional limits		without
WF-O	will follow in office	WOP	without pain
WFR	wheel-and-flare reaction	W.P.	whirlpool
WH	walking heel (cast)	WPFM	Wright peak flow meter
WHO	World Health Organization	WPP	Welcher Preschool Primary Scale of Intelligence
	wrist-hand orthosis		
WHPB	whirlpool bath	WPPSI	Wechsler Preschool and Primary Scale of Intelligence
WHV	woodchuck hepatitis virus		
WHVP	wedged hepatic venous pressure		
		WPW	Wolff-Parkinson-White
WI	ventricular demand pacing	WR	Wasserman reaction
	walk-in		wrist
W/I	within	WRAT	Wide Range Achievement Test
W+I	work and interest		
WIA	wounded in action	WS	ward secretary
WIC	women, infants, and children		watt seconds
			work simplification
WID	widow	W&S	wound and skin
	widower	WSepF	white separated female
WISC	Wechsler Intelligence Scale for Children	WSepM	white separated male
		WSF	white single female
WISC-R	Weschler Intelligence Scale for Children-revised	WSM	white single male
		WSP	wearable speech processor
		WT	walking tank
wk	week		weight (wt)
WL	waiting list		wisdom teeth
	weight loss	WTS	whole tomography slice
WLS	wet lung syndrome	W/U	workup
WLT	waterload test	WV	whispered voice
WK	week	W/V	weight-to-volume ratio
	work	WW	Weight Watchers
WKS	Wernicke-Korsakoff syndrome	W/W	weight-to-weight ratio
		WWAC	walk with aid of cane
WM	white male	WWidF	white widowed female
WMA	wall motion abnormality	WWidM	white widowed male
WMF	white married female		
WMM	white married male		
WMP	weight management program		

X

X	break
WMX	whirlpool, massage, and exercise
	cross
	crossmatch
WN	well nourished	except
WND	wound	start of anesthesia
WNL	within normal limits	ten
WNLS	weighted nonlinear least squares	times
	xylocaine
WO	weeks old	$\overline{X}$	except

X^2	chi-square		**Y**	
X+#	xyphoid plus number of fingerbreadths	YACP	young adult chronic patient	
X3	orientation as to time, place and person	YAG	yittrium aluminum garnert (laser)	
XBT	xylose breath test	Yb	ytterbium	
XC	excretory cystogram	Yel	yellow	
XD	times daily	YF	yellow fever	
X&D	examination and diagnosis	YFI	yellow fever immunization	
X2d	times two days			
XDP	xeroderma pigmentosum	YJV	yellow jacket venom	
Xe	xenon	YLC	youngest living child	
XeCT	xenon-enhance computed tomography	Y/N	yes/no	
		YO	years old	
X-ed	crossed	YOB	year of birth	
XKO	not knocked out	YORA	younger-onset rheumatoid arthritis	
XL	extra large			
X-leg	cross leg	YPLL	years of potential life lost before age 65	
XLH	X-linked hypophos-phatemia			
XLJR	X-linked juvenile retinoschisis	yr	year	
		YSC	yolk sac carcinoma	
XM	crossmatch	YTD	year to date	
X-mat.	crossmatch			
XMM	xeromammography		**Z**	
XOM	extraocular movements			
XP	xeroderma pigmentosum	Z-E	Zollinger-Ellison (syndrome)	
XR	x-ray			
XRT	radiation therapy	ZEEP	zero end-expiratory pressure	
XS	excessive			
XS-LIM	exceeds limits of procedure	ZES	Zellinger-Ellison syndrome	
XT	exotropia	Z-ESR	zeta erythrocyte sedimentation rate	
X(T)	intermittent exotropia			
XU	excretory urogram	ZIG	zoster serum immune globulin	
XULN	times upper limit of normal			
		ZIP	zoster immune plasma	
XV	fifteen	ZMC	zygomatic	
XX	normal female sex chromosome type	Zn	zinc	
		ZnO	zinc oxide	
	twenty	ZnOE	zinc oxide & eugenol	
XX/XY	sex karyotypes	ZPC	zero point of charge	
XXX	thirty		zopiclone	
XY	normal male sex chromosome type	ZPO	zinc peroxide	
		ZPT	zinc pyrithione	
XYL	Xylocaine	ZSB	zero stools since birth	
XYLO	xylocaine	ZSR	zeta sedimentation rate	

Miscellaneous

↑	above		(this is a dangerous
	alive		symbol as it is
	elevated		mistaken for a one)
	greater than	±	either positive or
	high		negative
	improved		no definite cause
	increase		plus or minus
	rising		very slight trace
↓	dead		right lower quadrant
	decrease	⌐	right upper quadrant
	falling	⌐	left upper quadrant
	lowered	⌐	left lower quadrant
	normal plantar reflex	>	greater than
	restricted	≥	greater than or
→	causes to		equal to
	progressing	<	caused by
	results in		less than
	showed	≤	less than or equal to
	to the right	◁	not less than
←	resulted from	▷	not more than
	to the left	∧	above
⟷	stable		diastolic blood
	to and from		pressure
	unchanging		increased
↓↓	flexor	∨	below
	testes descended		systolic blood
↑↑	extensor		pressure
	positive Babinsky	≠	not equal to
	testes undescended	≅	approximately equal
‖	parallel		to
	parallel bars	≈	approximately
✔	check	×	left ear-air conduction
	flexion		threshold
#	fracture	>	left ear-bone
	number		conduction threshold
	pound	☐	left ear-masked air
∴	therefore		conduction threshold
Δ scan	delta scan (computed	⌐	left ear-masked bone
	tomography scan)		conduction threshold
+	plus	○	right ear-air
	positive		conduction threshold
	present	<	right ear-bone
−	absent		conduction threshold
	minus	△	right ear-masked air
	negative		conduction threshold
/	slash mark signifying	⌐	right ear-masked
	per, and, or with		bone conduction

⊖	threshold	♀ (sitting)	sitting position
	threshold reversible		
♥	heart		
?	questionable	A α	alpha
∅	no	B β	beta
	none	Γ γ	gamma
@	at	Δ δ	anion gap
1°	first degree		change
	primary		delta
2°	second degree		delta gap
	secondary		prism diopter
3°	tertiary		temperature
	third degree		trimester
i	one (Roman numerals are dangerous expressions and should not be used)	E ε	epsilon
		Z ζ	zeta
		H η	eta
		Θ θ	negative
			theta
ii	two		
iii	three	I ι	iota
iiii	four	K κ	kappa
iv	four (this is a dangerous abbreviation as it is read as intravenous, use 4)	Λ λ	lambda
		M μ	micro
			mu
		N ν	nu
		Ξ ξ	xi
		O o	omicron
v	five	Π π	pi
vi	six	P ρ	rho
vii	seven	Σ σ	sigma
viii	eight		sum of
ix	nine	T τ	tau
x	ten	Υ υ	upsilon
xi	eleven	Φ φ	phenyl
xii	twelve		phi
♂	male		thyroid
♀	female	X χ	chi
■	deceased male	Ψ ψ	psi
●	deceased female		psychiatric
□	living male	Ω ω	omega
○	living female	′	feet
◇	sex unknown		minutes (as in 30′)
(□)	adopted living male	″	inches
*	birth		seconds
†	dead	⊙	start of an operation
	death	⊗	end of anesthesia
		3×	three times
♀	standing	2×2	gauze dressing folded 2″ x 2″
○—<	recumbent position	4×4	gauze dressing folded 4″ x 4″

$$\begin{array}{c|c|c} 140 & 101 & 17 \end{array}$$
Na = 140, Cl = 101,
BUN = 17

$$\begin{array}{c|c|c} 3.4 & 25 & 140 \end{array}$$
K = 3.4, CO_2 = 25,
glucose = 140

$$\begin{array}{c|c} 16 & 85 \\ 5.0 & \\ 45 & 30 \end{array} 35$$

red blood cell count, hemoglobin, mean corpuscular volume, mean corpuscular hemoglobin concentration, hematocrit, mean corpuscular hemoglobin

$$\frac{2\ cm\ |\ 80\%}{-2\ Vtx}$$

2 cm = dilation of cervix
80% = degree of cervix effacement
Vtx = vertex; presentation of fetus, (breech = Br)
−2 = station; distance above (−) or below (+) the spine of the ischium measured in cm

sodium	chloride	BUN	
potassium	bicarbonate	creatinine.	glucose

calcium	protein	AST	LDH	
phosphorus	albumin	ALT	Alkaline phos	bilirubin

segmented neutrophils	lymphocytes	eosinophils
banded neutrophils	monocytes	basophils

hemoglobin	WBC
hematocrit	platlets

Note: there are many individual variations as to how these are arranged

Reflexes[6]

Reflexes are usually graded on a 0 to 4+ scale:

- 4+   may indicate disease
  often associated with clonus
  very brisk, hyperactive
- 3+   brisker than average
  possibly but not necessarily indicative of disease
- 2+   average
  normal
- 1+   low normal
  somewhat diminished
- 0   may indicate neuropathy
  no response

Muscle strength[6]

0—No muscular contraction detected
1—A barely detectable flicker or trace of contraction
2—Active movement of the body part with gravity eliminated
3—Active movement against gravity
4—Active movement against gravity and some resistance
5—Active movement against full resistance without evident fatigue. This is normal muscle strength

Pulse[6]

  0   completely absent
+1   markedly impaired
+2   moderately impaired
+3   slightly impaired
+4   normal

Gradation of intensity of heart murmurs[6]

1/6 or I/VI	may not be heard in all positions very faint, heard only after the listener has "tuned in"
2/6 or II/VI	quiet, but heard immediately upon placing the stethoscope on the chest
3/6 or III/VI	moderately loud
4/6 or IV/VI	loud
5/6 or V/VI	very loud, may be heard with a stethoscope partly off the chest (thrills are associated)
6/6 or VI/VI	may be heard with the stethoscope entirely off the chest (thrills are associated)

Apothecary symbols

The symbols presented below are for informational use. The apothecary system should *not* be used. Only the metric system should be used. The methods of expressing the symbols, the meanings, and the equivalences are not the classic ones, nor are they accurate, but reflect the usual intended meanings when used by some older physicians in writing prescription directions.

℥ or ℥ī	dram, teaspoonful, (5 mL)	℥ or ℥i	ounce, (30 mL)
		gr	grain (approximately 60 mg)
℥ii	two drams, 2 teaspoonfuls, (10 mL)	♏	minim (approximately 0.06 mL)
℥ss	half ounce, tablespoonful, (15 mL)	gtt	drop

References

1. CBE Style Manual, 5th ed. Bethesda, MD: Council of Biology Editors; 1983.

2. Gennaro AR, ed. Remington's Pharmaceutical Sciences. 17th ed. Easton, PA: Mack Publishing Co; 1985; 1780.

3. Davis NM, Cohen MR. Medication errors: causes and prevention. Huntingdon Valley, PA: Neil M. Davis Associates; 1981.

4. Cohen MR. Medication error reports. Hosp Pharm (appears monthly from 1975 to the present).

5. Cohen MR. Medication errors. Nursing 90 (appears monthly, starting in Nursing 77, to the present).

6. Bates B. A guide to physical examinations. 4th ed. Philadelphia: J.B. Lippincott; 1987.

Please forward additional meanings for these abbreviations, additional abbreviations and their meanings, or corrections to the author so that the list can be updated. Thank you. Dr. Neil M. Davis, 1143 Wright Drive, Huntingdon Valley, PA 19006. FAX (215) 938 1937

Please forward additional meanings for these abbreviations, additional abbreviations and their meanings, or corrections to the author so that the list can be updated. Thank you. Dr. Neil M. Davis, 1143 Wright Drive, Huntingdon Valley, PA 19006.

Additions

Additions

Additions

Additions

Additions

Additions

PRICE

1-4 copies	**$9.95 each**	When check or money order *accompanies* the order.
		If payment is not included, a $2.00 fee per order will be added to cover the cost of invoicing
5-19 copies	**$9.95 each**	Purchase order accepted. No invoicing fee.
20 or more	**$7.10 each**	Purchase order accepted. No invoicing fee.

United States—Postage cost is included in the price. Pennsylvania residents add 6% sales tax.

Outside the United States—Prices as shown above plus postage. Pay in U.S. dollars through a correspondent U.S. bank.

Order from
    Neil M. Davis Associates
    1143 Wright Drive
    Huntingdon Valley, PA 19006
    Phone (215) 947-1752
    FAX (215) 938-1937

ISBN 0-931431-15-0

"Tu mue[rte] [será] placer para ambos, Raquel Mariana Morgan. Qué forma tan contradictoria de morir—con placer."

WITHDRAWN

Todo era borroso frente mí. Quedé pasmada al ver que esa cosa se transformaba de nuevo en un hombre alto, elegante, de levita. ¿Era un vampiro? ¿Un vampiro realmente viejo?

"¿Tal vez le temes al dolor?" dijo la visión de hombre elegante, hablando con tanta propiedad como el mismo profesor Henry Higgins. Sonriendo, me levantó lanzándome hacia el otro lado de la habitación.

Mi espalda golpeó el armario con tanta fuerza que perdí el aire y mi cuchillo sonó al caer al suelo. Me deslicé por el gabinete roto luchando por respirar, impotente frente a la cosa que me levantaba por el vestido.

"¿Qué eres?," dije carraspeando.

Sonrió. "Todo lo que te asusta."

"Divertido viaje a través de una fascinante versión de nuestro mundo."
Charlaine Harris

"No es fácil crear una protagonista que combine las cualidades de Anita Blake y Stephanie Plum, pero Kim Harrison lo hace con estilo."
Jim Butcher

Próximamente por Kim Harrison

EL REGRESO DE LOS MUERTOS VIVIENTES

LA NOCHE DE LA BRUJA MUERTA

KIM
HARRISON

Traducido del inglés por Felipe Cárdenas

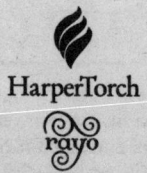

HarperTorch

rayo

Una rama de HarperCollinsPublishers

HARPERTORCH/RAYO
Una rama de HarperCollins*Publishers*
10 East 53rd Street
New York, New York 10022-5299

Copyright © 2004 por Kim Harrison
Traducción © 2005 por Felipe Cárdenas
Extracto de *El Regreso de Los Muertos Vivientes*
© 2005 por Kim Harrison
Traducción © 2005 por Felipe Cárdenas
ISBN-13: 978-0-06-083750-1
ISBN-10: 0-06-083750-0

Primera edición Rayo, Octubre 2005
Primera edición en inglés de HarperTorch: Mayo 2004
Primera edición especial de HarperTorch: Diciembre 2003

*Al hombre que dijo que le gustaba
mi sombrero.*

Agradecimientos

Quisiera darle las gracias a la gente que sufrió conmigo durante las reescrituras de este libro. Ustedes saben quienes son, y les agradezco mucho. Pero antes que nada, quisiera agradecer a mi editora, Diana Gill, por sus maravillosas sugerencias que me abrieron las puertas a muchos pensamientos, y a mi agente, Richard Curtis.

LA NOCHE
DE LA BRUJA
MUERTA

Uno

A la sombra de una tienda desierta, frente a la taberna Sangre y Pociones, me acomodé los pantalones de cuero tratando de pasar inadvertida. *Esto es patético,* pensé, mientras le echaba una mirada a la calle mojada y vacía. Soy demasiado buena como para esto.

Normalmente mi trabajo consistía en apresar brujas sin licencia y brujas negras: se necesita una bruja para atrapar a otra. Pero esta semana las calles estaban más calladas que de costumbre. Los que podían estaban en la costa oeste, en la reunión anual, pero yo estaba aquí con este caso de pacotilla. ¡Una carga! La suerte de estar aquí en la oscuridad bajo la lluvia se la debo al Giro.

"¿A quién estoy engañando?" murmuré, acomodándome la correa del bolso sobre el hombro. Hace un mes que no me mandaban a atrapar brujas sin patente, brujas blancas, brujas negras, nada. Tal vez no fue buena idea atrapar al hijo del alcalde por andar de hombre lobo en una noche sin luna llena.

Un auto elegante dobló la esquina. Era negro, iluminado por la luz de mercurio de la calle. Esta era la tercera vez que pasaba por la cuadra. Fruncí el ceño cuando se aproximó lentamente. "¡Maldición!," dije. "Necesito un sitio más oscuro."

"Él piensa que eres una prostituta, Raquel," me dijo mi asistente al oído. "Te dije que ese corpiño rojo era demasiado llamativo."

"¿Alguna vez te han dicho que hueles a murciélago borracho, Jenks?," gruñí entre dientes, mis labios apenas moviéndose. Mi asistente estaba incómodamente cercano esta noche aferrándose a mi arete—una cosa grande, colgante— el arete, no el duende. Jenks era pretencioso, con mala actitud e igual temperamento. Claro, eso sí, sabía en qué jardín estaba el néctar. Lo mejor que me daban de asistentes eran duendes, desde aquél incidente que tuve con un sapo. Habría jurado que las hadas eran demasiado grandes para caber en la boca de un animal de esos.

Me acerqué a la esquina mientras el auto se detenía chapoteando en el asfalto mojado. Escuché el típico sonido de la ventanilla automática cuando se bajó el vidrio oscuro. Me incliné acompañada de mi mejor sonrisa al tiempo que mostraba mi identificación de trabajo. Ahí desapareció la mirada lasciva del mirón y su cara se puso pálida. El auto arrancó de una vez con un chirrido de llantas. "Debe ser un dominguero," pensé con desdén, pero *No*, corregí de inmediato. Parecía normal. Era humano. A pesar de ser correctos, términos como dominguero, empleado, blandengue, desquiciado y—mi favorito, marrano—no eran bien vistos; pero si el tipo andaba buscando prostitutas en los andenes de Los Hollows, podríamos llamarlo muerto.

El auto ni siquiera paró en el semáforo rojo. Yo me di vuelta al oír los maullidos de las prostitutas que desplacé al atardecer. Con su pose descarada del otro lado de la esquina, no parecían muy contentas conmigo. Hice un gesto para saludarlas, pero la más alta me maldijo antes de mostrarme su pequeño trasero. La prostituta y su "amigo" fornido hablaban fuerte, ocultando el cigarrillo que compartían. Eso sí, no olía a tabaco corriente. *Ese no es mi problema esta noche,* pensé, y me metí de nuevo entre las sombras.

Me recosté contra la piedra fría del edificio con los ojos puestos en las luces rojas del auto que frenaba y alcé las cejas al verme a mí misma. Soy una mujer alta, aproximadamente de un metro setenta, pero no tengo tanta pierna como la ramera que estaba en el pozo de luz cercano. Tampoco estaba tan maquillada como ella. Mis caderas angostas y mi busto casi plano no contribuyen mucho para hacerme material de calle. Antes de buscar en las tiendas para duendes, estuve mirando en la sección "tu primer sostén." Es imposible encontrar algo sin corazones y unicornios estampados.

Mis ancestros emigraron a este país querido, Estados Unidos, en el siglo diecinueve. No se cómo, pero de generación en generación las mujeres se las arreglaron para conservar los típicos cabellos rojos y los ojos verdes de nuestra tierra irlandesa. Eso sí, mis pecas están ocultas gracias a un hechizo que papá me regaló el día que cumplí trece años. Metió el diminuto amuleto en un anillo de meñique. Nunca salgo de casa sin él.

Suspiré y me reacomodé el bolso sobre el hombro. Los pantalones de cuero, las botas rojas y el corpiño de tiras delgadas no eran tan diferentes de la indumentaria que usaba los viernes para martirizar a mi jefe; pero salir así a la calle por la noche... "mierda," le dije a Jenks, "parezco una ramera."

Un gruñido fue su única respuesta. Me esforcé por no reaccionar mientras regresaba a la taberna. Llovía demasiado y aun faltaba tiempo para que hubiera más gente, pues aparte de mi asistente y aquellas "damas," la calle estaba desierta. Había estado ahí parada casi una hora y no veía señales de mi objetivo. Lo mejor sería entrar y esperar. Además, adentro no daría la sensación de ser una callejera.

Respiré hondo y me decidí a entrar. Me solté el moño de cabellos rizados hasta los hombros. Unos instantes para ordenarlos artísticamente sobre la cara, tirar la goma de mascar y listo. El taconeo de mis botas produjo un elegante contrapunto con las esposas que colgaban de mi cintura mientras cruzaba la calle mojada en dirección de la taberna. Las argollas de acero parecían un accesorio de utilería barata, pero eran reales y destinadas a buen uso. Sonreí. Con razón se detuvo el mirón. Sí. Son para trabajar; pero no exactamente para lo que estás pensando.

Me mandaron a Los Hollows en medio de la lluvia para

atrapar a un hada por evadir impuestos. ¿Cuánto más bajo puedo llegar?, pensé. Tal vez fue por atrapar a ese perro la semana pasada. ¿Cómo podía saber que era un hombre lobo? Correspondía a la descripción que me habían dado.

Una vez que entré al pequeño vestíbulo y me sacudí el agua, le eché un vistazo a las típicas porquerías de las tabernas irlandesas: gaitas colgadas de las paredes, letreros verdes de cerveza, sillas de vinilo negro y un escenario diminuto donde una futura estrella organizaba sus instrumentos y gaitas en medio de montañas de amplificadores. Había un tufillo a azufre de contrabando que despertó mis instintos depredadores. Olía a viejo de tres días, pero no lo suficientemente fuerte para poder seguir su rastro. Si tan solo lograra clavar al que lo abastecía, tal vez podría borrarme de la lista negra de mi jefe. Tal vez me daría una misión digna de mi talento.

"Oye," gruñó una voz. "¿Estás reemplazando a Toby?"

Olvidé el azufre, abrí bien los ojos y me di vuelta, hallándome a boca de jarro ante una camiseta verde brillante. Mis ojos recorrieron a un hombre tan grande como un oso. Un gorila. El nombre en la camiseta decía CLIFF. ¡Vaya! "¿Quién?" murmuré, mientras secaba las gotas de agua en mi escote con la manga de su camisa. No se alteró. Fue deprimente.

"Toby, una ramera estatal. ¿Volverá otra vez?"

Escuché una vocecilla que provenía de mi arete, casi cantando. "Te lo dije."

Sonreí a medias. "No lo sé," repuse entre dientes. "No soy una ramera."

Gruñó de nuevo observando mi atuendo. Busqué en mi bolso y le di mi identificación de trabajo. Cualquiera que estuviera mirándonos pensaría que estaba cerciorándose de mi edad. Con tantos hechizos para ocultar la edad, era obligatorio hacerlo, como también lo era el amuleto para rechazar hechizos que llevaba él alrededor del cuello. Resplandecía de un rojo pálido reaccionando a mi anillo del dedo meñique. Claro que eso no era suficiente razón para investigarme del todo. Todos los hechizos que llevaba en mi bolso estaban sin invocar, pero no porque no los necesitara esta noche.

"Seguridad Entremundos," proseguí, mientras le entregaba mi identificación. "Estoy de ronda buscando a alguien. No vengo a acosar a sus clientes. Por eso llevo este...eh... disfraz."

"Raquel Morgan," dijo en voz alta, casi cubriendo mi carné por completo con sus gruesos dedos. "Agente de Seguridad de Entremundos. ¿Eres agente de Entremundos?" Sus ojos pasaron del carné a mí y de nuevo al carné. Hizo una mueca con sus grandes labios. "¿Qué le pasó a tu cabello? ¿Te peinaste con un soplete?"

No le contesté. La foto en mi carné ya tenía tres años. Y no había sido un soplete sino una broma, una especie de iniciación informal como agente de tiempo completo. ¡Vaya broma!

El duendecillo saltó y dejó mi arete oscilando en el aire. "Yo cuidaría más mis palabras," le dijo, girando la cabeza y fijando los ojos en mi carné. "El último grandulón que se burló de su foto pasó la noche en la sala de urgencias con una sombrilla atravesada en la nariz."

Ya me estaba calentando. "¿Cómo sabes eso?" le pregunté, arrebatándole mi carné al grandulón.

"Todos en el Comité de Asignaciones lo saben" rió gustosamente el duende; "y también saben de tu intento por atrapar al Lobo con un hechizo para la comezón, pero que lo dejaste escapar por el retrete."

"Ya quisiera verte tratando de atrapar a un Lobo la víspera de luna llena y lograrlo sin que te muerda," argumenté en mi defensa. "No es tan fácil como parece. Tuve que usar una poción y son costosas, ¿sabes?"

"Y luego hechizaste un autobús lleno de gente." Sus alas de libélula se tornaron rojas de risa. Parecía Peter Pan en miniatura, vestido de seda negra y pañoleta roja, posando como uno de esos miembros de pandilla de centro de ciudad: eran diez centímetros de fastidio y mal humor.

"No fue culpa mía," dije frunciendo el ceño. "El conduc-

tor pasó encima de un bache. Además, alguien había trasto-
cado los hechizos. Trataba de enredarle las patas, pero terminé por quitarle el cabello al conductor y a todos los que
estaban sentados en las tres filas de adelante. Por lo menos
logré atraparlo, aun cuando malgasté mi sueldo pagando taxis las tres semanas siguientes hasta que el autobús decidió
volver a llevarme."

"¿Y el sapo?" dijo Jenks que salió disparado con un golpecillo que el grandulón le propinó con los dedos. "Yo fui el
único que se atrevió a acompañarte esta noche y me pagan
por alto riesgo." Sacó el pecho orgulloso.

Pero a Cliff no parecía importarle. Yo estaba consternada.
"Escuche," le dije. "Solo quiero sentarme allá a tomarme un
trago, tranquila y calladamente." Le hice un gesto indicando
el escenario donde el post adolescente seguía enredando los
cables de los amplificadores. "¿A qué hora empieza la función?"

El grandote encogió los hombros. "Es nuevo. Creo que
en una hora." De pronto se sintió un estruendo seguido de
aclamaciones y un amplificador cayó del escenario. "Tal
vez dos."

"Gracias." Ignoré la aguda risa de Jenks y me abrí paso
por las mesas desocupadas hasta un lugar un poco más
oscuro. Me senté debajo de una cabeza de alce, hundiéndome un par de centímetros en el mullido cojín. Era una
afrenta. Llevaba tres años con la S.E.—siete, contando los
cuatro que hice de clínica—¡pero estaba haciendo trabajo
de práctica! Sólo hacíamos el trabajo de base. Vigilábamos
Cincinnati, incluido el suburbio más grande de la ciudad
del otro lado del río, conocido cariñosamente como Los
Hollows. Nos encargábamos de las cosas sobrenaturales
que los humanos de la AFE—sigla de la Agencia Federal
Entremundos—no podían manejar: solucionar problemas
secundarios creados por hechizos o sacar familiares de
adentro de los árboles, eran el tipo de labores que hacían
los internos. Pero yo era agente, ¡maldición! Yo era más que
esto. Y había hecho *mejores cosas*.

Yo sola perseguí y atrapé a la banda de brujas negras que burló los conjuros de seguridad del zoológico de Cincinnati para robarse a los monos. Los vendían luego a los laboratorios biológicos clandestinos. Y... ¿alguno me agradeció por ese trabajo? No.

Yo fui quien se dio cuenta que el pájaro bobo que desenterraba cadáveres en los cementerios de las iglesias tenía que ver con esa avalancha de muertes en la unidad de transplantes de uno de los hospitales administrados por humanos. Todos pensaron que sólo estaba recogiendo ingredientes para fabricar hechizos ilegales; pero nadie pensó que hechizaba los mismos órganos infundiéndoles salud pasajera para luego venderlos en el mercado negro.

¿Y qué me dicen de los robos a los cajeros electrónicos que acosaron a la ciudad la Navidad pasada? Tuve que aplicarme seis hechizos simultáneos para tomar el aspecto de un hombre... ¡pero atrapé a la bruja! Usaba un encantamiento de amor y olvido para asaltar a los humanos incautos. Ese objetivo fue especialmente gratificante. La perseguí por tres calles pero no tuve tiempo de lanzarle mis hechizos, pues se devolvió para atacarme con un conjuro que pudo ser fatal. Hice bien poniéndola fuera de combate con una patada de gancho. Mejor todavía, la AFE venía siguiéndola hacía tres meses, pero yo la atrapé en dos días. Quedaron como unos tontos; pero, ¿acaso me dijeron "bien Raquel, ¡buen trabajo!"? ¿Se ofrecieron a llevarme con mi pie hinchado al edificio de la S.E.? No. Claro que no.

Últimamente me han asignado menos aún: chicos universitarios que usan hechizos para ver televisión por cable gratis, robos familiares, hechizos en broma; y, ¿cómo olvidar mi preferido? Perseguir gnomos por puentes y alcantarillas antes de que se coman el cemento. Me sumí en suspiros mirando el bar. Patético.

Jenks eludió mis indiferentes manotazos para alejarlo y se acomodó de nuevo en mi arete. Que le pagaran triple por acompañarme no era buen síntoma.

Una camarera vestida con ropas ligeras de color verde

llegó a mi mesa. Estaba demasiado alegre para ser tan temprano. "¡Hola!" dijo, mostrando los dientes y los hoyuelos de las mejillas. "Me llamo Dottie. Seré tu camarera esta noche." Sin dejar de sonreír, puso tres bebidas sobre la mesa: un Bloody Mary, una tradicional y un Shirley Temple. Qué tierno.

"Gracias linda," le dije con un suspiro de desgano. "¿Quién las manda?"

Dirigió una mirada de chica difícil hacia la barra, pero solo logró parecer una colegiala el día del gran baile. Miré a la altura de su cintura delgada donde llevaba amarrado el delantal y ví a tres cuerpos con ojos rebosados de lujuria. Era una vieja costumbre: aceptar un trago era aceptar la invitación que portaba. Algo más de qué ocuparte, Raquel. Parecían normales, pero eso en realidad nunca se sabe.

Al ver que la conversación no iría más lejos, Dottie se fue a la barra a seguir con sus labores. "Chequéalos, Jenks," susurré, y el duende salió veloz con las alas rosadas de emoción. Nadie lo vio partir: pura vigilancia de duendes.

El bar estaba tranquilo pero noté que había dos cantineros detrás de la barra—un viejo y una chica. Más tarde habría más ambiente. Sangre y Pociones era un sitio caliente donde los normales se mezclaban con Entremundos. Después regresaban al otro lado del río con las ventanillas del auto bien cerradas, animados y convencidos de que estuvieron irresistibles. Eso sí, un humano solitario brilla entre Entremundos como un grano en la cara de una colegiala en la fiesta de graduación; en cambio los Entremundos se mimetizan fácilmente con los humanos. Se trata de una destreza de supervivencia que perfeccionaron desde antes de Pasteur. Por eso me acompañaba el duende. Las hadas y los duendes son capaces de olfatear a los Entremundos en un abrir y cerrar de ojos.

Pasé una aburrida mirada por la taberna casi vacía, cuando de repente cambié el malhumor por una sonrisa. Acababa de reconocer una cara familiar del trabajo. Era Ivy.

Ivy era un vampiro, la agente estrella de la S.E. Nos conocimos varios años atrás, durante mi último año de práctica, e hicimos un par de rondas juntas. Recientemente la habían contratado como agente de tiempo completo. Ivy había estudiado seis años de universidad en lugar de los dos años de universidad y cuatro de práctica que hice yo. Pensé que hacernos trabajar juntas era una especie de broma.

Trabajar con un vampiro vivo o muerto me daba terror. Después me enteré que Ivy no era un vampiro activo y que había jurado abstenerse de la sangre. Éramos tan diferentes como se puede ser: ella era fuerte donde yo era débil. Me gustaría agregar que sus flaquezas eran mis fortalezas; pero Ivy no tenía flaquezas—aparte de su habilidad para acabar con la diversión.

Hacía años que no trabajábamos juntas; pero a pesar de que yo obtuve un ascenso—a regañadientes, por supuesto—ella me superaba. Ivy sabía decir todas las cosas correctas a las personas correctas en el momento correcto. También la ayudaba el hecho de pertenecer a la familia Tamwood, un apellido tan antiguo como la ciudad de Cincinatti. Era el último miembro vivo de los Tamwood que tenía alma, tan viva como lo estaba yo, a pesar de haber recibido la infección del virus vampiro de su madre quien aun vivía en aquel entonces. El virus moldeó a Ivy mientras ella crecía en las entrañas maternas, dándole un poco de ambos mundos: el de los vivos y el de los muertos.

Le hice una seña y enfiló hacia mí. Los tipos de la barra se codearon volviéndose al tiempo para admirarla. Ella les devolvió una mirada de desprecio y podría jurar que oí a uno de ellos suspirar.

"¿Cómo van las cosas, Ivy?" pregunté. Se acomodó y se sentó frente a mí.

El asiento de plástico sonó al recostar la espalda contra la pared. Colocó los largos tacones de sus botas en el descanso y sus rodillas sobresalían del borde de la mesa. Me llevaba una cabeza de estatura y, a pesar de que yo también era alta, ella gozaba de un porte y una figura elegantes. Su aspecto ligeramente oriental le daba cierto aire enigmático, lo que confirmaba mi teoría de que casi todas las modelos son vampiros. También vestía como una modelo: falda modesta de cuero y blusa de seda fina al estilo vampiro: todo negro, naturalmente. Su cabello era suave, oscuro y ondulado lo que hacía resaltar su piel pálida y las facciones ovaladas de su cara. No importa lo que hiciera con su cabellera, la hacía ver exótica. Yo podía pasar horas con la mía pero siempre me quedaba roja y crespa. El tipo del auto negro no hubiera parado por Ivy. Ella tiene demasiada clase.

"Hola Raquel," repuso Ivy. "¿Qué haces en Los Hollows?" Su voz era suave y melodiosa y fluía con la sutileza de la seda. "Pensé que estarías tomando un poco de cáncer de la piel en la playa esta semana," agregó. "¿Denon sigue molesto por lo del perro?"

Encogí los hombros tímidamente. "No." En realidad, el jefe casi revienta. Estuve a un milímetro de que me mandara a barrer las oficinas.

"Fue un error." Ivy tiró la cabeza suavemente hacia atrás dejando ver la extensión total de su cuello. No tenía ni una sola cicatriz. "Le puede suceder a cualquiera."

A cualquiera menos a ti, pensé agriamente. "¿Cierto?" dije en voz alta acercándole el Bloody Mary. "Pues... adivina mi misión." Hice tintinear los hechizos contra mis esposas con el trébol labrado de madera de olivo.

Sus dedos delgados se enroscaron en el vaso como si quisieran acariciarlo; pero esos mismos dedos podían romperme la muñeca si les aplicaba un poco más de fuerza. Ella tendría que estar muerta antes de tener la fuerza para destrozarlo sin querer, pero, por ahora, seguía siendo más fuerte que yo. La mitad de la bebida roja bajó por su garganta. "¿Desde cuándo se interesa la S.E. por los duendes?," me preguntó mirando los otros hechizos.

"Desde la última vez que el jefe se puso de mal humor."

Se estiró un poco para sacar un crucifijo que llevaba detrás de la blusa y sostuvo provocativamente el aro metálico entre los dientes. Sus colmillos eran afilados como los de un gato pero no más grandes que los míos. Los más largos le saldrían después de morir. Les retiré la mirada y me concentré en la cruz de metal. Era tan larga como mi mano y hermosamente fabricada de plata. Empezó a llevarla recientemente para fastidiar a su madre. No estaban en muy buenos términos.

Con los dedos acaricié la diminuta cruz de mis esposas, pensando lo difícil que debe ser tener a la madre muerta viviente. Yo sólo conocía a unos pocos vampiros muertos. Los más viejos hablaban poco y los nuevos terminaban generalmente estacados, a menos que aprendieran a cuidarse a sí mismos.

Los vampiros muertos no tienen la más mínima conciencia: son el instinto cruel encarnado. La única razón por la que obedecen las reglas sociales es porque piensan que son un juego; y los vampiros muertos sí que saben de reglas. Su existencia perenne depende de ellas, pero si las desafían, terminan encontrando muerte o dolor. Por supuesto, la más importante de todas es ocultarse del sol. Necesitan sangre a diario para estar bien. Cualquier sangre. Su único placer es tomarla de los vivos. Son poderosos. Su fuerza y resistencia son increíbles y sanan con velocidad asombrosa. Es difícil destruirlos, excepto cortándoles la cabeza o enterrándoles una estaca en el corazón.

Alcanzan la inmortalidad a cambio del alma y la pérdida de la conciencia. Los vampiros viejos dicen que eso es lo mejor: pueden satisfacer sus necesidades carnales sin sentir culpa cuando una persona muere para darles un día más de placer.

Ivy portaba el virus vampiro, pero también tenía alma. Estaba atrapada en un mundo intermedio hasta que la muerte la convirtiera en una muerta viviente. A pesar de no poseer ni el poder ni el peligro de un vampiro muerto, sus hermanos muertos la envidiaban porque podía caminar bajo el sol y creer en Dios sin dolor.

Los aros metálicos del collar de Ivy sonaban al golpear

rítmicamente sus dientes nacarados. Yo traté de ignorar su sensualidad con falsa compostura. Me gustaba más de día, cuando controlaba más su imagen de depredadora sexual.

Mi duendecillo regresó para aterrizar en las flores plásticas que había en un florero lleno de colillas de cigarrillos. "Santo cielo," dijo Ivy dejando caer el crucifijo. "¿Un duende? ¡Denon debe estar cabreado de verdad!"

Jenks detuvo sus alas antes de reactivar el movimiento. "Vete al Giro, Tamwood" le dijo con desprecio. "¿Acaso crees que sólo las hadas tienen buen olfato?"

Hice un gesto de dolor cuando Jenks aterrizó pesadamente en mi arete. "Sólo lo mejor para la señora Raquel," agregué sarcásticamente. Ivy rió pero a mí se me pararon los pelos del cuello. Echaba de menos el prestigio de trabajar con ella, pero aun así me ponía nerviosa. "Puedo regresar más tarde. No quiero echar a perder tu objetivo," le dije.

"No. Está bien. Tengo a un par de adictos acorralados en el baño. Los pillé vendiendo animales fuera de estación." Se deslizó hasta el borde del asiento con el vaso en la mano, poniéndose sensualmente de pie con un leve suspiro. "Se ven muy ordinarios como para estar ocultos tras un hechizo de disfraz," dijo mientras se paraba. "En todo caso, mi búho está afuera por si tratan de escapar como murciélagos por una ventana rota. Se convertirán en comida para pájaros. Sólo estoy esperando." Tomó un sorbo mirándome por encima del vaso con sus ojos pardos. "Si encuentras a tu objetivo temprano podríamos compartir el taxi de regreso."

Presentí peligro en su voz y dije que sí evasivamente. Ivy se alejó. Mis dedos empezaron a jugar nerviosamente con los rizos rojos de mi cabello y decidí fijarme en su aspecto antes de meterme en un taxi con ella a esta hora de la noche. Tal vez Ivy no necesitaba beber sangre para sobrevivir, pero era obvio que la deseaba sin importarle su promesa pública de no hacerlo.

Se oyeron pésames en la barra pues ahora sólo quedaban dos tragos frente a mí. Jenks seguía alborotado con su pataleta. "Cálmate, Jenks," le dije, con la esperanza de que no me desgarrara la oreja con el arete. "Me gusta tener a un duendecillo como apoyo. Las hadas no hacen espionaje, a menos que obtengan permiso de su sindicato."

"¿Te diste cuenta?" gruñó, produciéndome cosquillas en la oreja cuando batía las alas. "Se creen más que nosotros sólo porque un escritor mantecoso escribió esa porquería de poesía antes del Giro. Publicidad, Raquel. No es más que publicidad. ¿Sabías que a las hadas les pagan más que a los duendes por hacer el mismo trabajo?"

"¿Jenks?," interrumpí, soplándome el pelo de los hombros. "¿Qué averiguaste en la barra?"

"¡Y esa foto!," siguió, haciendo columpiar el arete. "¿La viste? La del mocoso humano colándose en la fiesta de la fraternidad. Las hadas estaban tan borrachas que ni siquiera se dieron cuenta de que bailaban con humanos. ¡Y encima les dan regalías!"

"¡Cálmate ya Jenks!," le dije con firmeza. "¿Qué sucede en la barra?"

Rezongó y yo sentí que mi arete daba vueltas. "El concursante número uno es entrenador personal de atletismo" gruñó. "El concursante número dos es técnico de aire acondicionado; y el concursante número tres es periodista de un diario. Todos son de vida diurna."

"¿Y el tipo en el escenario?" susurré mirando hacia otro lado. "La S.E. sólo me suministró una descripción superficial, pues nuestro objetivo probablemente esté oculto tras un hechizo de disfraz."

"¿*Nuestro* objetivo?" preguntó Jenks. El movimiento de sus alas cesó y su voz cambió de tono. Ya no estaba enojado.

Aproveché eso. Tal vez sólo necesitaba sentirse partícipe. "¿Qué tal si lo chequeamos?" sugerí en lugar de darle una orden. "Creo que ni siquiera sabe de qué lado soplar la gaita."

Jenks dejó escapar una risilla y se fue zumbando de buen humor. No se fomentaba el confraternizar entre agentes y acompañantes; pero ¡qué demonios! Jenks se sentiría mejor y tal vez eso haría que mi oreja se mantuviera intacta hasta el amanecer.

Los tipos de la barra se tocaron con los codos y yo frotaba el borde de mi vaso con el dedo índice para que sonara mientras esperaba. Estaba aburrida y pensé que coquetear un poco le vendría bien a mi alma.

Unos tipos entraron hablando fuerte comentando que la lluvia arreciaba. Se acomodaron en el fondo del bar y hablaban al mismo tiempo. Estiraban los brazos reclamando sus tragos y exigían que los atendieran. Les eché un vistazo, pero un leve retorcijón de estómago me dijo que al menos uno de ellos era un vampiro muerto. Difícil saberlo con tanto disfraz encima.

Pensé que sería el tipo joven callado del fondo. Era el de aspecto más normal de todos esos cuerpos tatuados y perforados y vestía jeans con camisa de botones en lugar de cuero mojado por la lluvia. De seguro le iba bien con esa banda de humanos que lo acompañaban, sus cuellos llenos de cicatrices y los cuerpos flacos y anémicos. Pero parecían contentos y satisfechos con su cercanía tan familiar. Eran especialmente amables con una rubia bonita a quien trataban de convencer de comer un poco de maní. Se veía cansada. A lo mejor iba a ser su desayuno.

Como atraído por mis pensamientos, el tipo atractivo se dio la vuelta. Bajó los lentes de sol sobre su nariz y mi cara se puso lívida cuando nuestros ojos se encontraron. Respiré profundo mientras observaba las gotas de lluvia en sus pestañas. De pronto, me invadió la urgencia de limpiárselas. Casi sentía las húmedas gotas en mis dedos, su frescura. Sus labios se movían susurrando algo y me parecía oír sus palabras sin entenderlas: me envolvían y me empujaban hacia él.

Mi corazón martillaba. Le regalé una mirada de aprobación al tiempo que movía mi cabeza suavemente. Una leve sonrisa apareció en los extremos de su boca, pero volteó la mirada.

Mi respiración contenida escapó cuando le quité los ojos

de encima. Sí. Era un vampiro muerto. Un vampiro vivo no hubiera podido contrarrestar mi hechizo, ni siquiera por unos segundos. Si él realmente lo hubiera querido, yo hubiese quedado a su disposición. Pero para eso estaban las leyes ¿verdad? Los vampiros muertos podían atrapar novicios dispuestos sólo después de firmar papeles. Pero, ¿qué testigos había para demostrar que los habían firmado antes o después? Brujas, brujos y otros Entremundos eran inmunes a volverse vampiros: un pequeño consuelo si por alguna casualidad el vampiro perdía el control y uno moría degollado. Claro que contra eso también había leyes.

Agitada aún, levanté la cabeza para encontrarme con el músico que venía directamente hacia mí con ojos encendidos por el deseo. ¡Duende estúpido! Se dejó descubrir.

"¿Viniste a oírme tocar, preciosa?," dijo el chico parándose junto a mi mesa haciendo un esfuerzo por engrosar la voz.

"Mi nombre no es preciosa; me llamo Sue," mentí mientras observaba a Ivy que se reía de mí. ¡Muy gracioso! Sería el tema de conversación de la oficina.

"Mandaste a tu amigo hada a *che-quear-me*," agregó, cantando las sílabas.

"No es un hada; es un duende" repuse. Este tipo era un normal estúpido o un Entremundos inteligente aparentando ser un normal estúpido. Yo le apostaría a lo primero.

Abrió el puño y Jenks salió volando dando tumbos hacia mi arete. Tenía un ala torcida por donde le salía polvillo que regaba sobre la mesa y en mi hombro. Cerré los ojos y cogí fuerzas. Sabía que me llamarían la atención por esto. Seguro.

Los gruñidos de ira de Jenks no me dejaban oír y al mismo tiempo trataba de pensar. Por lo menos sabía que el chico era un normal.

"Si quieres te puedo mostrar la gaita grande que tengo en mi camioneta," dijo. "Apuesto que la harías cantar."

Lo miré de pies a cabeza. "¡Lárgate!" La propuesta del vampiro muerto me puso nerviosa.

"Llegaré muy lejos, Sue preciosa," alardeó. Tal vez pensó que mi hostilidad era una invitación para sentarse. "Iré a la costa apenas consiga suficiente dinero. Tengo un amigo que trabaja en el negocio de la música. Dice que conoce a un tipo que conoce a otro tipo que le limpia la piscina a Janice Joplin."

"Ya vete," repetí; pero se estiró hacia atrás con una mueca y se puso a cantar en voz alta: "Sue-Sue-Suessudio" golpeando la mesa con un ritmillo quebrado.

Era embarazoso. Estoy segura de que todos entenderían si lo cacheteaba. Pero no: yo era un buen soldado que luchaba contra los crímenes que se cometen contra los normales, aun cuando nadie más creía en esa lucha. Sonreí y me incliné para revelar mi escote. Eso siempre los hace reaccionar aun cuando no haya mucho que mostrar. Estiré el brazo sobre la mesa, lo agarré de los pelos del pecho y se los retorcí. Eso también los hace reaccionar y suele ser más satisfactorio.

Pegó un chillido y dejó de cantar. Fue como un postre: dulce. "Vete" susurré, poniéndole el vaso de la bebida tradicional en la mano y cerrándole los dedos alrededor. "Y termínate esto por mí." Le di un empujoncito y abrió los ojos asombrado. Lo solté y se marchó tomándose medio vaso de un solo trago.

En la barra sonaron ovaciones. Al darme vuelta vi que el viejo cantinero gruñía. Se tocó la nariz y yo bajé la vista. "Chico idiota," murmuré. No debería estar en Los Hollows. Alguien debería sacarle el trasero de este sitio y mandarlo al otro lado del río antes de que termine herido.

Aún tenía un trago delante y era seguro que ya estaban apostando si lo bebería o no. "¿Estás bien, Jenks?," le pregunté, aun cuando podía adivinar su respuesta.

"Ese gigante casi me vuelve picadillo, ¿y tú me preguntas si *estoy bien?*," gruñó. Su vocecilla sonó cómica y alcé las cejas. "Casi me rompe las costillas. Me dejó apestando a babas. *Por todos los cielos*, ¡apesto! ¡Y mira lo que le hizo a mi ropa! ¿Tienes idea de lo difícil que es quitarle este olor apestoso a la seda? Mi mujer me hará dormir en las macetas si regreso a casa oliendo así. ¡Al diablo con la paga triple! ¡Tú no la vales, Raquel!"

Jenks no se dio cuenta de que yo no lo escuchaba. No dijo nada sobre su ala y por eso supe que estaba bien. Me hundí deprimida en el asiento sintiendo que no avanzaba para ningún lado. Estaba cansada. Si regresaba con las manos vacías, solo me destinarían a disturbios de luna llena y reclamos por malos encantamientos, desde ahora hasta la primavera. No era mi culpa.

Como Jenks no podía volar sin ser visto, pensé que era mejor regresar a casa. Tal vez si le compraba unos hongos de Maitake no le contaría al tipo del Comité de Asignaciones cómo se dobló el ala. *Qué diablos,* pensé. *¿Por qué no mejor gozar?* Como última actividad antes de que mi jefe clavara de una vez por todas mi escoba en un árbol, podría ir al centro comercial a comprar un tratamiento de spa y un nuevo disco de jazz suave. Mi carrera iba en picada, pero no había razón para no gozar del vuelo.

Con perversa expectativa, tomé mi bolso y el Shirley Temple y me levanté para dirigirme a la barra. No es mi estilo dejar las cosas a medias. El concursante número tres estaba ahí parado haciendo muecas y moviendo la pierna para acomodarse. Ayúdame Señor. ¡Los hombres pueden ser tan repugnantes! Me sentía cansada, aburrida y despreciada. Sabía que todo lo que dijera lo tomaría como si estuviera haciéndome la difícil y me seguiría afuera del bar. Entonces dejé caer la bebida frente a él y seguí caminando.

Su furia por el ultraje me hizo reír. Puso una pesada mano sobre mi espalda pero me agaché y le lancé una pierna haciéndolo caer estruendosamente en los tablones del piso. Hubo una exclamación y luego el bar quedó en silencio. Me senté sobre su pecho antes de que se diera cuenta de que estaba tirado en el suelo.

Mis uñas rojas saltaban a la vista. Lo agarré del cuello y sus pelos se enredaban entre mis dedos. Tenía los ojos bien abiertos. Cliff estaba parado junto a la puerta cruzado de brazos disfrutando del espectáculo.

"Demonios, Raque," dijo Jenks saltando en mi arete. "¿Quién te enseñó esto?"

"Mi papá" repuse, inclinándome sobre la cara del tipo. "Cuánto lo siento," le susurré con el pesado acento de Los Hollows. "¿Quieres jugar duro?" Pude leer el miedo en sus ojos cuando me identificó como Entremundos y no como un bombón en busca de una noche de aventuras. Sí. Era un tipo rudo. Pero esto lo hacía por diversión y nada más. No le haría daño, pero eso él no lo sabía.

"Madre mía," exclamó Jenks apartando mi atención del lloriqueo del humano. "¿Hueles eso? ¡Trébol!"

Lo solté y el tipo gateó debajo de mi cuerpo. Se levantó tambaleándose, arrastrando a sus dos compinches hacia las sombras musitando insultos para cubrir las apariencias. "¿Es uno de los cantineros?" pregunté mientras me levantaba.

"La chica," dijo. Sentí que la emoción me recorría el cuerpo.

Levanté la mirada para verla mejor. Su cuerpo se ajustaba bien al apretado uniforme negro y verde y se movía con seguridad detrás de la barra. "¿Estás perdiendo el tino Jenks?" murmuré mientras me acomodaba de nuevo los pantalones. "No puede ser ella."

"Ya está," repuso al instante. *"Tú sí* estás en lo cierto. ¡Para qué escuchar al duende! Podría estar en casa mirando la televisión; pero no-o-o-o-o. Aquí me tienen con esta mujer que piensa que su intuición femenina funciona mejor que yo. Tengo frío, hambre y un ala torcida. Si se rompe tendré que esperar a que me vuelva a salir. ¿Tienes idea de cuánto se demora eso?"

Le eché un vistazo al bar y me tranquilicé al ver que todos charlaban normalmente otra vez. Ivy se había ido. A lo mejor se perdió todo. Mejor. "¡Cállate Jenks! Has de cuenta que eres un adorno."

Me dirigí sigilosamente hacia el viejo cantinero. Me incliné hacia adelante y él me lanzó una sonrisa que dejó ver los dientes que le faltaban. Las arrugas le cubrían el rostro de piel curtida y sus ojos revoloteaban por todas partes, pero no me miraba. "Dame algo" le dije; "algo dulce, algo que me haga sentir bien. Algo rico, cremoso, algo que no debería tomar."

"Necesito ver tu identificación, paloma," dijo el viejo con un fuerte acento irlandés. "No pareces tener edad como para estarte escapando de las faldas de tu mamita."

Falseaba el acento, pero le regalé una sonrisa auténtica por el cumplido. "Seguro, guapo." Escarbé en mi bolso buscando mi licencia de conducir, dispuesta a seguir el juego que evidentemente nos agradaba a los dos. "¡Oh!," exclamé dejando caer mi licencia del otro lado del mostrador. "¡Qué tonta soy!"

Me apoyé en el banco para inclinarme por encima de la barra y echar un buen vistazo atrás. Con el trasero al aire, no sólo logré distraer a los concurrentes sino lograr mi cometido. Tal vez era poco elegante, pero funcionaba. Cuando alcé la cabeza, el viejo me miraba mal: pensó que lo estaba chequeando. Pero quien me interesaba era la chica. Estaba parada encima de una caja.

Tenía la estatura indicada, estaba en el sitio indicado y Jenks la había detectado. Se veía más joven de lo que podía esperarse, pero si uno tiene 150 años de edad hay que conocer algunos secretos de belleza. Jenks resopló en mi oído y sentenció con petulancia: "Te lo dije."

Me acomodé otra vez en el banco y el cantinero me devolvió la licencia y me sirvió un Hombre-Muerto flotando con una cuchara. Era una porción de helado en un pequeño vaso de Bailey's. Ummm. Guardé la licencia y le guiñé el ojo. Luego dejé allí el vaso y me di la vuelta para mirar a los clientes que entraban. Mi pulso se aceleró y sentí cosquilleos en la punta de los dedos. Era hora de trabajar.

Sentí la adrenalina del cuerpo cuando la sonrisa condescendiente de la chica se topó con mi sonrisa tonta. Para mí, la emoción valía más que la paga semanal que me esperaba en el cajón de mi escritorio. Claro que la sensación menguaba tan rápido como llegaba. Mi talento estaba desperdiciado. Para este caso ni siquiera necesitaba usar hechizos.

Si esto es todo lo que S.E. tiene para mí, tal vez debería olvidarme del salario fijo y trabajar independiente, pensé. Pocos abandonaban la S.E., aun cuando existía un precedente: León Bairn. León fue una leyenda viviente antes de independizarse, pero desapareció al poco tiempo por un mal conjuro. Las malas lenguas dicen que la S.E. le puso precio a su cabeza por romper su contrato de treinta años. Pero eso ocurrió hace más de diez años. Los agentes desaparecían con frecuencia, algunas veces porque la presa era más astuta o tenía más suerte que ellos. Era malicioso eso de imputarles la culpa a los equipos de asesinos de la S.E. Nadie abandonaba la institución porque el salario era bueno y los horarios cómodos. Así de simple.

Sí, pensé, ignorando el sentimiento de peligro que sentí de repente. La muerte de León Bairn fue exagerada. Nunca comprobaron nada y el único motivo por el cual yo aún tenía trabajo era porque legalmente no podían despedirme. Tal vez debería trabajar independiente. Peor de lo que hacía ahora, imposible. Se alegrarían de verme partir. *Seguro,* pensé mientras sonreía: Raquel Morgan, agente privado. Se respetan los derechos. Se realizan venganzas honestas.

Sonreí forzadamente mientras la chica limpiaba lo derramado con una toalla junto a mis codos. Entonces comencé a respirar rápido. Con mi mano izquierda le arranqué la toalla y le enredé las manos. Mi brazo derecho voló hacia atrás buscando las esposas y luego hacia adelante para colocárselas alrededor de las muñecas. Fue en un instante y abrió los ojos asombrada. ¡Rayos, soy buena!

Sus ojos no podían creer lo sucedido. "¡Por todos los infiernos!" gritó con inconfundible y auténtico acento irlandés. "¿Qué demonios estás haciendo?"

Emití un suspiro mirando la última cucharada de helado que quedaba en mi bebida. "Seguridad Entremundos" repuse. "Se le acusa de conformar una red y luego falsear las ganancias obtenidas con dicha red, de no certificar las solicitudes correspondientes, de no informarle a las Autoridades sobre el propósito de dicha red, eso es todo."

"¡Mentira!" gritó la chica contorsionándose por las esposas. Pasaba salvajemente la mirada por todo el bar pues la atención se centró en ella. "¡Pura mentira! ¡Yo hice esa red legalmente!"

"Tiene derecho de mantener la boca cerrada," improvisé, mientras sacaba la cucharada de helado. Sentí frío en la boca y la pizca de alcohol no se comparaba con el calor que me produjo la adrenalina que empezaba a desvanecerse. "Claro que si no quiere mantener cerrada la boca, se la cerraré yo."

El cantinero golpeó la barra con la palma de la mano. "¡Cliff!"—esta vez bramó sin acento irlandés—"pon el aviso de 'se busca cantinero' en la ventana. Después ven acá y ayúdame."

"Sí jefe," repuso Cliff como a quien no le importa nada.

Dejé mi cuchara, me estiré hasta el otro lado del mostrador y jalé el hada hasta el suelo antes de que se hiciera más pequeña. Se estaba encogiendo, pero el poder de mis esposas contrarrestaba su débil hechizo. "Tiene derecho a un abogado," le dije guardando mi carné. "Si no puede pagar uno, entonces está en problemas."

"¡Tú no puedes atraparme!" amenazó luchando por soltarse. El público emocionado clamaba. "¡Unos aritos de acero no van a retenerme. He escapado de reyes, sultanes y de las redes de niños repugnantes!"

Traté de acomodar mi pelo húmedo mientras ella peleaba y luchaba. Poco a poco se dio cuenta de que estaba atrapada. Ella se encogía pero las esposas también, aprisionándola. "Ya me soltaré...es...cosa de...un instante." Pateó hasta que al fin se detuvo a mirar sus muñecas. "Ay no...por San Pedro." Se dio por vencida al ver la luna amarilla, el trébol verde y el corazón rosado que adornaban mis esposas. "Que el perro del mismísimo demonio te encorve las piernas. ¿Quién hay que se atreva a burlarse de estos hechizos?" Entonces miró más de cerca. "¿Me atrapaste con cuatro? *¿Cuatro?* Jamás hubiese creído que los hechizos viejos aún funcionan."

"Pueden llamarme anticuada," repuse tomando mi bebida, "pero cuando algo funciona yo lo sigo usando."

Ivy pasó caminando con dos vampiros de capa negra delante de ella, su elegancia encubría su lúgubre miseria. Uno tenía un moretón debajo del ojo; otro cojeaba. Ivy no era suave con los vampiros que asechaban a los menores de edad. Y yo estoy de acuerdo. Basta con recordar la atracción que sentí por el vampiro muerto del otro lado del bar. Una chica de dieciséis años no tendría defensa; o mejor aún, no *querría* defenderse.

"Escucha Raquel," me dijo muy alegre—se veía casi humana cuando no estaba trabajando. "Voy hacia el distrito residencial. ¿Compartimos el pasaje?"

Pensé en la S.E. y puse en la balanza el riesgo de convertirme en una pobre empresaria muerta de hambre o pasarme el resto de la vida persiguiendo ladronzuelos y vendedores ilegales de embrujos. La S.E. no me tenía en alta estima. No. Denon estaría feliz de hacer trizas mi contrato. Yo no podía darme el lujo de empezar una oficina en Cincinnati, pero ¿en Los Hollows? tal vez. Ivy pasaba bastante tiempo por aquí. De seguro sabría donde encontrar un lugar barato. "Está bien," le respondí, fijándome en sus hermosos ojos de color pardo. "Quisiera preguntarte algo."

Asintió y empujó a sus capturados hacia adelante. El gentío apretaba y el mar de ropas negras absorbía toda la luz. El vampiro muerto me hizo una señal respetuosa con la cabeza, como diciendo "Buena captura." El impulso de la emoción que me hacía sentir una falsa grandeza me hizo retribuirle el gesto en respuesta.

"Así se hace Raquel" dijo Jenks. Sonreí, pues hacía mucho que no escuchaba algo así.

"Gracias." Lo miré de reojo en el espejo del bar colgado de mi arete. Retiré el vaso con la mano para alcanzar mi bolso pero mi sonrisa fue aún mayor cuando el cantinero me dijo que era cortesía de la casa. Bajé del banco sintiendo una satisfacción que no provenía precisamente del alcohol y empujé al hada para que saliera caminando. Entonces comencé a soñar con una puerta de oficina y mi nombre en letras doradas. Libertad.

"¡Espera!" gritó el hada mientras yo tomaba mi bolso y le sacaba el trasero del bar. "¡Deseos! Tres deseos... ¿entiendes? Me dejas libre y te concedo tres deseos."

La saqué bajo la tibia lluvia que caía. Ivy había llamado un taxi y sus capturados estaban bien seguros en la cajuela. Así habría más espacio para nosotras. Aceptar deseos de un criminal era la forma más segura de hallarse del lado equivocado de la escoba... sólo si te atrapan.

"¿Deseos?" respondí, ayudándola a entrar al taxi. "Hablemos."

Dos

"¿Qué dijiste?" le pregunté girando en el asiento delantero para ver a Ivy. Me hizo un gesto de impotencia desde atrás. El ruido de los limpiaparabrisas gastados y el sonido de la música luchaban por sobresalir en una estrafalaria mezcla de guitarras agudas y chirridos de plásticos deshechos contra el vidrio. El grupo "Grito Rebelde" daba alaridos por los altoparlantes mientras Jenks trataba de bailar con la muñeca hawaiana giratoria encima del tablero. Yo no podía competir contra aquello. "¿Puedo bajar el volumen?," le pregunté al taxista.

"¡No tocar! ¡No tocar!" exclamó con un acento extraño. ¿Tal vez era de los bosques de Europa? Un ligero olor a almizcle lo identificó como hombre lobo. Tomé el botón del volumen pero me quitó con un golpe de su mano peluda.

El auto viró bruscamente hacia el carril siguiente. Sus hechizos—todos dañados por el aspecto que presentaban—rodaron por el tablero desparramándose sobre mí y cayeron al piso. El manojo de ajos que se balanceaba en el retrovisor me golpeó en un ojo. El olor que emanaban me produjo náuseas.

"Chica mala," me regañó. Viró otra vez para retomar su carril lanzándome contra él.

"Sí, soy buena chica ¿me dejas bajar el volumen?" le pregunté gruñendo deslizándome hacia mi asiento.

Hizo una mueca. Le faltaba un diente y le faltarían dos si me hacía enfadar. "Ta'bien. Ora'tan hablando." La música se había terminado y fue reemplazada por un anunciador que gritaba más que la misma música.

"Santo Dios," rezongué bajando el volumen. Mis labios se retorcieron al tocar la capa de grasa que había en el botón. Miré mis dedos y los limpié con los amuletos que estaban aún sobre mis muslos. De todas formas no servían para nada más. La sal que se había formado por su manipulación excesiva ya los había arruinado. Con una mirada de lástima los metí en un portavasos roto.

Miré a Ivy extendida en el asiento trasero. Con una mano agarraba al búho para evitar que saliera por la ventana con cada salto del auto. La otra la tenía detrás del cuello. Su negra silueta se iluminaba con las luces de los autos que pasaban y por las escasas luces de la calle. Tenía ojos oscuros. Sin pestañear, nuestras miradas se encontraron pero pronto regresaron a la ventanilla y a la noche. Sentí que se me erizaba la piel con su aire de tragedia antigua. No pretendía nada. Ivy era sólo Ivy, pero me ponía los pelos de punta. ¿No sonreía jamás esta mujer?

Mi prisionera estaba acurrucada en una esquina tan lejos de Ivy como le era posible. Sus botas verdes apenas llegaban al borde del asiento y parecía más bien una de esas muñecas que venden por la televisión: *¡Tres cómodos pagos de $49.95 por esta detallada réplica de Becky, la cantinera! Otras muñecas se han triplicado y cuadruplicado de valor.* Sólo que esta muñeca despedía un destello solapado en los ojos. Le hice una mueca maliciosa pero la mirada de sospecha de Ivy se cruzó con la mía.

El búho emitió un sonido lúgubre cuando pasamos sobre un bache, abriendo las alas para mantener el equilibrio. Ese era el último, pues habíamos cruzado el río y estábamos de nuevo en Ohio. Ahora el pavimento era liso como el cristal. El conductor disminuyó la velocidad y empezó a prestarle atención a las señales de tránsito.

Ivy soltó al búho y se pasó los dedos por la larga cabellera. "Dije 'nunca habías aceptado viajar conmigo'. ¿Sucede algo?"

"Eh... sí... sí," pasé el brazo por detrás del asiento. "¿Sabes dónde puedo alquilar un apartamento barato, tal vez en Los Hollows?"

Ivy me miró de frente con su perfecta cara ovalada, pálida por las luces de la calle. Ahora las había en todas las esquinas, tantas que parecía de día. Reglas de paranoicos. No es que los culpe. "¿Te mudas a los Hollows?" me preguntó con mirada burlona.

No pude evitar la sonrisa. "No. Pienso retirarme de la S.E."

Eso le llamó la atención. Lo sé por la forma como pestañó. Jenks dejó de bailar con la muñeca hawaiana en el tablero y se quedó mirándome. "No puedes incumplir tu contrato con la S.E." dijo Ivy. Le echó una mirada al hada que sonreía. "¿No estarás pensando..."

"¿Romper la ley? ¿Yo?" repuse suavemente. "Soy demasiado buena para romper la ley. Eso sí, no es mi culpa que ésta sea el hada equivocada," agregué sin sentir ni una pizca de culpa. La S.E. había dicho claramente que no requería más mis servicios. ¿Qué se supone que debía hacer? ¿Tirarme de espaldas con la panza al aire y lamerle el... eh... el hocico a alguien?

"Burocracia," interrumpió el taxista. Ahora hablaba con un acento tan plano como el pavimento. Hablaba y demostraba el comportamiento que se necesitaba para cobrar las tarifas de este lado del río. "Di que los documentos se perdieron. Siempre sucede así. Por aquí debo tener la confesión de Rynn Cormel, de cuando mi padre transportaba abogados que estaban en cuarentena hasta las cortes durante el Giro."

"Así es," dije, aprobando con una sonrisa. "Nombre equivocado en el documento equivocado. Q.E.D."

Ivy no parpadeó ni una sola vez. "León Bairn no estalló de repente, Raquel."

Dejé escapar un resuello. Yo no creía en esa historia. Era solo eso: una historia para evitar que los agentes de la S.E.

terminaran sus contratos una vez que aprendían todo lo que la S.E. tenía para enseñarles. "Eso fue hace diez años" repuse, "y la S.E. no tuvo nada que ver. No me van a matar por terminar mi contrato: ellos quieren que me vaya." Fruncí el ceño. "Además, debe ser más divertido trabajar sola y no hacer lo que hago ahora."

Ivy se inclinó hacia adelante. No se daba por vencida. "Dicen que les tomó tres días encontrar suficientes restos de León para llenar una caja de zapatos. Lo último lo rasparon del techo de su terraza."

"¿Y qué se supone que debo hacer?" repuse bajando el brazo. "No he recibido ni una sola misión decente en meses. Mira esto," dije gesticulando hacia mi prisionera. "Un hada por evasión de impuestos. Es un insulto."

La pequeña mujercita se puso seria. "Vaya vaya, dis-cúlpe-me usted."

Jenks abandonó a su nueva novia para sentarse en el ala de atrás del sombrero del taxista. "Sí," sentenció. "Raquel terminará barriendo con una escoba si yo me veo forzado a tomar tiempo libre para reponerme de esto."

Movió su ala torcida irregularmente ante lo cual mostré una sonrisa de lástima. "¿Maitake?"

"Un cuarto de libra" repuso. Yo lo aumenté automáticamente a media libra. Jenks no estaba tan mal para ser duende.

Ivy frunció el entrecejo. Sus dedos jugaban con la cadena del crucifijo. "Hay razones por las que nadie rompe el contrato. La última persona que lo hizo terminó succionada por una turbina."

Apreté los dientes y me di vuelta para mirar por la ventanilla. Lo recuerdo bien. Sucedió hace casi un año y lo habría matado si no estuviera ya muerto. El vampiro estaba por regresar a la oficina en cualquier momento. "No estoy pidiendo tu autorización" dije. "Sólo te pregunto si sabes de alguien que arriende un sitio barato." Ivy guardó silencio y yo giré para verla. "Tengo algo ahorrado. Puedo abrir una oficina, ayudar a la gente que necesita trabajo."

"¡Por amor a la sangre!" interrumpió Ivy. "Que te largues para abrir una tienda de hechizos, puede ser; ¿pero para abrir tu propia agencia?" Meneó la cabeza moviendo su pelo negro. "No soy tu madre, pero si lo haces eres mujer muerta. ¿Jenks? Dile que será mujer muerta."

Jenks asintió solemnemente. Yo di la vuelta para mirar por la ventana. Me sentí como una estúpida pidiendo ayuda. El taxista también asintió: "Muerta," dijo, "muerta, muerta, muerta."

Ahora sí que estaba hecha. Jenks y el taxista se encargarían de anunciarle a toda la ciudad que me retiraba antes de que yo personalmente le avisara a la S.E. "Mejor olvídenlo. No quiero hablar más de ello."

Ivy pasó el brazo por encima del asiento. "¿No te has detenido a pensar que tal vez alguien te tienda una trampa? Todos saben que las hadas buscan formas de comprar su libertad. Si te atrapan te dejarán el trasero como mantequilla."

"Sí, ya lo pensé" respondí. La verdad es que no lo había pensado, pero no quise decírselo. "Mi primer deseo será pedir que no me atrapen."

"Siempre es el primero" dijo el hada con picardía. "¿Es tu primer deseo?" En un arranque de excitación asentí y el hada sonrió de oreja a oreja. Estaba a medio camino de la libertad.

"Escucha Ivy. No necesito tu ayuda. Gracias por nada." Busqué mi billetera hurgando dentro del bolso. "Déjame aquí" le dije al taxista. "Necesito un café. ¿Jenks? Ivy te llevará a la S.E. ¿Me harías ese favor Ivy? ¿Por lo viejos tiempos?"

"¡Raquel!" exclamó, "¡no me estás escuchando!"

El taxista puso la señal de parar y se acercó a la orilla. "Cuídate la espalda, Candela."

Me bajé, abrí la puerta trasera con fuerza y saqué a mi hada por el uniforme. Mis esposas habían contrarrestado del todo su hechizo para hacerse más pequeña. Ahora parecía un niño regordete de dos años. "Toma" le dije a Ivy tirándole un billete de $20 en el asiento. "Eso cubre mi parte."

"Sigue lloviendo," gimió el hada.

"¡Cállate!" Las gotas me golpeaban arruinando el moño y hacían que los mechones se me pegaran al cuello. Tiré la puerta cuando Ivy se inclinaba para decirme algo. No tenía nada que perder. Mi vida se había convertido en una montaña de estiércol mágico, pero ni siquiera servía de fertilizante.

"¡Me estoy mojando!," se quejó el hada.

"¿Quieres regresar al auto?" le pregunté. Mi voz sonó calmada pero por dentro parecía un volcán. "Si quieres podemos olvidarlo todo. Estoy segura de que Ivy se encargará de tus papeles. Dos capturas en una noche, ¡le darán una bonificación!"

"No," dijo dócilmente.

Yo ya estaba fastidiada. Del otro lado de la calle había una cafetería Starbucks donde venden sesenta diferentes tipos de café, ninguno de los cuales satisface a los pelmazos de los barrios residenciales. A este lado del río—y a esta hora—lo más seguro es que estuviera casi desocupada. Era el lugar perfecto para escapar del malhumor y reorganizarme. Prácticamente tuve que arrastrar al hada hasta la puerta y traté de adivinar el precio de una taza de café mirando por encima de unos fulanos que estaban ahí parados frente a la ventana.

"Espera, Raquel." Ivy había bajado la ventanilla y pude oír otra vez la música en el taxi que retumbaba con una canción de Sting, "Mil años," como para regresar al auto.

Abrí la puerta del café y se escucharon unas campanillas. "Café negro" le grité al chico detrás del mostrador mientras me dirigía a la esquina más oscura con mi hada a cuestas. El chico parecía un tipo correcto, con delantal de rayas rojas y blancas y cabello perfecto. Seguro que era estudiante de universidad. Yo he debido asistir a la universidad por lo menos uno o dos semestres en lugar de ir a la escuela comunitaria. Había sido aceptada.

El asiento era suave y bien acolchado, la mesa tenía un mantel de verdad y mis zapatos no se quedaban pegados en el piso: punto a favor. El chico me miraba con interés, así que me quité las botas y crucé las piernas para provocarlo. Todavía seguía vestida de prostituta. Creo que el pobre no sabía si llamar a la S.E. o su homóloga humana, la AFE. ¡Vaya chiste!

Mi boleto para liberarme de la S.E. estaba delante de mí y no se quedaba quieta. "¿Me das un café con leche?" gimió.

"No."

De nuevo sonaron las campanillas de la puerta y entró Ivy con su búho en el brazo. El animal le apretaba el grueso brazalete con las garras. Jenks se había posado sobre su hombro tan lejos del búho como le era posible. Me quedé quieta mirando una foto de bebés disfrazados de ensalada de frutas que había encima de la mesa. Se supone que debía ser una foto bonita, pero a mí sólo me abría el apetito.

"Raquel, necesito hablar contigo."

Para el chico, eso fue demasiado. "Disculpe, señora," dijo con perfecta entonación. "No se admiten animales. El búho debe permanecer afuera."

¿Señora? pensé, haciendo un esfuerzo para no reventar de la risa.

Ivy se quedó mirándolo y él se puso blanco. Pasmado, por poco cae de espaldas cuando empezó a retroceder. Le estaba arrastrando el aura. Nada bueno.

Luego me dirigió la mirada. Acomodé la espalda en el sillón y exhalé. Sus depredadores ojos negros me clavaron contra el asiento de vinilo. Sentí que mi estómago se pegaba y que mis dedos temblaban.

La tensión de ese enlace era intoxicante. No podía dejar de mirarla. Esto no se parecía a la sugerencia amistosa del vampiro muerto en Sangre y Pociones. Esto era rabia, poder. A Dios gracias la rabia no era conmigo sino con el chico del mostrador.

Al darse cuenta de mi espanto hizo desaparecer la ira de sus ojos. Sus pupilas se contrajeron y sus ojos volvieron a ser de color pardo. En un instante la abandonó el velo de poder que regresó a las profundidades del infierno donde pertenecía. Tenía que venir de allá. Un poder tan salvaje no podía provenir de un encantamiento. Creo que mi rabia empezaba a disminuir, pues con rabia no habría sentido miedo.

Habían pasado años desde que Ivy me arrastró el aura. La última vez, discutíamos cómo atrapar a un vampiro de sangre baja sospechoso de atraer chicas menores de edad con juegos de cartas. Hice caer a Ivy con un hechizo para el sueño y escribí "idiota" en sus uñas con esmalte rojo. Luego la amarré a un asiento y la desperté. A partir de ese día fue una amiga modelo aunque a veces fuera un tanto fría. Creo que estaba agradecida porque no se lo conté a nadie.

El chico aclaró la garganta. "Señora…no puede…eh… eh…quedarse a menos que pida algo," dijo débilmente.

Guapo, pensé. *Debe ser un Entremundos.*

"Jugo de naranja" dijo Ivy con voz fuerte. "Sin pulpa."

Sorprendida, la miré de nuevo. "¿Jugo de naranja?" Fruncí el ceño. "Escucha," dije soltando las manos y poniendo mi bolso de hechizos sobre los muslos. "No me interesa si León Bairn terminó como una estampilla en el andén. Yo renuncio y nada de lo que digas me hará cambiar de opinión."

Ivy dio unos pasos preocupada. Eso me tranquilizó. ¿Ivy preocupada? Jamás la había visto así.

"Quiero irme contigo," dijo finalmente.

Me quedé mirándola un instante. "¡¿Qué?!"

Se sentó frente a mí con aire fingido dejando que el búho vigilara el hada. Aflojó ruidosamente los ajustadores del brazalete y lo dejó en el asiento de al lado. Jenks dio un salto hacia la mesa con los ojos bien abiertos y la boca por fin cerrada y el chico llegó con nuestras bebidas. Esperamos en silencio mientras ponía con manos trémulas todo en la mesa y luego desapareció en el cuarto de servicio.

Mi taza estaba descascarada y apenas a medio llenar. Contemplé la posibilidad de regresar más tarde para dejar un amuleto debajo de la mesa que arruinara toda la crema a un metro a la redonda, pero decidí que tenía cosas más importantes en qué pensar. Por ejemplo: ¿por qué Ivy quería tirar su brillante carrera por el inodoro?

"¿Por qué?," le pregunté sin saber qué decir. "El jefe te adora. Puedes escoger tus casos. El año pasado te dieron vacaciones pagadas."

Ivy miraba la foto eludiéndome. "¿Y qué?"

"¡Fueron cuatro semanas! Te fuiste a Alaska en el tren del sol de medianoche."

Sus cejas delgadas se juntaron y estiró el brazo para arreglarle las plumas al búho. "Yo pago la mitad del arriendo, de los servicios, la mitad de todo; tú pagas la otra mitad. Yo busco mi trabajo, tú buscas el tuyo. Si es necesario, trabajamos juntas. Como antes."

Me recosté en el espaldar y exhalé, pero no tan fuerte como hubiera querido. Los asientos eran bastante blandos.

"¿Por qué?," pregunté de nuevo.

Sus dedos dejaron el búho. "Soy buena en lo que hago," me dijo sin responder. Pero ahora su voz delataba algo vulnerable. "No voy a ser una carga para ti, Raquel. Ningún vampiro se atreverá contra mí. Puedo extenderte ese privilegio. Mantendré a los vampiros asesinos lejos de ti mientras consigues el dinero para pagar tu contrato. Con mis contactos y tus hechizos podremos sobrevivir hasta que la S.E. retire el precio que ponga por nuestra cabeza. Pero quiero un deseo."

"No hay precio por nuestra cabeza," me apresuré a agregar.

"Raquel" dijo coqueta. Sus ojos eran de un pardo suave cuando se preocupaba y eso me alarmó. "Lo habrá." Se inclinó hacia adelante y ya no pude alejarme. Respiré hondo tratando de percibir su olor a sangre pero sólo olía a jugo de naranja. Ivy estaba equivocada. La S.E. no le pondría precio a mi cabeza. Querían que me fuera. En cambio ella sí tenía de qué preocuparse.

"Yo también," dijo Jenks de repente saltando hasta el borde de mi taza. El polvillo iridiscente de su ala torcida cayó adentro formando una capa de grasa en el café. "Quiero que me incluyan. Quiero un deseo. Voy a retirarme de la S.E. y seré el apoyo de ustedes dos. Van a necesitarme. Raque, las cuatro horas antes de la medianoche son para ti; para Ivy las cuatro siguientes. Como prefieran. Cada cuarto día es libre, siete festivos pagados y un deseo. Además dejen que viva con mi familia en la oficina. ¿Sueldo? Lo mismo que gano ahora, pagadero cada dos semanas."

Ivy asintió y bebió un poco de jugo. "Suena bien. ¿Qué dices?"

Se me cayó la mandíbula. No podía creer lo que escuchaba. "No puedo darte mis deseos."

El hada meneó la cabeza. "Sí puedes."

"¡No!," repuse impaciente. "Quiero decir, los necesito." Sentí que la tensión me presionaba las tripas de pensar que Ivy tal vez tenía razón.

"Ya usé uno para que no me atrapen por dejarla libre. Ahora necesito otro para zafarme del contrato, así como para comenzar."

"Eh…" balbuceó el hada. "Si está por escrito, no puedo hacer nada al respecto."

Jenks resopló burlándose. "No fue tan buen trato, ¿verdad?"

"¡Cierra la boca, insecto!," le respondió con las mejillas rojas.

Esto no puede estar sucediendo, pensé. Lo único que quería era salirme, no convertirme en líder de una rebelión. "No estarás hablando en serio," dije. "Vamos Ivy, dime que este es el cruel sentido del humor que yo aún no conocía en ti."

Se quedó mirándome fijo. Nunca he sabido qué hay detrás de la mirada de un vampiro. Ivy habló haciendo un gesto de mano: "Por primera vez en mi carrera regresaré con las manos vacías. Dejé escapar a mis objetivos. Abrí la cajuela y los dejé huir. Rompí las reglas." Sonrió con los labios cerrados. "¿Te parece suficientemente grave?"

"Vas a tener que encontrar un hada" le dije mientras

me reponía alcanzando mi taza. Jenks todavía seguía ahí sentado.

Ivy rió. Hacía frío y esta vez estaba tiritando. "Yo selecciono mis casos" agregó. "¿Qué crees que pasaría si saliera por un hada, fallara la captura y luego tratara de largarme de la S.E.?"

Al otro lado el hada suspiraba. "Nadie lo va creer, ni deseándolo. De hecho, ya es difícil que este caso parezca coincidencia."

"¿Y tú Jenks?," pregunté con voz entrecortada.

Jenks encogió los hombros. "Yo quiero un deseo. Un deseo puede darme lo que la S.E. no puede. Quiero ser estéril para que mi esposa no me abandone." Voló haciendo curvas hasta el hada. "¿Es demasiado difícil para ti, chiquilla verde?" le preguntó sarcásticamente parado con las piernas abiertas y las manos en la cintura.

"Insecto," murmuró. Mis hechizos sonaban y ella amenazaba con aplastarlo. Las alas de Jenks se pusieron rojas de ira y hasta llegué a pensar que el polvillo que caía de sus alas estallaría en llamas.

"¿Esterilidad?," pregunté, tratando de continuar el tema.

Jenks se alejó del hada y vino hacia mí. "Sí. ¿Sabes cuántos mocosos tengo?"

Ivy también pareció sorprenderse. "¿Vas a arriesgar tu vida por eso?" le preguntó.

Jenks se rió. "¿Quién dice que voy arriesgar mi vida? A la S.E. le importa un rábano que me vaya. Los duendes no firmamos contratos. No nos investigan. Soy agente libre. Siempre lo he sido y siempre lo seré." Jenks me pareció demasiado astuto para ser tan pequeño. "Pienso que mi vida será más larga si solamente tengo que preocuparme de dos gigantes como ustedes."

Entonces le hablé a Ivy. "Sé que firmaste un contrato. Te adoran. Si alguien debería preocuparse por una amenaza de muerte, esa eres tú. No yo. ¿Por qué te arriesgas por... por—dudé en decirlo—por nada? ¿Qué deseo puede valer tanto la pena?"

Ivy se quedó estática. Una pizca de oscura sombra pasó tras ella. "No tengo que decírtelo."

"No soy una estúpida," dije tratando de ocultar mis nervios. "¿Cómo sé que no ejercerás de nuevo?"

Evidentemente, Ivy se ofendió, y fijó su mirada en mis ojos hasta que bajé la cara sintiendo escalofríos hasta la médula de los huesos. *Definitivamente esto no es buena idea,* pensé. "No practico el vampirismo" repuso finalmente. "Ya no. No más."

Bajé la mano al darme cuenta de que estaba jugando con mi pelo húmedo. Sus palabras a duras penas me alentaron. Su vaso estaba medio vacío y recuerdo que apenas había bebido un sorbo.

"¿Socias?" preguntó Ivy ofreciéndome la mano desde el otro extremo de la mesa.

¿Sociedad con Ivy? ¿Con Jenks? Ivy era la mejor agente de la S.E. Era más que halagador que quisiera trabajar conmigo de forma permanente; pero me preocupaba. Claro, tampoco se trataba de vivir con ella. Lentamente estiré la mano para encontrar la suya. Mis uñas rojas perfectamente pulidas se veían estridentes junto a las suyas sin arreglar. Todos mis deseos se esfumaron. Igual, a lo mejor los habría malgastado.

"Socias," repuse. Me estremecí al sentir su mano fría.

"¡Así se habla!" gritó Jenks, revoloteando hasta aterrizar en nuestras manos entrelazadas. El polvillo que despedía parecía calentar un poco la piel de Ivy.

"¡Socias!"

Tres

"**S**anto Dios," gemí. "No dejes que me enferme. Aquí no." Cerré los ojos esperando que no me dolieran mucho al abrirlos con la luz. Me hallaba en mi cubículo del piso 25 de la torre de la S.E. Los rayos del sol de la tarde entraban inclinados pero no me alcanzaban. Mi escritorio era un completo desorden. Alguien había comprado unas rosquillas y el olor del azúcar me producía ruidos en el estómago. Lo único que quería era regresar a casa y dormir.

Abrí el cajón de arriba buscando torpemente un amuleto para el dolor. Los había usado todos. Golpeé el borde metálico del escritorio con la frente y me quedé mirando el borde de mis botas encima de mis jeans. Me vestí más serio por respeto a mi renuncia: blusa de lino rojo y pantalón. No más cuero ajustado por ahora.

Lo de anoche fue un error. Bebí demasiado y fui lo suficientemente estúpida como para regalarles a Jenks e Ivy los dos deseos que me quedaban. En realidad estaba contando con ellos. Los que saben de deseos también saben que a uno no se le presentan así nomás. Lo mismo con los deseos de riqueza. El dinero no aparece así como así. Tiene que provenir de algún sitio. Y si uno no usa el primero para que no lo atrapen, entonces lo agarran a uno por hurto.

Los deseos son traicioneros. Por eso los Entretemundos casi siempre exigían un mínimo de tres para escapar. En retrospectiva, no me iría tan mal. El deseo de que no me atraparan por dejar libre al hada me permitiría al menos retirarme de la S.E. con una historia limpia. Y si Ivy tenía razón y querían liquidarme por terminar mi contrato, tendrían que hacerlo parecer un accidente. Pero, ¿para qué molestarse? Las amenazas de muerte eran costosas y de todas formas querían que me largara.

Ivy pidió un abalorio para portar su deseo y usarlo más adelante. Era una especie de moneda vieja con un agujero en la mitad. Lo amarró con una cinta púrpura y se lo colgó al cuello. Por otra parte, Jenks pidió su deseo ahí en el bar. Luego salió zumbando hacia su esposa para darle la noticia. Debí largarme cuando se fue Jenks, pero Ivy no tenía ganas de irse. Hacía mucho tiempo que no disfrutaba de una noche de chicas y pensé que encontraría valor para renunciarle a mi jefe en el fondo de un trago. Pero no fue así.

A los cinco segundos de decir mi discurso, Denon abrió un sobre de manila, sacó mi contrato y lo rompió en pedazos. Me dijo que quería que me fuera del edificio en media hora. Mi carné de identificación y las esposas estaban sobre su escritorio. Los hechizos que las adornaban estaban en mi bolsillo.

En mis siete años con la S.E. acumulé montañas de basura y memorandos vencidos. Con manos temblorosas agarré un grueso florero que no veía flores en meses. Lo tiré a la basura—donde también terminó el cretino que me lo regaló. Metí la vasija de disoluciones en la caja de cartón que tenía a mis pies. La cerámica azul cubierta con una costra de sal rayaba el cartón. Se había secado la semana anterior y quedaba un polvillo de sal como resultado de la evaporación.

Después de la vasija siguió una astilla de madera de secoya. Era demasiado gruesa para hacer una vara mágica, pero la verdad es que de todas formas no era suficientemente buena para convertirse en varita. La compré para fabricar un par de amuletos que detectan mentiras, pero nunca los hice. Era más fácil comprarlos. Me estiré y agarré mi lista telefónica de anteriores contactos. Eché un rápido vistazo para cerciorarme de que nadie me estaba observando y la escondí junto a mi vasija de disolución. Mi reproductor de CD's y mis audífonos les hicieron pronta compañía.

Tenía, además, unos pocos libros de referencia, que en realidad eran de Joyce. Ella estaba del otro lado del pasillo. Pero el recipiente de sal que usaba para apoyarlos había sido de papá. Lo metí en la caja pensando qué diría él por mi renuncia. "Estaría más que satisfecho," susurré apretando los dientes por la resaca.

Levanté la mirada por encima de las horribles divisiones amarillas. Lo que había para ver era muy poco, pues mis compañeros voltearon los ojos hacia otro lado. Todos chismorreaban en grupos fingiendo estar muy ocupados; pero sus cuchicheos me crisparon. Respiré profundo y cogí mi fotografía en blanco y negro de Watson, Crick y Rosalind Franklin, la mujer que estuvo detrás de todo. Estaban ahí, parados frente a su modelo de ADN; pero la sonrisa de Rosalind tenía el mismo humor oculto de la sonrisa de la Mona Lisa. Parecía saber lo que sucedería después. A veces me detuve a reflexionar si acaso Rosalind no era una Entremundos, pues muchas personas pensaban lo mismo. Conservé la foto para recordar cómo da vueltas el mundo por aquellos pequeños detalles que otros dejan pasar por alto.

Habían transcurrido casi cuarenta años desde que la cuarta parte de la humanidad murió por la mutación de un virus, el Ángel T4. Pero a pesar de la insistencia televisada de los eternos evangelistas, nosotros los Entremundos no tuvimos la culpa. Todo comenzó y terminó con la paranoia de siempre de los humanos.

En los años cincuenta, Watson, Crick y Franklin unieron sus cerebros y en seis meses resolvieron el misterio del ADN. Todo habría parado ahí, pero los soviéticos le echaron la mano a la tecnología. Y, por supuesto, el temor a una guerra hizo que le lloviera dinero a la ciencia genética en desarrollo. Al comenzar los años sesenta, ya estábamos produciendo insulina con bacterias y luego siguieron infinidad de drogas producidas con ingeniería biológica. Estas inundaron el mercado y fueron el resultado de las oscuras investigaciones de Estados Unidos con armas biológicas. No llegamos a la Luna. Más bien, nos dedicamos a hacer ciencia en secreto para tratar de aniquilarnos.

Y luego, hacia el final de la década, alguien cometió un error. Aún siguen debatiendo si fueron los norteamericanos o los soviéticos. El hecho es que una cadena mortal de ADN escapó de un laboratorio en algún lugar del Ártico, dejando un rastro moderado de muerte hasta Río, donde fue identificado y controlado. La mayoría de las personas nunca se enteró de lo sucedido. Pero el virus mutó a pesar de que los científicos ya habían escrito y archivado sus conclusiones de laboratorio.

El T4 se pegó a un tomate de ingeniería biológica en un punto débil de su cadena genética modificada, pero los científicos consideraron que aquello no revestía importancia suficiente para preocuparse. Ese tomate vino a conocerse oficialmente como Ángel T4—su identificación de laboratorio—y de ahí el nombre del virus: Ángel.

Ignorantes del hecho de que el virus usaba el tomate Ángel como huésped, las líneas aéreas lo transportaron. Pero dieciséis horas después era demasiado tarde. Los países del tercer mundo fueron arrasados en tres semanas de pánico y Estados Unidos cerró sus puertas a la cuarta semana. Las fronteras fueron militarizadas y se instituyó la política gubernamental de "Lo sentimos mucho, pero no podemos ayudarlos." Estados Unidos sufrió y murió gente; pero en comparación con el camposanto en que se convirtió el resto del mundo, lo nuestro fue un paseo.

Pero la razón principal por la que la civilización permaneció intacta es que la mayoría de las especies de Entremundos éramos resistentes al virus del Ángel. Las brujas, los muertos vivientes y las especies más pequeñas como los gnomos, duendes y hadas, no sufrieron en absoluto. Los hombres lobo y vampiros vivos simplemente contrajeron gripa. Pero todos los elfos murieron. Dicen que su práctica de procrear con humanos para multiplicar su población fracasó porque los infectó el virus Ángel.

Cuando pasó la tormenta y el virus fue erradicado, la cantidad de Entremundos de todo tipo y especie juntos era casi igual que la de humanos. Aquella fue una oportunidad que no dejamos pasar por alto. El Giro, como vino a conocerse después, comenzó al medio día. Cuando terminó a la media noche, la humanidad no podía aceptar la realidad de haber vivido con brujas, vampiros y hombres lobos desde antes de los tiempos de las pirámides.

La reacción instintiva de los humanos fue tratar de hacernos desaparecer de la faz de la Tierra. Pero se fue aplacando rápidamente cuando les hicimos ver que nosotros fuimos quienes salvamos a la civilización mientras el mundo se deshacía en pedazos. De no ser por nosotros, la mortandad habría sido peor.

Aun así, los años que siguieron al Giro fueron una locura. Los humanos temían atacarnos y además prohibieron las investigaciones médicas, pues las señalaban como culpables de todos sus males. Destruyeron los laboratorios de biología y los ingenieros biólogos que lograron escapar de la plaga fueron juzgados. Muchos murieron en lo que podríamos llamar asesinatos legales. Luego llegó la segunda ola de muerte cuando las fuentes de los medicamentos fueron destruidas por equivocación junto con la biotecnología.

Fue apenas cuestión de tiempo para que los humanos fundaran una institución ciento por ciento humana para controlar las actividades de los Entremundos. Entonces surgió la Agencia Federal Entremundos—AFE—que acabó y reemplazó a los organismos policiales y de seguridad en todo el país. Los policías y agentes federales Entremundos ahora desempleados, formaron su propia fuerza policial: La S.E. La competencia entre ambas es intensa inclusive hoy, lo cual ayuda a mantener bajo control a los Entremundos más agresivos.

Cuatro pisos del edificio principal de la AFE en Cincinnati se dedican a buscar y encontrar los laboratorios biológicos ilegales que aun persisten y en los cuales se consigue buena insulina a precios muy elevados y algo para conjurar la leucemia. La AFE de los humanos vive obsesionada con hallar tecnologías prohibidas, tanto como la S.E. lo está por erradicar de las calles la droga llamada azufre.

Y todo comenzó cuando Rosalind Franklin se dio cuenta de que alguien había movido su lápiz y de que alguien más estaba en el lugar equivocado, pensé, pasando las yemas de los dedos por mi adolorida cabeza. Pequeñas claves. Pequeñas pistas. Eso es lo que hace que el mundo de vueltas. Eso fue lo que me convirtió en buena agente. Le sonreí a Rosalind, limpié las huellas de mis dedos del marco y la metí en mi caja de cosas para conservar.

De pronto escuché un estallido de risa nerviosa a mis espaldas. Abrí el siguiente cajón moviendo papeles sucios, notas adhesivas y clips de papel. Encontré mi cepillo donde siempre lo dejaba, pero sobre todo sentí gran alivio cuando lo guardé en la caja. El pelo se puede usar para lanzar hechizos contra blancos específicos. Si Denon quisiera verme muerta, ya lo habría tomado.

Mis dedos se toparon con el pesado reloj de bolsillo de papá. Era mi única pertenencia y tiré el cajón para cerrarlo con fuerza. Sentí que mi cabeza iba a estallar. Las manecillas se habían detenido faltando siete minutos para la medianoche. Le gustaba tomarme del pelo diciendo que se había detenido la noche en que fui concebida. Lo metí en mi bolsillo de adelante escurriéndome en la silla. Casi podía verlo ahí parado bajo del umbral de la puerta de la cocina, paseando los ojos desde su reloj hasta el reloj encima del lavaplatos, con una sonrisa que le invadía la cara, como pensando adónde se habría ido el tiempo perdido.

Puse a Don Pez y su acuario—el pescadito que me habían regalado el año pasado en la fiesta navideña de la oficina—en la vasija de disoluciones, confiando en que agua y pez no se salieran a salpicones, y luego siguieron las latas de alimento para peces. De repente sentí un golpe acolchonado que venía del fondo de la oficina y que me hizo voltear la mirada por encima de las divisiones amarillas en dirección a la puerta cerrada de Denon.

"No te alejarás más de un metro de esta puerta, Tamwood," escuché que decía con su voz apagada, silenciando el murmullo de las conversaciones. Aparentemente, Ivy acababa de renunciar. "Tengo tu contrato. ¡Tú eres quien trabaja para mí, no al contrario! Si te largas ya verás lo que…" Se oyó un ruido detrás de la puerta. "¡Mierda!" exclamó en voz baja, "¿Cuánto dinero hay ahí?"

"Lo suficiente para pagar mi contrato," repuso Ivy con su frialdad de costumbre. "Suficiente para tí y para los muertos del sótano. ¿Trato hecho?"

"Sí," repuso Denon con asombro y codicia. "Sí…eh… estás despedida."

Sentí como si mi cabeza estuviera llena de papel higiénico y la recosté entre mis manos puestas en forma de cáliz. ¿Ivy tenía dinero? ¿Por qué no me lo dijo anoche?

"¡Vete a Girar, Denon!" le dijo Ivy con perfecta claridad en el silencio total que reinaba. "Yo renuncié. Tú no me has despedido. Puedes quedarte con el dinero, pero no te metas con sangre alta. Eres de segunda y ninguna suma de dinero podrá cambiarte. Aún si tuviera que vivir en los bajos fondos con las ratas, sería más que tú. Te estás muriendo porque ya no tendré que recibir tus órdenes."

"No creas que con esto estarás a salvo," rebuznó el jefe. Casi que podía verle las venas saliéndole del cuello. "Porque puede haber accidentes. Si te acercas demasiado, a lo mejor amaneces muerta."

La puerta de la oficina de Denon se abrió como empujada por una tormenta y por ahí salió Ivy. La cerró tan fuerte que hasta las luces titilaron. Estaba tensa y no creo que me haya visto cuando pasó frente a mi cubículo. Yo estaba totalmente convencida de que lo había hecho muy bien. Su falda larga se infló mientras cruzó el recinto con pasos mortíferos. Manchas de ira se reflejaban en su rostro. La tensión le fluía por el cuerpo y casi podía verse lo fuerte que era.

No se estaba transformando en vampiro, pero estaba iracunda. De todas formas, dejó una turbulencia gélida a su paso, tanto, que ni siquiera los rayos de sol que penetraban por la ventana la pudieron atravesar. Llevaba una bolsa vacía en el hombro y su deseo colgando alrededor del cuello. *Chica inteligente,* pensé. *Consérvalo para un día de lluvia.* Ivy se dirigió a las escaleras y yo cerré los ojos preparándome para el golpe de la puerta metálica contra la pared.

Jenks apareció en mi cubículo, zumbando alrededor de mi cabeza como una polilla trastornada y exhibiendo el remiendo que tenía en el ala. "Hola Raque," dijo con júbilo detestable. "¿Qué hay de nuevo?"

"Baja la voz," susurré. Habría dado lo que fuera por una taza de café, pero no estaba segura si valía la pena caminar los veinte pasos que me separaban del lugar donde estaba la cafetera. Jenks estaba vestido de civil, de colores fuertes y estridentes. El morado no va con el amarillo. Jamás. Nunca irá bien. Santo Dios, la venda de su ala también era morada. "¿No estás un poco mareado?" Respiré hondo.

Jenks se sentó en el vaso de los lápices haciendo muecas. "No. El metabolismo de los duendes es muy sofisticado. El alcohol se convierte en azúcar en cuestión de minutos. ¡Qué bueno! ¿No te parece?"

"Uhh, fantástico." Envolví la foto donde salgo junto a mamá con pañuelos de papel y la puse junto a la de Rosalind. Por un instante pensé contarle a mamá que estaba sin empleo, pero cambié de opinión por razones obvias. Decidí esperar hasta que tuviera otro. "¿E Ivy? ¿Está bien?" le pregunté.

"Sí. Estará bien." Jenks saltó hasta la maceta del laurel. "Solo está un poco fastidiada por haber usado todos sus ahorros para comprar su contrato y protegerse el trasero."

Asentí con la cabeza contenta de pensar que a mí me querían fuera. Todo sería más fácil si ninguna de las dos tuviera encima un precio por su cabeza. "¿Sabías que ella tenía dinero?"

Jenks desempolvó una hoja y se sentó con aire de superioridad. Claro que era un tanto contradictorio verlo así pues, apenas medía diez centímetros de altura y estaba vestido de mariposa malhumorada. "Pues…uhh…es obvio. Ivy es la última persona viva de sangre de su familia. Yo le daría un par de días. Está tan brava como una avispa mojada. Perdió su hacienda en el campo, la tierra, las acciones...todo. Lo único que le queda en la ciudad es la mansión junto al río, pero es de la mamá."

Me recosté en la silla, saqué mi última pastilla de chicle de canela y me la metí a la boca. Entonces escuché un traqueteo cuando Jenks aterrizó en mi caja de cartón y comenzó a hurgar. "Ah sí," exclamó. "Ivy dijo que ya alquiló un departamento. Aquí tengo la dirección."

"¡Sal de ahí!" Lo sacudí con un dedo y voló otra vez hacia el laurel, parándose en la rama más alta para observar el chismorreo de la gente. Mis sienes latían al agacharme a desocupar el cajón de abajo. *¿Por qué le dio Ivy todo lo que tenía a Denon? ¿Por qué no usó su deseo?*

"¡Atención!," exclamó Jenks rodando por la planta escondiéndose tras las hojas. "Aquí viene."

No acababa de enderezarme cuando me topé con Denon del otro lado de mi escritorio. Y detrás venía Francis, el hipócrita oportunista de la oficina. La mirada de mi ex jefe pasó por encima de las divisiones del cubículo y se detuvieron junto a mí. Por poco me trago el chicle.

Para ponerlo en palabras más sencillas, el jefe parecía luchador profesional con una especialización en coquetería: grande, músculos fuertes, piel morena perfecta. A lo mejor fue una roca en otra vida. Como Ivy, Denon era un vampiro viviente. Pero a diferencia de Ivy, nació humano y después cambió. Eso lo hacía de sangre baja, una segunda clase lejana en el mundo de los vampiros.

De todas formas Denon tenía poder y era persona de cuidado, pues había trabajado duro para sobreponerse a su origen innoble. Su exceso de músculos era más que atractivo: lo ayudaba a mantenerse con vida cuando frecuentaba la compañía de sus familiares adoptivos más fuertes que él. Poseía la mirada de eterna juventud de aquellos que se alimentan regularmente de zombies. Solamente un muerto viviente puede convertir a un humano en vampiro; y, dado su aspecto saludable, Denon era claramente uno de los preferidos de los vampiros. Por otro lado, la mitad del edificio soñaba con ser su juguete sexual. La otra mitad se mojaba en los pantalones de miedo. Yo era miembro orgulloso del segundo grupo.

Mis manos temblaban. Alcé la taza con el café del día anterior fingiendo tomar un sorbo. Sus brazos se movían como pistones cuando caminaba y su camisa deportiva amarilla contrastaba con sus pantalones negros. Estaban perfectamente planchados, mostrando la línea de los músculos de las piernas y su cintura delgada. La gente se quitaba a su paso y hubo varios que salieron corriendo por la puerta. Dios me proteja si me equivoqué con mi único deseo y me atrapaban.

El plástico crujió cuando se apoyó sobre el borde de mis cuatro paredes. No lo miré. Más bien fijé los ojos en los agujeritos que habían abierto las tachuelas en los separadores de corcho. Sentí cosquillas en la piel, como si Denon me estuviera tocando. Su presencia producía un torbellino a mi alrededor que azotaba las paredes del cubículo y ahora lo sentía detrás. Mi pulso se aceleró y fijé la mirada en Francis.

El tonto se detuvo en el escritorio de Joyce desabrochando su chaqueta azul de poliéster. Sonrió mostrándome sus dientes perfectos y lo miré mientras se subía las mangas de la chaqueta revelando sus brazos flacos. Su cara triangular estaba enmarcada por el cabello que le llegaba hasta las orejas y se quitaba de encima de los ojos cada segundo. Se creía juvenilmente atractivo, pero a mí me parecía como si acabara de despertar.

A pesar de que apenas eran las tres de la tarde, ya tenía una barbita que le cubría la cara. El cuello de su camisa hawaiana estaba intencionalmente volteado hacia arriba. El rumor en la oficina es que quería parecerse a Sonny Crockett, pero sus pequeños ojos eran bizcos y su nariz demasiado larga y delgada. Patético.

"Sé lo que está sucediendo, Morgan," dijo Denon forzándome a prestarle atención. Tenía esa voz baja y ronca que solo poseen los hombres de alma oscura y los vampiros. Es una regla que anda escrita por ahí. Voz ronca. Dulce. Persuasiva. La amenaza que transmitía me templó la piel y el temor recorrió mi cuerpo.

"¿Cómo?" respondí, satisfecha de que no me temblara la voz. Envalentonada, le sostuve la mirada. El aire me entró hasta los pulmones y me sentí tensa. Trataba de arrastrarme el aura a las tres de la tarde. *Maldición*.

Denon se inclinó sobre la división y descansó los brazos en el borde de arriba. Sus bíceps se encogieron inflamándole las venas. Los pelos de mi nuca se pararon y luché contra la urgencia que sentí de mirar hacia otro lado. "Todos creen que te largas por los casos de pacotilla que te he estado encargando" dijo con voz balsámica, acariciando las palabras a medida que salían de sus labios. "A lo mejor están en lo cierto."

Se enderezó y yo me sacudí con el sonido del plástico que se doblaba. El color pardo de sus ojos había desaparecido completamente tras sus pupilas dilatadas. *Doble maldición*.

"He tratado de librarme de ti durante los últimos dos años," continuó, "pero tú no tienes mala suerte." Sonrió mostrándome sus dientes humanos. "Me tienes atrapado. Malos refuerzos, mensajes indescifrables, filtraciones sobre tus objetivos. Pero apenas logro que te largues, te llevas a mi mejor agente contigo." Sus ojos se volvieron intensos. Hice un esfuerzo por soltar las manos pero fijó su mirada en ellas. "Mala cosa, Morgan."

No fui yo, pensé. No supe si debía alarmarme. No fui yo. Todos esos errores *no fueron* míos. Pero entonces Denon se acercó más.

De repente me hallé parada entre crujidos de plástico y metal apoyándome en el escritorio. Los papeles también crujieron y el ratón cayó de la mesa colgando como un péndulo. Los ojos de Denon se habían vuelto completamente negros y mi pulso me martillaba.

"No me gustas Morgan," dijo, envolviéndome con su aliento pegajoso. "Nunca me has gustado. Tus métodos son flojos y descuidados, igual que tu padre. Es increíble que no hayas sido capaz de agarrar a esa hada." Pero, de repente, su mirada se perdió en la distancia y me di cuenta de que yo estaba conteniendo la respiración. Sus ojos se volvieron vidriosos y pareció perder el entendimiento.

Por favor, funciona, pensé desesperada. *Funciona...funciona*. Dennon se acercó. Yo me clavé las uñas en la palma de la mano para no huir. Me forcé a respirar. "Absolutamente increíble" repitió, como si quisiera descifrar algo; pero luego batió la cabeza fingiendo estar consternado.

Mi respiración volvió a medida que él se retiraba. Rompimos el contacto visual y él fijó los ojos en mi cuello donde mi pulso se veía como un martillo. Lo cubrí con una mano pero él sonrió como solo lo habría hecho con su verdadero y único amor. Tenía una sola cicatriz en su cuello hermoso y me pregunté adónde tendría todas las demás. "Apenas pongas los pies en la calle todo vale," susurró.

Mi asombro y mi temor se mezclaron produciéndome náuseas. Le estaba poniendo precio a mi cabeza.

"No puedes hacerlo...," repuse tartamudeando. "Tú me pediste que me fuera."

No se movió, pero su inmovilidad me hizo temerle más. Mis ojos se fijaron en su respiración lenta y sus gruesos labios rojos. "Alguien va a morir por esto, Raquel." La forma como pronunció mi nombre me heló las entrañas. "No puedo matar a Tamwood, por eso tú recibirás su castigo. Felicitaciones." Denon me tenía entre cejas.

Bajé la mano del cuello apenas se alejó de mí. No era Ivy. Se notaba la diferencia entre la sangre alta y la sangre baja, entre los nacidos vampiros y aquellos humanos que cambiaron. Cuando llegó al pasillo, sus ojos amenazantes habían desaparecido. Denon sacó un sobre del bolsillo del pantalón y lo tiró en mi escritorio. "Disfruta tu último cheque, Morgan" dijo hablando fuerte para que los demás escucharan. No lo hacía por mí. Luego dio media vuelta y se fue.

"Pero tú querías que yo renunciara," murmuré mientras desaparecía en el ascensor. Las puertas se cerraron y la flechita roja que indica bajada se encendió. Ahora tenía que informarle a su jefe. De seguro tenía que estar bromeando. No podía ponerle precio a mi cabeza por algo tan estúpido como que Ivy y yo nos largábamos al mismo tiempo, ¿o sí?

"Buena esa Raquel." Alcé la cabeza reaccionando ante esa voz nasal. Me había olvidado de Francis. Se levantó del escritorio de Joyce y se recostó contra mi pared. Después de ver a Denon hacer lo mismo, la comparación con Francis era ridícula. Lentamente regresé a mi silla giratoria.

"He aguardado seis meses para que te desesperes y te largues" me dijo Francis. "Debí imaginar que lo único que te quedaba por hacer era emborracharte."

La ira terminó por quemar los restos de temor que me quedaban aun y seguí empacando. Mis dedos estaban fríos y traté de calentarlos frotándolos. Jenks salió de su escondite y regresó a la planta volando despacio.

Francis se bajó las mangas de la chaqueta hasta los codos, empujó mi cheque con un dedo y se sentó en mi escritorio con un pie en el suelo. "Te demoraste más de lo pensado," dijo con sorna. "O bien eres demasiado terca, o simplemente demasiado estúpida. De cualquier modo, estás muerta." Respiró con desdén carraspeando con su nariz delgada.

Entonces tiré duro un cajón para cerrarlo y casi le aplasto los dedos. "¿Estás tratando de demostrarme algo, *Francis?*"

"Me llamo Frank," respondió con tono de superioridad, pero en realidad sonó como si estuviera resfriado. "No te preocupes por desocupar los archivos de tu computadora. Ahora son míos. Y también tu escritorio."

Le eché un vistazo al protector de pantalla de mi computadora. Era un gran sapo verde con ojos saltones. ¡Más de mil veces lo había imaginado tragándose una mosca con la cara de Francis! "¿Y desde cuándo los duros de abajo permiten que un aprendiz de brujo se encargue de los casos?" le pregunté minimizando su posición. A Francis ni siquiera podía clasificarlo como brujo. No era suficientemente bueno. Era capaz de invocar un hechizo, pero no sabía cómo manipularlo. Yo sí podía, pero casi siempre compraba amuletos. Era más fácil y más seguro para mí y para mi objetivo. No era culpa mía que hubiéramos vivido durante miles de años con ese estereotipo de que las mujeres son brujas pero los hombres son magos.

Creo qué él mismo quería que le hiciera esa pregunta. "Tú no eres la única que sabe preparar, Raquel mi amiga. Obtuve mi licencia la semana pasada." Se inclinó, sacó un lapicero de mi caja y lo puso otra vez en el vaso de lápices. "Me habría convertido en brujo hace tiempo. Lo que pasa es que no quería ensuciarme las manos aprendiendo a hacer hechizos. Tal vez no debí aguardar tanto tiempo. ¡Es tan fácil!"

Saqué el lapicero de nuevo y lo metí en el bolsillo de mi pantalón. "Pues, qué bueno para tí." *¿Francis brujo?* pensé. *Tienen que haber recortado los requisitos.*

"Así es," dijo Francis limpiándose bajo las uñas con uno de mis puñales de plata. "Me dieron tu escritorio, tu archivo de casos...hasta tu auto de la compañía."

Le arrebaté el cuchillo de las manos y lo lancé a la caja. "No tengo auto de la compañía."

"Pero yo sí." Se acomodó el cuello de la camisa de palmeras, sintiéndose muy a gusto con sí mismo. Juré mantener la boca cerrada para no darle otra oportunidad de fanfarronear. "Así es," insistió con una sobredosis de volumen. "Lo voy a necesitar. Denon quiere que vaya el lunes a entrevistar al concejal Trenton Kalamack." Francis rió burlonamente. "Mientras que tú revoloteabas tratando de arrastrar a tu miserable captura, yo lideré la misión que confiscó dos kilos de azufre."

"No me digas" repuse, lista para ahorcarlo.

"No es la cantidad" dijo, quitándose el pelo de los ojos, "sino quién los portaba."

Eso me llamó la atención. ¿El nombre de Trent asociado con azufre? "¿Quién?" pregunté.

Francis se levantó de mi escritorio y tropezó con mis zapatillas rosadas. Por poco cae al piso. Logró reponerse y me apuntó con el dedo, imitando una pistola. "Cuídate la espalda Morgan."

Hasta ahí llegó mi paciencia. Apreté los dientes y estiré la pierna colocándola certeramente debajo de la suya. Francis cayó aullando. Luego le puse mi rodilla detrás de su asquerosa chaqueta de poliéster y mi mano buscó automáticamente mis esposas, ¡pero ya no estaban! Jenks gritó un par de vivas revoloteando encima. Después de un grito ahogado de alarma, la oficina volvió a quedar en silencio. Ninguno se entrometía. Ni siquiera me dirigían la mirada.

"Escucha chiquillo, no tengo nada que perder" gruñí, inclinándome hasta que olí su sudor. "Tal como lo dijiste, yo ya estoy muerta; así es que lo único que me detiene de arrancarte los ojos ahora es una simple curiosidad. Te lo preguntaré de nuevo: ¿a quién atrapaste con azufre?"

"¡Raquel!" exclamó. Podía golpearme el trasero pero se moría de miedo. "Estás hundiéndote en m…¡ay! ¡ay!," gritó al sentir mis uñas que se enterraban en sus ojos. "¡Yolin! ¡Yolin Bates!"

"¿El secretario de Trent Kalamack?" preguntó Jenks volando sobre mi hombro.

"Sí," dijo Francis, raspando la alfombra con la cara, tratando de voltear la cabeza para mirarme. "O mejor, su ex secretario. ¡Maldición Raquel, quítate de encima!"

"¿Está muerto?" pregunté, sacudiéndome el polvo de los jeans mientras me levantaba.

Francis se puso de pie. Alguna satisfacción sacaba de contarme todo esto; de lo contrario ya se habría largado.

"Era una mujer, no un hombre," continuó mientras se ajustaba el cuello de la camisa hacia arriba. "Ayer la encontraron tiesa como una roca en un calabozo de la S.E. Literalmente como una roca. Era aprendiz."

Dijo lo último con tono condescendiente pero yo le devolví una sonrisa agria. Cómo podía sentir desprecio por algo que él era hasta hace apenas una semana. *Trent,* pensé, fijando la mirada a lo lejos. Si yo lograba demostrar que Trent estaba traficando con azufre y lo entregaba a la S.E. en bandeja de plata, Denon se vería obligado a dejarme en paz. La S.E. estaba tras él desde hacía años, desde que la red del azufre empezó a extenderse. Nadie sabía si Trent era humano o Entremundos.

"Demonios Raquel," gimió Francis frotándose la cara. "Me partiste la nariz."

Mi mente estaba clara y me volteé mirándolo con sorna.

"Tú eres brujo. Ve a preparar un hechizo." Yo sabía que no podía hacerlo. Tendría que pedir uno prestado, como cuando era aprendiz, y yo sabía que eso lo irritaba. Sonreí con satisfacción cuando empezó a abrir la boca para decir algo; pero pensó dos veces, se tapó la nariz y se fue.

Sentí un golpecito seco al aterrizar Jenks en mi arete. Francis caminó afanosamente por el pasillo con la cabeza ladeada en un ángulo extraño. Su chaqueta deportiva se movía según su extraño caminar y no pude contener la risa al oír que Jenks cantaba el tema musical de *Miami Vice*.

"Qué pedazo de trapo sucio" dijo Jenks mientras yo regresaba a mi escritorio.

Volví a fruncir el ceño y traté de meter mi maceta y el laurel en la caja ahora repleta de cosas. Me dolía la cabeza y quería irme a casa a dormir la siesta. Pasé una última mirada por el escritorio y levanté mis zapatillas para guardarlas con todo lo demás. Le dejé los libros a Joyce sobre su silla con una nota diciéndole que la llamaría luego. *¿De manera que quieres mi computadora?* pensé mientras abría un archivo. Bueno, tres clics...y ya está: ahora le sería imposible cambiar el protector de pantalla sin arruinar todo el sistema.

"Me voy a casa, Jenks" susurré, mirando el reloj de la pared. Las tres y media. Había estado en la oficina solo media hora, pero me pareció un siglo. Una última mirada a todo el piso. Solo cabezas y espaldas volteadas. Era como si yo no existiera. "¡Quién los necesita!" mascullé. Tomé mi chaqueta del espaldar de la silla y mi cheque.

"¡Ey!" le grité a Jenks que me jalaba de la oreja. "¡Diablos, Jenks...ya deja eso!"

"¡El cheque!" exclamó, "Demonios, mujer...¡ha hechizado tu cheque!"

Me quedé inmóvil. Dejé caer la chaqueta en la caja y observé el sobre aparentemente inofensivo. Cerré los ojos y respiré profundo buscando identificar el olor de secoya.

Luego traté de sentir en la garganta el persistente sabor de azufre de magia negra. "No huele a nada."

Jenks soltó una carcajada. "¡Pero yo sí! Tiene que ser el cheque. Es lo único que te dio Denon. Ten cuidado Raquel: ¡es negra!"

Tuve una sensación de malestar. Denon no podía estar hablando en serio. No era posible.

Le eché otro vistazo a la oficina pero no había nadie que quisiera ayudarme. Saqué mi vasija del cesto de la basura que tenía agua del acuario de Don Pez. Le agregué una porción de sal, la probé con el dedo y luego le agregué un poco más. Muy bien. La misma salinidad del mar. Luego la vertí sobre el cheque. Si estaba hechizado, la sal rompería el hechizo.

Del sobre salió un humillo amarillo. "Relámpagos" dije, sintiendo temor repentinamente. "¡Cuidado con la nariz, Jenks!" y me resguardé debajo del escritorio.

El hechizo negro se disolvió formando burbujas. Una ola amarilla de humo sulfúrico se alzó y salió por los respiraderos, acompañado de varios lamentos. Hubo una pequeña estampida, pues todos se levantaron buscando puertas. Aun estando preparada para ello, el fétido olor a huevo podrido me irritó los ojos. El hechizo era inmundo y dirigido a mí, pues tanto Denon como Francis habían tocado el sobre. No podía creerlo.

Aún agitada, salí de debajo del escritorio. La oficina estaba desierta. "¿Está todo bien?," dije con algo de tos. Jenks asintió parado en mi arete. "Gracias Jenks."

Tenía revuelto el estómago pero tiré mi cheque empapado en la caja y salí pasando junto a todos los cubículos desocupados. Parecía que la amenaza de muerte de Denon iba en serio. ¡Maldición!

Cuatro

"**R**a-a-a-queeel-l-l-l" dijo cantando una vocecilla irritante que cortó el traqueteo de los cambios del autobús y el desfogue del motor diesel. La voz de Jenks chirrió adentro de mi oído peor que una tiza sobre el pizarrón. Tuve que hacer un esfuerzo por no lanzarle la mano para agarrarlo. Yo nunca lo había tocado. El pequeño fastidioso era muy rápido.

"No estoy dormida" le dije antes de que lo hiciera otra vez. "Solo descanso los ojos."

"Pues vas a descansarlos más allá de tu parada, Candela." Me llamó con el mismo apodo que me había dado el taxista y lo miré por una rendija del párpado.

"No me llames así." El bus dobló una esquina y tuve que sostener la caja con fuerza para equilibrarla sobre mis muslos. "Faltan aún dos cuadras" dije entre dientes. La náusea había desaparecido pero persistía la jaqueca. Sabía que faltaban dos cuadras por el ruido que hacían los de la liga de béisbol infantil. Los niños practicaban en el parque junto a mi apartamento y después del atardecer habría otra práctica.

Sentí el rasgueo de las alas de Jenks que descendía de mi arete hasta la caja. "¡Madre mía! ¡¿Ese era tu sueldo?!" exclamó.

Abrí los ojos como un relámpago. "¡Fuera de ahí!" Agarré mi cheque húmedo y lo metí en un bolsillo de la chaqueta. Jenks se burló haciendo muecas y yo froté mis dedos pulgar e índice como diciéndole que lo iba a triturar. Parece que entendió. Se alejó con sus pantalones de seda amarillo y morado y se sentó en el asiento frente a mí. "¿No deberías estar en algún lugar?" le pregunté, "¿por ejemplo, ayudando a tu familia a mudarse?"

Jenks soltó una carcajada. "¿Ayudarlos a mudarse? ¡Por nada del mundo!" Sus alas temblaron. "Además, debería darle una olfateada a tu sitio, sólo para asegurarnos de que todo esté en orden antes de que vueles en mil pedazos cuando quieras entrar al baño." Rió estruendosamente y varias personas voltearon a mirarme. Me encogí de hombros, como diciendo: "Duendes."

"Gracias," le respondí agriamente. Un duende guardaespaldas. Denon se moriría de la risa. Estaba agradecida con Jenks por detectar el hechizo en el cheque, pero la S.E. no tenía tiempo de perpetrar nada más. Pensé que a lo mejor tendría que cuidarme un par de días si la amenaza iba en serio. Pero yo creo que lo que quiso decir fue "no dejes que el hechizo te mate cuando vayas de salida" o algo así.

Me levanté y el autobús se detuvo. Bajé las escalerillas y me encontré con el último sol de la tarde. Jenks seguía fastidiando dando vueltas a mi alrededor. Era peor que un zancudo. "Bonito lugar" dijo sarcásticamente, mientras yo esperaba a que pasara el tráfico antes de cruzar la calle hacia mi apartamento. Asentí con la cabeza en silencio. Vivía en el distrito residencial de Cincinnati, en lo que fue un buen vecindario hace veinte años. El edificio de cuatro pisos era de ladrillo, construido originalmente para universitarios de clase alta. Había disfrutado de su elegancia hacía muchos años pero ahora quedaba reducido a esto.

Los buzones negros del porche eran feos y estaban abollados y se notaba que los habían forzado. La dueña me llevaba el correo, aun cuando sospechaba que era ella quien forzaba los buzones para escudriñar a sus anchas la correspondencia de los inquilinos. Había una pequeña franja de césped y dos arbustos desaliñados a cada lado de las escaleras. El año pasado sembré las semillas de milenrama que recibí de una promoción por correo de la revista *Hechizo Semanal;* pero el perro chihuahua de la dueña, el Sr. Dinky, las escarbó junto con el resto del jardín. Había pequeños terrones por todas partes, lo que le daba el aspecto de un campo de batalla de hadas.

"Y yo que pensaba que mi casa era mala," susurró Jenks cuando salté por encima del escalón podrido.

Mis llaves tintinearon mientras balanceaba la caja con una mano y trataba de abrir la puerta con la otra. Una vocecita en la cabeza me decía siempre lo mismo, año tras año. El olor a comida frita me asaltaba tan pronto entraba en el vestíbulo haciéndome fruncir la nariz. Una alfombra verde desaliñada y deshilachada adornaba las escaleras. La Sra. Baker había aflojado la bombilla de nuevo, pero la luz del atardecer que entraba por la ventana sobre el papel de botones de rosas de la pared me bastaba para encontrar el camino.

"Oye," dijo Jenks mientras subía las escaleras, "esa mancha en el techo tiene forma de pizza."

Miré hacia arriba. Tenía razón. Es gracioso. Jamás la había notado antes.

"¿Y esa abolladura en la pared?" continuó apenas alcanzamos el primer piso; "es justo del tamaño de una cabeza. Demonios, ¡si las paredes hablaran!"

Aun podía sonreír. Esperemos a que vea mi apartamento. Había una abolladura en el piso de la sala donde alguien había encendido una hoguera.

Pero la sonrisa desapareció tan pronto pisé el segundo descanso: todas mis cosas estaban en el pasillo.

"¿Qué demonios?" susurré. Asombrada, dejé la caja en el piso y miré por el pasillo buscando la puerta de la Sra. Talbú. "¡Ya pagué el alquiler!"

"¿Raque?," llamó Jenks desde el techo. "¿Dónde está tu gato?"

La rabia iba aumentando. Miré mis muebles y me pareció que ocupaban más espacio amontonados en el pasillo, sobre la ordinaria alfombra plástica. "¿Pero...por qué? ¡Maldición!"

"¡Raquel!" gritó Jenks. "¿Dónde está tu gato?"

"No tengo gato" gruñí. Ese era uno de mis puntos débiles.

"Pensé que todas las brujas tenían un gato."

Recorrí el pasillo con los dientes apretados. "Los gatos hacen estornudar al Sr. Dinky."

Jenks volaba junto a mi oreja. "¿Quién es el Sr. Dinky?"

"Es él" le dije, señalando una fotografía gigante de un chihuahua blanco que colgaba de frente a la puerta de la propietaria. El cochino perro de ojos saltones tenía uno de esos lazos que las mamás les ponen a las bebitas para que se sepa que es una niña. Golpeé en la puerta. "¿Sra. Talbú? ¿¡Sra. Talbú!?"

Se escuchaban los chillidos secos del Sr. Dinky y de alguien que clavaba detrás de la puerta. Luego... los gritos de la propietaria tratando de hacer callar al bendito animal. El Sr. Dinky multiplicó sus ladridos, arañando el piso y tratando de excavar un camino para salir.

"¡Sra. Talbú!" grité, "¿Qué hacen mis cosas en el pasillo?"

"¿Tus cosas, Candela?," dijo Jenks desde el techo. "Querrás decir mis desbaratadas cosas."

"¡Ya te dije que no me llames así!" grité, golpeando la puerta de nuevo.

Oí que adentro se cerraba una puerta y los ladridos del Sr. Dinky se hicieron más lejanos y desesperados. "¡Vete! ¡Aquí no puedes vivir más!"

Me dolía la palma de la mano y comencé a masajearla. "¿Usted piensa que no voy a pagarle el alquiler?" le dije sin importarme que todos los vecinos se enteraran. "Tengo dinero, Sra. Talbú. No puede sacarme así. Aquí mismo tengo el dinero del arriendo del próximo mes." Saqué mi húmedo cheque y lo agité frente a la puerta.

"Cambié la cerradura," dijo la Sra. Talbú con voz trémula. "Vete antes de que te maten."

Incrédula, me quedé inmóvil mirando la puerta. ¿Sabía de la amenaza de la S.E.? Además, esa actitud de señora anciana era pura comedia. Gritaba claro y duro a través de la pared cuando pensaba que tenía muy alta la música. "¡No puede desalojarme!" le dije desesperada. "¡Tengo mis derechos!"

"Las brujas muertas no tienen derechos" dijo Jenks parado en la instalación eléctrica.

"¡Maldita sea, Sra. Talbú!," grité frente a la puerta. "¡No estoy muerta aún!"

No hubo respuesta. Me quedé ahí parada pensando. No tenía mayor opción y ella lo sabía. Tal vez podía quedarme en mi nueva oficina hasta encontrar algo. Mudarme a vivir con mamá estaba descartado y no había hablado con mi hermano desde que empecé a trabajar con la S.E.

"¿Y mi depósito de garantía?" le pregunté. Seguía el silencio. Mi rabia se convirtió en fuego lento que podía arder durante días. "Sra. Talbú," dije calmadamente. "Si usted no me devuelve el saldo de este mes de alquiler y mi depósito de garantía, no me moveré de este sitio." Hice una pausa a ver si la escuchaba. "Me quedaré aquí sentada hasta que me atrapen y me hechicen. A lo mejor voy a explotar aquí mismo y dejaré una gran mancha de sangre en su alfombra que jamás podrá sacar. Y tendrá que verla todos los días. ¿Me escucha? ¿Sra. Talbú?," amenacé. "¡Encontrará pedazos míos en el techo de su pasillo!"

Escuché un jadeo. "Oh, mi pobre Dinky" dijo la Sra. Talbú. "¿Dónde está mi chequera?"

Miré a Jenks sonriendo agriamente y me respondió con un gesto de triunfo.

Se escucharon unos crujidos seguidos de un momento de silencio. Luego, el típico sonido de un cheque que se arranca de la chequera. No entiendo para qué continuaba con esa comedia de viejecita. Todos sabían que era más dura que la boñiga petrificada de dinosaurio y seguramente viviría más que todos nosotros. ¡No la quería ni la muerte!

"¡Desfachatada! Voy a asegurarme de que todos se enteren de esto. No encontrarás sitio para arrendar en toda la ciudad."

Jenks bajó como un dardo tan pronto vio que un papel blanco se asomaba debajo de la puerta. Luego de girar a su alrededor unos instantes, me indicó que estaba bien. Lo levanté y leí la suma. "¿Y mi depósito de garantía?" pregunté. "¿Quiere venir a mi apartamento para inspeccionarlo? ¿Quiere asegurarse de que no hay agujeros de clavos en las paredes o malos augurios debajo de la alfombra?"

Se oyó una maldición apagada seguida de más rasguños. Apareció otro papel. "¡Lárgate de mi edificio!" gritó la Sra. Talbú. "¡Lárgate antes de que te ataque el Sr. Dinky!"

"Yo también la quiero mucho, vieja murciélago." Saqué la llave de mi llavero y la tiré. Enfadada pero satisfecha, agarré el segundo cheque.

Regresé donde estaban mis cosas y reconocí el revelador olor a azufre que salía de ellas. Mis hombros estaban tensos de los nervios al observar mi vida arrimada contra las paredes. Todo estaba hechizado. No podía tocar nada. ¡Oh Dios, ayúdame! Estaba bajo amenaza de muerte de la S.E.

"No puedo empapar todo con sal" dije, al tiempo que oí una puerta que se cerraba.

"Conozco a un tipo que tiene un depósito," dijo Jenks con ánimo inusualmente comprensivo. Miré hacia arriba cruzando los brazos. "Si se lo pido, vendrá por todo esto y lo guardará. Luego podrás disolver los hechizos." Dudó un instante observando los discos compactos tirados de cualquier manera en mi gran cuenco de cobre para hechizos.

Asentí poniendo mi espalda contra la pared dejándome escurrir lentamente hasta quedar sentada en el piso. Mi ropa, mis zapatos, mi música, mis libros... ¿mi vida?

"Ay, no..." dijo Jenks suavemente. "Hechizaron tu disco de los *Éxitos de Takata*"

"Está autografiado" susurré. El ronroneo de sus alas disminuyó. El plástico sobreviviría al baño en agua salada, pero el catálogo de papel quedaría arruinado. ¿Me mandaría otro si se lo pedía? A lo mejor se acordaba de mí. Pasamos juntos una noche salvaje, persiguiendo sombras entre las ruinas de los viejos laboratorios biológicos de Cincinatti. Creo que escribió una canción sobre eso: "Nueva luna naciente perdida al amanecer / las sombras de la muerte son

de temer." Estuvo entre los veinte primeros éxitos durante
dieciséis semanas seguidas. Fruncí el ceño. "¿Habrán dejado
algo sin hechizar?"

Jenks aterrizó sobre el directorio telefónico encogiéndose
de hombros. Les habían dado todo a los forenses.

"Vaya." Me levanté sintiendo un nudo en el estómago.
Recordé lo que había dicho Ivy sobre León Bairn. Pedacitos
de brujo esparcidos por todo el porche. Tragué con dificultad. No podía ir a casa. *¿Cómo demonios iba a pagarle a
Denon?*

Volvió el dolor de cabeza. Jenks se acomodó en el arete
con la bocota cerrada mientras yo levantaba mi caja de cartón. Bajé las escaleras. Primero lo primero. "¿Cómo se
llama el tipo ese que conoces?" le pregunté cuando llegué al
vestíbulo. "El del depósito. ¿Crees que si le pago extra me
ayudará a diluir mis cosas?"

"Tendrías que explicarle cómo hacerlo. . . . no es brujo."

Me quedé pensando tratando de componerme. Mi teléfono celular estaba en el bolso, pero la pila estaba muerta y
el cargador en algún lugar entre mis cosas hechizadas.
"Puedo llamarlo desde la oficina," dije.

"No tiene teléfono" dijo Jenks saltando de mi arete y volando en reverso a nivel de mis ojos. La venda de su ala se
había soltado y pensé ofrecerle ayuda para ponérsela de
nuevo. "Vive en Los Hollows," concluyó Jenks. "Hablaré
con él. Es un poco tímido."

Agarré la perilla de la puerta pero dudé un instante. Con
la espalda contra la pared, levanté ligeramente la cortina
amarilla desteñida por el sol para echar un vistazo por la
ventana. El estropeado jardín estaba en silencio bajo el sol
de la tarde, quieto y vacío. El ruido de una cortadora de
pasto y el zumbido de los autos que pasaban era amortiguado por el vidrio. Con los labios apretados, decidí aguardar allí hasta el próximo autobús.

"Prefiere efectivo" dijo Jenks, bajando para detenerse en
el umbral. "Lo llevaré a la oficina cuando haya guardado tus
cosas."

"Querrás decir, todo lo que aun no ha desaparecido" repuse, a pesar de que creía que todo estaba relativamente a salvo. Se supone que los hechizos tienen un blanco determinado, sobre todo si son magia negra; pero nunca se sabe. Nadie se arriesgaría a morir por mis cosas. "Gracias Jenks." Me había salvado el trasero por segunda vez. Me sentía incómoda, y un poco culpable.

"Oye, para eso están los socios," respondió. Pero con eso no mejoró nada.

Apenas sonreí al ver su entusiasmo. Puse mi caja en el piso y esperé.

Cinco

El autobús estaba en silencio, pues a esa hora del día casi todo el tráfico salía de Los Hollows. Jenks había salido por la ventana poco después de que cruzamos el río hacia Kentucky. Era de la opinión de que la S.E. no intentaría atacarme en un autobús con testigos. Yo no estaba tan segura, pero tampoco le pediría que se quedara conmigo.

Le di la dirección al chofer y acordamos que me avisaría cuando llegáramos. Era un humano flaco. Su desteñido uniforme azul le quedaba grande, a pesar de todas las galletas waffers que se metía a la boca como si fueran dulces.

Casi todos los choferes del sistema de transporte público de Cincinatti se llevaban bien con los Entremundos. Pero no todos. Las reacciones que los humanos tenían hacia nosotros variaban mucho. Algunos sentían miedo. Otros no. Algunos nos querían. Otros nos querían muertos. Unos pocos aprovechaban las tarifas de los impuestos y se iban a vivir a Los Hollows, pero eran la minoría.

Poco después del Giro se presentó una emigración inesperada. Casi todos los humanos que podían, decidieron mudarse a las ciudades. Los sicólogos de entonces la bautizaron "el síndrome de hogar; y, en retrospectiva, ese fenómeno nacional tenía sentido. Los Entremundos estaban más que dispuestos a tomarse las propiedades de las afueras, atraídos por la perspectiva de poseer un poco más de tierra que po-

dían considerar suya. Y eso sin contar siquiera la gran deva-
luación de las casas.

Apenas ahora la población empieza a equilibrarse a medida que los Entremundos ricos regresan a las ciudades y los
humanos con menos suerte—pero más inteligentes—prefieren vivir en un bonito vecindario de Entremundos y no en un
basurero humano. Pero, por lo general, aparte de una pequeña sección alrededor de la universidad, los humanos vivían en Cincinatti y los Entretemundos en Los Hollows del
otro lado del río. A nosotros no nos importa que los humanos rechacen nuestros vecindarios viéndolos como ghettos
anteriores al Giro.

Los Hollows se han convertido en el bastión de la vida de
los Entremundos, cómoda y casual en la superficie, pero con
problemas potenciales ocultos. Muchos humanos se asom-
bran de ver lo normales que se ven Los Hollows. Y, pensán-
dolo bien, tiene sentido. Nuestra historia es la historia de la
humanidad. No caímos del cielo en el 66. Emigramos por
Ellis Island. Combatimos en la Guerra Civil, en la Primera
Guerra Mundial, en la Segunda Guerra Mundial—algunos
de nosotros en las tres. Sufrimos la Depresión y todos juntos
esperamos para saber quién le disparó a JR.

Pero existen diferencias peligrosas y todos los Entremundos mayores de cincuenta años han pasado la primera parte
de su vida ocultándolas—tradición que se mantiene aún hoy.

Las casas son modestas, pintadas de blanco, amarillo o
rosado. No hay casas embrujadas, con la excepción del cas-
tillo Loveland en el mes de octubre. Entonces se convierte
en la peor de las casas encantadas a ambos lados del río. Hay
columpios, piscinas, bicicletas en los jardines y autos estacionados en las calles. Hay que tener entrenada la vista para
darse cuenta de que las flores están organizadas en hechizos
contra la magia negra y que las ventanas de los sótanos generalmente están cementadas. La peligrosa y salvaje realidad sólo florece en las profundidades de la ciudad, donde la
gente se encuentra y la emotividad corre desenfrenada: par-

ques de diversión, clubes de baile, bares, iglesias. Pero en nuestros hogares, *jamás*.

Es silencioso—incluso de noche, cuando sus moradores andan despiertos. El silencio era lo que primero que hacía reaccionar a los humanos y los inquietaba haciendo volar sus instintos.

Sentí que no estaba tan tensa mientras miraba por la ventana y contaba las persianas negras a prueba de luz. La tranquilidad del vecindario parecía apoderarse del autobús. Hasta los pocos pasajeros que iban conmigo estaban inmóviles. Algo había en Los Hollows que me hacía sentir "en casa."

Mi cabello cayó hacia adelante cuando el autobús se detuvo. Salté nerviosamente cuando el tipo que venía atrás me rozó el hombro al levantarse. Bajó apresuradamente por la escalerilla con un ruido metálico de botas y se perdió en dirección del atardecer. El chofer me dijo que la siguiente parada era la mía. Aguardé de pie mientras el buen hombre se acercaba al andén para dejarme bajar. Descendí hacia las sombras que ya caían, envolviendo la caja con mis brazos y tratando de no respirar los gases del autobús que se alejaba. Desapareció tras una esquina llevándose consigo los últimos vestigios de ruido y humanidad.

Me fui quedando en silencio oyendo el cantar de algunos pájaros. En algún lugar cercano unos niños llamaban... no; gritaban... y un perro ladraba. Algunos augurios en tiza de colores decoraban los andenes rotos y una muñeca olvidada con colmillos pintados me recibió con su sonrisa. Del otro lado de la calle había una pequeña iglesia de piedra con su campanario que sobresalía por encima de los árboles.

Giré sobre mis tacones para ver lo que había arrendado Ivy para nosotras: era una casa de un piso que podía convertirse fácilmente en oficina. El techo parecía nuevo, pero el cemento de la chimenea se caía a pedazos. Al frente el pasto estaba tan crecido que necesitaba una podada. Hasta tenía garaje. Y, adentro, una máquina oxidada de cortar césped.

Estaremos bien, pensé, mientras abría la reja encadenada a la cerca que cerraba el patio. Un hombre viejo negro estaba sentado en el porche, meciéndose al ritmo del atardecer. ¿El dueño? cavilé sonriendo. Pensé si acaso sería un vampiro, pues usaba lentes oscuros frente al sol de la tarde. Su aspecto era descuidado, a pesar de estar afeitado. Junto a las sienes, su cabello rizado se tornaba gris. Tenía barro en los zapatos y otro tanto en las rodillas de sus jeans. Se veía muy gastado y cansado—desechado como un caballo de arado al que ya no quieren, pero que aun puede trabajar otra temporada más.

Colocó un vaso largo en la baranda del porche a medida que yo subía las escaleras. "No gracias" dijo, quitándose los lentes y guardándolos en el bolsillo de la camisa. Su voz era áspera.

Vacilante, lo miré parada en el primer escalón. "¿Disculpe?"

Tosió para despejar la garganta. "Lo que sea que esté usted vendiendo de esa caja, no lo quiero. Tengo suficientes velas de maleficio, caramelos, revistas; y no tengo dinero para un nuevo revestimiento exterior, purificador de agua o cuarto de sol."

"No vendo nada," le dije. "Soy su nueva inquilina."

Se enderezó, lo que lo hizo verse más descuidado aun. "¿Inquilina? Querrá decir...del otro lado de la calle."

Confundida, cambié mi caja de pierna. "¿No es éste el 1597 de la calle Oakstaff?"

Rió. "Queda del otro lado de la calle."

"Disculpe que lo haya incomodado." Me di vuelta para salir, subiendo mi caja un poco más.

"Así es," dijo el hombre. Me detuve, pues no quise ser descortés. "En esta calle los números están invertidos. Los números impares están en el lado equivocado de la calzada." Sonrió de nuevo plegando las arrugas alrededor de los ojos. "Pero a mí no me preguntaron cuando pusieron los números." Me extendió la mano. "Yo soy Keasley," dijo, esperando a que yo subiera por las escaleras para darle la mano.

Vecinos, pensé, rotando los ojos mientras subía. *Más vale ser amable.* "Raquel Morgan" repuse, con un sólo apretón de manos. Se sonrió dándome unas palmaditas paternales en el hombro. La fuerza de su mano era sorprendente, lo mismo que el olor de secoya que despedía. Era un brujo, o por lo menos aprendiz. Incómoda por su exceso de confianza, di un paso atrás y me soltó la mano. El porche estaba más fresco y me sentía más alta parada bajo el techo.

"¿Tus amigos están con la vampiro?" dijo, indicando con el mentón hacia el otro lado de la calle.

"¿Ivy? Sí."

Asintió lentamente, como si se tratara de algo importante. "¿Las dos renunciaron juntas?"

Parpadeé. "Las noticias vuelan."

Rió otra vez. "Así es. Vuelan de verdad."

"¿No le da miedo que me hechicen delante de su puerta y que lo arrastre conmigo?"

"No." Se recostó en su mecedora y tomó el vaso. "Este te lo quité de encima." Tomó un diminuto amuleto autoadhesivo entre el pulgar y el índice. Yo quedé con la boca abierta mientras que él lo dejaba caer en el vaso. Lo que pensé que era limonada comenzó a formar espuma a medida que el hechizo se disolvía. Salió humo amarillo mientras él movía su mano dramáticamente. "¡Cáspita! . . . Era feo."

¿Agua salada? Sonrió al ver mi conmoción. "Él tipo del autobús . . . ," tartamudeé retirándome del porche. El azufre amarillo se arremolinó en las escaleras, como si me estuviera buscando.

"Un gusto conocerla, Srta. Morgan" dijo el hombre. Salí a trompicones hasta la acera. "Una vampiro y un duende pueden ayudarla a seguir con vida un par de días, pero de nada servirá si no tiene más cuidado."

Volteé los ojos buscando calle abajo el autobús que obviamente ya no estaba. "El tipo del autobús . . ."

Keasley asintió con la cabeza. "Es verdad que no intentarán nada cuando haya testigos, menos aun al principio; pero tiene que cuidarse de los amuletos que sólo se activan cuando está sola."

Había olvidado los hechizos de acción retardada. Pero, ¿de dónde sacaba Denon el dinero? Fruncí el ceño tratando de pensar en el dilema; el dinero de soborno de Ivy estaba financiando mi pena de muerte. ¡Qué bien!

"Estoy en casa todo el día," dijo Keasley. "Venga si quiere hablar. Ahora salgo muy poco. Artritis." Se dio una palmadita en la rodilla.

"Gracias por encontrar ese hechizo."

"Un gusto," respondió con la mirada fija en el techo del porche y el ventilador que giraba lentamente.

Sentía un nudo en el estómago mientras me dirigía hacia la acera. ¿Acaso toda la ciudad se había enterado de mi despido? Tal vez Ivy habló con él.

Me sentía vulnerable en la calle vacía. "Mil quinientos noventa y tres" musité, observando una pequeña casa amarilla con dos bicicletas en el césped. "Mil seiscientos uno," dije mirando para el otro lado, hacia una casa de ladrillo bien cuidada. Me mordí los labios. Lo único que había en medio de ambas era la iglesia de piedra. Quedé helada. ¿Una iglesia?

Un zumbido áspero pasó por mis oídos y me agaché instintivamente.

"¡Hola Raque!" Jenks se detuvo en el aire justo fuera de mi alcance.

"¡Diablos, Jenks!" grité, enojándome más al oír la risa del viejo. "¡No hagas eso!"

"Tus cosas ya están organizadas" dijo Jenks. "Lo hice colocar todo encima de bloques."

"Es una iglesia."

"No me digas, Sherlock. Espera a que veas el jardín."

Permanecí inmóvil. "Es una *iglesia*."

Jenks flotaba en el aire esperándome. "Atrás hay un jardín inmenso; buenísimo para hacer fiestas."

"Jenks," le dije con los dientes apretados, "es una iglesia y el jardín es un *cementerio*."

"No todo," dijo flotando con impaciencia; "y, además, ya no es iglesia. Es una guardería infantil desde hace dos años. Ahí no han enterrado a nadie desde el Giro."

Lo miré fijamente. "¿Sacaron los cuerpos?"

Dejó de revolotear y quedó suspendido, inmóvil. "Naturalmente que sacaron los cuerpos. ¿Me crees *estúpido*? ¿Crees que viviría donde hay *humanos* muertos? Dios me ayude. ¡Los gusanos, las enfermedades, los virus y toda esa mierda filtrándose por el piso infectándolo todo!"

Acomodé de nuevo la caja y crucé la calle en sombras. Luego subí por las amplias escaleras de la iglesia. Jenks no tenía la más mínima idea si los cuerpos habían sido trasladados o no. Los escalones de piedra gris estaban hundidos en el centro por tantos años de uso y además estaban resbalosos. Tenía dos puertas dobles de madera rojiza más altas que yo aseguradas con metal. Una tenía una placa atornillada que decía: "Guardería Infantil de Donna." Rezongué leyendo la placa. Empujé una de las puertas y me asombré de la fuerza que se necesitaba para moverla. Ni siquiera tenía candado, tan sólo un pasador interior.

"Claro que sacaron los cuerpos" dijo Jenks, revoloteando por toda la iglesia. Apostaría cien dólares a que se dirigía hacia el jardín para investigar.

"¿Ivy?" grité, tratando de cerrar la puerta a mis espaldas. "Ivy, ¿estás aquí?" El eco de mi voz resonó por el santuario que aun no había visto. Era un sonido grave en un espacio cerrado rodeado de vitrales de colores. El vestíbulo estaba oscuro. No tenía ventanas y había unos paneles negros de madera. Era cálido y tranquilo y se sentía la atmósfera de las antiguas liturgias. Dejé la caja en el piso de madera y contemplé el resplandor verde y ámbar que provenía del santuario.

"¡Enseguida bajo!," llegó el grito distante de Ivy. Sonaba casi alegre; pero, ¿dónde demonios estaba metida? Su voz venía de todas partes, pero a la vez de ninguna en especial.

Escuché el suave sonido de un pestillo e Ivy apareció detrás de un panel. A sus espaldas había una escalera angosta en espiral. "El búho está en el campanario" dijo, sus ojos pardos más vivos que nunca. "Es perfecto como almacén. Cantidades de repisas y estantes. Sólo que alguien dejó sus cosas. ¿Quieres que echemos un vistazo juntas más tarde?"

"Ivy, estamos en una iglesia."

Ivy se detuvo. Cruzó los brazos y me miró, su cara súbitamente vacía.

"Hay gente muerta en el jardín" agregué. Entonces se dirigió al santuario. "Se pueden ver las lápidas desde la calle," continué diciendo mientras la seguía.

Los bancos habían desaparecido, lo mismo que el altar. Sólo quedaba un cuarto desocupado y una tarima ligeramente elevada. Esa misma madera negra formaba el revestimiento que quedaba debajo de los altos ventanales con vitrales de colores que no podían abrirse. Una sombra descolorida en la pared indicaba el lugar donde alguna vez colgó una cruz inmensa sobre el altar. El techo tendría unos tres pisos de altura y yo fijé mis ojos en la talla de la madera. Pensé que sería difícil mantener el calor en el lugar durante el invierno. No era otra cosa que un espacio desnudo y vacío, pero la fría desolación lo proveía de una sensación de paz.

"¿Cuánto cuesta?" pregunté, acordándome de que debería estar enojada.

"Setecientos al mes, servicios incluidos" dijo Ivy secamente.

"¿Setecientos?" dije sorprendida y algo escéptica. Es decir, mi parte son tres cincuenta. Pagaba cuatrocientos cincuenta en los suburbios por mi propio castillete de una habitación. No estaba mal. Nada mal. Sobre todo si tenía jardín. *No,* pensé, de vuelta con mi mal humor. Es un *cementerio.*

"¿Adónde vas?" le pregunté a Ivy que se alejaba. "Te hablo a ti."

"Voy por una taza de café. ¿Quieres una?" Desapareció por la puerta que estaba detrás de la tarima elevada.

"Está bien. El alquiler es barato" dije. "Eso fue lo que dije que quería, ¡pero es una iglesia! ¡No puedes administrar un negocio desde una iglesia!" Molesta la seguí, pasando junto a los baños para hombres y mujeres. Más adelante, a la derecha, había una puerta. Eché un vistazo al pasar y me hallé con un cuarto desocupado de buen tamaño, piso y paredes respondiendo a mi respiración con un eco. Una ventana con un vitral de santos estaba abierta con una vara para ventilarlo y podía escuchar a los gorriones cantando afuera. El cuarto daba la impresión de haber sido una oficina, adaptado luego para acomodar cunas de bebés. El piso estaba polvoriento pero la madera se veía bien y no tan rayada.

Satisfecha, eché otro vistazo por la puerta del otro lado del pasillo. Había una cama arreglada y cajas abiertas. Antes de que pudiera ver más, Ivy se paro de frente y cerró la puerta.

"Son tus cosas" le dije mirándola.

Ivy se quedó inmutable, helándome más que si hubiese tratado de arrastrarme el aura. "Tendré que quedarme aquí hasta que pueda arrendar una habitación en algún lugar." Dudó por un instante acomodándose el cabello negro detrás de la oreja. "¿Algún problema?"

"No" repuse suavemente, cerrando mis párpados unos instantes. Por el amor de Santa Filomena. Tendría que vivir en la oficina mientras encontraba otro lugar. Abrí los ojos y me llamó la atención la extraña mirada de Ivy. Era una mezcla entre temor y ¿expectativa?

"Parece que yo también voy aterrizar aquí" le dije, a pesar de que esto no me gustaba para nada. Pero no tenía otra opción. "Me sacaron del apartamento. La caja que hay adelante es todo lo que tengo hasta que logre conjurar el hechizo de mis cosas. La S.E. embrujó todo mi apartamento con magia negra y por poco me clavan en el autobús. Además, gracias a la dueña, nadie me alquilará un apartamento dentro de los límites de la ciudad. Denon le puso precio a mi cabeza, tal como tú dijiste." Traté de que mi voz no sonara quejumbrosa, pero era imposible.

Los ojos de Ivy aun destellaban esa extraña luz y pensé si acaso me habría mentido respecto a que no era un vampiro activo. "Puedes quedarte en la habitación desocupada" dijo asegurándose de que la voz le sonara inexpresiva.

Asentí ligeramente. *Está bien*, pensé, al tiempo que respiraba profundo. Estaba viviendo en una iglesia con cuerpos en el jardín, con una amenaza de la S.E. y con un vampiro al otro lado del pasillo. Me pregunto si se dará cuenta si pongo un candado en la puerta. Me pregunto si haría alguna diferencia.

"La cocina queda atrás" dijo. La seguí, atraída por el aroma del café. Dimos la vuelta por la galería y de nuevo olvidé que estaba molesta.

El tamaño de la cocina era aproximadamente la mitad del santuario, tan bien equipada y moderna, mientrar que el santuario era medieval y vacío. El metal de cromo relucía y las luces fluorescentes brillaban. El refrigerador era inmenso. De un lado del cuarto había una estufa y un horno de gas. Del otro, un reverbero eléctrico. El centro era una isla de acero inoxidable con estantes desocupados abajo. La estantería superior estaba engalanada con utensilios metálicos, sartenes y ollas. Era una cocina de ensueño para una bruja: ¡ahora no tendría que revolver mis hechizos y la cena en la misma estufa!

Aparte de la mesa y los asientos de madera medio desbaratados de la esquina, la cocina parecía una de esas que salen en los programas de televisión. Un extremo de la mesa estaba organizado como un escritorio para computadora, con la pantalla titilando incesantemente en busca de enlaces de red. Era un programa costoso y eso me dejó pensando.

Ivy aclaró la garganta mientras abría un armario al lado del fregadero. Había tres tazas diferentes en la repisa de abajo. Por lo demás, estaba desocupado. "Instalaron la cocina nueva hace cinco años a petición del Departamento de Sanidad" dijo atrayendo mi atención. "La congregación no era muy grande y cuando terminaron de instalarla, no tenían como pagar. Por eso la están alquilando. Para pagarle al banco."

El sonido del café cayendo en las tazas llenó la habitación mientras yo pasaba mis dedos por la intachable isla de acero. Jamás habían preparado allí un pastel de manzana o galletas para la escuela de domingo.

"Quieren recuperar su iglesia" dijo Ivy apoyándose contra el mostrador con la taza bien acomodada entre sus manos pálidas. "Pero se están muriendo. Quiero decir, la iglesia" agregó, cuando mis ojos y los suyos se encontraron. "No hay nuevos miembros. Es triste, de verdad. La sala queda acá detrás."

No supe qué responder, prefiriendo mantener la boca cerrada. La seguí por el pasillo y por una puerta angosta al final del corredor. La sala era acogedora y dispuesta con tan buen gusto que no dudé ni un instante de que estas eran las cosas de Ivy. Era la primera cosa cálida y suave que había visto en este lugar, aun cuando todo fuera en tonos grises y las ventanas apenas simples vidrios transparentes. Celestial. Sentí que disminuía mi tensión. Ivy oprimió un control remoto y sonó música de jazz. Tal vez no estaba del todo mal.

"¿Por poco te atrapan?" preguntó Ivy lanzando el control sobre la mesita de centro y acomodándose en uno de los voluptuosos sillones de gamuza gris junto a la chimenea vacía. "¿Estás bien?"

"Sí," repuse agriamente, hundiéndome hasta los tobillos en la alfombra. "¿Todas estas cosas son tuyas? Un tipo se topó conmigo pegándome un hechizo que solo invocaría cuando no hubiera testigos presentes...además de mí. No puedo creer que Denon haga esto en serio. Tú tenías razón." Me esforcé para sonar despreocupada, pues no quería que Ivy se diera cuenta de lo nerviosa que estaba. ¡Demonios! Yo tampoco quería darme cuenta de lo preocupada que estaba. Conseguiría el dinero de alguna manera para pagar mi contrato. "Tuve mucha suerte de que ese viejo del otro lado de la calle me lo quitara." Levanté una fotografía de Ivy con un perro labrador. Sonreía mostrando los dientes y yo oculté mi estremecimiento.

"¿Qué viejo?" preguntó Ivy de inmediato.

"Al otro lado de la calle. Te ha estado observado." Dejé el marco metálico en la mesa y acomodé el cojín de la silla frente a ella antes de sentarme. Muebles que hacen juego; qué bien. Un viejo reloj de repisa sonaba suave y melódicamente. Había una pantalla grande de televisión con un reproductor de discos compactos en una esquina y muchos botones. Ivy sabía de aparatos electrónicos.

"Traeré mis cosas una vez que las haya disuelto" dije, pensando cómo se verían mis cosas ordinarias junto a las suyas. "Al menos lo que sobreviva a la sumergida," agregué.

¿Sobrevivir a la sumergida? pensé de repente cerrando los ojos y frotándome la frente. "Ay no," dije suave, "no puedo disolver mis hechizos."

Ivy equilibró su taza en una rodilla mientras pasaba las páginas de una revista. "Ummmm...¿qué?"

"Hechizos," dije a media voz. "La S.E. recubrió mi colección de hechizos con magia negra. Sumergirlos en agua salobre para romper el encantamiento los arruinará y no puedo comprar más." Hice una mueca observando su mirada en blanco. "Si la S.E. llegó hasta mi apartamento, estoy segura que también fueron al almacén. Debí traer unos cuantos ayer antes de renunciar, pero nunca pensé que les importaría que me fuera." Ajusté con desgano la pantalla de la lámpara de mesa. Nunca les importé, hasta el día en que Ivy se fue conmigo. Deprimida, tiré la cabeza hacia atrás y fijé los ojos en el techo.

"Pensé que ya sabías preparar hechizos," comentó Ivy extrañada.

"Sí puedo, pero es como una patada en el trasero; además ¿dónde consigo los materiales?" Cerré los ojos con amargura. Tendría que preparar mis hechizos.

Hubo un sonido de páginas y alcé la cabeza para ver a Ivy que ojeaba su revista. En la portada salía Blanca Nieves y una manzana. El corsé de Blanca Nieves estaba abierto y dejaba ver su ombligo. En un extremo de la boca, una gota de sangre brillaba como una joya. Le daba otro sentido a ese cuento del hechizo para dormir. El Sr. Disney se habría horrorizado; a menos, claro está, que hubiese sido un Entremundos. Eso explicaría muchas cosas.

"¿Y no puedes simplemente comprar lo que necesitas?," preguntó Ivy.

Reaccioné ante los destellos de sarcasmo en su voz. "Sí, pero tendré que sumergir todo en agua salobre para asegurarme de que no lo hayan alterado. Será virtualmente imposible deshacerme de toda la sal y con eso las mezclas quedarían mal."

Jenks salió zumbando de la chimenea con un chillido irritante, dejando una nube de hollín a su paso. Quién sabe cuánto tiempo habría estado ahí escuchando. Aterrizó sobre una caja de pañuelos de papel y se limpió un poco las alas. Parecía una mezcla de libélula con gato en miniatura. "Vaya vaya…parece que estamos obsesionadas," dijo respondiendo a mi pregunta sobre su posible espionaje.

"Tienes a la S.E. tratando de acabarte con magia negra y te pones un tanto paranoica." Le di un porrazo a la caja donde estaba sentado y salió por los aires. Se quedó volando estático en medio de las dos. "Aun no has visto el jardín ¿verdad Sherlock?"

Le lancé un cojín pero ágilmente se quitó. El cojín golpeó la lámpara junto a Ivy, pero ella la alcanzó con indiferencia antes de que cayera al piso. No levantó la mirada de su revista ni derramó una sola gota del café que balanceaba en la rodilla. Se me pararon los pelos de la nuca. "No me llames así tampoco" le dije tratando de ocultar mi molestia. Se veía realmente petulante ahí suspendido en el aire frente a mí "¿Y entonces?" le pregunté maliciosamente, "¿el jardín tiene algo más aparte de maleza y gente muerta?"

"Tal vez."

"¿Verdad?" Esto podría ser la primera cosa buena en sucederme hoy. Me levanté para mirar por la puerta trasera "¿Vienes?," le pregunté a Ivy mientras le daba la vuelta a la perilla.

Su cabeza estaba doblada mirando una página con cortinas de cuero. "No," repuso desinteresadamente.

Así es que quien me acompañó a salir por la puerta trasera del jardín fue Jenks. El sol poniente era fuerte y excitante y los olores se hacían más fuertes por la humedad que salía de la tierra mojada. En algún lugar había un árbol de serbal y respiré profundo. También un abedul y un roble. Aquellos chiquillos que de seguro eran los hijos de Jenks, revoloteaban ruidosamente por todos lados, persiguiendo a una mariposa amarilla encima de los montículos de vegetación. Hileras de matas adornaban las paredes y el muro de piedra alrededor de la iglesia. Una muralla de la altura de una persona le daba la vuelta completa a la propiedad, aislando diplomáticamente a la iglesia de sus vecinos.

Otro muro menos alto, tanto que se podía saltar por encima, separaba el jardín de un pequeño cementerio. Entrecerré los ojos y vi algunas plantas que sobresalían entre el pasto alto y de las lápidas, pero solo aquellas que crecían más entre los muertos. Cuanto más me acercaba, más me asombraba. El jardín estaba completo. Hasta las cosas fuera de lo común estaban allí.

"Es perfecto" susurré, paseando mis dedos por el limoncillo. "Todo lo que yo necesitaba, ¿cómo llegó todo esto aquí?"

La voz de Ivy sonó a mis espaldas. "Según la vieja…"

"¡Ivy!," dije girando para verla ahí parada, quieta, silenciosa, en medio de un haz de luz color ámbar. "¡No hagas eso!" *Vampiro escalofriante,* pensé, *debería colgarle una campana.*

Prosiguió con la palma de la mano de frente al sol poniente. "Dijo que el último pastor fue brujo. Él hizo el jardín. Puedo hacer que nos rebajen cincuenta del arriendo si alguien se encarga de mantenerlo como está."

Echándole una mirada al tesoro escondido dije: "Yo lo haré."

Jenks voló de entre un grupo de violetas. Sus pantalones morados tenían manchas de polen que hacían juego con su camisa amarilla. "¿Trabajo manual?" preguntó, "¿con esas uñas tuyas?"

Miré los óvalos perfectos de mis uñas rojas. "Esto no es trabajo; esto es terapia."

"Lo que sea." Volvió la atención hacia sus niños y zumbó por el jardín para rescatar a la mariposa que era su víctima.

"¿Crees que aquí habrá todo lo que necesitas?" preguntó Ivy al tiempo que daba la vuelta para entrar de nuevo.

"Casi todo. La sal no se puede hechizar, así que mi provisión va a estar bien; pero necesito mi caldera de buenos hechizos y todos mis libros."

Ivy se detuvo en el camino. "Yo creía que era necesario saber preparar las pociones de memoria para obtener licencia de bruja."

Sentí vergüenza y me incliné para arrancar una hoja de pasto detrás de una mata de romero. Nadie preparaba sus propios hechizos si podía comprarlos. "Sí," repuse, dejando caer la hojita y sacando la tierra debajo de mis uñas. "Es que he perdido la práctica" suspiré. Esto sería más difícil de lo que parecía.

Ivy se encogió de hombros. "Podrías descargarlas de la red... me refiero a las recetas."

La miré con recelo. "¿Confiar en la red? No creo que sea buena idea."

"Hay algunos libros en el desván."

"Sí, claro," repuse sarcásticamente. "Ciento un hechizos para principiantes. Todas las iglesias tienen un ejemplar."

Ivy se puso seria. "No te des aire de superioridad" me dijo. El color pardo de sus ojos comenzó a desaparecer tras sus pupilas dilatadas. "Solo pensé que si alguno del clero era brujo y con las plantas adecuadas aquí, a lo mejor podría haber dejado sus libros. La vieja dijo que huyó con una feligresa joven. Es probable que esas cosas en el desván sean suyas. A lo mejor tiene agallas para regresar."

Lo último que necesitaba era a un vampiro molesto durmiendo al otro lado del pasillo. "Disculpa" le dije. "Echaré un vistazo. Si tengo suerte, cuando pase por el cobertizo en busca de un serrucho para cortar mis amuletos me toparé con una bolsa de sal de las que se usan para descongelar el hielo en el invierno."

Ivy comenzó a caminar y luego volteó a mirar el cobertizo que más parecía un armario. La pasé, deteniéndome bajo el umbral. "¿Vienes?" le pregunté, decidida a no dejarla creer que encender y apagar el vampiro me estaba poniendo nerviosa. "¿O tus búhos me dejarán tranquila?"

"No...digo...sí." Ivy se mordió el labio. Ese fue sin duda un gesto humano que me hizo alzar las cejas. "Te dejarán subir. No hagas demasiado ruido. Yo...yo subiré pronto."

"Como quieras," musité girando para buscar el camino hacia el campanario.

Tal como lo prometió Ivy, los búhos me dejaron tranquila. Resultó que en el desván había un ejemplar de todo lo que había perdido en mi apartamento. Algunos libros eran tan antiguos que se deshacían. En la cocina había un conjunto de ollas de cobre, probablemente usadas, que Ivy había encargado para sus competencias de cocina. Eran perfectas para preparar hechizos pues no habían sido selladas para disminuir las manchas. El hecho de encontrar todo lo necesario resultaba un tanto misterioso, tanto que cuando salí a buscar un serrucho en el cobertizo, me tranquilicé al no encontrar sal. Así es...pero estaba en el piso de la despensa.

Todo marchaba demasiado bien. Algo debía estar mal.

Seis

Me senté encima de la antigua mesa de cocina de Ivy: con las piernas cruzadas y mis pies en mis pantuflas rosadas de peluche. Los trozos de verdura estaban cocidas en su punto, crujientes aun, y les di vuelta con mis palillos chinos buscando más pollo en la cajita blanca. "Fantástico," dije mascullando todavía con la boca llena. El ají rojo me quemó la lengua y mis ojos se aguaron, así que me tomé casi todo el vaso de leche. "Picante" dije. Ivy alzó la mirada de su cajita que acomodaba muy bien entre sus manos largas. "¡Demonios, sí está picante!"

Ivy arqueó sus negras cejas delgadas. "Me alegro que estés de acuerdo." Estaba sentada a la mesa en el espacio que había despejado delante de la computadora. Inclinándose sobre su cajita de comida, una ola de cabello negro le caía hacia adelante formando una cortina sobre su cara. Se lo pasó detrás de la oreja y me quedé mirándole el contorno de la mandíbula mientras comía.

Yo tenía poca experiencia con palillos, apenas lo suficiente como para no parecer tonta, pero Ivy los usaba con gran precisión, llevándose a la boca los trozos pequeños de comida con ritmo sensual. Por eso cambié la mirada, porque me sentí incómoda.

"¿Cómo se llama?" pregunté, buscando en mi cajita de cartón.

"Pollo al curry rojo."

"¿Eso es todo?" pregunté extrañada mientras ella movía la cabeza afirmativamente. Recuerdo que hice un ruido y encontré otro trozo de pollo. El curry estalló en toda mi boca y lo pasé con un sorbo de leche. "¿Dónde lo compraste?"

"Piscary."

Abrí los ojos asombrada. Piscary era un hueco de pizzería y un sitio donde se reunían los vampiros. Buena comida en una atmósfera más bien particular. "¿Esto viene de Piscary?" pregunté, recalcando bien la pregunta mientras masticaba un vegetal. "No sabía que prepararan cosas que no fueran pizza."

"No lo hacen . . . por lo general."

De inmediato, me puse en alerta cuando escuché su voz ronca, pero la ví muy concentrada en su comida. Alzó la cabeza al percatarse de que yo no me movía y me guiñó sus ojos de almendra. "Mi madre le dio la receta. Piscary lo prepara especialmente para mí. No es nada del otro mundo."

Me invadió una sensación de desazón al verla comer. Escuchaba los grillos y el ruido que hacían nuestros palillos. Don Pez nadaba en su pecera sobre la repisa de la ventana, y los sonidos nocturnos de Los Hollows no se podían oír por el rítmico golpeteo de mi ropa dando vueltas en la secadora.

No me acostumbraba a la idea de tener que vestirme mañana con la misma ropa, pero sabía por Jenks que su amigo no podría desembrujar mi ropa sino hasta el domingo. Ahora sólo podía lavar lo que tenía y esperar a no toparme con nadie conocido. Tenía puesta la pijama y la bata de Ivy. Todo negro, naturalmente, pero ella insistía en que me quedaban bien. El ligero olor a ceniza de madera no era desagradable y parecía adherirse a mí.

Mis ojos se posaron en el espacio vacío encima del fregadero donde debería haber un reloj. "¿Qué hora será?"

"Más de las tres" repuso Ivy sin mirar su reloj. Seguí escarbando y caí en la cuenta de que ya me había comido la piña. "Ojalá que mi ropa esté lista pronto. Estoy agotada."

Ivy cruzó las piernas y se inclinó sobre la comida. "Ve

a acostarte. Yo la sacaré. Estaré despierta hasta eso de las cinco."

"No. Me quedo." Bostecé cubriéndome la boca con la mano. "No tengo que madrugar mañana para ir al trabajo" concluí sarcásticamente. Ivy dejó escapar un murmullo de aprobación y yo dejé de escarbar en la cajita. "Ivy, puedes decirme que no es asunto mío, pero... ¿por qué entraste a la S.E. si no querías trabajar para ellos?"

Pareció sorprenderse y me miró respondiéndome con un tono de voz indiferente que lo decía todo. "Lo hice para quitarme de encima a mi madre." Un destello de dolor pasó por sus ojos; ocurrió tan rápidamente que no supe si fue real. "Mi padre no está contento con mi renuncia" agregó. "Piensa que debí quedarme... o matar a Denon."

Dejé mi comida a un lado. No sabía si me asombraba más oír que su padre vivía o su original consejo sobre cómo ascender en el trabajo. "Eh... Jenks dice que tú eres el último miembro viviente de tu casa."

Ivy asintió moviendo la cabeza lentamente. Fijó sus ojos pardos en mí mientras movía rítmicamente los palillos de la cajita a la boca. Aquella demostración de sensualidad sutil me confundió y me acomodé nerviosamente en mi sitio. Nunca la había visto mal cuando trabajamos juntas; pero, claro, generalmente abandonábamos el trabajo antes de la medianoche.

"Mi padre se casó en la familia" dijo entre bocado y bocado. No creo que Ivy tuviera idea de lo atractiva que era en ese momento. "Soy el último miembro vivo de mi linaje. El dinero de mi madre ahora es mío. Bueno... era. Está furiosa porque renuncié. Quiere que consiga un buen vampiro vivo de sangre alta, que asiente cabeza y produzca tantos hijos como sea posible, para garantizar que su linaje no desaparezca. Me mataría si muero antes de tener un hijo."

Moví la cabeza como si hubiera entendido. Pero no entendí. "Yo entré a la S.E. gracias a mi padre" dije. Volví la atención a mi comida un tanto apenada. "Papá trabajaba para la S.E. en la división de misterios. Todas las mañanas regresaba a casa con alguna historia extraña de gente a la que había ayudado o atrapado. Lo hacía ver todo tan emocionante" dije sonriendo. "Nunca habló de la parte burocrática. Cuando murió, pensé que de esa manera tendría su recuerdo más cerca. Qué tontería ¿verdad?"

"No."

Subí la mirada al tiempo que masticaba una zanahoria. "Tenía que hacer algo. Pasé un año viendo cómo mi mamá perdía el juicio. No está loca, pero no quiere aceptar que mi padre murió. No puedes hablarle sin que te diga cosas como 'Hoy hice budín de banano; era el preferido de tu padre.' Ella sabe que está muerto, pero no lo deja ir."

Ivy fijó la mirada en la oscuridad afuera de la cocina, reflexionando sobre sus recuerdos. "Mi padre es así. Se la pasa pensando en mi madre. No lo tolero."

Mastiqué lentamente. Pocos vampiros continuaban con vida después de morir. Las sofisticadas precauciones para evitar la luz del sol y el valor del seguro bastaban para arruinar a cualquier familia. Y para qué hablar del suministro permanente de sangre fresca.

"No lo veo casi nunca" agregó casi suspirando. "No entiendo Raquel. A él le queda toda la vida por delante, pero no deja que ella tome la sangre que necesita de nadie más. Si no está con ella, está tirado en el suelo de tanta sangre que ha perdido. Se está muriendo para mantenerla viva. Una sola persona no puede mantener a un vampiro muerto. Ambos lo saben."

La conversación tomó un giro incómodo, pero ahora no podía retirarme así nada más. "Tal vez lo hace porque la ama" sugerí suavemente.

Ivy frunció la frente. "Y... ¿qué clase de amor es ese?" Se puso de pie y sus piernas largas se enderezaron con elegancia. Luego desapareció por el pasillo con su cajita de cartón en la mano.

El silencio repentino me golpeó los oídos y me sorprendí a mí misma mirando su asiento vacío. Se había marchado. ¿Cómo podía marcharse así? La conversación era demasiado interesante como para abandonarla. Me levanté de la mesa con mi cajita de comida y la seguí hasta la sala.

Se había recostado en uno de los sillones de gamuza gris, extendida, con mirada desinteresada. Recostó la cabeza en uno de los gruesos brazos del sillón y sus pies colgaban del otro. Por un instante dudé confundida frente a la puerta con esta imagen que me mostraba Ivy. Era una leona satisfecha en su madriguera después de la matanza. *Pues bien,* pensé, *después de todo es un vampiro.* ¿Cómo se supone que debería verse?

A mi mente volvió el hecho de que ella no era un vampiro activo. Yo no tenía nada que temer. Me acomodé despacio en la silla delante de ella. La mesita de centro estaba en el medio. Solamente una de las lámparas de mesa estaba encendida, de manera que la sala estaba en penumbra. Sólo brillaban las luces de su equipo electrónico. "¿De manera que la S.E. fue idea de tu padre?" le pregunté.

Ivy se había colocado la cajita blanca sobre el estómago. Sin mirarme, se recostó y siguió comiendo perezosamente un vegetal con los ojos fijos en el techo mientras masticaba. "Originalmente fue idea de mi madre. Ella quería que yo trabajara en la parte administrativa." Comió un poco más. "Se supone que iba a ser un puesto seguro. Pensaba que tenía que mejorar mis relaciones sociales." Se encogió de hombros. "Pero yo quería ser agente."

Me quité las pantuflas y me senté con los pies cruzados. La miré mientras se sacaba los palillos de la boca. Casi todos los que estaban en la alta administración de la S.E. eran muertos vivientes. Siempre pensé que era un trabajo ideal para los que no tienen alma.

"Ella no podía detenerme" continuó Ivy con la mirada fija en el techo, "y para castigarme por hacer lo que yo quería en lugar de lo que ella quería, se aseguró de que Denon fuera mi jefe. Pensó que me fastidiaría tanto que aceptaría el primer cargo administrativo que hubiera. Pero jamás imaginó que daría mi herencia para librarme de mi contrato. Pero ahora ya lo sabe," dijo sarcásticamente.

Dejé a un lado una mazorca en miniatura para comerme un trozo de tomate.

"¿Así que tiraste todo tu dinero porque no te gustaba el jefe? A mi tampoco me gusta pero..."

Ivy se puso tensa. El poder de su mirada me dejó fría. Mi boca enmudeció apenas noté el odio en su expresión. "Denon es un demonio." Las palabras de Ivy helaron todo el cuarto. "Sólo un día más bajo su órdenes y le hubiera rajado el pescuezo."

Dudé un momento antes de hablar. "¿Un demonio?" pregunté confundida. "Pensé que era un vampiro."

"Lo es." Al ver que yo no le respondía se enderezó y puso sus botas en el piso. "Mira" dijo algo molesta. "Habrás notado que Denon no parece un vampiro. Sus dientes son humanos, ¿no es así? No puede arrastrar un aura al mediodía y camina tan fuerte que lo oyes venir a dos kilómetros de distancia."

"No estoy ciega, Ivy."

Acomodó su cajita de cartón blanco y me miró. El aire de la noche que entraba por la ventana era muy fresco para ser final de primavera y me acomodé mejor la bata sobre los hombros.

"A Denon lo mordió un muerto viviente y por eso tiene el virus vampiro" continuó. "Eso le permite hacer un par de trucos y parece muy mono, pero no me cabe duda alguna de que puede ser más temible que el mismo infierno si te dejas intimidar. Pero Denon no pasa de ser el sirviente de alguien, Raquel. Es una marioneta. Siempre lo será."

Puso su cajita blanca en el borde de la mesa que nos separaba y se acomodó en el sillón de manera que pudiera alcanzarla. "Incluso si muere y alguien se toma la molestia de convertirlo en un muerto viviente, siempre será de segunda clase. La próxima vez que lo veas, míralo a los ojos. Verás que tiene miedo. Cada vez que se deja morder de un vampiro para alimentarlo, debe confiar en que lo regresarán como muerto viviente... si en algún momento pierden el control y lo matan por…accidente." Respiró pausadamente. "Tiene de qué tener miedo."

El curry rojo perdió todo el picante. El corazón me latía fuerte pero busqué su mirada y recé que fuera Ivy quien me devolviera la mirada. Sus ojos todavía eran pardos, pero tenían algo; algo del lejano pasado que yo no lograba entender. Mi estómago se puso tenso y de repente me sentí insegura de mí misma. "No le temas a los demonios como Denon" susurró. Yo pensé que esas palabras eran para tranquilizarme, pero sólo lograron templarme la piel hasta que sentí un hormigueo. "Hay cosas más peligrosas."

¿Como tú? pensé para mis adentros. Su repentino aire de depredadora reprimida hizo que sonaran las alarmas en mi cabeza. Pensé levantarme y largarme. Tal vez era mejor meter mi escuálido trasero de bruja en la cocina, donde le correspondía estar. Ivy se volvió a acomodar con la comida en su sillón y yo no quería que se diera cuenta que me ponía los pelos de punta. No es que nunca la hubiera visto con actitud de vampiro. Pero jamás después de la medianoche. En su sala. Solas las dos.

"¿Cosas como tu madre?" dije, con la esperanza de no ir demasiado lejos.

"Cosas como mi madre" respiró. "Por eso estoy viviendo en una iglesia."

Recordé mi pequeño crucifijo, aquél que llevo en mi pulsera junto con mis otros hechizos. Nunca ha dejado de admirarme cómo algo tan pequeño puede detener fuerzas tan poderosas. La cruz no disminuía la actividad de un vampiro vivo, solo la de un vampiro muerto viviente. Pero yo estaba dispuesta a defenderme como fuera.

Ivy colocó los tacones de sus botas al borde de la mesita de centro.

"Mi madre ha sido una muerta viviente desde hace unos diez años, más o menos" dijo, sacándome de mis oscuros pensamientos. "Detesto eso."

Sorprendida, no pude más que preguntarle. "¿Por qué?"

Empujó la comida hacia un lado con gesto de evidente molestia. Su expresión se volvió aterradoramente vacía y no quiso mirarme a los ojos. "Yo tenía dieciocho años cuando mi madre murió" susurró. Su voz era distante, como si no se diera cuenta de que hablaba.

"Algo había perdido, Raquel. Cuando no puedes caminar bajo el sol, pierdes algo tan difuso que ni siquiera sabes qué es. Pero ya lo has perdido. Ella tenía un patrón de conducta del que no podía escapar, pero no sabía por qué. Todavía me ama, pero no se acuerda de por qué me ama. Lo único que le da vida es tomar sangre, y cuando lo hace se vuelve totalmente salvaje. Una vez saciado su deseo, entonces la veo como mi madre... lo que queda de ella. Pero nunca dura. Nunca es suficiente."

Ivy levantó la mirada. "Tú tienes un crucifijo... ¿no es así?"

"Aquí está" repuse con un tono de alegría forzada. No iba a dejar que viera que me estaba poniendo muy nerviosa. No lo permitiría. Alcé la mano dejando caer la manga de la bata hasta el codo mostrando mi pulsera de hechizos.

Ivy puso las botas en el suelo. Yo me tranquilicé al ver que asumía una posición menos provocativa, pero entonces se inclinó sobre la mesita. Su mano cruzó hacia la mía con una velocidad inesperada, tomándome de la muñeca antes de que me percatara que se había movido. Me recorrió un frío a pesar de sentir el calor de sus dedos. Estudió con cuidado el hechizo de metal que llevaba incrustado en la madera mientras yo luchaba contra el impulso de retirar la mano. "¿Está bendecida?" me preguntó.

Pálida, asentí. Ella me soltó retirando la mano con sobrecogedora lentitud. Aun sentía su puño aferrándome con firmeza. No apretaría más, a menos que tratara de soltarme. "La mía también" repuso, sacándola de adentro de la blusa.

Más asombrada todavía, dejé mi cena a un lado y me acerqué. No pude resistir la tentación de tomarla en mis manos. Era como si la plata pidiera que la tocaran. Ivy se inclinó sobre la mesa para que pudiera alcanzarla. Estaba labrada con antiguos augurios y otras bendiciones más tradicionales. Era hermosa y me pregunté cuán antigua sería.

De repente sentí el aliento cálido de Ivy en la mejilla. Me senté un poco más derecha con su crucifijo aun entre mis manos. Sus ojos estaban oscuros y su cara no mostraba sensación alguna. Estaba vacía. Asustada, pasé de mirar sus ojos a mirar el crucifijo. No podía soltarlo así. La golpearía en el pecho. Pero tampoco podía soltarlo lentamente contra su cuerpo.

"Ten," le dije sintiéndome muy incómoda ante su mirada vacía. "Toma."

Ivy estiró la mano y sus dedos rozaron los míos mientras agarraba el viejo metal. Tragué y me acomodé de nuevo en el asiento tapándome las piernas con su bata prestada.

Con lentitud provocadora, Ivy se quitó el crucifijo. La cadena de plata se enredó en su lustroso cabello negro. Lo soltó dejándolo caer hacia atrás. Era una cascada de resplandores. Puso el crucifijo en la mesita delante nuestra y se escuchó el duro sonido del metal golpeando la madera. Se acurrucó en el sillón frente a mí sin pestañear, sentada sobre los pies, y me miró fijamente.

¡Mierda!, pensé con un repentino destello de claridad y pánico. ¡Yo le gustaba! Eso era lo que sucedía. ¿Cómo pude ser tan ciega?

Apreté los dientes mientras que mi cabeza volaba buscando la manera de salirme de esto. Yo era heterosexual. Nunca pensé lo contrario. Me gustaban los hombres más altos que yo, pero no tan fuertes que no pudiera lanzarlos al suelo en caso de una sobrecarga pasional. "Eh…Ivy…," comencé.

"Yo nací vampiro" dijo Ivy suavemente.

Su voz grave recorrió mi médula espinal y me obstruyó la garganta. Casi sin respirar, mis ojos se toparon con el negro de sus ojos. No dije nada temiendo que se moviera. ¡Yo sólo quería que no se moviera! Algo había cambiado, pero no estaba del todo segura de qué estaba sucediendo.

"Mi padre y mi madre son vampiros" dijo. Aun cuando no

se movió, sentí como aumentó la tensión en toda la sala, tanto que ya no escuchaba los grillos. "Fui concebida y nací antes de que mi madre se convirtiera en una muerta viviente. ¿Sabes lo que eso significa... Raquel?" Sus palabras fueron lentas y precisas, salieron de sus labios como un rumor de salmos.

"No," repuse, respirando a duras penas.

Ivy inclinó la cabeza. Su pelo parecía una ola de obsidiana que brillaba con la luz de la sala. Entonces me miró diciendo: "El virus no esperó a que yo muriera para moldearme. Me moldeó a medida que crecí dentro de mi madre. Me dio un poco de dos mundos: el de los vivos y el de los muertos."

Abrió los labios y sus dientes afilados me hicieron estremecer. No quería sudar, pero por mi espalda comenzó a correr el agua. Ivy contuvo la respiración. Creo que eso la hizo reaccionar. "Para mí es fácil arrastrar un aura," me dijo soltando el aire. "En realidad, el truco está en suprimirla."

Se estiró en su asiento. Yo solté el aire por la nariz con un suave silbido y ella trató de sonreír cuando me oyó. Lenta y metódicamente, puso los pies en el suelo. "Y aunque mis reflejos y mis fuerzas no son tan buenos como los de un muerto viviente, al menos son mejores que los tuyos" concluyó.

Yo sabía todo eso, pero ¿por qué me lo estaba diciendo? Mi preocupación se triplicó. Luchando por no mostrar mis nervios, decidí quedarme donde estaba mientras ella se inclinaba hacia adelante con las palmas de las manos sobre la mesa, una a cada lado del crucifijo.

"Más aun, ya es seguro que voy a ser una muerta viviente, así me muera sola en el campo con la sangre en el cuerpo. No tengo de qué preocuparme, Raquel. Ya soy eterna. La muerte sólo me hará más fuerte."

Mi corazón martillaba. No podía quitarle la mirada de los ojos. ¡Maldición! Esto era más de lo que necesitaba.

"Y... ¿sabes lo mejor?" me preguntó.

Agité la cabeza temiendo que mi voz se quebrara. Caminaba en el filo de un cuchillo tratando de conocer su mundo, pero sin penetrar en él.

Sus ojos relucían. Con el torso inmóvil, levantó una rodilla y la puso sobre la mesita...y luego la otra. Dios, ayúdame. ¡Viene por mí!

"Los vampiros vivos pueden deshechizar a la gente...si la gente quiere" susurró. La suavidad de su voz recorrió mi piel hasta erizarla. ¡Doble maldición!

"¿De qué te sirve si sólo funciona con las personas que lo permiten?" pregunté con voz carrasposa comparada con la fluidez de la suya.

Los labios de Ivy se abrieron dejando ver la punta de sus dientes. No podía dejar de mirarla. "Sirve para tener relaciones sexuales maravillosas...Raquel."

"¡Oh!" Fue todo lo que pude decir. Sus ojos se llenaron de lujuria.

"Tengo el gusto de mi madre por la sangre" dijo arrodillándose sobre la mesa que nos separaba. "Es como el ansia por el azúcar que tienen algunas personas. No es la mejor analogía, pero lo que más se le parece....si pruebas."

Ivy exhaló moviendo todo el cuerpo y su respiración reverberó por el mío. Tenía los ojos muy abiertos de asombro y desconcierto, pues sentía deseos. ¿Qué demonios estaba sucediendo? Yo era heterosexual. ¿Por qué de repente quería sentir la suavidad de su cabello?

Solo tenía que estirar la mano. Estábamos a centímetros. Listas, preparadas. En el silencio escuchaba los latidos de mi corazón. Su sonido producía un eco en mis oídos. Entonces observé con horror cómo Ivy retiraba su mirada de mis ojos y miraba mi cuello donde sabía que me latía el pulso.

"¡No!" grité sintiendo pánico.

Pataleé ahogada de susto al sentir todo su peso sobre mí, aprisionándome contra el sillón.

"¡No Ivy!" grité. Tenía que quitármela de encima. Luché por moverme. Tomé una bocanada de aire y la solté en un inútil grito de desamparo. ¡Cómo pude ser tan estúpida! ¡Era un vampiro!

"Quieta Raquel."

Su voz era suave y calmada. Con una mano me tomó del cabello, lanzando mi cabeza hacia atrás para exponer el cuello. Dolía y me escuché gemir a mí misma.

"Estás complicando las cosas" dijo, mientras que yo me movía, jadeando, su mano apretando mi muñeca hasta lastimarme.

"¡Suéltame!" dije ya casi sin aire como si hubiera estado corriendo. "¡Dios, ayúdame! Suéltame Ivy. Por favor. ¡No quiero esto!" le rogué. No pude evitarlo. Estaba aterrada. Había visto fotos. Dolía. Oh Dios, esto sí que iba a doler.

"Quédate quieta" repitió. Su voz era tensa. "Raquel, estoy tratando de soltarte, pero tienes que quedarte quieta. Estás haciendo todo más difícil. Tienes que creerme."

Respiré jadeando y contuve el aire. Moví los ojos tratando de verla. Su boca estaba a milímetros de mi oreja. Tenía los ojos negros, con un apetito que contrastaba con el suave sonido de su voz. Su mirada estaba fija en mi cuello. Sentí una gota cálida de saliva que tocaba mi piel. "¡Oh Dios, no!," susurré.

Ivy se estremeció y su cuerpo temblaba junto al mío. "Quieta Raquel," repitió de nuevo. Esta vez el terror me invadió hasta el pánico. Mi respiración se volvió irregular y muy fuerte. En verdad ella estaba tratando de retirarse, pero según parece, perdía la batalla.

"¿Qué hago?" susurré.

"Cierra los ojos" dijo. "Necesito tu ayuda. No pensé que sería tan difícil."

Sentí la boca seca al escuchar su voz de niña derrotada. Tuve que usar toda mi fuerza de voluntad para cerrar los ojos.

"No te muevas."

Su voz tenebrosa y suave al mismo tiempo. La tensión me golpeaba. Sentí náuseas en el estómago y el pulso que se estrellaba contra mi piel. Tal vez estuve debajo de Ivy un minuto. Todos mis instintos me ordenaban correr. Escuché los grillos y sentí que me corrían las lágrimas mientras que su aliento se acercaba y alejaba de mi cuello.

Al fin lloré cuando sentí que aflojaba su mano de mi cabello. Poco a poco me volvió el aliento a medida que retiraba su peso de mi cuerpo. Ya no sentía su olor. Quedé paralizada, helada. "¿Puedo abrir los ojos?" susurré.

No hubo respuesta.

Me senté y vi que estaba sola. Escuché el sonido lejano de la puerta del santuario que se cerraba y la rápida cadencia de sus tacones en la acera. Después, nada. Entumecida y agitada, me sequé primero las lágrimas y luego la saliva del cuello. Mis ojos escudriñaron la habitación pero no encontraron familiaridad en el ambiente gris. Se había marchado.

Me levanté sin fuerzas y sin saber qué hacer. Me agarré tan fuerte con los brazos que me dolió. Mi mente regresó al terror y, antes de eso, al destello de deseo que me invadió, poderoso y embriagante. Había dicho que solamente podía deshechizar a los que estaban dispuestos. ¿Me mintió, o yo realmente quería que me atrapara contra el sillón y me destrozara?

Siete

El sol ya no entraba por la ventana de la cocina, pero aun hacía calor. Pero no lo suficientemente caliente para llegar al centro de mi alma, aunque agradable. Estaba viva. Aun tenía todas las partes de mi cuerpo. Era una buena tarde.

Estaba sentada en el extremo despejado de la mesa de Ivy, estudiando el libro más destrozado que hallé en el desván. Era lo suficientemente viejo como para haber sido impreso antes de la Guerra Civil. Nunca había oído hablar de algunos de sus hechizos y por eso su lectura me resultaba fascinante. Debo admitir que la posibilidad de probar uno o dos de ellos me despertó una peligrosa excitación. Ninguno hacía referencia al ocultismo, lo cual me alegró sobremanera. Lastimar a la gente con la magia era repugnante y equivocado. El ocultismo iba en contra de mis principios, y el riesgo que representa no valía la pena.

Toda magia tenía su precio, que se paga con la muerte en diferentes niveles de gravedad. Yo era estrictamente una bruja terrestre. Mi fuente era un poder proveniente de las plantas de la tierra que se aceleraba con el calor, la sabiduría y mi herencia de bruja. Puesto que solamente trabajaba con magia blanca, el costo se pagaba con la vida de las plantas. Hasta ahí, estaba bien conmigo. No profundizaba en la moralidad o inmoralidad de matar plantas, de lo contrario me volvería loca cada vez que cortaba el césped de mamá. Esto no significa que no hubiera brujas terrestres de magia negra: las había; pero los que ejercían la magia negra en la Tierra usaban ingredientes inmundos, como por ejemplo pedazos de cuerpos y hacían sacrificios. La sola actividad de recolectar los ingredientes para fabricar un hechizo negro, bastaba para que casi todas las brujas terrestres hicieran magia blanca.

Sin embargo, las brujas de línea ley eran historia aparte. Obtenían su poder directamente de la materia prima, de la fuente cruda, sin el filtro de los seres vivos. Ellas también dependían de la muerte; pero era una muerte más sutil: la lenta muerte del alma. Y no necesariamente la suya. La muerte del alma que necesitaban las brujas de línea ley no era tan severa como la que sostenía a las brujas negras. En lugar de cortar el césped degollaban carneros en el sótano. Pero la creación de un poderoso hechizo diseñado para lastimar o matar, deja una herida profunda en el ser.

Las brujas negras de línea ley evitaban esto desviando el pago hacia otro ser. Generalmente iba adherido al hechizo. Pero si la persona era "pura de espíritu" o más poderosa, el costo—no el hechizo—volvía hacia su creador. Se dice que si uno tiene mucha magia negra en el alma les facilita a los demonios el arrastrarlo a uno involuntariamente hacia el nunca jamás.

Tal como era papá, pensé mientras frotaba mi dedo pulgar en la página que tenía en frente. Yo sabía con absoluta certeza que él fue un brujo blanco hasta el final. Sé que habría podido encontrar el camino hacia la realidad, a pesar de que no vivió para ver el nuevo amanecer.

Un pequeño ruido llamó mi atención. Me puse tensa al ver a Ivy vestida con una bata de seda negra recostada contra el marco de la puerta. El recuerdo de la noche anterior me envolvió formando un nudo en mi estómago. No logré detener la mano que se arrastraba hacia mi cuello, pero sí cambié el movimiento como si me acomodara el arete, simulando estudiar el libro que tenía al frente. "Buenos días," dije con cautela.

"¿Qué hora es?" preguntó Ivy con un susurro ronco.

Le eché una mirada. Su pelo, que normalmente era lacio estaba desarreglado, dejando ver las huellas de los dobleces de su almohada. Tenía sombras oscuras debajo de los ojos y su cara ovalada estaba flácida. La lasitud de la tarde temprana le había aplastado su aire de depredadora al acecho. Sostenía en una mano un librito delgado encuadernado en cuero y no pude menos que pensar si habría pasado la noche en blanco, como yo.

"Son casi las dos," repuse con cautela, empujando con el pie la silla hacia el otro lado de la mesa para que no se sentara junto a mí. Se veía bien, pero yo no sabía cómo tratarla. Llevaba puesto mi crucifijo—que no servía para detenerla— y mi cuchillo de plata en el tobillo—que tampoco servía de mucho más. Un amuleto de sueño la haría caer, pero estaba en mi bolso, en una silla lejos de mi alcance. Me tomaría unos cinco segundos invocar uno. Pero, sinceramente, en ese momento no parecía tan amenazante.

"Hice muffins," dije. "Fue con tus provisiones. Espero que no te moleste."

"Uh," dijo, cruzando el suelo brillante con sus pantuflas negras hasta la cafetera. Se sirvió una taza de café tibio, recostándose luego en el mostrador para beberlo. Su deseo había desaparecido de su cuello. No podía imaginar qué habría deseado. Pensé si tendría que ver con lo sucedido anoche. "Estás vestida," susurró, a la vez que se dejaba caer en la silla que yo acababa de empujar frente a su computadora. "¿A qué hora te despertaste?"

"Mediodía." *Mentirosa,* pensé. Estuve despierta toda la noche fingiendo dormir en el sofá de Ivy. Decidí comenzar el día oficialmente al vestirme. Pasé la página amarillenta ignorándola. "Veo que ya usaste tu deseo," murmuré cuidadosamente. "¿Qué deseaste?"

"Eso no te incumbe," respondió. La advertencia era obvia.

Suspiré lentamente y seguí con la mirada baja. Nos envolvió un incómodo silencio que dejé crecer, resistiéndome a romperlo. Anoche estuve a punto de irme, pero la muerte segura que me acechaba afuera lejos de la protección de Ivy pesaba más que mi posible muerte en manos de Ivy. Tal vez quería saber lo que sentiría si la dejara hundir sus dientes en mi cuello.

Pero *no* quería que mis pensamientos se encaminaran en esa dirección. Ivy me había propinado un susto de mil demonios, pero en la luz brillante de la tarde parecía humana. Inofensiva. ¿Malhumorada?

"Quiero que leas algo," dijo. Alcé la mirada y vi que ponía sobre la mesa que nos separaba el librito que traía en la mano. No había nada escrito en la cubierta, el adorno casi desgastado por completo.

"¿Qué es?" pregunté secamente sin tomarlo.

Bajó la mirada y se lamió los labios. "Siento mucho lo de anoche," dijo. Sentí que mis tripas se tensaron. "Tal vez no me creas, pero yo también estaba asustada."

"No tanto como yo." El haber trabajado con ella durante un año no me había preparado para lo de anoche. Yo sólo conocía su lado profesional y jamás pensé que fuera diferente fuera de la oficina. La miré primero y luego aparté la mirada hacia otro lado. Parecía completamente humana. Buen truco ese.

"Hace tres años que no soy vampiro activo," dijo suavemente. "No estaba preparada...no caí en la cuenta." Me miró con sus ojos pardos suplicantes. "Tienes que creerme Raquel. Yo no quería que eso sucediera. Lo que pasa es que tú me mandabas señales equivocadas. Luego te asustaste y sentiste pánico, y fue peor."

"¿Peor?" repuse, convencida de que la rabia es mejor que el temor. "¡Por poco me atraviesas el cuello!"

"Lo sé," me dijo casi implorando. "Perdóname. Afortunadamente no lo hice."

De nuevo, tuve que luchar contra el estremecimiento al recordar el calor de su saliva goteando en mi cuello.

Acercó más el libro. "Sé que podemos evitar una repetición de lo de anoche. Yo quiero que esto funcione y no hay ninguna razón para que no sea así. Te debo algo por haber tomado uno de tus deseos. Si te vas, no podré protegerte de los vampiros asesinos. No querrás morir en sus manos."

Apreté la mandíbula. No. No quería morir por la mano de un vampiro, mucho menos un vampiro que me pide perdón mientras me asesina.

Encontré su mirada al otro lado de la mesa abarrotada. Se había sentado ahí con su bata y sus pantuflas, tan peligrosa como una esponja. Su necesidad de que le aceptara las disculpas era tan obvia y básica que me pareció dolorosa. Pero no podía. Todavía no. Estiré un dedo para acercar el libro un poco más. "¿Qué es?"

"Eh…hmm…una guía para…parejas," dijo vacilante.

Tomé aire y retiré la mano como si me hubieran aguijoneado.

"No Ivy."

"¡Espera!," repuso. "No es eso lo que quiero decirte. Tú me estás enviando señales contradictorias. Mi mente entiende que no lo haces a propósito, pero mis instintos…" Arrugó la frente. "Es vergonzoso, pero los vampiros, vivos o muertos, se mueven por instintos provocados especialmente por…olores," concluyó casi disculpándose. "Sólo lee la sección de las cosas que excitan ¿sí? ¡y no las hagas!"

Me acomodé de nuevo en mi silla. Lentamente, acerqué el libro. Podía darme cuenta de lo antiguo que era por la encuadernación. Habló de instintos, pero creo que apetito era la palabra adecuada. Tan sólo el hecho de lo difícil que le resultaba admitir que podía ser manipulada por algo tan estúpido como los olores, evitó que le lanzara el libro a la cara. Ivy se enorgullecía de su autocontrol. El que me haya confesado esa debilidad me decía que verdaderamente lo sentía, mucho más que cien disculpas. "Está bien," dije secamente. Ella me respondió con una sonrisa con los labios cerrados.

Tomó un muffin y la edición vespertina del *Enquirer* de Cincinatti que encontré frente a la puerta principal. El ambiente seguía algo tenso, pero al menos era un comienzo. No quería abandonar la seguridad de la iglesia, aun cuando la protección de Ivy era una espada de doble filo. Había reprimido su apetito de sangre por tres años. Si lo quebrantaba, yo estaría muerta.

" 'El concejal Trenton Kalamack acusa a la S.E. de negligencia por la muerte de su secretaria'," leyó, evidentemente buscando cambiar el tema.

"Así es," comenté con cautela. Puse su libro con el montón de libros que tenía para leer después. Sentí que tenía los dedos sucios y los limpié con mis jeans. "Mira lo que logra el dinero. Hay otra noticia que lo declara inocente de traficar con azufre."

No dijo nada, pasando las páginas y mordiendo el muffin hasta encontrar el artículo. "Escucha esto," dijo suavemente. "Dice: 'Me sorprendí al enterarme de la otra vida de la Sra. Bates. Parecía ser la empleada ejemplar. Naturalmente, yo pagaré la educación de su hijo'." Ivy dejó escapar una risa amarga. "Típico." Pasó a las tiras cómicas. "Entonces ¿hoy te dedicarás a tus hechizos artesanales?"

Negué con cabeza. "Hoy voy a la bóveda de los archivos antes de que cierren por el fin de semana. Esto..." golpeé el diario con el dedo, "no sirve para nada. Yo quiero saber qué fue lo que realmente sucedió."

Ivy dejó el muffin y levantó las cejas en señal de asombro.

"Si logro demostrar que Trent está traficando azufre y lo entrego a la S.E., se olvidarán de mi contrato. En este momento tiene en contra una orden de registro" *y así podré largarme de esta iglesia,* concluí para mis adentros.

"¿Demostrar que Trent trafica azufre?" se mofó Ivy. "Ni siquiera se ha podido demostrar si es humano o Entremundos. Su dinero lo hace más resbaloso que babas de sapo en un aguacero. El dinero no compra la inocencia, pero sí compra el silencio." Mordió el muffin. Vestida así de bata y con el pelo desarreglado, se parecía a cualquiera de mis compañeras esporádicas de cuarto de los últimos años. Era desconcertante. Todo era diferente cuando salía el sol.

"Están deliciosos," dijo Ivy agitando un muffin. "Te propongo una cosa: yo compro la comida si tu cocinas. Puedo solucionar mi desayuno y mi almuerzo, pero no me gusta cocinar."

Puse cara de estar de acuerdo—tampoco disfrutaba mucho el arte de cocinar, pero luego me puse a pensar. Me tomaría tiempo, pero me gustaba la idea de no tener que ir a la tienda. Ivy lo decía para que yo no tuviera que arriesgarme la vida por una lata de frijoles, y yo encantada. De todas formas, tenía que cocinar, y es más fácil cocinar para dos que para uno. "Está bien," repuse. "Podemos tratar por un tiempo."

Hizo un sonido suave. "Trato hecho."

Miré mi reloj. Era la una y cuarenta. Mi silla chirrió en el linóleo al levantarme por otro muffin. "Pues bien, ya me voy. Tengo que conseguir un auto, o algo. Esto de andar en autobús es terrible."

Ivy dejó las tiras cómicas encima del revoltijo que había alrededor de su computadora. "La S.E. no te dejará entrar así como así."

"Tiene que dejarme. Los archivos son públicos; y nadie me atrapará con tantos testigos a quienes tendrían que sobornar. Les costaría demasiado," concluí sarcásticamente.

Ivy arqueó las cejas y con ello entendí claramente que no estaba del todo convencida.

"Escucha," le dije mientras agarraba mi bolsa y organizaba mis cosas. "Usaré un hechizo de disfraz y saldré de inmediato a la primera señal de problemas."

Agité un amuleto en el aire que pareció satisfacerla, pero regresando su atención a las tiras cómicas dijo: "Llevarás a Jenks . . . ¿verdad?"

Eso no sonó como una pregunta y le repuse con una mueca. "Sí, claro." Yo sabía que él estaba de niñero, pero tan pronto saqué la cabeza por la puerta trasera y grité llamándolo, pensé que no era mala idea ir acompañada . . . así fuera de un duende.

Ocho

Me apretujé contra la esquina en el asiento del autobús, tratando de asegurarme de que nadie pudiera ver por encima de mis hombros. Estaba repleto y no quería que vieran lo que estaba leyendo: "Si su amante vampiro está saciado y usted no logra estimularlo, intente ponerse algo suyo. No tiene que ponerse demasiado, tal vez algo tan insignificante como un pañuelo o una corbata. El olor de ambos sudores mezclados es algo que ni siquiera los vampiros más controlados pueden resistir."

Muy bien. No volveré a usar la bata ni la pijama de Ivy.

"Muchas veces, el hecho de lavar la ropa junta impregna suficiente aroma. Su amante entenderá que él es importante para usted."

Arreglado. Lavaremos la ropa separada.

"Si su amante vampiro se instala en un lugar más privado en medio de una conversación, tenga por seguro que no la está rechazando. Se trata de una invitación. Déjese llevar. Relájese. Lleve algo de comer o de beber para aflojar la mandíbula y fomentar la salivación. No coquetee. El vino rojo está pasado de moda. Pruebe con una manzana o algo igualmente crujiente."

¡Maldición!

"No todos los vampiros son iguales. Averigüe si a su amante le gusta conversar en la cama. La estimulación erótica tiene muchas formas. Charlar acerca de lazos antiguos y ancestros de sangre pueden dar la nota y sacar a relucir el orgullo, a menos que su amante provenga de una línea de segunda."

¡Doble maldición! Me comporté como una ramera. ¡Una maldita perra vampira!

Cerré los ojos y recosté la cabeza contra el espaldar del asiento. Sentí un leve calorcillo en el cuello y salté, volteando a mirar. Mi mano golpeó la palma de la mano de un hombre atractivo. Él rió al sentir el sonido sordo del golpe y alzó las dos manos conciliatoriamente; pero lo que me hizo detener fue el asombro que reflejaban sus ojos.

"¿Ha leído la página cuarenta y nueve?," me preguntó al tiempo que descansó sus brazos en el espaldar de mi asiento.

Lo miré con indiferencia, pero su sonrisa era aun más seductora. Era demasiado atractivo y la suavidad de sus rasgos dejaba entrever un entusiasmo casi infantil. Su mirada fue directa al librito que sostenía en mis manos. "Cuarenta y nueve," repitió, su voz un poco más baja. "Nunca volverá a ser la misma."

Pasé hasta esa página nerviosamente. ¡Oh, Dios mío! El libro de Ivy era ilustrado; pero entonces dudé, y me arrinconé confusa. ¿Eran tres personas? ¿Y qué diablos era aquello atornillado a la pared?

"Míralo así," dijo, estirando el brazo por encima del asiento y haciendo girar el libro en mis manos. Su colonia tenía un nítido olor a bosque. Era tan agradable como su voz tranquila y su mano que intencionalmente me rozaba con suavidad. Era el clásico vampiro lacayo: bien fornido, vestido de negro y con una necesidad innata de ser querido. Y ni hablar de su falta de respeto por el espacio personal.

Le quité la mirada cuando tocó el libro. "Oh," dije, tan pronto entendí; y acto seguido exclamé "¡oh!," cerrando el libro. Eran dos personas…tres, contando a la otra que portaba esa cosa…lo que fuera eso.

Alcé los ojos buscando los suyos. "¿Y usted sobrevivió a eso?," pregunté, sin saber si debería estar consternada, horrorizada o impresionada.

Su mirada se tornó casi reverente. "Sí. No pude mover las piernas durante dos semanas, pero valió la pena."

El corazón me latía apresuradamente y metí rápidamente el libro en mi bolso. Se levantó con una sonrisa y avanzó tranquilamente para descender. No pude dejar de notar que cojeaba. Me sorprendía que pudiera caminar. Me miró sin retirar sus ojos profundos al bajar por la escalerilla.

Tragué fuerte y miré para otro lado. Pero la curiosidad no me abandonó y antes que de las últimas personas hubieran descendido del autobús, saqué de nuevo el libro de Ivy. Mis manos estaban frías. No miré la ilustración. Leí lo escrito en letra pequeña bajo las instrucciones de "Cómo hacerlo." Mi expresión se heló y sentí un nudo en el estómago.

Era una advertencia para no permitir que su amante vampiro la obligue a hacerlo sin antes haber sido mordida tres veces; de lo contrario podría no tener suficiente saliva de vampiro en el sistema para sobrecargar los receptores de dolor, haciéndole creer a su cerebro que el dolor es placer. También había instrucciones sobre cómo evitar perder el conocimiento si no se tenía suficiente saliva de vampiro y se hallaba agonizando de dolor. Aparentemente, si la presión sanguínea descendía también disminuía el placer de su amante vampiro. Pero ni una palabra sobre cómo detenerse.

Cerré los ojos y mi cabeza daba golpecillos contra el vidrio. El cuchicheo de los demás pasajeros me hizo abrir los ojos, dirigiendo la mirada hacia la acera. Ahí estaba ese hombre parado mirándome. Me sujeté fuertemente con un brazo, temblando. Sonreía como si nunca le hubieran rajado cuidadosamente la entrepierna y chupado la sangre, consumiéndola como en comunión. Lo había disfrutado, o al menos eso era lo que él creía.

Alzó tres dedos, haciendo el saludo de los Boy Scouts, se los llevó hasta los labios y luego me mandó un beso. El autobús se sacudió al arrancar de nuevo y él se fue caminando, con el dobladillo de su saco colgando.

Miré por la ventana y sentí náusea. ¿Habría participado Ivy alguna vez de algo así? A lo mejor había matado accidentalmente a alguien. Tal vez por eso ya no era activa. Debería preguntarle. O, tal vez debería mantener la boca cerrada para poder dormir de noche.

Cerré el libro y lo puse en el fondo de mi bolso, pero encontré una hoja de papel en medio de las páginas con un número telefónico. Lo arrugué y lo metí en el bolso junto con el libro. Cuando alcé la cabeza vi que Jenks venía zumbando hacia mí. Había estado hablando con el chofer.

Aterrizó en el espaldar del asiento delante del mío. Aparte de una correa color rojo chillón, vestía de negro de la cabeza a los pies: su atuendo de trabajo. "Los pasajeros recientes no tienen hechizos contra ti," dijo alegremente. "¿Qué quería ese tipo?"

"Nada." Saqué de mi mente el recuerdo de esa imagen. ¿Dónde estaba Jenks anoche cuando Ivy me tenía atrapada? Eso es lo que yo quería saber. Se lo habría preguntado, pero temía que me contestara que todo había sido por culpa mía.

"Es en serio," insistió Jenks. "¿Qué quería?"

Lo miré fijamente. "Nada, en serio. Nada. Ya olvídalo," repuse, agradecida de tener mi hechizo de disfraz. *No* quería que el Sr. Página Cuarenta y Nueve me reconociera en la calle un día de estos.

"Está bien, está bien," dijo, volando como un dardo hacia mi arete. Estaba cantando "Strangers in the Night." Suspiré, pues sabía que la llevaría prendida en la mente todo el día. Saqué mi espejo de mano pretendiendo arreglarme el cabello, asegurándome de golpear por lo menos dos veces el arete donde estaba sentado Jenks.

Me había convertido en una morena de nariz grande. Tenía el cabello asegurado con una hebilla en una trenza. Aun era largo y crespo. Algunas cosas son más difíciles de hechizar que otras. Llevaba volteada mi chaqueta de jeans con estampado de flores y tenía puesta una gorra de cuero de Harley-Davidson. Se la devolvería a Ivy disculpándome tan pronto la viera y no volvería a usarla. Después de todos los errores que cometí anoche, no quisiera que Ivy perdiera de nuevo el control.

El autobús pasó bajo las sombras de los grandes edificios. La próxima parada era la mía, así que tomé mis cosas y me levanté. "Tengo que encontrar algún medio de transporte," le dije a Jenks tan pronto aterricé en la acera. Exploré la calle. "Tal vez una moto," rezongué, calculando el tiempo necesario para no tocar las puertas de vidrio del edificio de archivos de la S.E.

De mi arete llegó un gruñido. "Yo no haría eso," advirtió. "Una moto es muy fácil de alterar. Yo seguiría usando el transporte público."

"Podría estacionarla adentro," protesté, observando nerviosamente a las pocas personas que había en el vestíbulo.

"Entonces, no podrías conducirla, Sherlock," dijo con su acostumbrado sarcasmo. Llevas una bota desamarrada."

Miré y no era cierto. "Muy gracioso Jenks."

El duende murmuró algo que no pude entender. "No," dijo impacientemente. "Quise decir que hagas como que vas a amarrar tu bota mientras me aseguro que estarás segura."

"Ah." Obedecí. Fui hasta una silla en una esquina y amarré de nuevo mis botas. Casi no podía verlo mientras volaba encima de varios agentes, detectando con su olfato los hechizos lanzados contra mí. La sincronización había sido precisa. Era sábado y abrían la bóveda por cortesía, apenas durante unas horas. Pero aun así había gente buscando información, poniendo archivos al día, fotocopiando o tratando de dar una buena impresión por trabajar el fin de semana.

"Huele bien," dijo Jenks al regresar. "No creo que pensaran que vendrías aquí."

"Bien." Con más confianza de la que merecía, me dirigí al mostrador de la recepción. Tenía suerte. Lo atendía Megan. Le sonreí y abrió los ojos asombrada. Rápidamente trató de ajustarse los lentes. El marco de madera estaba hechizado para ver a través de casi todo. Equipo estándar de las recepcionistas de la S.E. Hubo un movimiento agitado delante de mí y me detuve bruscamente.

"¡Atención mujer!," gritó Jenks, pero era demasiado tarde. Alguien me rozó. Logré mantener el equilibrio instintivamente cuando un pie se deslizó entre mis piernas para hacerme caer. Aterrada, giré para terminar de cuclillas. El miedo me invadió mientras aterrizaba en posición de defensa.

Era Francis. *¿Qué diantre hacía aquí?* pensé, levantándome para verlo agarrarse el estómago de la risa con las manos. Debí deshacerme de mi bolso. No esperé encontrarme con alguien que pudiera reconocerme bajo mi hechizo de disfraz.

"Bonita gorra, Raquel," dijo Francis casi aullando, subiéndose el cuello de su brillante camisa. Hablaba con un desagradable tono de bravucón, perdiendo el temor por el ataque que estuve a punto de lanzarle. "Escucha, compré cuatro suertes de la lotería ayer. ¿Habrá alguna esperanza de que te mueras mañana, entre las siete y la medianoche?"

"Por qué no me atrapas tú mismo," le dije con desdén. O bien no tenía orgullo o no se daba cuenta de lo ridículo que se veía ahí parado con una de sus botas desamarradas y su horrible cabello perdiendo ya el hechizo de ondulación. ¿Y cómo tenía esa barba a estas tempranas horas del día? Debió pintársela con un atomizador.

"Si te atrapara yo mismo saldría perdiendo." Francis adoptó su aire usual de superioridad. "No tengo tiempo de hablar con una bruja muerta," dijo. "Tengo una cita con el concejal Trenton Kalamack y necesito investigar unos asuntos. ¿Entiendes? Investigaciones. ¿Alguna vez lo has hecho ...investigar?" Aspiró por su nariz aguileña. "No que yo sepa."

"Vete a rellenar tomates, Francis," le dije suavemente.

Le echó un vistazo al pasillo que conducía hacia la bóveda. "Oh," dijo arrastrando las palabras. "Qué miedo. Es mejor que te vayas ya si quieres llegar con vida a tu iglesia. Si Meg no hizo sonar la alarma, yo lo haré."

"Deja la palabrería. Estás empezando a hartarme."

"Nos vemos luego, Ra-quel-mi-Ra-quel…en un obituario." Su risa fue demasiado alta.

Le eché una mirada fulminante y firmó el libro de entrada que estaba frente a Megan con elegancia exagerada. Se volteó y dijo: "Corre, bruja, corre." Sacó su teléfono celular y oprimió algunos botones mientras pasaba frente a las oficinas oscuras de los funcionarios de mayor jerarquía. Megan me hizo un gesto de disculpa a la vez que oprimía el botón de acceso de la puerta.

Cerré los ojos durante unos segundos. Tan pronto los abrí le hice una señal a Megan diciéndole "espera un minuto," y me senté en una de las sillas del vestíbulo, hurgando en mi bolso como buscando algo. Jenks aterrizó en mi arete. "Vámonos," dijo preocupado. "Regresaremos esta noche."

"Está bien." El embrujamiento que ordenó Denon de mi apartamento era puro acoso, pero contratar a una pandilla de asesinos era demasiado costoso. Yo no valía la pena. Pero, ¿para qué arriesgarse?

"Jenks," susurré, "¿puedes entrar a la bóveda sin que te detecten las cámaras?"

"Naturalmente mujer. Jugar a las escondidas es lo que mejor sabemos hacer nosotros los duendes. ¿Que si puedo burlar las cámaras? ¿Quién crees que les da mantenimiento? Te lo diré: los duendes. ¿Y alguien les reconoce algo? No-o-o-o-o. Sólo se lo reconocen al técnico grandulón que está ahí sentado debajo de las escaleras; el que maneja el camión, abre la caja de herramientas y se come todas las rosquillas. ¿Pero qué si hace algo? No-o-o-o-o."

"Excelente Jenks. Cállate y escucha." Miré a Megan. "Anda a ver los documentos que estudia Francis. Yo esperaré todo lo que pueda, pero si hay señas de peligro, me largo. Puedes llegar a casa desde aquí, ¿verdad?"

Jenks aleteó, produciéndome cosquillas en el cuello con

un mechón de mi cabello. "Sí, puedo hacerlo. Y si quieres podría echarle algún hechizo por tí, ya que estaré adentro."

Levanté las cejas. "¿Hechizarlo? ¿Puedes hacerlo? Yo pensé que eran...eh...cuentos de hadas."

Se detuvo en el aire frente a mí con cara de suficiencia. "Le mandaré la rasquiña. Es la segunda cosa que mejor saben hacer los duendes." Dudó haciendo una mueca. "No... es más bien la tercera."

"¿Por qué no?" dije suspirando. Jenks se alzó para estudiar las cámaras. Las observó unos instantes para medir el tiempo de sus movimientos. Luego se elevó hasta el techo, cruzó el pasillo, pasó las oficinas y entró por la puerta de la bóveda. Si no lo hubiera estado observando, jamás lo habría visto entrar.

Saqué un lapicero, cerré el bolso y me dirigí hacia Megan. El gigantesco mostrador de caoba separaba completamente el vestíbulo de las oscuras oficinas del fondo. Era el último bastión entre el público y el meticuloso personal que conservaba los archivos en orden. Se escuchó una voz de mujer que reía del otro lado del pasillo abovedado. La gente no trabajaba mucho los sábados. "Hola Meg," le dije acercándome.

"Buenas tardes Srta. Morgan," dijo demasiado fuerte mientras se acomodaba los lentes. *¿Srta. Morgan?* pensé. *¿Desde cuándo soy señorita Morgan?* "¿Qué hay Meg?," dije, mirando el vestíbulo vacío a mis espaldas.

Me respondió con total seriedad. "Gracias a Dios que sigues con vida," susurró entre dientes y sonriendo. "¿Qué haces aquí? ¡Deberías estar oculta en un sótano!" Antes de que pudiera responder, agitó la cabeza en señal de colaboración, sonriendo. "¿Qué puedo hacer por tí, Srta. Morgan?"

Puse una cara burlona y Megan dirigió una mirada muy elocuente por encima de mi hombro. Su cara se puso un poco tensa. "La cámara, idiota," murmuró. "La cámara."

Suspiré en señal de haber entendido. Me preocupaba más el celular de Francis, pues nadie revisaba las grabaciones a menos que sucediera algo. Pero ya para entonces era demasiado tarde.

"Todos estamos luchando por ti," susurró Megan. "Las probabilidades son de doscientos contra uno a que logras sobrevivir la primera semana. Personalmente, te doy cien a uno."

Me sentí enferma. Su mirada se fijó de nuevo por encima de mí y otra vez se puso tensa. "Hay alguien detrás de mí, ¿no es así?," pregunté y ella hizo un gesto. Suspiré. Acomodé mi bolso contra mi espalda para poder quitarlo del camino antes de darme vuelta muy lentamente.

Vestía un elegante traje negro, camisa blanca almidonada y corbata negra muy angosta. Llevaba los brazos cruzados a sus espaldas y no se quitó los lentes oscuros. Percibí un leve olor a almizcle que junto con su suave barba roja me hizo pensar que se trataba de un hombre zorro.

Se le unió otro hombre parado entre la puerta principal y yo. Tampoco se quitó los lentes oscuros. Los miré para calcular su estatura. Tenía que haber un tercer hombre en alguna parte, a lo mejor a mis espaldas. Los asesinos siempre trabajan en trío. *Ni uno más, ni uno menos. Siempre tres,* pensé con el estómago tenso. Tres contra uno. No era justo. Miré al fondo del pasillo. "Nos vemos en casa Jenks," susurré, sabiendo que no podía oírme.

Las dos sombras se pusieron firmes. Uno desabrochó su chaqueta exhibiendo una cartuchera. Alcé las cejas. No irían a acribillarme a sangre fría delante de un testigo. Denon estaba molesto, pero no era un estúpido. Estaban esperando a que yo saliera corriendo.

Me paré con las manos en los muslos y las piernas abiertas para equilibrarme. "No creo que podamos dialogar, ¿no es cierto muchachos?," dije ásperamente sintiendo los latidos de mi corazón.

El que se había desabrochado su chaqueta sonrió socarronamente. Sus dientes eran pequeños y afilados y una capa de fino pelo rojo le cubría el dorso de la mano. Sí señor. Un hombre zorro. Grandioso. Tenía mi cuchillo, pero trataría de mantener la distancia para no tener que usarlo.

A mis espaldas se escuchó el grito airado de Meg. "Ah, no en mi vestíbulo, no. Este lío se lo llevan para afuera."

Mi pulso aceleró. ¿Será que Meg me estaba ayudando? *Tal vez*—pensé, saltando por encima del mostrador—*no quiere manchas en su alfombra*.

"Allá," dijo Megan apuntando hacia los arcos que conducían a las oficinas de atrás.

No había tiempo para dar las gracias. Entré disparada como un dardo por la puerta hallándome en un gran salón de oficinas. Detrás escuché golpes secos y maldiciones. El recinto del tamaño de una bodega tenía espacios de oficina formados por paneles divisorios de un metro con veinte. ¡Un laberinto de proporciones bíblicas!

Sonreí y agité la mano saludando a los asombrados ocupantes mientras mi bolso golpeaba los paneles al pasar. Tropecé volteando un botellón de agua, ofreciendo falsas disculpas a mi paso. No se rompió, pero sí se abrió. El sonido del borboteo del agua pronto fue superado por el clamor de los presentes pidiendo un trapeador.

Eché un vistazo hacia atrás y vi a una de las sombras enredado con tres oficinistas que trataban de colocar el botellón de nuevo. El arma la llevaba escondida. Hasta ahora todo marchaba bien. Ví la puerta trasera. Corrí hacia la pared del fondo y empujé la puerta de emergencia saboreando el aire fresco.

Alguien estaba aguardando y me apuntaba con un arma de gran calibre.

"¡Mierda!," exclamé retrocediendo. Cerré la puerta otra vez, pero antes de que cerrara del todo, algo húmedo la golpeó dejando una mancha gelatinosa. Sentí que me ardía el cuello. Me toqué con las manos y sentí una ampolla del tamaño de una moneda de medio dólar. Mis dedos ardieron al tocarla.

"Maravilloso," musité, quitándome esa cosa pegajosa de la chaqueta. "Ahora no tengo tiempo para esto." Activé el mecanismo de emergencia de una patada y me dirigí de nuevo hacia donde estaba la acción. Ya no usaban hechizos de acción retardada sino que los preparaban y los metían en estos pegotes. Vaya idea. Pensé que se trataba de un hechizo incendiario instantáneo. Si me hubiera pegado de lleno ya estaría muerta, convertida en un montoncito de ceniza sobre la alfombra. Jenks jamás habría podido oler esto, así hubiera estado a mi lado.

Yo personalmente, preferiría morir con una bala. Al menos era algo más romántico. Pero claro, es más difícil descubrir al fabricante de un hechizo fatal que al fabricante de una bala convencional de pistola. Además, un buen hechizo no deja rastros. Un hechizo incendiario instantáneo no deja casi ningún rastro. Sin rastro, no hay crimen, no hay condena.

"¡Ahí está!" gritó alguien. Me metí debajo de un escritorio golpeándome un codo. Sentía que mi cuello ardía. Tenía que ponerle sal para neutralizar el hechizo antes de que se extendiera.

Mi corazón parecía estallar. Me quité la chaqueta cubierta de salpicaduras de esa cosa pegajosa. Sin ella tal vez estaría muerta. La metí en el cesto de la basura que había allí.

La gente pedía traperos. Entre tanto, busqué una ampolla de agua salada en mi bolso. Mis dedos me ardían y el dolor en el cuello me estaba torturando. Con las manos temblorosas, mordí la tapa de goma del frasco. Contuve la respiración y lo vacié sobre mis manos y luego en el cuello. Respiré con alivio al sentir el repentino ardor y el tufillo de azufre que siempre sale cuando se rompe un hechizo negro. El agua salada goteaba en el suelo. Por un instante disfruté la gloriosa sensación del dolor que desaparece.

Temblando, me froté el cuello con la manga de la blusa. Me dolía la ampolla que tenía debajo de los dedos, pero los latidos que me producía el agua salada eran tranquilizantes en comparación con el ardor. Me quedé sentada como una idiota tratando de encontrar una manera de salir de ahí. Yo era una bruja buena y por eso todos mis hechizos eran defensivos, no de ataque. Mi técnica era dar palizas y dejar al enemigo trastornado para luego atraparlo. Siempre había sido la cazadora, pero nunca la presa. Fruncí el ceño al darme cuenta que no tenía nada para salir de esto.

El escándalo de Megan me ayudó para enterarme de dónde estaban todos. Toqué la ampolla de nuevo. Había dejado de crecer. Tuve suerte. Mi respiración se detuvo cuando sentí pasos silenciosos a unos cuantos cubículos de donde yo estaba. No quería sudar demasiado pues los hombres zorros tienen un gran olfato pero sólo tienen una idea en la cabeza. El olor a azufre seguramente les impedía encontrarme. No podía quedarme aquí. Un golpe seco en la puerta trasera me decía que era hora de largarme.

Al asomarme cautelosamente por encima de los paneles, sentía que la tensión me haría estallar la cabeza. Vi que la sombra número uno removía algunas cosas para dejar entrar a la sombra número tres. Tomé aire y avancé agachada en la dirección opuesta. Podría apostar mi vida a que los asesinos habían dejado a la otra sombra parada en la puerta principal, de manera que no me toparía con el tipo antes de llegar a ella.

Gracias a la constante gritería de Megan por el agua en el suelo, logré avanzar hasta el pasadizo abovedado sin toparme con nadie. Miré a mi alrededor para cerciorarme de que no hubiera nadie en el mostrador de la recepción. Había papeles tirados por todas partes. Los lápices se habían caído y el teclado de Megan colgaba del cable oscilando. Casi sin respiración me dirigí hacia la entrada del mostrador, la tabla que sube y se vuelve a bajar. Aún acurrucada, eché un vistazo hacia la puerta principal.

Ahí había una sombra, inquieta, un tanto hosca porque no la habían dejado entrar en acción. La probabilidad de escaparmele a uno era mayor que la de escaparmele a dos.

De la bóveda llegó la voz quejumbrosa de Francis. "¿Aquí? ¿Denon los mandó aquí contra ella? Debe estar cabreado. Esto hay que verlo. Será para reír."

Su voz se aproximaba cada vez más. *Tal vez Francis*

quiera venir de paseo conmigo, pensé. Las esperanzas me regresaron y dejé de temblar. Una cosa era cierta: Francis era curioso y estúpido, una combinación peligrosa en nuestra profesión. Aguardé con la adrenalina corriendo por mis venas, hasta que levantó la tabla y entró detrás del mostrador.

"Qué desorden" dijo, más concentrado en el reguero en el piso que en mi presencia. No vio que me acercaba. Estaba muy ocupado rascándose. Como un mecanismo de relojería, le pasé un brazo por la nuca y le doblé uno de los suyos detrás de la espalda, casi levantándolo del suelo.

"¡Ay! ¡Demonios, Raquel!," gritó, demasiado imbécil para saber lo fácil que sería codearme en el estómago para soltarse. "¡Suéltame! ¡Esto no es chistoso!"

Tragué saliva y dirigí la mirada hacia la sombra en la puerta, su arma presta y apuntando. "No, no lo es lindura," le dije respirándole en el oído y pensando lo cerca que estábamos de la muerte. Francis ni siquiera se daba cuenta pero la idea de que hiciera algo estúpido me asustaba más que la pistola. Mi corazón se estrellaba en mi pecho y sentí que se me aflojaban las rodillas. "¡Quédate quieto!," le dije. "Si él cree que puede dispararme, lo hará."

"¿Y a mí qué me importa?," gruñó.

"¿Ves alguien más aquí, además de tú, yo y la pistola?" dije suavemente. "Sería muy fácil deshacerse de un testigo, ¿no crees?"

Francis se quedó quieto. Escuché un ruido cuando Megan entró por la puerta de las oficinas del fondo. Había más gente que miraba por encima de su hombro, hablando alto. Eché un vistazo y sentí pánico. Demasiada gente. Demasiadas probabilidades de que algo saliera mal.

Me tranquilicé un poco cuando la sombra se levantó de su posición de cuclillas y guardó la pistola. Colocó los brazos a los lados pretendiendo estar conforme. Atraparme delante de tantos testigos le saldría caro. Estábamos mano a mano.

Mantuve a Francis delante de mí. Era mi escudo. Entonces se escuchó un murmullo cuando las otras dos sombras salieron como fantasmas de la zona de las oficinas. Tenían las espaldas contra la pared de la oficina de Megan. Uno desenfundó el arma pero al entender la situación la guardó en la cartuchera.

"Muy bien Francis," dije. "Es hora de tu paseo de la tarde. Lento, despacio."

"Vete al diablo, Raquel," repuso con voz temblorosa y sudando copiosamente.

Caminamos pegados al borde del mostrador. Tuve que luchar para que Francis caminara erguido pues se resbalaba al pisar los estilógrafos en el suelo. El hombro zorro parado junto a la puerta se retiró amablemente del camino. Con su actitud lo dijo todo. No tenían apuro. Tenían tiempo. Bajo sus ojos vigilantes, Francis y yo salimos de espaldas por la puerta hacia la libertad.

"¡Suéltame!," dijo Francis forcejeando. Los peatones nos observaban atónitos y los autos disminuían la velocidad para mirar. Detesto a los mirones, pero a lo mejor podía usarlos a mi favor. "Vamos, corre," dijo Francis. "Es lo que mejor sabes hacer Raquel."

Lo apreté más hasta oírlo lamentarse. "Tienes razón. Cuando tengo que correr para atrapar a alguien, lo hago mejor que cualquiera. Tú jamás podrás igualarme." Los curiosos comenzaron a alejarse al darse cuenta que esto era más que una pelea entre amantes. "Tal vez tú también quieras empezar a correr," agregué, esperando confundirlo aún más.

"¿De qué demonios estás hablando?" El olor a sudor ocultaba su colonia.

Arrastré a Francis hacia el otro lado de la calle, haciendo zigzag en medio de los autos que se detenían. Las tres sombras estaban afuera observándonos. Estaban parados, tensos, metidos en sus trajes negros y ocultándose tras sus lentes oscuros. "Imagino que estarán pensando que me ayudas. Qué más van a pensar. ¿Un brujo grande y fuerte como tú incapaz de zafarse de una niña menuda y frágil como yo?"

Sentí que respiraba profundo indicando que había entendido. "Buen chico," dije. "Ahora, ¡corre!"

Con el tráfico que me separaba de las sombras, solté a Francis y corrí para desaparecer entre la multitud. Francis corrió en sentido contrario. Yo sabía que no me seguirían hasta la casa si lograba sacarles una buena ventaja. Los zorros son supersticiosos y jamás violarían mi refugio en camposanto. Por ahora estaría a salvo, hasta que Denon decidiera enviar alguna otra cosa a buscarme.

Nueve

"**O**tra cosa," cavilé, pasando la delicada y descolorida página que olía a éter y gardenias. Un hechizo para pasar inadvertida sería lo mejor, pero necesitaba semillas de helecho. No solamente no había tiempo para recolectarlas, sino que no era la estación. Las vendían en el mercado de Findlay, pero no tenía suficiente tiempo. "Aterriza Raquel." Cerré el libro y estiré la espalda sintiendo dolor. "No puedes preparar una poción tan complicada."

Ivy estaba del otro lado, en la mesa de la cocina, completando los formularios del cambio de dirección y mordisqueando su último tallo de apio con salsa. Esa era toda la cena que tuve tiempo de preparar, pero a ella no pareció importarle. A lo mejor pensaba salir más tarde y comer alguna cosa. Si lograba conservarme con vida hasta mañana, prepararía una cena de verdad. Tal vez pizza. Pero esta noche la cocina no era apta para preparar alimentos.

Estaba haciendo hechizos y todo estaba en completo desorden. Había plantas a medio triturar, tierra, cuencos manchados de verde con restos cernidos enfriándose y pailas de cobre sucias arrumadas en el fregadero. Parecía la cocina de estudiantes de primer año de universidad. Había preparado amuletos para identificación, pociones para provocar sueño, e inclusive unos hechizos de disfraz para verme más vieja en lugar de joven. No pude evitar sentir cierta satisfacción por el hecho de haberlos preparado yo misma. Tan pronto hallé un hechizo lo suficientemente fuerte para permitirme entrar a la bóveda de archivos de la S.E., Jenks y yo salimos de inmediato.

Esa tarde, Jenks venía acompañado de un hombre greñudo como un lobo. Era su amigo, el que tenía mis cosas. Le compré un catre que olía a viejo y le di las gracias por traer las pocas prendas que no estaban hechizadas: mi abrigo de invierno y un conjunto deportivo para el entrenamiento que estaban metidos en una caja en el fondo del armario. Le dije que no se preocupara de nada más por ahora, sólo de mi música, mi ropa y mis utensilios de cocina. Se fue con cien dólares en la mano prometiendo traerme mañana la ropa, por lo menos.

Con un suspiro, levanté los ojos del libro y pasé la mirada por Don Pez que descansaba en la repisa de la ventana. De ahí, dirigí los ojos al jardín oscuro. Me toqué la ampolla del cuello con la mano y puse a un lado el libro haciendo espacio para otro. Denon debía estar realmente molesto para enviar a esos zorros contra mí en plena luz del día, pues me daba algo de ventaja. De haberlo hecho de noche, ahora estaría muerta—con luna nueva o sin ella. El hecho de que estaba gastando tanto dinero decía mucho de lo que le dolió perder a Ivy.

Luego de deshacerme de los Zorros tomé un taxi de regreso a casa. Me dije que lo hacía para evitar a algún posible asesino en el autobús, pero la verdad es que lo hice para que nadie se diera cuenta de que temblaba. Comencé a sentir escalofríos tres cuadras después de haber subido y no pararon hasta que terminé con toda el agua caliente de la ducha. Nunca había estado en la posición de presa y no me gustaba. Pero lo que más me asustaba era la posibilidad de tener que usar un hechizo negro para seguir con vida.

Buena parte de mi trabajo había consistido en atrapar fabricantes de "hechizos grises"—brujas que convertían un hechizo bueno, por ejemplo un hechizo de amor, en un hechizo malo. Claro que también había atrapado a unos cuantos brujos peligrosos de magia negra, aquellos que se especializan en las formas más ocultas de hacer el mal, como por ejemplo, hacerlo desaparecer a uno y, luego, por unos cuantos dólares más, hechizar a la familia para que se olviden de su existencia. Un puñado de Entremundos manejaban el poder del ocultismo ilegal. A veces lo único que podía hacer era tapar la sucia realidad para que los humanos no se dieran cuenta de lo difícil que era controlar a los Entremundos, quienes veían a la humanidad como un hato de vacas. Pero jamás había sido perseguida de esta forma. No sabía cómo hacer para mantenerme a salvo y al mismo tiempo conservar mi karma limpio.

Había pasado las últimas horas del día en el jardín. El hecho de jugar en la tierra con niños duendes husmeando todo el tiempo a mi alrededor, era una buena forma de calmarme, y me di cuenta que le estaba muy agradecida a Jenks. En realidad, no me di cuenta hasta que volví a entrar a la casa con mis materiales para preparar hechizos del motivo de la gritería y movimiento de los niños: no estaban jugando a las escondidas sino interceptando proyectiles gelatinosos.

Quedé aterrada al ver la pirámide de proyectiles que habían formado junto a la puerta de atrás. Cada uno portaba mi sentencia de muerte y yo ni me había dado cuenta. Cuando los vi ahí amontonadas se me encendió no el temor sino la rabia. ¡Juré estar preparada la próxima vez que los cazadores me encontraran!

Luego del torbellino de la preparación de hechizos, mi bolso estaba repleto con lo usual. La astilla de secoya que traje de la oficina fue mi salvavidas. Los hechizos se pueden guardar en cualquier madera, pero en la secoya duran más. Los amuletos que no estaban en mi bolso colgaban de los ganchos para las tazas en el aparador vacío de la cocina. Todos eran buenos hechizos, pero necesitaba algo más poderoso. En medio de suspiros abrí el siguiente libro.

"¿Transmutación?" dijo Ivy dejando los formularios a un lado y acercando el teclado. "¿Así de buena eres?"

Me saqué la tierra de una uña con la uña del pulgar. "La

necesidad es la madre del valor," musité. Examiné el índice sin dirigirle la mirada a Ivy. Necesitaba algo pequeño, preferiblemente algo que pudiera defenderse a sí mismo.

Ivy continuó con su búsqueda en la pantalla mientras comía apio. Yo la venía observando cuidadosamente desde la puesta del sol. Era la compañera perfecta. Se le notaba el esfuerzo por mantener al mínimo sus reacciones normales de vampiro. Tal vez sirvió el hecho de volver a lavar mi ropa. Tan pronto viera que se estaba poniendo seductora le pediría que se fuera.

"Aquí hay uno," dije en voz baja. "Un gato. Necesito una onza de romero, media taza de menta, una cucharadita de extracto de algodoncillo recolectado después de la primera helada... bueno, pues ya está, esta receta tengo que descartarla. No tengo extracto y ahora no puedo ir a la tienda."

Ivy pareció contener la risa y yo volví al índice. ¿Un murciélago? No. No tenía árbol cenizoso en el jardín y se necesitaba parte de la corteza interna. Además, no pensaba pasarme el resto de la noche aprendiendo a volar por radar. Lo mismo con las aves. La mayoría de las que aparecían en el libro no vuelan de noche. ¿Un pez? Absurdo... pero a lo mejor...

"Un ratón," dije buscando la página y revisando la lista de ingredientes. Nada exótico. Ya tenía casi todo lo necesario en la cocina. Había una nota escrita a mano en el margen de abajo y entrecerré los ojos para poder leer la borrosa letra masculina: *puede adaptarse con seguridad a cualquier roedor.* Miré la hora. Funcionaría.

"¿Un ratón?" preguntó Ivy. "¿Vas a hacer un hechizo para convertirte en ratón?"

Me levanté dirigiéndome hacia la mesa de acero inoxidable en medio de la cocina y abrí el libro. "Seguro. Tengo todo menos el pelo del ratón." Subí las cejas. "¿Puedo tomar una bolita de tu búho? Necesito cernir la leche con un pelaje."

Ivy dejó caer su pelo negro sobre el hombro. "Claro. Te traeré una." Meneó la cabeza y cerró el sitio que estaba visitando. Se levantó estirándose de tal modo que dejaba ver su estómago al descubierto. Ví la joya roja que llevaba incrustada en el ombligo y luego alejé la mirada. "De todas formas tenía que limpiar," concluyó.

"Gracias." Volví a mi receta repasando exactamente todo lo que necesitaba y colocándolo en la mesa del centro de la cocina. Cuando Ivy regresó del campanario, todo estaba listo y medido. Sólo faltaba revolver.

"Todo tuyo," me dijo. Dejó la bolita en la mesa y fue a lavarse las manos.

"Gracias," susurré. Con un cuchillo abrí la masa y saqué tres pelos de entre los huesos diminutos. Hice una mueca pensando que no había pasado completamente por el búho. Solo lo había regurgitado.

Luego, tomé una manotada de sal y mirándola le dije: "Voy a hacer un círculo de sal. No intentes cruzarlo." Me fijó la mirada y agregué: "Este hechizo puede ser peligroso. No quiero que caiga algo accidentalmente en la vasija. Puedes quedarte en la cocina; pero por favor, no cruces el círculo."

Incrédula, asintió con la cabeza. "Está bien."

Me gustaba verla fuera de base. Hice el círculo más grande que lo usual, llenando toda la mesa del centro de la cocina con mis cosas. Ivy se apoyó con las manos para sentarse en una esquina del mostrador. Abrió los ojos con curiosidad. Si pensaba hacer esto frecuentemente, más bien debía olvidarme del depósito de seguridad del arriendo y abrir una ranura recta en el linóleo del piso. ¿De qué sirve el depósito de seguridad si muero por causa de un hechizo mal orientado?

El corazón me latía con fuerza. Hacía tiempos que no cerraba un círculo pero la presencia de Ivy me ponía nerviosa. "Muy bien," murmuré. Tomé aire lentamente, cerré los ojos y despejé la mente. Gradualmente me concentré en mi objetivo.

No solía hacer esto con frecuencia pues confunde más

que otra cosa. Sentí un viento del otro lado de la realidad que levantaba mi cabello. Hice un gesto con la nariz al sentir el olor de ámbar quemado. Inmediatamente sentí que estaba afuera. Las paredes a mi alrededor desaparecieron y apenas las podía percibir. Ivy desapareció. Sólo veía el paisaje y las plantas. Sus siluetas se movían con un resplandor rojo que llenaba el aire. Era como estar parada en este lugar antes de que hubiera sido descubierto por la humanidad. Se me electrizó la piel al notar que las lápidas existían también en este mundo, blancas y sólidas como la luna en el firmamento.

Con los ojos cerrados, traté de mirar buscando la línea ley más cercana. "Mierda," dije sorprendida al encontrar una marca roja de poder que cruzaba por el jardín. "¿Sabías que hay una línea ley que cruza el jardín?"

"Sí," repuso Ivy suavemente. Su voz parecía provenir de un lugar indefinido. Empujé toda mi voluntad hasta alcanzarla. Mi olfato se abrió y me invadió una fuerza que repercutió en mis extremidades hasta que el poder se equilibró. La universidad estaba construida en una línea ley tan grande que podía alcanzarse casi desde cualquier lugar de Cincinnati. Casi todas las ciudades están construidas sobre una línea. Manhattan tiene tres grandes. La línea ley más grande de la costa del este pasa por una granja en las afueras de Woodstock. ¿Coincidencia? No lo creo.

La línea de mi jardín era muy pequeña, pero estaba tan cerca y subutilizada que me producía más fuerza de la que me dio la universidad. Aun cuando nunca me tocó la brisa real, la piel se me erizó por el viento que soplaba del más allá.

Meterse en una línea ley era un asunto peligroso. No me gustaba hacerlo. Su poder me recorría como el agua que va dejando residuos. Ya no podía mantener cerrados los ojos y los abrí.

La roja visión surrealista del más allá fue reemplazada por la rutina de la cocina. Ví la versión terrenal de Ivy sentada en el mostrador. A veces la gente se ve tan diferente, pero me tranquilicé al verla normal. Su aura—su verdadera aura, no su aura de vampiro—destellaba. Qué extraño.

"¿Por qué no me dijiste que había una línea ley tan cerca?" le pregunté.

Ivy me dirigió la mirada. Se encogió de hombros, cruzó las piernas y dejó caer los zapatos debajo del mostrador. "¿Qué importaba?"

No tenía ninguna importancia. Cerré los ojos para reforzar mi segunda visión que se desvanecía mientras cerraba el círculo. La vertiginosa inundación de poder me hacía sentir incómoda. Con mi voluntad transporté la delgada franja de sal desde esta dimensión hasta el más allá y fue reemplazada por un círculo igual de la otra realidad.

El círculo se cerró con una sacudida que me hizo saltar. "Diablos," musité. "Tal vez utilicé demasiada sal." Buena cantidad de la fuerza que atraje del más allá se movía en mi círculo. Lo que se arremolinaba a mi alrededor me ponía la piel de gallina. El residuo seguiría aumentando hasta que yo rompiera el círculo y me desconectara de la línea.

Podía sentir la barrera de la realidad del más allá como una presión lejana. Nada podía atravesar las bandas de realidades que cambiaban. Con mi segunda visión podía ver la borrosa oleada de rojo brillante que me rodeaba desde los pies hasta la cabeza. La media esfera recorría mi espalda a la misma distancia. Más adelante haría un examen más de cerca para asegurarme de no estar cruzando tuberías o cables eléctricos que harían que el círculo pudiera romperse, si acaso algo activo cruzara por ese lado.

Ivy me estaba observando cuando abrí los ojos. Le sonreí amargamente y me di vuelta. Muy pronto, mi segunda visión se redujo a nada quedando sólo mi visión normal.

"Está bien cerrado," le dije al ver que su aura comenzaba a desaparecer. "No intentes cruzar. Duele."

Asintió solemnemente. "Tú mandas . . . bruja."

Sonreí complacida. ¿Por qué no dejar que por una vez la bruja le muestre los dientes al vampiro? Tomé el cuenco de cobre más pequeño de todos, aproximadamente del tamaño de mis dos manos juntas, y lo puse encima de la estufita de gas de excursionista que Ivy me había comprado hacía poco. La había usado para preparar mis hechizos menores. La conexión corriente de gas hubiera abierto el círculo. "Agua," murmuré, llenando mi tubo de vidrio graduado con agua de manantial, agachándome para cerciorarme de la medida exacta. La vasija crepitó cuando la agregué. Luego, la quité de la llama. "Ratón, ratón, ratón," musité, luchando por no dejar ver mi nerviosismo. Este era el hechizo más difícil que había probado fuera de clase.

Ivy bajó del mostrador y me puse tensa. Los pelos de la nuca se me pararon cuando se paró detrás de mí, pero aun fuera del círculo. Detuve lo que estaba haciendo y me volteé a mirarla. Sonrió avergonzada y regresó al mostrador.

"No sabía que podías pasar al más allá," dijo antes de sentarse frente a su pantalla.

Levanté la mirada de la receta. "Soy una bruja terrestre y no lo hago con mucha frecuencia. Este hechizo me cambiará físicamente y no sólo me dará la apariencia de un ratón. Si algo llegara a meterse accidentalmente en la vasija, tal vez no logre romperlo o puede que apenas cambie a medias... o algo así."

Su actitud se tornó evasiva. Yo, mientras tanto, puse el pelo de ratón en un cernidor para agregarle luego la leche. Existe todo una rama de brujería que usa líneas ley en vez de pociones. Había pasado dos semestres limpiando el laboratorio de uno de mis profesores pues así no tendría que tomar más que el curso básico. A todos les dije que era porque aun no tenía un familiar (es un requisito de seguridad), pero la verdad es que no me gustaba. Perdí a un amigo muy querido que decidió especializarse en líneas ley pero terminó rodeado de mala compañía. Y para qué mencionar la muerte de papá, que estuvo relacionada con las líneas. Para nada sirvió que las líneas ley fueran la puerta hacia el más allá.

Se dice que el más allá era un paraíso donde vivían los elfos que entraban en nuestra realidad con tiempo suficiente para robar niños humanos. Pero cuando los demonios se apoderaron del sitio destrozándolo, los elfos se vieron forzados a quedarse aquí para siempre. Naturalmente, eso sucedió mucho antes de que Grimm escribiera sus cuentos de hadas. Todo está explicado en los cuentos más antiguos. Casi todos terminan con la frase "y vivieron felices por siempre." Bueno, así se supone que era. Grimm debió agregar "en el más allá." Puesto que algunas brujas usan líneas ley, es probable que por ello se piensa erróneamente que están del lado de los demonios. Me estremecí de sólo pensar cuántas vidas había costado ese error.

Yo era una bruja terrestre exclusivamente. Trabajaba con amuletos, pociones y hechizos. Los gestos y conjuros formaban parte del mundo de la magia ley. Las brujas que se especializan en esta rama se meten a las líneas para obtener su poder directamente de ellas. Era una magia más ruda, menos estructurada y no tan hermosa, pues no contaba con la disciplina de la hechicería terrestre. La única ventaja que yo le veía es que se podía invocar instantáneamente con la palabra adecuada. La desventaja es que uno tiene que portar un trozo del más allá en el chi. No me importa que haya formas de aislarlo de los chakras. Estoy convencida de que la mancha demoníaca del más allá deja una acumulación de inmundicias en el alma. He visto a muchos amigos perder su destreza de ver con claridad en qué lado del campo está su magia.

La magia de línea ley tenía el potencial más grande de volverse magia de ley negra. Si era difícil seguir el rastro de un hechizo hasta hallar a su fabricante, hallar al responsable de un hechizo ley era casi imposible. Esto no quiere decir que todas las brujas de línea ley sean malas. Sus destrezas tenían gran demanda para el entretenimiento, el control del tiempo y la seguridad de las industrias; pero debido a su relación cercana con el más allá y con más poder en las manos, era fácil volverse inmoral.

El motivo por el cual no me ascendieron en la S.E. podría deberse a que me negué a usar magia ley para capturar a los grandes capos del mal. Pero, ¿qué diferencia había si los atrapaba con un hechizo en lugar de hacerlo con un conjuro? Yo había perfeccionado la lucha contra la magia ley usando elementos terrestres, aun cuando nadie tenía porqué saberlo con sólo mirar mi promedio de capturas por misión.

El recuerdo de esa pirámide de proyectiles explosivos junto a la puerta me producía punzadas en el cuerpo. Vertí la leche en la vasija sobre el pelo de ratón. La mezcla estaba hirviendo. La alcé aun más en el trípode revolviéndola con una cuchara de madera. No era buena idea usar madera para preparar un hechizo y todas mis cucharas de barro tenían conjuros. Usar metales era provocar una catástrofe. Las cucharas de madera actuaban como amuletos pues absorbían el hechizo y se podían cometer errores vergonzosos; pero si al terminar las lavabas con agua salada, todo estaría bien.

Puse las manos en la cintura, programé el tiempo y leí de nuevo el hechizo. La mezcla hirviente empezó a soltar un olor almizclado. Ojalá estuviera bien.

"Entonces…" dijo Ivy mientras escribía en su teclado. "Vas a meterte en los archivos como ratón. ¿Cómo piensas abrir los cajones?"

"Jenks dice que ya tiene copias de todo. Sólo tenemos que echar una mirada."

La silla de Ivy crujió cuando se recostó hacia atrás y cruzó las piernas. Era obvia su duda de que dos enanos fueran capaces de hacer funcionar el teclado. "¿Por qué no vuelves a tu forma de bruja cuando estés allá?"

Sacudí la cabeza negativamente mientras revisaba de nuevo la receta. "Las transformaciones invocadas mediante una poción duran hasta que te empapes bien con agua salada. Si quisiera, podía transformarme con un amuleto, forzar mi entrada a la bóveda, quitármelo, buscar lo que necesito en forma de humano y luego ponerme el amuleto para salir. Pero no lo haré."

"¿Por qué no?"

Me abrumaba con preguntas. Alcé la cabeza en medio del sonido que producía una de las plantas al disolverse. "¿Nunca has usado un hechizo de transformación?" inquirí. "Creí que los vampiros los usaban todo el tiempo para transformarse en murciélagos y cosas así."

Ivy bajó la mirada. "Algunos lo hacen," repuso en voz baja.

Era evidente que Ivy jamás se había transformado. Me pregunto por qué. El dinero no era problema. "No es buena idea usar amuletos para transformarse. Tendría que amarrarme el amuleto o llevarlo en el cuello, y todos mis amuletos son más grandes que un ratón. Se vería algo extraño. ¿Y qué pasaría si estoy trepada en una pared y se me cae? Algunas brujas han muerto al volver a la normalidad cuando se rompe el hechizo al quedar incrustadas en paredes o rejas." Me estremecí a medida que revolvía la poción rápidamente en el sentido de las manecillas del reloj. "Además" agregué, "no voy a tener ropa puesta cuando regrese."

"¡Oh, vaya!" rió Ivy. "Esa es la verdadera razón, Raquel, ¡eres tímida!"

¿Que podía responder ante eso? Un poco avergonzada, cerré el libro y lo puse debajo de la mesa, junto con el resto de mi nueva biblioteca. El reloj sonó y soplé la llama para apagarla. Quedaba apenas un poco de líquido y en breve alcanzaría la temperatura del cuarto.

Me limpié las manos en los jeans y me incliné sobre el desorden de la mesa hasta alcanzar un punzón de sangre. Antes del Giro, muchas brujas fingían sufrir de diabetes con el fin de obtener una de estas valiosas herramientas gratis. Los odiaba, pero era preferible que usar un cuchillo para cortarse una vena como lo hacían en épocas más nebulosas. Lista para pincharme, me asaltó la duda un instante. Ivy no podía cruzar el círculo, pero la noche anterior estaba fresca en mi mente. Si pudiera dormiría dentro de un círculo de sal, pero tal vez me volvería loca estando permanentemente conectada con el más allá sin un familiar que absor-

biera las toxinas mentales que expedían las líneas. "Yo...eh
...necesito tres gotas de mi sangre para acelerar el hechizo,"
le dije.

"¿Verdad?" Su mirada carecía de aquella expresión decidida que generalmente se observaba antes del aura depredadora de los vampiros pero, aun así, no confiaba en ella.

Hice una señal con la cabeza y agregué: "Tal vez sea mejor que te vayas."

Ivy rió. "Tres gotas sacadas con un punzón de sangre no
causan nada."

Aun así dudé. Sentí la tensión en el estómago ¿Cómo podía estar segura de que ella conocía sus límites? Sus ojos se
volvieron menos circulares y en sus pálidas mejillas aparecieron unas manchas rojas. Si le insistía para que se fuera se
ofendería, lo sabía. Pero tampoco estaba dispuesta a demostrarle miedo. Estaba totalmente segura adentro del círculo.
Podía parar a un demonio, así que parar a un vampiro no
era nada.

Tomé aire y me pinché el dedo. Hubo un destello negro en
sus ojos y un escalofrío me recorrió el cuerpo. Luego, nada.
Mis hombros se relajaron. Decidida, le agregué las tres gotas
a la mezcla. El líquido pardo lechoso se veía igual, pero sentía un olor distinto. Cerré los ojos y respiré hondo hasta que
el olor a pasto y grano penetrara en mis pulmones. Necesitaría otras tres gotas de mi sangre para preparar cada dosis antes de usarlas.

"Huele diferente."

"¿Cómo?" dije, maldiciendo mi reacción. Olvidé que ella
estaba allí.

"Tu sangre huele diferente," dijo Ivy. "Huele a madera. A
especias. Huele a tierra, a tierra viva. Ni la sangre humana ni
la de vampiro huelen así."

"Umm," musité, totalmente segura de que no me gustaba
nada el hecho de ella pudiera oler mi sangre desde el otro
lado del cuarto a través de una barrera con el más allá. Al
menos me reconfortaba saber que jamás había desangrado a
una bruja.

"¿Serviría mi sangre?" preguntó con curiosidad.

Agité la cabeza mientras que revolvía nerviosamente la poción. "No. Tiene que ser sangre de bruja o de aprendiz. No es la sangre sino las enzimas que tiene. Actúan como catalizadores."

Asintió, dejando su computadora y dedicándose a observarme.

Froté la punta de los dedos para no untar nada con restos de mi sangre. Esta receta, al igual que casi todas las demás, me daba siete hechizos. Los que no usara esta noche los guardaría en pociones. Si quisiera, podía ponerlos en amuletos para que duraran un año. Pero no me transformaría por nada del mundo con un amuleto.

Ivy no me quitaba los ojos de encima mientras yo vertía cuidadosamente la mezcla en frascos del tamaño del dedo pulgar y luego los tapaba firmemente. Listo. Ahora sólo quedaba romper el círculo y mi conexión con la línea ley. Lo primero era fácil. Lo segundo un poco más difícil.

Le sonreí a Ivy y abrí una brecha en la sal con mis pantuflas rosadas. El sonido de fondo del poder del más allá se hizo más intenso. Mi respiración silbaba por la nariz pues toda la fuerza que antes fluía por el círculo ahora fluía por mi cuerpo.

"¿Qué está sucediendo?," preguntó Ivy desde su silla, alerta y preocupada.

Hice un esfuerzo conciente por respirar pensando en que podía hiperventilarme. Me sentía como un globo excesivamente inflado. Con los ojos fijos en el piso, le agité la mano pidiéndole que no se acercara. "El círculo está roto. Aléjate. Aún no he terminado," le dije, sintiéndome un tanto aturdida y fuera de la realidad.

Tomé aire y empecé a separarme de la línea. La lucha se presentaba entre el deseo de poder que siente el sujeto y la certidumbre de que tal poder termina por enloquecerlo. Tenía que sacarlo de mí, expulsarlo de la cabeza a los pies hasta que volviera a la tierra.

Mis hombros saltaron a medida que me abandonaba y caminé a trompicones hacia el mostrador.

"¿Te encuentras bien?" preguntó Ivy preocupada y curiosa.

Jadeante, levanté la mirada. Me sostenía de un codo ayudándome a parar. No la vi moverse y eso me produjo escalofríos. Sentía sus dedos cálidos a través de mi blusa. "Puse demasiada sal. La conexión era muy fuerte. Estoy…eh… estoy bien. Suéltame."

Su preocupación desapareció. Era evidente que sintió una afrenta y me soltó. Se sintió el crujir de la sal bajo sus pies y regresó a su esquina a sentarse en su silla, herida. Yo no me disculparía. No hice nada mal.

El pesado e incómodo silencio me afectó mientras guardaba todos los frascos en el mueble con mis amuletos, excepto uno. No pude evitar sentir una pizca de orgullo al verlos. Los hice yo. Y aunque el seguro para venderlos costaba más que mi viejo sueldo anual de la S.E., los podía usar.

"¿Necesitas ayuda esta noche?," preguntó Ivy. "No me importaría cubrir tu espalda."

"No," solté la respuesta. Fue muy prematuro y su expresión se tornó agria. Meneé la cabeza, sonriendo para suavizar mi rechazo, esperando que pudiera obligarme a mí misma a decir "sí, por favor." Pero aun no confiaba en ella y no quería estar en posición de tener que confiar de alguien. Papá murió porque confió en que alguien le cubriera la espalda. "Trabaja sola, Raquel," me dijo cuando me senté a acompañarlo en su cama del hospital, tomando su mano temblorosa en las mías mientras su sangre perdía la capacidad de transportar oxígeno. "Trabaja siempre sola."

Sentí un nudo en la garganta cuando encontré los ojos de Ivy. "Si no soy capaz de escabullirme de un par de sombras merezco que me atrapen," le dije tratando de evadir la realidad del asunto. Metí la vasija retractable y una botella de agua salada en mi bolso, además de un nuevo amuleto de disfraz que nadie en la S.E. conocía.

"¿No piensas probar uno primero?" me preguntó cuando vio que ya me iba.

Acomodé nerviosamente hacia atrás un mechón de mi pelo crespo. "Se hace tarde. Estoy segura de que funcionará."

Ivy no parecía convencida. "Si no has regresado al amanecer, iré a buscarte."

"Está bien." Si no regresaba antes del amanecer es porque estaba muerta. Agarré mi abrigo de invierno que colgaba de un asiento y me lo puse. Le sonreí nerviosamente a Ivy y salí por la puerta trasera. Cruzaría el cementerio y tomaría el autobús una calle más allá.

El aire de esta noche de primavera era frío y tirité al cerrar la puerta de anjeo. El espectáculo de ese montón de plastas explosivas era un recuerdo desagradable. Me sentí vulnerable y decidí refugiarme a la sombra de un roble a la espera de que mis ojos se acostumbraran a la noche sin luna. Apenas había pasado la luna nueva de modo que no se veía hasta despuntar el amanecer. *Gracias, Dios mío, por estos pequeños favores.*

"¡Eh...señorita Raquel!" dijo una vocecita zumbadora y volteé pensando que era Jenks. Era Jax, el hijo mayor de Jenks. El duendecillo preadolescente me había acompañado toda la tarde y estuvo a punto de que yo lo cortara varias veces por su curiosidad y sentido del "deber" que lo pusieron demasiado cerca de mis podadoras mientras su padre dormía.

"Hola Jax. ¿Tu papá está despierto?," le pregunté ofreciéndole una mano para que aterrizara.

"¿Srta. Raquel? La están esperando."

Mi corazón palpitó. "¿Cuántos? ¿Adónde?"

"Son tres." Se puso verde de excitación. "Adelante. Son tipos grandes. De su tamaño. Apestan a zorro. Los ví cuando el viejo Keasley los sacó corriendo de su acera. Yo le habría informado antes," dijo diligentemente, "pero no alcanzaron a cruzar la calle y ya nosotros les habíamos robado todos sus proyectiles explosivos. Papá nos dijo que no la molestáramos, a menos que alguien saltara por la pared."

"Está bien. Hiciste lo correcto." Jax salió volando y yo comencé a andar. De todas formas iba a cruzar el jardín para tomar el autobús al otro lado de la cuadra. Miré forzadamente en la oscuridad y le propiné un golpecillo al pequeño bulto diciendo: "Jenks, vamos a trabajar." Y se escuchó un rugido de irritación casi subliminal que provenía del bulto.

Diez

La mujer bonita que estaba sentada frente a mí en el autobús se levantó para bajarse. Hizo una pausa pero estaba demasiado cerca, tanto como para hacerme subir la guardia. Alcé la mirada del libro de Ivy. "Tabla 6.1" dijo, al tiempo que nuestras miradas se encontraron. "Es *todo* lo que necesitas saber." Cerró los ojos y se estremeció como si hubiera sentido placer.

Un poco avergonzada, pasé las páginas hacia atrás. "Vaya," susurré. Se trataba de una tabla de accesorios y sugerencias para usarlos. Me sonrojé y, aunque no soy ninguna mojigata... algunas de estas cosas ¿y con un vampiro? Tal vez con un brujo, y solo tan bien parecido como para quitarle a uno la respiración. Sin la sangre, naturalmente. *Tal vez*.

Me sacudí y ella se agachó en el pasillo. Se inclinó demasiado dejando caer una tarjeta de negocios negra en el libro abierto. "En caso de que quiera invitar a otra persona," susurró, sonriendo con una rápida familiaridad que no logré entender. "Los principiantes brillan como las estrellas, expresando lo mejor que llevan por dentro. No me disgustaría tocar el segundo violín en tu primera noche, y podría ayudarte... después. A veces se les olvida." Un destello de temor cruzó por su cara, veloz pero real.

Me dejó con la boca abierta. No pude decir ni una palabra. Ella se levantó, se alejó y bajó por la escalerilla.

Jenks volaba cerca y cerré el libro inmediatamente. "Raque," dijo, a la vez que aterrizaba en mi arete. "¿Qué lees? Tienes la nariz enterrada en ese libro desde que subimos al autobús."

"Nada," repuse, con el pulso latiendo fuerte. "Esa mujer. Era humana, ¿verdad?"

"¿La que hablaba contigo? Sí. Por su olor, es un vampiro lacayo. ¿Por qué?"

"Por nada," respondí, mientras guardaba el libro en el fondo de la bolsa. No volvería a leer esta cosa en un sitio público. Afortunadamente, la próxima parada era la nuestra. Me dirigí a los restaurantes del centro comercial ignorando el interrogatorio permanente de Jenks. Mi abrigo largo golpeaba contra mis tobillos mientras que ingresaba en el bullicio de una tarde de domingo. En el baño invoqué mi disfraz de mujer anciana esperando engañar a cualquiera que me hubiera reconocido. Aun así, me pareció prudente relajarme un poco entre la multitud antes de dirigirme a la S.E.: matar el tiempo un poco, reunir fuerzas, comprar un sombrero para reemplazar el que le perdí a Ivy en la mañana—comprar un poco de jabón para eliminar cualquier rastro de su olor en mí.

Pasé frente a una tienda de amuletos con mi usual actitud de duda. Podía preparar todo lo que quisiera y si alguien me buscaba, este sería el primar lugar que estaría vigilando. *Pero a nadie se le ocurriría pensar que compraría un par de botas,* pensé, disminuyendo el paso tan pronto ví la vitrina. Las cortinas de cuero y las luces tenues, más que su nombre, decían que este negocio estaba concebido para vampiros.

¡Qué diablos! pensé. *Yo vivo con un vampiro.* El vendedor no podía ser peor que Ivy. Además, creo que yo ya era lo suficientemente sabia como para no dejar rastros de sangre. Así es que no le presté atención a los reclamos de Jenks y entré. Mis pensamientos saltaron de la Tabla 6.1 al atractivo y coqueto vendedor que alejó a los otros vendedores y me miró por encima de los aros de madera de sus lentes.

El nombre impreso en su etiqueta de identificación decía VALENTINO. Capturé su atención como un imán, mientras que me ayudaba a escoger un buen par de botas y suspiraba sobre mis medias de seda, acariciando mis pies con sus dedos fuertes y vigorosos. Jenks aguardaba en el pasillo metido en una maceta, resentido y malhumorado.

Dios me perdone, pero Valentino era atractivo. Estoy segura de que ese era un requisito para obtener el empleo, como lo debía ser el vestirse de negro y saber cómo coquetear sin alarmar. Mirar no cuesta nada...¿verdad? Podía mirar sin tener que entrar al club, ¿no es así?

Pero cuando salía caminando con mis botas demasiado costosas, reflexioné acerca de mi repentina curiosidad. Ivy había admitido que se sentía atraída por los olores. A lo mejor los vampiros exhalan feromonas para tranquilizar y atraer a los desprevenidos. Así era mucho más fácil seducir a la presa. Yo había disfrutado concientemente con Valentino, tan tranquila como si se hubiese tratado de un viejo amigo, dejándolo tomarse algunas libertades coquetas con sus palabras y manos que normalmente no permitiría. Pero traté de olvidar esa incómoda sensación y seguí con mis compras.

Tenía que entrar a la Gran Cereza por salsa para pizzas. Los humanos boicoteaban todas las tiendas que vendían tomates, así la variedad Ángel T-4 se hubiera extinguido hace tiempos, de tal modo que el único lugar donde se podían conseguir era en alguna tienda de especialidades donde no importaba si medio mundo tomaba la decisión de no entrar por la puerta.

El nerviosismo era lo que me hacía detenerme en la confitería. Todos saben que el chocolate relaja los nervios; y me parece que alguien realizó un estudio sobre eso. Entonces Jenks estuvo silencioso durante cinco minutos que me parecieron la gloria mientras comía el caramelo que le compré.

Luego, no podía dejar de entrar a Bath and Body: no volvería a usar el champú ni el jabón de Ivy. Y eso me condujo a una tienda de fragancias. Con la ayuda y los gruñidos de Jenks, elegí un nuevo perfume que me ayudara a tapar el persistente aroma de Ivy. La lavanda era lo único que serviría. Jenks dijo que apestaba como una explosión en una fábrica de flores. No es que me gustara tanto, pero si me ayudaba a no provocar los instintos de Ivy ¡y para eso hasta sería capaz de tomármela, no solo de bañarme en ella!

Dos horas antes del alba estaba de regreso en la calle en dirección hacia la bóveda del archivo. Mis nuevas botas eran deliciosamente silenciosas, pues sentía que flotaba sobre el pavimento. Valentino tenía razón. Me lancé a la calle vacía sin dudarlo. Mi hechizo de mujer anciana aun conservaba su efecto, lo cual seguramente explica las miradas curiosas en la tienda de cueros; pero si nadie me veía, mejor.

La S.E. cerraba bien los edificios. Casi todas las oficinas en esta cuadra tenían horarios humanos y habían estado cerradas desde la noche del viernes. El tráfico zumbaba a dos cuadras de distancia, pero aquí estaba en silencio. Miré hacia atrás antes de meterme al callejón que había en medio del edificio de archivos y la torre de seguros. Mi corazón comenzó a galopar tan pronto pasé frente a la puerta de incendios donde por poco me atrapan. Pero no pensaba entrar por ese lado. "¿Ves un tubo de desagüe Jenks?" pregunté.

"Voy a revisar," respondió, y voló hacia adelante para hacer un pequeño reconocimiento.

Yo lo seguí más lentamente agachándome un poco para escuchar el sonido sordo de los golpecillos sobre el metal. Disfrutando a fondo la explosión de adrenalina, me deslicé en medio de un gran bote de basura y una plataforma de carga. Sonreí al ver a Jenks sentado sobre el extremo curvado de una canal, dándole golpecitos con los tacones de las botas. "Gracias Jenks," le dije, quitándome el bolso y colocándolo encima del cemento cubierto de rocío fresco.

"Seguro." Voló para sentarse encima de un contenedor de basura. "Madre mía, Campanita," protestó, tapándose la nariz. "¿Sabes lo que hay aquí adentro?" Lo observé. Entonces continuó. "Lasagna de hace tres días, cinco variedades de yogurt, palomitas de maíz quemadas..." Dudó unos instantes cerrando los ojos mientras olfateaba..."tipo sureño, un millón de papelitos de caramelos...y alguien vive obsesionado con los burritos de carne de cerdo."

"¿Jenks? ¡Cállate!" El suave ruido de llantas contra el pavimento me advirtieron que me quedara inmóvil, pero hasta la mejor visión nocturna tendría problemas para detectarme aquí atrás. El callejón apestaba tanto que no tendría que preocuparme por los zorros. Pero aun así, aguardé hasta que la calle quedara en silencio antes de buscar un hechizo antidetección y un punzón de sangre en mi bolso. El fuerte pinchazo me hizo saltar. Dejé caer las tres gotas requeridas sobre el amuleto que inmediatamente brilló de un verde pálido. Dejé escapar el aire que retenía sin darme cuenta. El único ser viviente a cien pies de distancia era Jenks—y yo tenía mis duda sobre él. Pero estaba segura y podía transformarme en ratón.

"Ten, mira esto y dime si se torna rojo," le dije a Jenks a la vez que equilibraba el disco sobre el contenedor.

"¿Por qué?"

"¡Sólo haz lo que te digo!," susurré. Sentada encima de un montón de cartones, me desamarré las botas, me quité las medias y puse un pie descalzo sobre el cemento. Estaba frío y húmedo por la lluvia de anoche y dejé escapar un leve quejido de desagrado. Le eché un vistazo rápido al fondo del callejón y escondí mis botas y mi abrigo detrás de un contenedor de papeles machacados. Me sentía como una adicta al azufre. Me acurruqué en el canal y saqué mi frasco de poción. "Así se hace, Raquel," susurré, recordando que aún no había preparado la vasija de disolución.

Confiaba en que Ivy sabría que hacer si regresaba a casa como un ratón, pero jamás dejaría de recalcármelo. El agua salada formaba burbujas al llenar la vasija. Luego escondí el frasco. La tapa de rosca cayó en el contenedor haciendo el típico ruido metálico y me estremecí mientras presionaba otras tres gotas de sangre del dedo palpitante. Sin embargo, la incomodidad desapareció cuando mi sangre tocó el líquido y se elevó una suave fragancia.

Mi estómago se templó a medida que mezclaba la solución con unos golpecitos en el vidrio. Me limpié una mano nerviosamente en los jeans y miré a Jenks. Hacer un hechizo es fácil. Lo difícil es confiar en que quedó bien hecho. A la hora de la verdad, lo único que diferenciaba a una bruja de un aprendiz era el valor. *Yo soy una bruja,* me dije a mí misma. *Esto está bien preparado. Seré un ratón y podré regresar si me sumerjo en agua salada.*

"¿Me prometes que no le dirás nada a Ivy si no funciona?" le pregunté a Jenks que hacía muecas y bajaba su gorro casi tapándole los ojos.

"¿Qué me darás a cambio?"

"No te cubriré las alas con veneno para hormigas."

Suspiró. "Házlo ya," me dijo. "Quisiera llegar a casa antes de que el sol sea nova. Los duendes duermen de noche, ¿sabes?"

Me lamí los labios demasiado nerviosa para responderle. Jamás me había transformado antes. Había tomado clases, pero el valor de la matrícula no cubría el costo de comprar un hechizo profesional de transformación y los seguros contra terceros no les permitía a los estudiantes ensayar con sus propias pociones. ¡Seguros contra terceros! ¡Qué tontería!

Apreté los dedos alrededor del frasco y sentía mi pulso martillar. Esto iba a doler de verdad.

De repente cerré los ojos y lo tomé. Era amargo, pero lo tragué de un solo golpe tratando de no pensar en los tres pelos de ratón. ¡Qué asco!

Sentí calambres en el estómago y me doblé aun más. Jadeé y perdí el equilibrio. El frío del cemento me invadió el cuerpo y estiré un brazo para detener mi caída. Estaba negro y velludo. *¡Funciona!* Pensé en la felicidad y en el temor. No estaba del todo mal.

Entonces, un dolor agudo cruzó por mi columna vertebral. Me recorrió desde el cráneo hasta los pies como si fuera fuego. Grité aterrorizada al tiempo que un chirrido gutural me reventaba los oídos. Una sensación de frío y calor me corrió por mis venas.

Estaba convulsionando, la agonía me dejaba sin aire. Tuve pánico cuando la vista se tornó negra. A tientas, estiré los brazos y escuché un terrible ruido. "¡No!," chillé. El dolor se agigantó, se envolvió, me devoró.

Once

"**R**aquel! ¡Raquel! Despierta. ¿Estás bien?"

Una voz baja y desconocida me devolvió poco a poco a la realidad. Me estiré sintiendo los músculos diferentes. Abrí los ojos y ví una gama de sombras grises. Jenks estaba parado frente a mí con las manos en la cintura y las piernas abiertas. Me pareció que medía un metro ochenta. "¡Mierda!," maldije. ¡Soy un maldito ratón!

De nuevo me invadió el pánico cuando recordé el intenso dolor que sentí en la transformación. Además, tendría que experimentarlo todo de nuevo cuando regresara. Con razón la transformación era un arte en vías de extinción. Dolía como rayo.

Mis temores comenzaron a desaparecer y logré salir de entre mi ropa. Mi corazón latía muy rápido y el olor de lavanda era intenso. Me asfixiaba. Arrugué la nariz y traté de controlar mi reacción al sentir que podía oler el alcohol de las aromáticas flores. Podía detectar el olor de incienso y ceniza con el que identificaba a Ivy y pensé si acaso el olfato de los vampiros era tan sensible como el de los ratones.

Bamboleándome en cuatro patas, me senté un instante para ver el mundo con mis nuevos ojos. El callejón era del tamaño de una bodega y el cielo sobre mí se veía negro y amenazante. Lo veía todo en sombras grises y blancas: no podía ver los colores. El sonido del tráfico distante era fuerte y el hedor del callejón era abrumador. Jenks tenía razón: había alguien que le encantaban los burritos.

Ahora que estaba metida de lleno en esto, la noche parecía más fría. Giré hacia la montaña que formaba mi ropa para tratar de esconder mis joyas. La próxima vez dejaría todo en casa, menos mi cuchillo.

Miré a Jenks riendo de asombro. *¡Vaya chico!* Jenks se veía fantástico. Era todo un atleta con alas. Sus hombros eran fuertes y bien desarrollados para el vuelo. La cintura era delgada, pero el cuerpo musculoso. El pelo le caía artísticamente encima de las cejas dándole aire de autosuficiencia. Una red de destellos le cubría las alas. Mirándolo desde la misma perspectiva de su tamaño, ahora ya entendía por qué Jenks tenía más hijos que tres parejas de conejos.

Y sus ropas... ¡eran impactantes inclusive en blanco y negro! Las mangas y el cuello de su camisa estaban bordados como dedaleras y helechos. El pañuelo negro que llevaba amarrado a la frente y que yo antes veía rojo, estaba adornado con pequeños resplandores muy llamativos.

"Eh... oye, Candela" me dijo de buen humor con una voz sorprendentemente baja y grave para mis oídos de roedor. "Funcionó. ¿Dónde encontraste un hechizo de visón?"

"¿Visón?," pregunté, oyendo tan solo un chirrido. De inmediato dirigí la mirada hacia mis manos. Mis pulgares eran pequeños, pero mis dedos eran tan ágiles que no tenía necesidad de los pulgares. En la punta tenía unas pequeñas uñas puntiagudas. Me toqué la nariz y sentí el hocico corto y triangular. Luego, di la vuelta y pude ver mi cola larga y hermosa. Todo mi cuerpo mostraba una línea elegante. Nunca había sido así de flaca. Levanté una pata y me di cuenta de que mis pies eran blancos y con almohadillas blancas. Era difícil calcular los tamaños, pero de seguro era mucho más grande que un ratón, más bien como una ardilla grande.

¿Un visón? pensé, sentándome mientras que frotaba las patas delanteras en mi piel. ¿Y ahora qué? Abrí la boca y sentí los dientes afilados y peligrosos. Al menos no tendría que preocuparme de los gatos, pues era casi tan grande

como uno de ellos. Los búhos de Ivy eran mejores cazadores de lo que pensé. Cerré los ojos mirando al cielo. Búhos. Aun tendría que preocuparme de los búhos. Y de los perros. Y de todo lo que fuera más grande que yo. ¿Qué andaría haciendo un visón en la ciudad?

"Te ves muy bien Raque," dijo Jenks.

Mis ojos regresaron a Jenks. *Y tú también, hombrecito*. Pensé desinteresadamente si existiría un hechizo para convertir a la gente al tamaño de los duendes. Por lo que podía apreciar en Jenks, valdría la pena tomarse unas vacaciones como duende y gozar de lo mejor de Cincinnati. Me llamaría Tumbelina y sería una chica feliz.

"Nos vemos en el techo, ¿está bien?" agregó sonriendo al ver cómo lo devoraba con los ojos. Asentí viendo cómo se elevaba. *Tal vez exista un hechizo para agrandar duendes*.

Mi nostálgico suspiro sonó como un chirrido extraño mientras corrí hacia el canal de desagüe. Al fondo había un pozo con la lluvia de anoche y mis bigotes lo rozaron cuando comencé a subir con gran agilidad. Me di cuenta de que mis uñas eran afiladas mientras trepaba por el metal. Eran un arma tan buena como mis dientes.

Cuando alcancé el techo plano estaba jadeando. Salí del canal como un chorro de agua, trotando alegremente hasta la sombra que producía el extractor del aire acondicionado del edificio y oí el ¡hurra! de Jenks.

"Acá, Raque," llamó. "Alguien dobló la malla."

Mi sedosa cola se sacudía alegremente mientras me dirigía hacia el aire acondicionado. Faltaba un tornillo en una de las esquinas de la malla. Mejor todavía, estaba doblada. No fue difícil entrar con Jenks abriéndola un poco más para mí. Una vez adentro, aguardé a que mis ojos se acostumbraran a la oscuridad mientras que Jenks revoloteaba por todas partes. Muy pronto nos topamos con otra malla. Mis cejas de roedor se levantaron al ver que Jenks cortaba una tajada triangular en el metal. Sin duda habíamos descubierto la puerta trasera secreta para entrar a la S.E.

Llenos de confianza, Jenks y yo exploramos nuestra ruta

de ingreso por los conductos de aire del edificio. Jenks nunca cerró la boca. Sus comentarios sobre lo fácil que era perdernos y morir de hambre no eran muy alentadores. Era evidente que la maraña de conductos de aire eran usados frecuentemente. Los excrementos estaban duros y el olor viejo a animal era muy penetrante. Sólo había un sentido para movernos: hacia abajo; y, luego de un par de vueltas equivocadas, nos hallamos de pronto ante el paisaje familiar de la bóveda de archivos.

El respiradero en el cual estábamos quedaba directamente encima de las terminales de las computadoras. Nada se movía en las fotocopiadoras. La fea alfombra roja estaba cubierta de mesas rectangulares y asientos de plástico. Los archivos estaban empotrados en la pared. Se trataba de archivos activos, una diminuta fracción de la basura que la S.E. guardaba sobre las poblaciones de humanos y Entremundos, de vivos y muertos. Casi todo estaba archivado electrónicamente, pero si alguien sacaba un archivo se dejaba una copia de papel durante diez años en los archivadores, o cincuenta, si se trataba de un vampiro.

"¿Listo Jenks?" dije, olvidando que mi voz sonaba como un chillido. Podía oler el café quemado y el azúcar junto a la puerta. Mis tripas bramaron. Me acosté y estiré un brazo entre las rejas del respiradero doblando extrañamente el codo para alcanzar la palanca de apertura. Se abrió con inesperada velocidad, meciéndose por las bisagras con un fuerte chirrido. Me quedé inmóvil acurrucada en las sombras, esperando a que mi pulso se normalizara antes de sacar la nariz.

Jenks me detuvo cuando estaba a punto de empujar un rollo de soga del conducto de aire. "Aguarda," susurró. "Déjame alterar las cámaras." Dudó por un instante y sus alas se tornaron oscuras. "No le dirás a nadie esto ¿verdad? es un... eh...es algo que hacemos los duendes para pasar inadvertidos." Hizo una mueca de desilusión y yo asentí con la cabeza.

"Gracias," dijo, y se lanzó al aire. Contuve la respiración y aguardé un instante mientras regresó como un relámpago y se acomodó sentado en la rejilla que colgaba. "Todo listo. Van a grabar un lapso de quince minutos. Ven. Te mostraré lo que miraba Francis."

Empujé la soga del respiradero y bajé hasta el suelo. Fue fácil con las uñas.

"Hizo una copia extra de todo lo que necesitaba" dijo Jenks parado junto a la basura de reciclables al lado de la fotocopiadora. Hizo una mueca cuando volteé la basura y comencé a hurgar entre los papeles. "Yo alteré la fotocopiadora desde adentro y él no entendía por qué la máquina le estaba dando dos copias de todo. Seguramente su ayudante pensó que era un idiota."

Alcé la mirada muriéndome de ganas de decir: "Francis es un idiota."

"Yo sabía que estarías bien," continuó Jenks a medida que organizaba los papeles en el suelo. "Pero fue muy difícil tener que quedarme aquí sin hacer nada cuando oí que corrías. No me pidas que lo haga de nuevo, ¿oíste?"

Tenía los dientes apretados y no supe qué responder, de manera que solo asentí con la cabeza. Jenks me ayudaba más de lo que yo había anticipado. Me sentí mal por haberlo dejado de lado tantas veces y me dediqué a colocar los papeles en orden. No había mucha información, y cuanto más leía más me desilusionaba.

"Según esto," dijo Jenks parado encima de la primera página con las manos en la cintura, "Trent es el último miembro de su familia. Sus padres murieron en circunstancias con olor a magia. Casi todos los habitantes de la casa estaban bajo sospecha. Pasaron tres años antes de que la AFE y la S.E. se dieran por vencidas y decidieran hacerse los ciegos oficialmente."

Repasé rápidamente el manifiesto del investigador de la S.E. pero mis bigotes se retorcieron cuando reconocí su nombre: León Bairn—el mismo que acabó como una mancha en la acera. Interesante.

"Sus padres negaron tener ascendencia humana o Entremundos," continuó Jenks, "lo mismo que Trent. No quedó nada de ellos para realizar las autopsias. Tal como lo hacían sus padres, Trent contrata tanto a Entremundos como a humanos. De todo, menos duendes y hadas."

Eso no me sorprendía. ¿Para qué arriesgarse a una demanda por discriminación?

"Sé lo que estás pensando," dijo Jenks; "pero no parece que él se inclina hacia un lado o el otro. Sus secretarias personales siempre son aprendices de brujería. Su niñera fue una humana de buena reputación y cuando asistió a la Universidad de Princeton compartió su habitación de estudiante con una manada de lobos." Jenks se rascó la cabeza analíticamente. "Pero no ingresó a la fraternidad estudiantil. Al menos no se ve en su archivo; pero, de hecho, no es lobo ni vampiro, nada de eso." Me encogí de hombros y Jenks continuó. "Trent no huele bien. Hablé con un hada que una vez sospechó de Trent cuando trabajó como refuerzo de un agente que lo vigilaba en sus establos. No es que Trent no huela a humano, sino que tiene algo muy sutil que lo desenmascara como Entremundos."

Pensé en el hechizo que había usado esta noche para esconderme. Comencé a abrir la boca para preguntarle algo a Jenks al respecto, pero la cerré de inmediato. Lo único que podía decir sonaba como un chillido. Jenks refunfuñó y luego sacó un lápiz del bolsillo. "Tendrás que escribirlo," me dijo, escribiendo el alfabeto en la parte de abajo de una hoja.

Le mostré mis dientes y todo lo que hizo fue reír. No tenía otra opción. Resbalando el lápiz sobre el papel señalé las letras que escribía "¿hechizo?"

Jenks se encogió de hombros. "Tal vez. Sin embargo, una hada podría atravesar un hechizo con el olfato, tal como yo puedo olfatear una bruja detrás del hedor de visón. Pero, si se trata de un disfraz, eso explicaría lo de las secretarias aprendices. Cuanto más uses la magia, más hueles." Lo miré burlonamente, y agregó: "Todas las brujas huelen parecido, pero las que practican más la magia huelen más intenso, menos terrestre. Tú, por ejemplo, apestas por tu reciente hechizo. Además, esta noche convocaste al más allá ¿cierto?"

Jenks no me estaba formulando una pregunta. Sorprendida, me senté en mis ancas. ¿Jenks podía saber eso gracias a mi olor?

"Tal vez Trent hace que otra bruja le haga sus conjuros. Así puede cubrir su olor con un hechizo. Lo mismo sucede con los lobos y los vampiros."

De pronto me vino una idea, y deletreé: "¿Ivy olor?"

Jenks revoloteó nerviosamente en el aire antes de que hubiera terminado. "Eh…sí…Ivy apesta. O bien es una diletante que dejó de chupar sangre la semana pasada o una activa apasionada que dejó el vicio hace un año. No podría asegurarlo. Tal vez sea un punto intermedio—tal vez."

Fruncí el ceño—tanto como podría hacerlo un visón. Ella había dicho que habían pasado tres años. Debió ser muy intenso. ¡Vaya vaya!

Miré el reloj de la bóveda. Nos quedaba poco tiempo. Ya impaciente, tomé el escaso archivo de Trent. Según la S.E., él vivía y trabajaba en una gran propiedad, en las afueras de la ciudad. Criaba caballos de carreras en su propiedad, pero casi todos sus ingresos provenían de la agricultura: naranjales y arboledas de nuez pacana en el sur, fresas en la costa y trigo en el Medio Oeste. También tenía una isla cerca de la costa este donde sembraba té. Eso ya lo sabía. Era noticia de todos los días en los diarios.

Trent era hijo único. Perdió a su madre cuando tenía diez años y a su padre cuando cursaba el primer año de universidad. Sus padres tuvieron dos hijos más que no sobrevivieron a la infancia. El médico no quiso entregar los documentos sin una citación judicial; y poco después de la solicitud, su oficina fue incendiada y reducida a cenizas. Fue trágico: el médico estaba adentro y no logró salir. *Vaya*, pensé. *Los Kalamack guardan sus secretos.*

Me levanté y crují los dientes. Aquí no había nada que pudiera usar. No sé por qué tenía el presentimiento de que inclusive los archivos de la AFE—si es que milagrosamente lograba verlos—me serían de poca ayuda. Alguien se había tomado la molestia de asegurarse de que no se supiera nada sobre los Kalamack.

"Lo siento," dijo Jenks. "Sé que estabas contando con estos archivos."

Me encogí de hombros metiendo de nuevo los papeles en la basura. No podría levantarlo, pero al menos parecería que se había volteado sin haber sido hurgado.

"¿Quieres acompañar a Francis a la entrevista que sostendrá con Trent con respecto a la muerte de su secretaria? Es el lunes al mediodía."

Mediodía, pensé. Es una hora bastante segura. No era demasiado temprano para la mayoría de Entremundos. A lo mejor podía seguirlos. Sentí que mis labios de visón trataban de sonreír. No creo que a Francis le importara. Podía ser mi única oportunidad para averiguar algo sobre Trent. Si lograba atraparlo como traficante de azufre pagaría con eso mi contrato.

Jenks voló y se paró sobre el borde de la basura, sus alas moviéndose rítmicamente para conservar el equilibrio. "¿Te importaría si te acompaño para darle una buena olfateada a Trent? Te apuesto que puedo averiguar qué es."

Mis bigotes escudriñaron el aire mientras pensaba en la respuesta. Un segundo par de ojos no me vendrían nada mal. Además, podía viajar en el auto de Francis. Claro que no como un visón. Seguro se pondría a chillar como una bebita y echaría todo a perder si me descubría escondida en el asiento trasero. "Hablamos después," deletreé. "Casa."

Jenks hizo una sonrisa maliciosa. "Antes de irnos...¿te gustaría ver tu archivo?"

Negué con la cabeza. Había visto mi archivo mil veces. "No," escribí. Quiero triturarlo.

Doce

"**N**ecesito un auto," murmuré mientras descendía por la escalerilla. Tiré de mi abrigo que había quedado atrapado entre las puertas y contuve el aire mientras que el motor diesel arrancaba de nuevo y el autobús se alejaba. "Pronto," agregué, colgándome el bolso.

Llevaba varios días durmiendo mal. La sal se había secado por todas partes y sentía que me picaba el cuerpo. Además, no transcurrían cinco minutos sin golpearme la ampolla del cuello. Jenks estaba de mal humor, seguramente porque se le terminó el efecto del azúcar del caramelo. En pocas palabras, éramos los compañeros ideales.

Un falso amanecer trataba de asomarse iluminando el cielo del este, produciendo un hermoso azul traslúcido. Los pájaros cantaban a todo pulmón y las calles estaban en silencio. El frío del aire me hizo dar gracias por el abrigo. Calculé que el sol aún tardaría una hora en salir. Las cuatro de la mañana en el mes de junio era hora dorada. Todos los buenos vampiros estaban acurrucados en sus camas y los humanos sabios aun no asomaban las narices para recoger la edición matutina del periódico. "Yo estoy lista para irme a la cama," murmuré.

"Buenos días, Srta. Morgan," dijo una voz baja. Giré rápidamente y me agaché.

Jenks soltó una carcajada sarcástica desde mi arete. "Es el vecino," dijo secamente.

Me enderecé, pero el corazón me latía fuerte y me sentía tan vieja como debería ser mi aspecto por el hechizo de disfraz. ¿Por qué no está en la cama?

"Buenos días" respondí, avanzando hasta la reja de Keasley. No se mecía en su mecedora, su cara oculta por las sombras.

"¿De compras?" dijo moviendo el pie dándome a entender que había visto mis botas nuevas.

Cansada, me apoyé sobre la reja que estaba asegurada con un candado. "¿Le gustaría un chocolate?" pregunté, y él me hizo señas para que lo siguiera.

Jenks habló algo preocupado. "El alcance de una plasta explosiva es mayor que mi sentido del olfato, Raque."

"Es un hombre viejo solitario," dije, mientras retiraba el candado de la reja. "Quiere un chocolate, y además, yo parezco una vieja arpía. Cualquiera que esté observando pensará que soy su novia." Dejé caer el candado suavemente y me pareció que Keasley escondía una sonrisa detrás de unos bostezos.

Jenks dejó escapar un suspiro dramático. Yo dejé mi bolso en el porche y me senté en el escalón de arriba. Con un movimiento inusual, saqué una bolsita del bolsillo de mi abrigo y se la ofrecí.

"¡Ah!" exclamó, la mirada puesta en el sello del caballito con el jinete. "Hay algunas cosas por las que vale la pena arriesgar la vida." Tomó un chocolate oscuro, tal como yo lo esperaba. Un perro ladró a la distancia. Él masticaba lentamente dirigiendo la mirada hacia la calle silenciosa.

"Estuvo en el centro comercial."

Me encogí de hombros. "Entre otros lugares"

Jenks me ventiló el cuello con sus alas. "Raquel"

"Ya cálmate Jenks," le dije fastidiada.

Keasley se puso de pie con dolorosa lentitud. "No. Él tiene razón. Es tarde."

Definitivamente, los comentarios frívolos de Keasley y el instinto de Jenks me hicieron alarmarme. El perro ladró de nuevo y yo salté. Mi mente regresó a esa montaña de plastas explosivas junto a la puerta. Tal vez debí entrar por el cementerio, disfrazada o no.

Keasley se movió lentamente hacia la puerta. "Tenga cuidado por donde camina, Srta. Morgan. Una vez que se dan cuenta que se les puede escabullir, cambiarán de táctica." Abrió la puerta y entró. El anjeo se cerró sin hacer ruido. "Gracias por el chocolate."

"No hay de qué," susurré mientras me daba vuelta. Se que podía oírme.

"Viejo escalofriante," dijo Jenks, haciendo columpiar mi arete mientras cruzaba la calle en dirección a la motocicleta que estaba estacionada frente a la iglesia. El tenue amanecer brillaba en el cromo y pensé si acaso era la de Ivy que había enviado al taller.

"A lo mejor me deja usarla," dije en voz alta echándole una mirada provocativa al pasar junto a ella. Era brillante y negra, de líneas estilizadas y cuero satinado. Una nave de la noche. ¡Qué ganas! Pasé mi mano envidiosa por el asiento dejando una huella donde antes la cubría el rocío.

"¡Raquel, abajo!" gritó Jenks.

Me tiré y mis manos golpearon el pavimento. El corazón me latía aceleradamente. Algo zumbó por el aire donde yo estaba hacía menos de un segundo. Me subió la adrenalina y me empezó a doler la cabeza. Rodé por el suelo cubriéndome con la moto.

Contuve el aire. Nada se movía entre los arbustos y la maleza crecida. Puse el bolso frente a la cara y con las manos hurgué adentro.

"Quédate abajo," dijo Jenks entre dientes. Su voz era grave y las alas se tornaron color púrpura.

Sin darme cuenta me pinché con el punzón que me hizo saltar de dolor. Luego, invoqué en 4 segundos y medio mi hechizo para hacer dormir—tiempo récord. En realidad no me serviría de mucho si el que me atacaba se quedaba metido entre los arbustos. Tal vez podría lanzarlo. Vaya. Si la S.E. pensaba convertir sus ataques en rutina, a lo mejor valdría la pena invertir en una pistola de plastas. En realidad, mi estilo era enfrentar y dejar a mis enemigos inconscientes y eso de esconderse entre los arbustos me parecía de segunda categoría. Claro que si tienes que atacarlos con sus propias armas...

Sostuve el hechizo de la cuerda para que no me afectara y esperé.

"Guárdalo para otro día," dijo Jenks más tranquilo, a medida que quedamos completamente rodeados por una hueste de niños duendes que zumbaban. Volaban encima de nosotros tan alto y hablaban tan rápido que no logré entender lo que decían.

"Ya se fueron," dijo Jenks. "Discúlpame. Sabía que estaban allí pero..."

"¡¿Sabías que estaban allí?!" exclamé mirándolo desde el piso, sintiendo un fuerte dolor en el cuello. Oí ladrar a un perro y bajé la voz. "¿Y qué demonios se supone que estabas haciendo?"

Hizo una mueca. "Tenía que hacerlos salir."

Me levanté muy molesta. "¡Qué bien! Gracias. Avísame la próxima vez que me uses como carnada." Sacudí mi largo abrigo y me di cuenta de que los chocolates estaban aplastados.

"Vamos, Raque" comenzó diciendo con voz acaramelada zumbándome al oído. "Si te hubiera avisado habrías reaccionado mal y las hadas habrían esperado hasta que yo no estuviera en guardia."

Mi cara se relajó. "¿Hadas?" dije asombrada. A Denon le debe faltar un tornillo. Las hadas son cos-to-sí-si-maaas. A lo mejor le hicieron un descuento por el incidente con el sapo.

"Ya se fueron," siguió Jenks, "pero yo no me quedaría aquí afuera más tiempo. El rumor es que los zorros quieren una nueva oportunidad para atraparte." Se sacó el pañuelo rojo para dárselo a su hijo. "Jax, tú y tus hermanas tendrán la catapulta."

"¡Gracias pa!" El pequeño duendecillo saltó de alegría. Se

amarró el pañuelo rojo a la cintura y junto con otros seis duendecillos zumbaron hacia el otro lado de la calle.

"¡Tengan cuidado!," gritó Jenks. "¡Puede ser una trampa!"

Hadas, pensé, cruzando los brazos y mirando hacia la acera opuesta. ¡Mierda!

Los otros hijos de Jenks flotaban a su alrededor hablando todos al mismo tiempo, jalándolo para que les prestara atención.

"Alguien está con Ivy," dijo Jenks a medida que se elevaba, "pero registra bien. ¿Te importa si lo dejamos así por hoy?"

"No…para nada," repuse mirando la moto. Al fin de cuentas, no era de Ivy. "Ah, y gracias."

Se elevaron como una nube de luciérnagas. Muy cerca estaban Jax y sus hermanas, trabajando juntos transportando una catapulta tan pequeña como ellos. Volaron por lo alto encima de la iglesia con un seco repiqueteo de alas y gritos dejando tras de sí la calle sumida en el silencio del amanecer.

Me di vuelta y subí por las escaleras de piedra. Del otro lado de la calle cayó una cortina frente a la única ventana iluminada. *Se terminó la función. Vete a dormir, Keasley,* pensé, tirando de la pesada puerta para abrirla y deslizándome adentro. La cerré con cuidado y coloqué el pasador. Al menos me sentía mejor a pesar de que estaba segura de que los asesinos de la S.E. no usarían una puerta. *¿Hadas? Denon tenía que estar realmente cabreado.*

Exhalé con preocupación recostándome contra los gruesos maderos, queriendo bloquear el amanecer. Sólo quería tomar un baño y acostarme a dormir. Al cruzar por el santuario vacío escuché el sonido de una suave música de Jazz y la voz enfadada de Ivy que provenían del salón.

"Maldita sea, Kist" oí cuando entraba a oscuras a la cocina. "Si no levantas el trasero de ese asiento ahora mismo, voy a lanzarte al espacio."

"Tranquilízate Tamwood. No voy hacer nada," dijo una

nueva voz. Era masculina, profunda, quejumbrosa, como si quien hablara tuviera derecho a todo. Hice una pausa para remojar mis amuletos usados en la vasija de agua salada que había junto al refrigerador. Aun servían, pero tenía el buen juicio de no dejar amuletos activos dando vueltas por ahí.

La música dejó de sonar repentinamente. "Fuera," dijo Ivy suavemente. "Ahora."

"¿Ivy?," llamé, dejando que la curiosidad me tomara la delantera. Jenks dijo que quienquiera que estuviera aquí estaba limpio. Dejé mi bolso en el mostrador de la cocina y me dirigí hacia el salón. A pesar del cansancio, me sentía un poco molesta. No lo habíamos discutido, pero yo pensaba que mientras hubiera un precio por mi cabeza, trataríamos de llamar poco la atención.

"Ooooh," se burló el invisible Kist. "Ha regresado."

"Compórtate," amenazó Ivy cuando entré al salón, "o te desollaré."

"¿Lo prometes?"

Di tres pasos en el salón y me detuve en seco. Mi ira desapareció arrastrada por una sobrecarga instintiva natural. Un vampiro vestido de cuero se encontraba despatarrado encima del asiento de Ivy, como si estuviera en su casa. Sus botas inmaculadas estaban sobre la mesa de centro y Ivy las empujó molesta. Nunca la había visto moverse tan rápido. Se alejó dos pasos echando chispas, la cintura firme y los brazos cruzados agresivamente. Se escuchaba el tic tac del reloj de la repisa.

Kist no podía ser un vampiro muerto, pues estaba en campo santo y ya casi despuntaba el sol; pero que me parta un rayo si no era fácil confundirlo. Sus pies tocaron el suelo con exagerada lentitud. La mirada indolente que me propinó me llegó hasta la médula y me tensó las tripas. Y, era bien parecido. Peligrosamente hermoso. Mi mente voló hasta la Tabla 6.1 y tragué saliva.

Tenía una barba de tres días que le daba cierto aspecto tosco. Se enderezó quitándose los mechones de pelo rubio de los ojos con tanta gracia que seguramente llevaba años perfeccionando ese movimiento. Su chaqueta de cuero abierta dejaba ver una camiseta negra de algodón apretada sobre el pecho musculoso y atractivo. Aretes colgaban de una oreja. La otra tenía un solo arete y una cicatriz. Aparte de esa, no tenía más cicatrices a la vista. Pensé si acaso podría sentirlas si pasara mi mano por su cuello.

Mi corazón latió aceleradamente y bajé la mirada, prometiéndome no mirarlo de nuevo. Ivy no me asustaba tanto como este. Se movía por instinto salvaje, según su capricho.

"Wow," dijo Kist acomodándose mejor en el asiento. "Es bonita. Debiste decirme que era así de lii-nnn-daa." Sentí como respiraba profundo, saboreando la noche. "Y apesta a tí, Ivy bella... ¿no es dulce?"

Helada, agarré el cuello de mi abrigo y retrocedí hasta detenerme bajo el umbral.

"Raquel, este es Kisten. Ya se va. ¿Verdad Kist?"

Aquello no era una pregunta. Contuve el aire mientras que se levantaba con la fluidez y gracia de un animal. Kist se estiró, sus manos buscando el techo. Su cuerpo delgado se movía como una cuerda mostrando la hermosura de cada uno de sus músculos. No pude evitar mirarlo. Sus brazos cayeron y nuestros ojos se encontraron. Los suyos eran pardos. Sonrió levemente, pues sabía que lo estaba observando. Tenía los dientes afilados, como Ivy. No era un demonio. Era un vampiro vivo. Miré para otro lado, a pesar de que los vampiros vivos no pueden arrastrar a quienes son precavidos. "¿Te gustan los vampiros, brujita?," suspiró.

Su voz era agradable y mis rodillas flaquearon ante la coacción con la que dijo esas palabras. "No puedes tocarme," respondí, sin dejar de mirarlo. Trataba de arrastrarme. Mi voz sonaba como si me saliera de la cabeza. "No he firmado papeles."

"¿No?," susurró, alzando las cejas con confianza seductora. Se acercó más con paso silencioso. Con el corazón martillándome, miré hacia la puerta buscando el marco con las manos. Él era más fuerte y más rápido que yo; pero un rodillazo en la entrepierna lo haría caer al suelo como a cualquier hombre.

"A las cortes no les importa," dijo mientras seguía acercándose. "Ya estás muerta."

Abrí grande los ojos cuando lo tuve a mi lado. Su fragancia me invadió—húmeda fragancia a tierra. Me estallaba el pulso y di un paso al frente. Su mano cálida me tomó la quijada. Una descarga me recorrió el cuerpo doblándome las rodillas. Me agarró el codo y me apretó contra el pecho. La expectativa de una promesa desconocida me aceleró la sangre. Me incliné hacia él, y esperé. Sus labios se movieron y musitó unas palabras que no pude entender, bellas y oscuras.

"¡Kist!," gritó Ivy sorprendiéndonos a ambos. Un relámpago de ira cruzó por sus ojos y luego desapareció.

Mi voluntad empezó a retornar dolorosamente. Traté de zafarme, pero estaba atrapada. Olía a sangre. "¡Suéltame!"

Me soltó y se volteó hacia Ivy, olvidándose de mí por completo. Retrocedí pasando por el umbral, temblando, incapaz de irme voluntariamente hasta que me di cuenta de que ya no estaba.

Kist estaba parado frente a Ivy, calmado y sereno, indiferente a la agitación de Ivy. "Ivy, amor, ¿por qué te atormentas? Tu aroma la cubre a ella, pero su sangre aun está pura. ¿Cómo puedes resistir? Lo está pidiendo. Lo está pidiendo a gritos. Se quejará y gemirá la primera vez, pero al final te lo agradecerá."

Su expresión se volvió tímida. Suavemente, se mordió el labio y los recorrió deliberadamente con su lengua tentadora. Mi respiración sonó áspera, inclusive a mis oídos, y la contuve.

Ivy estaba furiosa. Sus ojos se convirtieron en esferas negras. La tensión no me dejaba respirar. Los grillos del jardín chirriaban más rápidamente. Con exagerada lentitud, Kist se inclinó cuidadosamente hacia Ivy. "Si no quieres abrirla" dijo con voz suave y llena de expectativa, "dámela a mí. Te la devolveré." Sus labios se abrieron dejando ver sus brillantes colmillos. "Palabra de scout."

La respiración de Ivy era agitada. Su cara era una mezcla irreal de odio y lujuria. Podía ver su lucha por sobreponerse al apetito y observé fascinada y aterrada cómo se desvanecía, permaneciendo tan sólo el odio. "¡Fuera de aquí!" dijo, con la voz ronca y temblorosa.

Kist suspiró lentamente. Yo pude respirar otra vez. Tomé rápidas y cortas bocanadas de aire mientras que mis ojos saltaban del uno al otro. Ya había pasado. Ivy ganó. ¿Estaría yo a salvo?

"Es una estupidez, Tamwood," dijo Kist mientras se ajustaba su chaqueta de cuero negro con movimientos cuidadosamente serenos. "El desperdicio de algo bueno a cambio de algo que no existe."

Con pasos abruptos y veloces, Ivy se dirigió a la puerta trasera. Un hilillo de sudor bajó por mi espalda al sentir la brisa que formó a su paso. El frío aire de la mañana inundó el salón reemplazando a la oscuridad que pareció haberse instalado adentro. "Es mía," dijo Ivy, como si yo no estuviera allí. "Está bajo mi protección. Lo que yo haga o no haga con ella es asunto mío. Dile a Piscary que si vuelvo a ver a una de sus sombras en mi iglesia, asumiré que está poniendo en tela de juicio lo que me pertenece. Pregúntale si quiere guerra conmigo, Kist. Pregúntale eso."

Kist pasó en medio de las dos, deteniéndose un instante bajo el umbral. "No puedes ocultar tu apetito por ella para siempre," dijo Kist. Ivy apretó los labios. "Una vez que ella te vea, correrá; entonces será presa libre." Instantáneamente pareció desanimarse. Sus facciones se suavizaron con su cara de niño regañado. "Regresa," dijo con inocencia dulzona. "Puedes volver a tu antiguo lugar, pero solamente si accedes a una pequeña concesión. Ella es sólo una bruja. Ni siquiera sabes si ella…"

"¡Fuera!" interrumpió Ivy, señalando hacia afuera.

Kist salió por la puerta. "Una oferta rechazada trae enemigos funestos."

"Y una oferta semejante, avergüenza a quien la hace."

Encogiéndose de hombros, sacó un gorro de cuero del bolsillo trasero y se lo puso. Me miró con ojos hambrientos. "Hasta pronto, mi amor," suspiró. Me estremecí como si hubiera rozado mi mejilla con su mano. No sabría decir si sentí repulsión o deseo. Ya se había marchado.

Ivy tiró la puerta. Con la misma gracia escalofriante, cruzó la sala y se tumbó en un asiento. Su cara estaba llena de ira y me quedé mirándola. *Mierda, estaba viviendo con un vampiro.* Activa o no, ella era un vampiro. ¿Qué dijo Kist? ¿Que Ivy estaba desperdiciando el tiempo? ¿Que yo saldría corriendo cuando viera su apetito? ¿Que yo era suya? *¡Mierda!*

Lentamente, salí del salón caminando de espaldas. Ivy me miró y me quedé estática. La ira desapareció de su cara y la reemplazó por alarma cuando se dio cuenta de mi temor.

Parpadeé. Mi garganta se cerró y le di la espalda, dirigiéndome hacia el pasillo.

"Raquel, espera," me dijo con voz dulce. "Lamento lo de Kist. Yo no lo invité. Simplemente apareció."

Seguí hacia el pasillo, tensa y lista para explotar si llegaba a tocarme. ¿Fue por eso que Ivy decidió renunciar conmigo? No podía cazarme legalmente pero, como dijo Kist, a las cortes no les importa.

"Raquel..."

Estaba justo detrás de mí y giré súbitamente. Mi estómago dio un vuelco. Ivy dio tres pasos hacia atrás. Fueron tan veloces que no estaba segura si realmente se había movido. Alzó las manos para apaciguarme y demostraba su preocupación con el ceño fruncido. Sentí el pulso dandome martillazos, jaqueca. "¿Qué quieres?" le pregunté, esperando que me mintiera diciendo que todo había sido una equivocación. Desde afuera llegó el ruido de la moto de Kist. La observé mientras el ruido del motor se hacía cada vez más distante.

"Nada," dijo, sus ojos pardos fijos en los míos. "No escuches a Kist. Él solo te quiere confundir. Coquetea con lo que no puede obtener."

"¡Así es!," grité para no comenzar a temblar. "Yo soy tuya. Eso fue lo que tú dijiste, que soy tuya. ¡Yo no soy de nadie, Ivy! ¡Maldición, aléjate de mí!"

Sorprendida, movió los labios. "¿Oíste eso?"

"¡Claro que lo oí!" grité. La ira pudo más que mi temor y di un paso adelante. "¿Es así como tú eres de verdad?" le dije, señalando el salón. "¿Como ese…ese animal? ¿Eres así? ¿Me estás cazando Ivy? ¿El juego es llenarte la panza con mi sangre? ¿Acaso sabe mejor cuando lo haces traicionando? ¿Sí?"

"¡No!" exclamó turbada. "Raquel…yo"

"¡Me mentiste!" le grité. "Él me arrastró. Me dijiste que un vampiro vivo no podía hacerlo, a menos que yo quisiera …y por todos los infiernos…¡ten la seguridad de que yo no quería!"

No respondió. Su sombra se reflejaba en las paredes del pasillo. Podía oír su respiración y percibir su agridulce y penetrante olor a ceniza húmeda y madera de secoya: nuestros aromas se mezclaban peligrosamente. Su postura era tensa y su inmovilidad me electrizaba el cuerpo. Sentí la boca seca y di un paso hacia atrás al caer en la cuenta de que le estaba gritando a un vampiro. La adrenalina se fue extinguiendo. Sentí náusea y frío. "Me mentiste," dije entre suspiros retrocediendo hacia la cocina. Sí, me había mentido. Papá tenía razón. No confíes en nadie. Ahora empacaría mis cosas para irme.

Los pasos de Ivy resonaban fuertemente a mis espaldas. Era obvio que golpeaba el suelo lo suficientemente duro para hacer ruido, pero yo estaba demasiado airada para prestarle atención.

"¿Qué haces?" me preguntó al ver que abría un gabinete para descolgar un manojo de hechizos de un gancho y meterlos en mi bolso.

"Me voy."

"¡No puedes! Ya oíste a Kist. ¡Te están esperando!"

"Prefiero morir conociendo a mis enemigos que morir durmiendo inocentemente junto a ellos," repliqué, dándome cuenta de que era una de las frases más estúpidas que había dicho. No tenía sentido.

Me detuve de repente cuando ella se deslizó frente a mí y cerró el gabinete.

"Quítate de mi camino," dije amenazante pero con voz baja para que no se diera cuenta que temblaba.

Se veía consternada y frunció el ceño. Me pareció totalmente humana y eso me asustaba hasta la médula. Justo cuando comenzaba a entenderla, comenzaba a actuar de esta manera.

Con mis hechizos y punzones fuera de mi alcance, estaba indefensa. Ella podía lanzarme contra la pared del otro lado del cuarto y romperme la cabeza contra el horno. Podía romperme las piernas para que no pudiera correr. Podía atarme a una silla y desangrarme. Pero todo lo que hizo fue quedarse ahí parada con una mirada de dolor y frustración en su cara pálida y perfectamente ovalada. "Puedo explicarlo," dijo en voz baja.

Luché contra el temblor al encontrarme con su mirada. "¿Qué es lo que quieres de mí?" susurré.

"No te he mentido," siguió, sin responder mi pregunta. "Kist es el descendiente elegido por Piscary. Casi siempre Kist es sólo Kist; pero Piscary puede..." Dudó. La miré y cada músculo de mi cuerpo pedía a gritos salir corriendo. Pero si yo me movía, ella se movería. "Piscary es más viejo que el polvo," dijo secamente. "Es lo suficientemente poderoso para hacer que Kist vaya a los lugares donde él ya no puede ir."

"Es un sirviente," solté. "El maldito lacayo de un vampiro muerto. Le hace las compras a la luz del día y le lleva humanos a papi Piscary para que se alimente."

Ivy hizo un gesto. Estaba menos tensa y asumió una actitud más relajada—aun entre mis hechizos y yo. "Es un gran honor que le pidan ser sirviente de un vampiro como Piscary. Pero no todo es unilateral. Gracias a ello, Kist tiene más poder del que debe tener un vampiro vivo. Por eso pudo arrastrarte. Pero Raquel" se apuró a continuar cuando quise decir algo, "yo no se lo hubiera permitido."

¿Y se supone que por eso debería estar contenta? ¿Porque no me quieres compartir? Mi pulso se había calmado y me hundí en un asiento. No creo que mis rodillas me aguantaran más. No sabía si mi debilidad se debía a la adrenalina usada o al aire cargado de feromonas que exhalaba Ivy. *¡Maldición, maldición, maldición!* Estaba hundida hasta la coronilla, especialmente si Piscary estaba metido en esto.

Se decía que era uno de los vampiros más viejos de Cincinnati. No se metía en problemas y mantenía a su gente a raya. Trabajaba dentro del sistema, ni más ni menos, y cumplía con toda la documentación, asegurándose de que cada captura hecha por su gente fuese legal. Era mucho más que el simple propietario de un restaurante. La política de la S.E. con este vampiro mayor era "no preguntes, no hables." Era uno de esos personajes que mencioné antes que se movía en los círculos ocultos de poder; pero mientras que pagara cumplidamente los impuestos y mantuviera al día su licencia para comprar de licores, no había nada que se pudiera hacer—y que nadie quisiera hacer. Pero si un vampiro parecía inofensivo, era sólo porque era más inteligente que los demás.

Miré a Ivy, parada con los brazos cruzados como si estuviera molesta. *Dios santo . . . ¿qué estaba haciendo aquí?*

"¿Cuál es tu relación con Piscary?," le pregunté con vos trémula.

"Ninguna," respondió. Hice una mueca de burla. "Es cierto," insistió. "Es un amigo de la familia."

"El tío Piscary ¿eh?," dije sarcásticamente.

"A decir verdad, eso es más preciso de lo que te imaginas. Piscary fundó la línea de sangre de vampiros vivos de mi madre en el siglo dieciocho."

"Y los ha estado desangrando lentamente desde entonces," agregué de nuevo con sarcasmo.

"No es así," repuso un poco molesta. "Piscary nunca me ha tocado. Es como un segundo padre."

"A lo mejor está dejando añejar la sangre en la botella."

Ivy pasó una mano por su pelo con inusual preocupación. "No es así. Créeme."

"Qué bueno," dije poniendo mis codos sobre la mesa. ¿Ahora tenía que preocuparme por un lacayo que poseía el poder de su maestro invadiendo mi iglesia? ¿Por qué no me lo dijo antes? Yo no iba a jugar este juego si las reglas iban a cambiar constantemente.

"¿Qué quieres de mí?," pregunté de nuevo, temiendo que me respondiera y me viera obligada a irme.

"Nada."

"Mentirosa," repuse; pero cuando levanté la cabeza ya no estaba.

Volví a respirar normalmente. El corazón me latía fuertemente dentro del pecho y me quedé allí parada, con los brazos cruzados, observando las paredes y los gabinetes vacíos. Odiaba que me hiciera eso. Don Pez movía sus aletas en el agua. Tampoco estaba a gusto.

Lentamente y de mala gana, guardé mis hechizos de nuevo. Pensé en el reciente ataque de las hadas en las escalinatas de la iglesia, las plastas explosivas de los zorros arrimadas junto a la puerta trasera y en las palabras de Kist sobre vampiros que esperaban a que estuviera sin la protección de Ivy. Estaba atrapada e Ivy lo sabía.

Trece

Le di unos golpecitos desde afuera a la ventana del pasajero del auto de Francis llamando a Jenks. "¿Qué hora es?" pregunté en voz baja, pues hasta los suspiros formaban eco en el estacionamiento. Seguramente las cámaras me estaban grabando pero nadie revisaba las películas, a menos que alguien se quejara de algún robo.

Jenks saltó de la visera y oprimió el botón que abría la ventanilla automática. "Las once y quince," dijo mientras bajaba la ventana. "¿Crees que hayan reprogramado la entrevista con Kalamack?"

Giré la cabeza y miré por encima de los autos hacia las puertas del ascensor. "No, pero si me demoran, me voy a cabrear." Me acomodé un poco la falda. Por fortuna el amigo de Jenks me había traído mi ropa y algunas joyas ayer. Todo estaba colgado ordenadamente en hileras o en montoncitos bien organizados dentro del clóset. Verla ahí me hacía sentirme un poco mejor. El tipo había hecho un buen trabajo lavando, secando y doblando todo y me puse a pensar cuánto cobraría por lavarme la ropa todas las semanas.

Encontrar ropa que fuera conservadora pero a la vez provocativa había sido más difícil de lo que imaginaba. Al final me decidí por una faldita roja, mallas sencillas y una blusa blanca de botones que podía abrirse o cerrarse, según la necesidad. Mis aretes de argolla eran demasiado pequeños para que Jenks pudiera posarse. Naturalmente, se quejó de su tamaño por media hora. Tenía el pelo recogido encima de la cabeza y un par de zapatos rojos de tacones. Parecía una estudiante desenfadada. El hechizo de disfraz servía de alguna ayuda. De nuevo era una morena de nariz grande apestando a perfume de lavanda. Francis me reconocería... y justamente quería que sucediera eso.

Me saqué nerviosamente la tierra de las uñas, prometiéndome cuidarlas. El esmalte rojo había desaparecido cuando me transformé en visón. "¿Me veo bien Jenks?," le pregunté mientras coqueteaba con mi collar.

"Sí. Muy bien."

"Ni siquiera me miraste," me quejé. Sonó la campana del ascensor. "A lo mejor es él," dije. "¿Tienes lista la poción?"

"Sólo tengo que darle vuelta a la tapa y le caerá encima."

Jenks subió la ventanilla y voló a esconderse. Yo había colocado un frasco de "hora de dormir" entre la visera y el techo. Sin embargo, Francis pensaría que se trataba de algo más siniestro. Era para ayudarlo a convencerse de dejarme a mí adelantar la entrevista con Kalamack. Secuestrar a un hombre adulto, por más tonto que fuera, era un asunto complicado. No podía sencillamente dejarlo sin sentido y meterlo en el maletero. Si lo dejaba ahí tirado inconsciente, cualquiera lo encontraría y me atraparían.

Jenks y yo habíamos aguardado una hora en el estacionamiento haciéndole algunas modificaciones pequeñas pero significativas a su auto deportivo. Jenks se demoró apenas unos instantes cortando la alarma y "arreglando" el seguro de la puerta del conductor y de la ventanilla. Y, aun cuando yo tenía que esperar a Francis afuera del auto, mi bolso ya se encontraba metido debajo del asiento del pasajero.

A Francis le habían dado un lindo auto: un convertible rojo con asientos de cuero. Tenía doble control de clima. Los vidrios podían polarizarse—lo sé porque los probé. Hasta tenía un teléfono celular—cuyas pilas ahora estaban en mi bolso. La placa personalizada decía: ATRAPADO. El bendito auto tenía mil cosas. Sólo le hacía falta despegar. Y todavía olía a nuevo. ¿Un soborno o dinero por su silencio?, pensé sintiendo celos.

La luz indicadora del ascensor se apagó. Me agaché detrás de un pilote esperando que fuera Francis. Lo último que quería era llegar tarde. Mi pulso se estabilizó en un ritmo rápido que ya me era familiar y sonreí al reconocer los pasos rápidos de Francis. Venía solo. Sacó un ramillete de llaves y luego se sorprendió cuando el auto no produjo su acostumbrado pito de bienvenida al desactivarse la alarma. Sentí un cosquilleo de emoción en la punta de los dedos. Esto sería divertido.

La puerta del auto se abrió y yo le di la vuelta por un lado. Simultáneamente, Francis y yo nos sentamos cada uno a un lado, cerrando las puertas al mismo tiempo.

"¿Qué demonios?" exclamó Francis, cayendo en la cuenta que tenía compañía. Sus pequeños ojos me miraban y se quitaba el pelo que le caía en la cara. "¡Raquel!" dijo, asombrado y perdiendo toda la confianza. "Estás muerta."

Trató de abrir la puerta pero yo estiré el brazo tomándolo por la muñeca y mandándole una señal a Jenks. El duende hizo una mueca. Agitaba las alas emocionado acariciando el frasco de poción. Francis se puso lívido. "Atrapado," susurré soltándolo y cerrando las puertas con seguro desde mi lado. "Te tengo."

"¿Qué…eh…qué estás haciendo?" tartamudeó Francis, pálido tras su sucia barbilla.

Sonreí. "Me estoy apoderando de tu misión…la entrevista de Kalamack; y tú acabas de ofrecerte de voluntario para conducir."

Se puso serio y dejó exhibir algo de su petulancia. "Por qué no te vas de Giro" repuso, con la mirada fija en Jenks y la poción. "Por ejemplo, haz magia negra y comete algún error fatal. Ahora mismo te voy a atrapar."

Jenks emitió un sonido de disgusto e inclinó el frasco. "¡Aguarda Jenks!" grité, arremetiendo sobre el asiento, casi encima de Francis. Pasé mi brazo derecho alrededor de la escuálida tráquea del hombre y lo presioné contra el asiento en una llave que no le permitía moverse. Sus dedos me apretaron el brazo, pero no me hacía daño. Comenzó a sudar mojando su chaqueta y el olor me pareció peor aun que el de mi perfume. "¡Idiota!," le dije entre dientes a Francis en el oído y mirando a Jenks. "¿Sabes qué es eso colgando encima de tus piernas? ¿Se te ha ocurrido pensar que podría ser irreversible?"

Sudando, agitó la cabeza. Yo me acerqué aún más, a pesar de que la palanca de cambios se me enterraba en la cintura. "Tu no prepararías nada fatal," me dijo, su voz más aguda que de costumbre.

Jenks se quejó desde el retrovisor. "Vamos Raque, déjame hechizarlo. Yo te puedo indicar cómo manejar un auto de cambios."

Me apretó más fuerte el brazo con los dedos. El dolor me hizo reaccionar apretándolo más todavía contra el asiento. "¡Insecto!" exclamó Francis, "¡eres un…" Sus palabras se cortaron pues le apreté el cuello con el brazo.

"¿¡Insecto!?" exclamó Jenks enfurecido. "Apestoso… mis pedos huelen mejor que tú. ¿Te crees mejor que yo? ¿Pastelito de manzanas? ¡Llamarme insecto! ¡Déjamelo Raquel! ¡Déjamelo ya!"

"No," respondí suavemente. El fastidioso de Francis ya empezaba a hartarme de verdad. "Estoy segura de que Francis y yo podemos llegar a un acuerdo. Todo lo que quiero es que me lleve hasta la hacienda de Trent y a la entrevista. Francis no se meterá en problemas. Es una víctima ¿verdad?" Le sonreí socarronamente a Jenks esperando que aguantara su ira por haber sido insultado y que no le aplicara el somnífero a Francis todavía. "No lo harás desaparecer después Jenks, ¿me oyes? No matas al buey después de arar el campo. A lo mejor puedes usarlo la próxima primavera." Me recosté contra Francis respirándole en el oído. "¿No es cierto, muñeco?"

Asintió como pudo y lo solté lentamente. No le quitaba de encima la mirada a Jenks. "Atrévete a tocar a mi socio y ese frasco caerá sobre ti. Manejas demasiado aprisa, el frasco caerá. Tratas de llamar la atención..."

"y haré que te bañes en él" interrumpió Jenks, su voz juguetona ahora grave y rabiosa. "Repítelo y te hechizaré de lo lindo" dijo riendo y con malicia, "¿oíste *Francina?*"

Francis cerró los ojos un instante y se acomodó de nuevo en el asiento, arreglándose el cuello de su camisa blanca antes de arremangarse la chaqueta hasta los codos y tomar el volante. Le di gracias a Dios porque Francis había dejado su camisa hawaiana en casa por respeto a Kalamack.

Con la cara tensa, metió las llaves en la ranura del arranque y encendió el motor. La música retumbó y me hizo saltar. La brusquedad con la que giró el volante e hizo el cambio indicaba obviamente que no se había rendido aun. Iba a jugar el juego hasta que hallara la manera de salirse. A mí no me importaba. Todo lo que necesitaba era sacarlo de la ciudad. Después, Francis dormiría una buena siesta.

"No te saldrás con la tuya," me dijo, sonando como una película mediocre. Agitó su permiso de parqueo frente a la rejilla automática y salimos a la luz brillante y el tráfico del mediodía con la canción "Boys of Summer" de Don Henley a todo dar. Si no estuviera metida en este lío, tal vez lo estaría disfrutando.

"¿No podías ponerte un poco más de ese perfume, Raquel?" dijo Francis con tal desprecio que se le retorcía la cara, "¿o lo usas para tapar el hedor de tu insecto mascota?"

"¡Cállalo!" gritó Jenks. "Si no lo haces, lo haré yo."

Esto era estúpido. "Haz lo que quieras, Jenks," le dije mientras bajaba el volumen de la música. "Lo único que no dejes que esa poción lo toque."

Jenks hizo una mueca y comenzó a volar alrededor de Francis. El polvillo de duende comenzó a caer sobre Francis. él no lo veía, pero yo si podía verlo desde mi puesto pues se reflejaba con el sol. Francis comenzó a rascarse detrás de la oreja.

"¿Cuánto dura?" le pregunté a Jenks.

"Unos veinte minutos."

Jenks tenía razón. Cuando salimos de entre los edificios y pasamos por los suburbios directo hacia el campo, Francis no daba pie con bola. No se quedaba quieto. Sus comentarios eran cada vez peores y la rasquiña cada vez más intensa. Finalmente, saqué la cinta adhesiva y lo amenacé con sellarle la boca. Le habían salido verdugones rojos donde la ropa le tocaba la piel y supuraban un líquido transparente, como si padeciera de envenenamiento con hiedra venenosa. Cuando llegamos a campo abierto se rascaba tanto que mantener el auto sobre la vía era un verdadero reto. Lo estuve observando cuidadosamente. Manejar un auto mecánico no parecía tan difícil.

"Tú, *insecto*" dijo gruñendo, "también me hiciste esto el sábado, ¿verdad?"

"Lo voy a conjurar," dijo Jenks. Sentí el agudo timbre de su voz hasta en los ojos.

Cansada de todo esto le hablé a Francis. "Muy bien muñeco, acércate a la orilla."

Francis parpadeó. "¿Qué?"

Idiota, pensé. "¿Cuánto más crees que puedo controlar a Jenks si continúas insultándolo? ¡A la orilla!" Francis miró nerviosamente hacia mi lado. No habíamos visto ningún auto durante las últimas cinco millas. "¡Dije *a la orilla!*" grité. Condujo el auto a la orilla y manejó sobre la polvorienta gravilla. Apagué el motor y saqué las llaves. Nos detuvimos con una fuerte sacudida y mi cabeza golpeó el retrovisor. "¡Afuera!" ordené, desactivando el seguro de las puertas.

"¿Qué? ¿Aquí?" Francis era un niño de ciudad. Pensó que lo haría regresar caminando. Claro, la idea era tentadora, pero no podía correr el riesgo de que alguien lo recogiera o que lograra encontrar un teléfono. Se bajó rapidamente y entendí por qué cuando comenzó a rascarse. Abrí la cajuela y la carita delgada de Francis se puso blanca.

"Olvídalo," dijo, alzando sus brazos escuálidos. "No voy a meterme ahí."

Sentí un chichón en la frente por el golpe que acababa de darme. "Métete a la cajuela o te voy a enseñar cómo te transformo en visón para luego hacer una orejeras contigo." Vi como pensaba en lo que acababa de decirle preguntándome si se echaría a correr. Tal vez me hubiera gustado que lo hiciera. Sería un placer vencerlo otra vez. La última vez había sido hace dos días. De alguna forma lo metería en esa cajuela.

"Corre," dijo Jenks volando en círculos encima de él con el frasco. "Vamos. Atrévete, apestoso."

Francis se desinfló. "Vaya, cuánto te gustaría eso, ¿verdad insecto?," dijo con sorna. Pero se acercó mucho a mí y ni siquiera tuve problemas para inmovilizarle las manos con cinta adhesiva. Ambos sabíamos que podía soltarse con suficiente tiempo; pero su actitud prepotente desapareció tan pronto vio que yo alzaba la mano y que Jenks aterrizaba sobre ella con el frasco.

"Dijiste que no lo harías," tartamudeó. "¡Dijiste que me convertiría en un visón!"

"Te mentí. Las dos veces."

Francis me lanzó una mirada que parecía una bomba. "Esto no lo olvidaré," me dijo apretando los dientes. Así se veía más ridículo que con sus botas chillonas y sus pantalones anchos. "Yo mismo te atraparé."

"Eso espero," le dije sonriendo, y dejé caer el contenido del frasco en su cabeza.

"Felices sueños."

Abrió la boca para agregar algo pero su mandíbula quedó inmovibilizada tan pronto lo tocó el fragante líquido. Observé fascinada cómo se dormía en medio del aroma de hojas de lilas y laurel. Satisfecha, cerré la cajuela.

Luego me senté un poco tensa tras el volante acomodando bien el asiento y los retrovisores. Nunca antes había conducido un auto mecánico, pero si Francis podía hacerlo, era obvio que yo también podía.

"Pon primera," dijo Jenks, sentado en el retrovisor y modelando los movimientos que tenía que hacer. "Luego, aprieta el acelerador más de lo que creas necesario y suelta el embrague."

Con cuidado moví la palanca de cambios y arranqué el motor.

"¿Y? ¿Qué esperamos?"

Apreté el acelerador y solté el embrague. El auto saltó hacia atrás golpeando un árbol. Asustada, quité los pies de los pedales y el auto se apagó. Estaba confundida, pero Jenks estalló en risas. "Pusiste reverso, bruja" dijo, saltando por la ventana.

Lo observé a través del retrovisor mientras evaluaba los daños. "¿Es grave?" le pregunté.

"Está bien," repuso. Me sentí un poco mejor. "En un par de meses ni siquiera podrás ver dónde le pegaste. Eso sí, rompiste una de las luces traseras."

"Oh," dije, al darme cuenta que la primera frase se refería al árbol, no al auto. Estaba nerviosa pero moví la palanca hacia adelante, encendí el motor y arrancamos. Estábamos en camino.

Catorce

Jenks resultó ser un maestro relativamente pasable, gritando advertencias por la ventanilla mientras yo practicaba arrancando con el auto detenido hasta adquirir algo de habilidad. Pero mi seguridad desapareció tan pronto giré para entrar a la hacienda de Kalamack y tuve que reducir la velocidad en la garita de seguridad de la entrada. Era baja con el aspecto de una cárcel. Arbustos de muy buen gusto y un muro bajo escondían el sistema de seguridad que evitaba entrar sin ser visto.

"¿Y cómo has pensado pasar por aquí?" preguntó Jenks, volando para esconderse encima del visor.

"Eso no es problema," repuse, mi mente dando vueltas. De repente me acordé de que Francis venía en la cajuela, así es que le regalé al guardia mi mejor sonrisa y detuve el auto delante de la barrera blanca que nos cerraba el paso. El amuleto junto al reloj del guardia permaneció en verde. Era un control de hechizos mucho más barato que los lentes con aros de madera que dejaban ver a través de los encantamientos. Tuve la precaución de usar poca magia en mi hechizo de disfraz. Mientras que su amuleto estuviera verde, pensaría que mi hechizo era simplemente un maquillaje vanidoso, pero no un disfraz.

"Soy Francine," le dije. Alcé la voz sonriendo como una estúpida, como si hubiera pasado toda la noche sembrando azufre. "Tengo una cita con el Sr. Kalamack." Para parecer más tonta, empecé a jugar con un mechón de pelo. Hoy era morena. "¿Llegué atrasada?," pregunté, zafándome el dedo del nudo que accidentalmente me había hecho en el pelo. "No pensé que me tomara tanto tiempo llegar. ¡Vive tan lejos!"

El guardia no se inmutó. A lo mejor ya estaba perdiendo mi atractivo. O tal vez debí desabotonar otro botón más de la blusa. A lo mejor le gustaban los hombres. Revisó su lista y luego me miró.

"Soy de la S.E.," le dije, con un tono entre petulante y fastidioso. "¿Quiere ver mi identificación?" Hurgue en mi bolso por la inexistente identificación.

"Sra., su nombre no está en la lista" dijo el guardia con cara de estatua.

Giré la cabeza. "Oh, no... ¿de nuevo ese tipo me inscribió como Francis? ¡Demonios!" exclamé, golpeando el volante con el puño. "Siempre hace lo mismo desde que me negué a salir con él. En serio. ¡Ni siquiera tenía auto! Quería llevarme al cine en autobús... por-fa-vo-o-o-o-r," gemí. "¿Me imagina en un autobús?"

"Un momento Sra." Alzó el teléfono y comenzó a hablar. Esperé, tratando de conservar mi estúpida sonrisa, y recé. Su cabeza asintió inconscientemente, pero su expresión parecía vacía cuando dio la vuelta.

"Siga directo," me dijo. Hice un esfuerzo por mantenerme tranquila. "Es el tercer edificio a su derecha. Puede estacionar en el estacionamiento de visitantes, justo al frente de las escalinatas."

"Gracias," repuse cantando alegremente. Arranqué con dificultad tan pronto se levantó la barrera blanca. Lo ví regresar a su garita por el retrovisor. "Como quitarle un dulce a un niño," murmuré.

"Salir puede ser más difícil," repuso Jenks secamente.

Debía conducir tres millas en medio de un bosque fantasmagórico. Mi buen humor se fue apaciguando a medida que el camino serpenteaba en medio de tantos centinelas silenciosos. A pesar de que todo me parecía muy antiguo, tuve la sensación de que todo estaba planeado, inclusive la cascada de agua que había junto a una curva. Un poco desilusionada, continué y el bosque artificial comenzó a ser menos denso hasta convertirse en un pastizal. Llegamos a un segundo camino, más concurrido. Aparentemente llegamos por la parte de atrás. Seguí el tráfico desviándome en el aviso que decía ESTACIONAMIENTO PARA VISITANTES. Una curva y ahí estaba. La hacienda Kalamack.

La gigantesca construcción que parecía una fortaleza era una extraña combinación de arquitectura moderna y tradicional, muy elegante, con puertas de vidrio y ángeles en los canalones. Las rocas grises estaban matizadas por árboles viejos y camas de flores. Otros edificios más pequeños la rodeaban, pero el principal tenía tres pisos de alto. Detuve el auto en uno de los espacios para visitantes. El elegante auto que estaba estacionada al lado hacía parecer el de Francis como un premio de caja de cereal.

Dejé caer el racimo de llaves de Francis en mi bolso y observé al jardinero que cuidaba los arbustos rodeando el estacionamiento. "¿Todavía quieres que nos separemos?," pregunté, acomodando el espejo retrovisor para arreglarme el pelo. "No me gustó lo que pasó allá en la entrada."

Jenks voló hasta pararse en la palanca de cambios, con las manos en la cintura como Peter Pan. "¿Tu entrevista dura los cuarenta minutos usuales?" preguntó. "Yo terminaré en veinte. Si no estoy aquí cuando termines, espérame más o menos a una milla de la entrada. Yo te alcanzo."

"Seguro," le dije, cerrando la cuerda de mi bolso. El jardinero usaba zapatos, no botas, y estaban limpios. ¿Qué jardinero tiene los zapatos limpios? "Ten cuidado," dije, señalando con la quijada al pequeño hombre. "Hay algo que huele mal."

Jenks rió. "El día que no pueda eludir a un jardinero me meteré a panadero."

"Bueno, entonces...deséame suerte." Le abrí la ventanilla a Jenks y salí del auto. Mis tacones sonaban rítmicamente al acercarme a revisar el golpe en la cajuela del auto de

Francis. Tal como lo dijo Jenks, una de las luces traseras se había roto y además estaba hundido. Di media vuelta sintiéndome culpable. Respiré profundamente y subí por las escalinatas angostas hacia las puertas dobles.

Un hombre apareció de un recoveco cuando me aproximaba y me detuve en seco. Era tan alto que se necesitaba mirarlo dos veces para verlo del todo. Y flaco. Me recordó a un refugiado europeo del post-Giro: formal, correcto y estirado. El hombre tenía nariz de halcón y el ceño permanentemente fruncido. Su pelo era gris en las sienes, aun cuando todo el resto era de color negro carbón. Su discreto pantalón gris y camisa blanca de oficina le venían perfectamente. Yo me acomodé el cuello de la blusa. "¿Srta. Francine Percy?," dijo con una sonrisa vacía y una voz ligeramente sarcástica.

"Sí. Hola," repuse adrede, dándole al hombre una buena sacudida de mano. Se estiró molesto. "Tengo una cita al mediodía con el Sr. Kalamack."

"Yo soy el asesor de publicidad del Sr. Kalamack, Jonathan," dijo el hombre. Además de cuidar exageradamente su pronunciación, no tenía acento alguno. "¿Tendría la amabilidad de acompañarme? El Sr. Kalamack la recibirá en su oficina al fondo." Parpadeó y sus ojos se aguaron. Pensé que sería el efecto de mi perfume. Tal vez me puse demasiado, pero por nada me arriesgaría a incitar los instintos de Ivy.

Jonathan me abrió la puerta indicándome que siguiera adelante. Caminé y me llamó la atención ver que el edificio era más claro adentro que afuera. Yo esperaba encontrarme en la residencia privada, pero esta no lo era. La entrada parecía la de cualquier negocio próspero, con el típico diseño de mármol y vidrio. El techo estaba sostenido por columnas blancas. Había un gran escritorio de caoba en medio de dos escaleras que conducían al segundo y tercer piso. La luz entraba por todas partes. O bien provenía del techo, o Trent gastaba una fortuna en bombillas de luz natural. Una suave y mullida alfombra verde silenciaba mis pasos. Se sentía el murmullo de conversaciones y un flujo lento pero permanente de personas en su rutina de costumbre.

"Por acá, Srta. Percy," me dijo suavemente mi acompañante.

Quité la vista de las gigantescas macetas con árboles de cítricos y fijé los ojos en los pasos medidos de Jonathan, pasando el escritorio de la recepción y luego por una serie de corredores. Cuanto más nos alejábamos, más bajo se hacía el techo y más agradables los colores y las texturas. De repente, oí el tranquilizante rumor del agua. No habíamos visto a nadie desde la entrada y eso me hizo sentir inquieta.

Era evidente que las oficinas habían quedado atrás y que ahora entrábamos a las áreas más privadas. ¿Qué es esto? me pregunté. Me alarmé cuando Jonathan se detuvo de repente y puso la punta de un dedo en su oído.

"Discúlpeme," murmuró, alejándose unos cuantos metros. Observé que llevaba un micrófono en el reloj de pulsera cuando alzó el brazo. Alarmada, traté de leer las palabras en sus labios pero se dio vuelta evitando que pudiera verlo.

"Sí Sh'an," susurró respetuosamente.

Contuve la respiración y esperé con la esperanza de oír lo que decía.

"Conmigo," dijo. "Me informaron que usted manifestó su interés y me tomé la libertad de acompañarla hasta su galería." Jonathan se dio vuelta un poco incómodo. "¿Ella?"

No supe si interpretar aquello como un insulto o un cumplido y fingí estar acomodando mis medias y dejando caer otro mechón de mi cabello junto a mi arete. Pensé si acaso alguien había examinado la cajuela. Mi pulso se aceleró cuando me di cuenta de lo rápido que esto podría volverse en mi contra.

Sus ojos se abrieron más que nunca. "Sa'han," dijo muy preocupado, "por favor, acepte mis disculpas. La garita de seguridad dijo que…" Sus palabras fueron cortadas y pude ver cómo se tensó ante lo que evidentemente era un llamado de atención. "Sí, Sa'han," dijo inclinando la cabeza en un acto inconsciente de respeto. "En su oficina principal."

El hombre alto retomó su compostura y se dio la vuelta mirándome. Yo le disparé una gran sonrisa. Sus ojos azules eran inexpresivos, como si yo fuera insignificante. "¿Si tuviera la gentileza de dar media vuelta?," dijo secamente, apuntando.

Sintiéndome más como una prisionera que como una invitada, obedecí las sutiles indicaciones de Jonathan y regresamos hacia el frente. Él caminaba detrás de mí. Esto no me gustaba para nada. No me ayudaba sentirme tan pequeñita junto a él y que mis pasos fueran los únicos que se escuchaban. Lentamente, los colores y las texturas suaves se convirtieron en paredes corporativas y eficiencia de oficina.

Siempre manteniendo una distancia de tres pasos atrás, Jonathan me indicó el camino a lo largo de un pasillo que salía del vestíbulo. A lado y lado había puertas de vidrios esmerilados. Casi todas estaban abiertas y había gente trabajando adentro, pero Jonathan me indicó que era la última oficina. La puerta era de madera y dudó antes de adelantarse a mí para abrirla. "Haga el favor de esperar aquí," me dijo con un ligero amago de amenaza en su voz. "El Sr. Kalamack la verá en breve. Yo estaré en el escritorio de su secretaria, si me necesita."

Me señaló un escritorio evidentemente desocupado, metido en una esquina poco notoria. Pensé en la Srta. Yolin Bates, muerta hace tres días. Sonreí forzadamente. "Gracias Jon," le dije vivazmente. "Eres una dulzura."

"Es Jonathan." Cerró la puerta secamente delante de mí, pero no sonó el click del cerrojo.

Me di la vuelta para examinar la oficina principal de Kamalack. Se veía normal, una oficina de un ejecutivo rico con mal gusto. En la pared junto a su escritorio habían empotrados toda suerte de aparatos electrónicos, con tantos botones e interruptores que un estudio de grabación envidiaría. En la pared opuesta había un gran ventanal por donde entraba la luz que brillaba sobre la alfombra. Sabía que estaba demasiado adentro del edificio para que esa ventana y la luz del sol fueran reales. Me parecía que ameritaba una exploración a fondo.

Puse mi bolso en la silla opuesta del escritorio y me acerqué a la "ventana." Con las manos en la cintura me fijé en los retoños y las manzanas caídas. Alcé las cejas. Los ingenieros estaban mal en sus cálculos. Era mediodía y el sol no estaba tan bajo para producir sombras tan grandes.

Satisfecha por descubrir el error, dirigí la atención a los peces que nadaban en el tanque junto a la otra pared detrás del escritorio. Estrellas de mar, doncellas azules, peces amarillos y hasta caballitos de mar convivían pacíficamente sin darse cuenta de que el mar quedaba a quinientas millas de allí. Recordé a Don Pez, nadando tranquilo en su pequeña pecera de vidrio. Fruncí el entrecejo, no con celos, sino molesta por la veleidad del futuro del mundo.

El escritorio de Trent tenía encima las cosas usuales, incluyendo una pequeña fuente de agua de piedra negra. El protector de pantalla de su computadora eran tres números que cambiaban: veinte, cinco, uno. Un mensaje enigmático. En una esquina, en el techo, había una cámara con una lucecilla roja que titilaba. Me estaban vigilando.

De nuevo pensé en la conversación que tuvo Jonathan con el misterioso Sa'han. Era evidente que mi historia de Francine había sido descubierta. Pero, si hubieran querido arrestarme, ya lo habrían hecho. Tenía la sensación de el Sr. Kalamack quería algo de mí. *¿Mi silencio?* Tendría que averiguarlo.

Sonreí a la cámara y me acomodé detrás del escritorio de Trent. Pude imaginar la conmoción que estaba produciendo cuando comencé a tocar las cosas. Primero, la agenda con sus citas estaba frente a mí, provocativamente abierta sobre el escritorio. El nombre de Francis estaba tachado con lápiz y con un punto de interrogación al frente. Haciendo una mueca de preocupación, pasé las hojas hacia atrás hasta el día en que la secretaria de Trent había sido atrapada con azufre. No había nada fuera de lo común. Una frase me llamó la atención: "Los Huntington a Ulrich." ¿Acaso estaba sacando gente ilegalmente del país? Buena pregunta.

El cajón de arriba no contenía nada inusual: lápices, lapiceros, notas adhesivas y un jaspe negro. No pude imaginar qué preocupaba tanto a Trent como para ameritar un objeto así. Los cajones laterales contenían archivos codificados por colores, relativos a la hacienda. Mientras esperaba a que alguien entrara a detenerme, me incliné para leer cómo su plantación de nuez pacana había sufrido por las heladas de este año, pero que sus fresas en la costa balanceaban la pérdida. Cerré el cajón sorprendida de que nadie hubiera entrado. ¿A lo mejor tenían curiosidad de saber qué estaba buscando? Al menos, yo sí lo sabía.

Trent tenía el gusto por los dulces de arce y por el whiskey del pre-Giro—por lo que encontré en el cajón inferior. Estuve tentada a destapar una botella de más de cuarenta años para probar su licor, pero pensé que eso haría que mis espías llegaran más rápido.

El siguiente cajón estaba lleno de discos compactos perfectamente bien organizados. *¡Bingo!,* pensé, abriéndolo más.

"Alzheimer," susurré, pasando un dedo sobre el rótulo escrito a mano. "Fibrosis cística, cáncer, cáncer..." En total, ocho estaban rotulados "cáncer." Depresión, diabetes ...seguí leyendo hasta que encontré "enfermedad de Huntintgon." Mis ojos regresaron a la agenda y cerré el cajón. *Ahhh...*

Cómodamente sentada en el asiento de Trent, tomé su agenda y la puse sobre los muslos. Comencé en enero pasando las páginas lentamente. Cada cinco días, más o menos, salía un envío. Comencé a respirar más rápido al notar un patrón. Huntington salía el mismo día todos los meses. Pasé las hojas adelante y atrás. Todos los envíos salían el mismo día de cada mes, apenas con días de diferencia entre uno y otro. Luego, miré el cajón con los discos. Segura de que había descubierto algo, metí uno en la computadora y moví el ratón. ¡Demonios! Necesitaba la palabra clave.

Sonó una manija que giraba. Salté para ponerme en pie y oprimí el botón para sacar el disco.

"Buenas tardes, Srta. Morgan."

Era Trent Kalamack. Traté de no sonrojarme mientras

introducía el pequeño disco en mi bolsillo. "¿Disculpe?" repuse, reforzando mi hechizo al máximo. Ya sabían quién era. Vaya sorpresa.

Trent cerró el último botón de su saco gris y cerró la puerta. Tenía una sonrisa paralizante que acompañaba a sus facciones y su cara bien afeitada, dándole el aspecto de una persona de mi edad.

Su cabello era rubio, casi blanco, y él se veía bronceado. Parecía sencillo y relajado. Su aspecto era demasiado agradable para ser tan rico como decían. No era justo ser adinerado y además bien parecido. Las dos cosas... no.

"¿Prefiere ser Francine Percy?" dijo Trent, mirándome por encima de sus lentes metálicos.

Acomodé un mechón de pelo por detrás de la oreja, luchando por mostrar una actitud despreocupada. "En realidad, no," acepté. A lo mejor aun me quedaban unas cartas para jugar o no se tomaría la molestia perdiendo tiempo conmigo.

Trent se dirigió hacia su escritorio mostrándose un tanto preocupado, obligándome a retroceder al otro lado. Acomodó su corbata azul oscura y se sentó. Alzó la cabeza y, asombrado de que yo aun seguía en pie, dijo con cortesía mostrando sus dientes blancos y pequeños: "Siéntese, por favor." Apuntó un control remoto hacia la cámara. La luz roja se apagó y guardó el control en un cajón.

Seguí de pie. No confiaba en su actitud relajada. Toda suerte de sospechas aparecieron en mi cabeza y me sentí mal del estómago. El año pasado, la revista *Fortune* había impreso su foto en la portada como el soltero más codiciado. Era una fotografía desde la cabeza hasta las rodillas, reclinado casualmente contra una puerta con el nombre de la compañía en letras doradas. Su sonrisa era una combinación de confianza y secreto. Algunas mujeres se sienten atraídas por una sonrisa de esas. ¿Yo? Yo me pongo en guardia. Siguió con su sonrisa, colocando la mano debajo de la quijada, apoyando el codo en el escritorio.

Ví como se movía su pelo corto por encima de las orejas y

pensé que debía ser increíblemente suave para tan solo moverse con el viento que producía el sistema de ventilación.

Trent se tensó al ver cómo lo observaba, pero luego volvió a sonreír. "Le pido disculpas por el error en la reja de entrada, y luego por Jon," dijo. "No la esperaba por lo menos hasta dentro de una semana."

Me senté y las rodillas me flaquearon. *¿Me esperaba?* "Ciertamente, no comprendo," le dije directamente, contenta de que mi voz no temblara.

El hombre tomó un lápiz casualmente, pero sus ojos saltaron cuando moví los pies. Me pareció que estaba tan amarrado como yo. Borró meticulosamente el signo de interrogación frente al nombre de Francis y escribió el mío. Dejó el lápiz y se pasó la mano por el pelo para alisarlo.

"Soy un hombre ocupado, Srta. Morgan," dijo con voz segura pero agradable. "Para mí resulta más rentable atraer a los empleados de otras compañías que entrenarlos desde cero; y, aun cuando me cuesta admitir que he competido con la S.E., debo decirle que sus métodos de entrenamiento y las destrezas que logran son conmensurables con mis necesidades. Con toda sinceridad, habría preferido constatar que usted posee el ingenio para sobrevivir a una sentencia de muerte de la S.E. antes de contratarla. Pero tal vez el hecho de que por poco logra entrar a mis aposentos privados es suficiente confirmación."

Crucé las piernas y alcé las cejas. "¿Me está ofreciendo empleo, Sr. Kalamack? ¿Le gustaría que fuera su nueva secretaria? ¿Escribir sus cartas? ¿Servirle el café?"

"Santo cielo, ¡no!" dijo, ignorando mi sarcasmo. "Usted huele muy fuerte a magia como para que trabaje de secretaria, a pesar de que hace el intento de ocultarlo con ese... ummm...¿perfume?"

Me hizo ruborizar, pero estaba determinada a no quitarle la mirada a sus ojos inquisidores.

"No," prosiguió Trent. "Usted es demasiado interesante como para ser secretaria...inclusive una de las mías. No solamente ha abandonado a la S.E.: la está retando. Salió de compras. Entró a la bóveda de archivos para destruir el suyo. Encerró inconsciente a uno de sus agentes en la cajuela de su propio auto" dijo con risa perfectamente calculada. "Me gusta. Pero, mejor aun, me gusta su lucha por mejorar. He aplaudido su motivación para ampliar sus horizontes, aprender nuevas destrezas. La voluntad para explorar opciones que las mayoría rechazarían, es una actitud que trato de inculcarles a mis empleados. Claro que el leer ese libro en el autobús demuestra cierta falta de…buen juicio" Un ligero brillo de humor negro se asomó en sus ojos. "¿A menos que su interés por los vampiros tenga una explicación más terrenal, Srta. Morgan?"

Mi estómago se había vuelto un gran nudo y pensé si tendría suficientes hechizos para salirme de esta. ¿Cómo averiguó Trent todo aquello si ni siquiera la S.E. podía controlar todos mis movimientos? Traté de pensar calmadamente al darme cuenta de lo profundo que estaba hundida en polvo de duende. ¿Qué diablos estaba pensando cuando me metí a este lugar? La secretaria del hombre estaba muerta. Él traficaba con azufre, no importa lo generoso que era con las colectas de beneficencia o que jugara al golf con el marido de la alcaldesa. Era muy inteligente y no le bastaba con controlar la tercera parte de la industria manufacturera de Cincinnati. Sus intereses ocultos formaban toda una red en los bajos fondos y estaba segura que deseaba conservarla.

Trent se inclinó hacia adelante con expresión resuelta y entendí que la cháchara inútil había terminado. "Mi pregunta, Srta. Morgan, es ¿qué quiere usted de mí?"

No dije nada. Toda mi confianza desapareció de repente.

Señalando su escritorio me preguntó: "¿Qué estaba buscando?"

"Chicle," respondí. Suspiró.

"Por favor, no perdamos más tiempo y esfuerzo. Sugiero que seamos honestos el uno con el otro." Se quitó los lentes dejándolos a un lado. "¿Por qué se arriesgó a morir para venir a verme? Le doy mi palabra que la historia de sus acciones hoy...¿desaparecerá? Sólo quiero saber con qué contar. ¿Qué hice yo para atraer su interés?"

"¿Saldré caminando libre de aquí?" le pregunté. Él se reclinó en el asiento asintiendo. Sus ojos tenían un color verde que jamás había visto. No eran azules. Ni por asomo.

"Todos quieren algo, Srta. Morgan," dijo con palabras claras que fluían como agua. "¿Qué es lo que quiere?"

Mi corazón latió ante su promesa de libertad. Seguí su mirada hacia mis manos y la tierra debajo de mis uñas. "A usted" repuse, doblando los dedos para esconderlos. "Quiero pruebas de que usted asesinó a su secretaria. Que está traficando con azufre"

"Oh..." exclamó con un suspiro conmovedor. "Usted quiere su libertad. Debí adivinarlo. Srta. Morgan, usted es más compleja de lo que pensé." Hizo un gesto y su traje de seda sonó con sus movimientos. "Entregarme a la S.E. ciertamente pagaría por su independencia. Pero usted comprenderá que no puedo permitirlo." Se enderezó de nuevo asumiendo su actitud de hombre de negocios. "Yo puedo ofrecerle algo tan valioso como su libertad. Tal vez mejor. Puedo pagar su contrato con la S.E. Podríamos llamarlo... eh...un préstamo. Usted podría trabajar conmigo. Yo le conseguiría un establecimiento decente, inclusive un pequeño personal de trabajo."

Primero sentí que se me helaba la piel, pero luego la sentí hervir. Quería comprarme. Sin notar mi rabia, abrió un archivo. Sacó un par de lentes con armadura de madera del bolsillo interior del saco y los equilibró sobre su pequeña nariz. Hice una mueca de molestia cuando me miró, cociente de que estaba observándome a través de mi disfraz. Hizo un leve ruido antes de doblar la cabeza para leer su contenido.

"¿Le gusta la playa?" preguntó suavemente. Me pregunté para qué fingía necesitar los lentes para leer. "Tengo un sembrado de nueces macadamia que me gustaría agrandar. Queda en los mares del sur. Usted podría, inclusive, elegir los colores de la casa principal."

"Puede irse a girar, Trent," le dije. Me miró por encima de sus lentes aparentemente sorprendido. Se veía atractivo y traté de alejar esa idea de mi mente. "Si quisiera que me tuvieran con correa de perrito me habría quedado en la S.E. En esas islas cultivan azufre. Más me valdría ser humana estando tan cerca del mar. Allá ni siquera funcionan los hechizos de amor."

"Sol," dijo persuasivamente guardando sus lentes. "Arena cálida. Dueña de su tiempo." Cerró el archivo y puso la mano encima. "Puede llevar a su nueva amiga ¿es Ivy? Un vampiro Tamwood. Qué amiguita." Concluyó con una sonrisa irónica.

Mi genio se encendió. Él pensaba que podía comprarme; pero el problema era que me tentaba y eso me enfurecía conmigo misma. Lo miré desafiante, mis manos tiesas sobre los muslos.

"Sea honesta," dijo Trent, jugando con un lápiz entre sus largos dedos con asombrosa destreza. "Usted es muy astuta, inclusive tendrá habilidades. Pero nadie puede eludir permanentemente a la S.E. sin ayuda."

"Yo tengo una forma mejor," dije luchando por quedarme sentada. No tenía adónde ir si no me dejaba libre. "Voy a amarrarlo contra un poste en el centro de la ciudad. Voy a demostrar que usted está involucrado en la muerte de su secretaria y que trafica con azufre. Abandoné mi empleo Sr. Kalamack, pero no mis principios."

La ira destelló en sus ojos verdes, pero su cara siguió tranquila mientras guardó de nuevo el lápiz con un golpecito sonoro. "Puede confiar en que mantengo mi palabra, promesas o amenazas." Sus palabras llenaron el cuarto como una inundación y yo luché contra la estúpida tentación de levantar los pies de la alfombra. "Así debe hacerlo un hombre de negocios," dijo con cierto énfasis. "de lo contrario, no durará mucho en el mundo de los negocios."

Tragué saliva pensando qué demonios era Trent. Tenía la gracia, la voz, la velocidad y la seguridad del poder de un vampiro. Y, a pesar de lo mucho que me disgustaba este hombre, tenía un atractivo natural que se acentuaba con su fuerte personalidad en lugar de hacerlo con coqueteos o insinuaciones sexuales. Pero no era un vampiro vivo. A pesar de ser cálido y agradable por fuera, contaba con una gran personalidad que la mayor parte de los vampiros no tenían. Mantenía a la gente a distancia, demasiado alejado para seducir con el toque. No, no era un vampiro, pero quiás... ¿un lacayo humano?

Me asombré. Trent parpadeó al ver que yo pensaba en algo sin saber qué era. "¿Decía, Srta. Morgan?," dijo, sintiéndose incómodo por primera vez.

El corazón me estallaba. "Su pelo está flotando de nuevo" le dije, tratando de confundirlo. Sus labios se abrieron ligeramente pero no encontraba palabras.

Salté de repente al sentir la puerta que se abría. Jonathan entró velozmente. Estaba tenso y disgustado, con actitud de protector encadenado por el mismo a quien había dado su palabra de proteger. Traía en las manos una bola de cristal del tamaño de una cabeza. Jenks estaba adentro. Asustada, me levanté apretando mi bolso contra el cuerpo.

"Jon," dijo Trent tranquilizándolo a medida que se ponía de pie. "¿Tendrías la amabilidad de acompañar a la Srta. Morgan y su socio?"

Jenks estaba tan furioso que de sus alas solo se percibía una nube negra. Lo veía gesticular algo, pero no podía oírlo; pero sus gestos eran inconfundibles.

"¿Mi disco, Srta. Morgan?"

Giré, jadeando, al darme cuenta que Trent había dado la vuelta a su escritorio y estaba detrás de mí. No lo sentí moverse.

"¿Su qué?" tartamudeé.

Tenía estirada la mano derecha. Era suave, pero con fortaleza. Portaba un sólo anillo de oro en un dedo y no pude evitar notar que apenas era unos cuantos centímetros más alto que yo. "¿Mi disco?" repitió. Yo tragué en seco.

Demasiado asustada para reaccionar, lo saqué de mi bolsillo y se lo devolví. Algo pasó sobre él. Fue como una sutil sombra azul tan difícil de distinguir como un copo de nieve entre miles, pero ahí estaba. En ese instante comprendí que a Trent no le preocupaba el azufre. Era algo que había en ese disco.

Mi mente regresó a ese cajón con todos esos discos bien organizados; pero mi determinación de mirarlo jamente a los ojos en lugar de volver la mirada hacia su escritorio fue más fuerte. Dios me ayude. El hombre no solamente traficaba con azufre, sino con drogas biológicas. Este tipo era un maldito capo de drogas biológicas. Mi corazón estuvo a punto de estallar y se me secó la boca. La pena por traficar con azufre era la cárcel. Pero la pena por traficar con drogas biológicas era la estaca, la hoguera y los restos esparcidos. ¡Y quería que trabajara para él!

"Usted ha demostrado una extraordinaria capacidad de planificación, Srta. Morgan," dijo Trent interrumpiendo mis rápidos pensamientos. "Los vampiros asesinos no la atacarán mientras se encuentre bajo la protección de un Tamwood. Además, organizar a un clan de duendes que mantengan alejadas a las hadas y vivir en una iglesia que les impide a los lobos acercarse es hermosamente simple. Avíseme cuando cambie de opinión y decida trabajar para mí. Aquí encontrará grandes satisfacciones y reconocimiento; algo en lo cual la S.E. ha sido negligente."

Yo mantuve mi actitud, concentrándome en evitar que mi voz temblara. Yo no había planeado nada. Había sido Ivy; y ni siquiera conocía sus motivos. "Con el debido respeto, Sr. Kalamack, váyase a Girar."

Jonathan se alteró, pero Trent simplemente agitó la cabeza y se dirigió a su escritorio.

Una mano gruesa me golpeó en el hombro. Instintivamente la agarré y me agaché para lanzar por los aires y derribar contra el suelo a quien me hubiera tocado. Jonathan cayó con un gruñido de asombro. Yo estaba arrodillada encima de su cuello antes de que siquiera me hubiera dado cuenta de mis propios movimientos. Asustada por lo que acababa de hacer, me levanté y retrocedí. Trent alzó la mirada totalmente despreocupado luego de guardar su disco en el cajón.

Tres personas más entraron al sentir la pesada caída de Jonathan. Dos me rodearon, y la tercera se acercó a él.

"Déjenla ir," dijo Trent. "El error fue de Jon," suspiró con un leve aire de desilusión. "Jon," agregó con actitud de cansancio, "ella no es la pelusa que aparenta ser."

El alto Jonathan se puso lentamente de pie. Se arregló la camisa y se acomodó el cabello con una mano. Me miró con odio. No solamente lo había superado frente a su jefe sino que le habían llamado la atención delante de mí. El pobre hombre alzó furioso a Jenks y me indicó la puerta.

Salí caminando libre bajo el sol más asustada por lo que acababa de rechazar que por abandonar la S.E.

Quince

Mordí la pizza descargando mi frustración por la extraordinaria tarde. De la mesa de madera de Ivy provino un crujido de papel. Volví mi atención hacia ella. Con la cabeza agachada y el ceño fruncido, centró la atención en un mapa. Sería una tonta si no hubiera caído en la cuenta de que su actividad se aceleraba al caer el sol. Se movía de nuevo con aquella gracia desconcertante, aun cuando estaba airada en lugar de amorosa. De todas formas, estaba pendiente de todos sus movimientos.

Ivy tiene una misión de verdad, pensé con amargura, parada en medio de la cocina mientras preparaba una pizza. Ivy tenía una vida. Ivy no estaba tratando de demostrar que el ciudadano más querido y destacado de la ciudad era un capo de las drogas biológicas y a la vez luchando por salvarse.

Sólo tres días trabajando independiente y Ivy ya tenía una misión para encontrar a un humano desaparecido. Me pareció extraño que un humano le solicitara ayuda a un vampiro, pero Ivy tenía sus propios hechizos, o mejor, la capacidad para intimidar. Había pasado toda la noche con las narices metidas en el mapa de la ciudad, indicando con un marcador de color los lugares que aquel hombre frecuentaba y señalando las vías que habría tomado para conducir de regreso del trabajo a casa y cosas por el estilo.

"No soy experta," dijo Ivy hablándole a la mesa, "pero ¿es así que se hace eso?"

"¿Quieres preparar la cena?" dije de inmediato, dirigiendo la mirada a la masa en mis manos. La circunferencia tenía más el aspecto de un óvalo, tan delgada en algunos sitios que ya tenía agujeros. Avergonzada, moví un poco de masa para cubrir el pequeño agujero. La observé de reojo mientras luchaba con los bordes de la masa. A la primera mirada seductora o movimiento inesperado, yo estaba lista para salir por la puerta y esconderme detrás de Jenks. Abrí el frasco de salsa con un sonoro "plop" y mis ojos saltaron hacia Ivy. No se movió. Desocupé casi todo en la pizza y cerré de nuevo el frasco.

¿Qué más puedo agregarle? pensé. Sería un milagro que Ivy me dejara cubrirla con todo lo usual. Decidí olvidarme de las castañas y más bien ponerle algo más mundano. "Pimientos," dije, "champiñones." La miré de nuevo. Me pareció que era una chica carnívora... "tocino que sobró del desayuno."

El marcador produjo un chirrido a medida que Ivy trazaba una línea desde la Universidad hasta la sección más peligrosa de clubes nocturnos de Los Hollows, frente al río. "Entonces..." dijo arrastrando las palabras. "¿Vas a decirme qué es lo que te molesta, o tendré que pedir una pizza cuando hayas quemado esa?"

Puse el pimiento en el lavaplatos apoyándome sobre el mostrador. "Trent es traficante de drogas biológicas," le dije, sintiendo de nuevo la misma sensación desagradable. "Si supiera que ahora lo quiero atrapar por eso, me mataría antes que la S.E."

"Pero no lo sabe," dijo Ivy casi de inmediato. "Sólo sabe que tu piensas que trafica con azufre y que ordenó asesinar a su secretaria. Si estuviera preocupado no te habría ofrecido ese trabajo."

"¿Trabajo?" repuse, dándole la espalda mientras lavaba el pimiento. "¿En los mares del sur, administrándole sus cultivos de azufre? Me quiere fuera de su camino. Eso es todo."

"Vaya vaya," dijo tapando el marcador golpeándolo contra la mesa. Giré alerta esparciendo gotas de agua por todas partes. "Piensa que eres una amenaza," concluyó, sacudiéndose exageradamente las gotas de agua que le cayeron accidentalmente encima.

Sonreí avergonzada, esperando que no se diera cuenta de que me tenía tensa. "No lo había pensado así."

Ivy volvió a su mapa, gruñendo por las manchas de agua sobre los nítidos dobleces. "Dame algo de tiempo para hacer una chequeo," dijo preocupada. "Si logramos hacernos con sus registros financieros y con los nombres de unos cuantos clientes suyos, podríamos tener alguna pista sobre el papel. Pero sigo pensando que se trata solo de azufre."

Abrí la refrigeradora para sacar el parmesano y el mozzarella. Si Trent no traficaba con drogas biológicas entonces yo era una princesa ninfa. Los marcadores de Ivy sonaron al meterlos en la taza de cerámica que tenía junto a su computadora. De nuevo me alarmé, puesto que le daba la espalda.

"Solo porque tiene un cajón lleno de discos rotulados con nombres de enfermedades que son tratadas con drogas biológicas, no significa que sea un capo," prosiguió, lanzando otro marcador en la taza. "A lo mejor son listas de clientes. El hombre es un filántropo. Media docena de hospitales funcionan gracias a sus donaciones."

"Puede ser," repuse poco convencida. Conocía las generosas contribuciones de Trent. El otoño pasado, su donación para la subasta de beneficencia para el programa Por los Niños sumó más de lo que me pagaban por un año de trabajo. Personalmente, pensaba que sus esfuerzos eran una máscara publicitaria. El hombre era una basura.

"Además," dijo Ivy reclinándose en el asiento y lanzando otro marcador a la taza en una extraordinaria demostración de coordinación, "¿para qué querría traficar con drogas biológicas? El hombre es muy rico. No necesita más dinero. Raquel, la gente tiene tres motivaciones: Amor…," Un marcador rojo cayó junto a los demás; "venganza," ahora uno negro, "y poder," terminó lanzando uno verde. "Trent tiene suficiente dinero para comprar las tres."

"Olvidaste una" dije, pensando si acaso era mejor mantener la boca cerrada. "Familia."

Ivy sacó los marcadores de la taza. Se sentó sobre los pies y comenzó a lanzarlos de nuevo. "¿Familia no va con amor?," preguntó.

No si los miembros están muertos, pensé, con mis recuerdos volando hacia papá. *En ese caso, iría con venganza.*

La cocina quedó en silencio mientras rociaba el queso parmesano sobre la salsa. Sólo el tableteo de los marcadores de Ivy rompían el silencio. Todos cayeron adentro. Los golpecillos ya me estaban poniendo nerviosa. De pronto, todo quedó en silencio y me quede inmóvil. Su cara quedó en sombras. No podía ver si sus ojos se habían puesto negros. Mi corazón latió más fuerte y me quedé quieta. Esperando.

"¿Por qué no me estacas, Raquel?" dijo exasperada, lanzando su pelo de medio lado para mostrarme sus iracundos ojos pardos. "No voy a atacarte. Ya te dije que lo del viernes fue un accidente."

Encogiéndome de hombros, hurgué ruidosamente en el cajón buscando un abrelatas para los champiñones. "Un accidente demasiado siniestro," murmuré para mí misma, mientras escurría los champiñones.

"Oí lo que dijiste," repuso con algo de duda. Sonó el ruido de un marcador cayendo en la taza. "Tú...eh...leíste el libro, ¿verdad?"

"Casi todo," admití; pero alarmada continué: "¿Por qué? ¿Estoy haciendo algo mal?"

"Me estás cabreando. Eso es lo que estás haciendo mal," dijo con voz fuerte. "Deja de vigilarme. No soy un animal. Puede que sea un vampiro, pero tengo alma."

Me mordí la lengua para no tener que responderle. De nuevo sonó la taza con los últimos marcadores que le quedaban en la mano. El silencio se hizo denso y tomó sus mapas. Yo le di la espalda para demostrarle que confiaba en ella. Pero no era cierto. Puse el pimiento en la tabla de cocina y abrí un cajón buscando ruidosamente hasta encontrar un gran cuchillo. Era demasiado grande para cortar pimientos, pero me sentía vulnerable. Ese era el cuchillo que usaría.

"Eh . . . No irás a ponerle pimiento a la pizza, ¿verdad?"

Dejé escapar el aire poniendo el cuchillo sobre la mesa. Según parece, nuestra pizza solo tendría queso. Sin decir otra palabra, guardé el pimiento en la refrigeradora. "¿Qué es una pizza sin pimientos?" murmuré.

"Algo comestible," fue su respuesta inmediata. Gurñí. Se supone que no debió oír eso.

Mis ojos pasaron revista a las delicias que había sobre la mesa. "¿Champiñones, ok?"

"No me imagino la pizza sin champiñones."

Puse capas de champiñones tajados sobre el parmesano. Ivy desdobló su mapa y yo la miré de reojo.

"Nunca me dijiste lo que hiciste con Francis," dijo.

"Lo dejé con la cajuela abierta. Alguien lo bañará con agua salada. Creo que le hice algo a su auto. No acelera, no importa la velocidad que pongas ni que tanto pises el acelerador."

Ivy se rió y se me erizó la piel. Se levantó y vino hacia mí, reclinándose sobre la mesa, como desafiándome a que objetara a su actitud. Mi nerviosismo regresó y se duplicó cuando Ivy se sentó encima de la mesa, a mi lado. "Entonces . . ." dijo, abriendo una bolsa de salchichón, metiéndose provocativamente una tajada en la boca, "¿qué crees que es?"

Estaba comiendo. Magnífico.

"¿Francis?" pregunté, sorprendida de que me lo preguntara ella.

"No. Trent."

Estiré la mano pidiéndole el salchichón y ella puso la bolsa en mi mano. "No lo sé. No es un vampiro. Pensó que mi perfume era para cubrir mi olor de bruja y no . . . eh . . . tu olor." Me sentía muy extraña con Ivy tan cerca de mí. Puse las tajadas de salchichón en la pizza como si fueran las cartas de un naipe. "Y sus dientes no son lo suficientemente afilados." Terminé y guardé la bolsa en la refrigeradora, lejos del alcance de Ivy.

"Podrían estar cubiertos." Ivy se quedó mirando a la refrigeradora y el salchichón guardado. "Le sería más difícil ser un vampiro activo, pero ha sucedido antes."

Mi mente volvió a la Tabla 6.1 y sus dos útiles diagramas. Sentí escalofríos que traté de ocultar estirándome para alcanzar un tomate. Ivy agachó la cabeza y mi mano pasó por encima. "No," dije con seguridad, "él entiende bien eso de respetar el espacio personal, cosa que ninguno de los vampiros vivos que he conocido—excepto tú—entienden."

Hubiera querido retirar mis palabras tan pronto como las dije. Ivy se puso tiesa. Pensé si acaso la distancia que ella establecía entre sí misma y todos los demás tenía que ver con el hecho de que ella no era un vampiro activo. Tenía que ser frustrante no saber si cada movimiento lo motivaba su cabeza o su apetito. Con razón Ivy tenía la tendencia a perder el control. Estaba luchando contra un instinto de mil años de antigüedad sin alguien que la ayudara a buscar el camino. Dudé antes de preguntarle: "¿Hay alguna forma de saber si Trent es un lacayo humano?"

"¿Lacayo humano?" repitió asombrada. "Esa es una posibilidad."

El cuchillo atravesó el tomate formando cuadraditos rojos. "Podría ser. Tiene la fortaleza interior, la gracia y el poder de un vampiro, pero sin ser un tocón. Y apostaría mi vida a que no es brujo ni aprendiz. No tiene ni el más mínimo rastro de olor a secoya. Son sus movimientos, la luz detrás de sus ojos..." Me quedé en silencio recordando sus ilegibles ojos verdes.

Ivy dio un pequeño salto bajándose de la mesa robándose de paso un salchichón de la pizza. La moví indiferentemente hacia el otro lado del fregadero para alejarla de la pizza. Acto seguido, tomó otro. De pronto sonó un zumbido y era Jenks que entraba por la ventana. Traía en los brazos un champiñón tan grande como él mismo, llenando la cocina de olor a tierra. Miré a Ivy y ella se encogió de hombros.

"Oye, Jenks," dijo Ivy dirigiéndose a su asiento en una esquina de la cocina. "Creo que ya superamos la prueba de 'puedo sentarme junto a tí sin morderte,' tú que piensas de Trent. ¿Crees que es un lobo?"

Jenks dejó caer su champiñón, aleteando furiosamente. "¿Cómo voy a saberlo? No estuve lo suficientemente cerca de él. Me atraparon. ¿Contenta?" Voló hacia la ventana junto a Don Pez, y se paró con las manos en la cintura mirando hacia la oscuridad.

Ivy movió la cabeza con molestia. "Así que te atraparon. Valiente cosa. Ellos sabían quién era Raquel, y sin embargo no la ves gimiendo por eso."

En verdad, yo le había dado vía libre a mi pataleta camino a casa. Tal vez eso fue lo que produjo ese ruido extraño que hacía el auto de Francis cuando lo estacioné debajo del árbol en el centro comercial.

Jenks comenzó a volar a 5 centímetros de la nariz de Ivy, sus alas rojas de rabia. "Veamos qué harías tú si te atrapara un *jardinero* en una bola de cristal. ¿Acaso no verías el mundo con otros ojos, Srta. Girasol?"

Mi mal humor desapareció de sólo ver a un duende de 10 centímetros retando a un vampiro. "Ya, déjate de renegar, Jenks" le dije suavemente. "No creo que fuera un jardinero de verdad."

"¿En serio?," dijo sarcásticamente volando hacia mí. "¿De verdad lo crees?" A sus espaldas, Ivy hacía un gesto como si fuera destriparlo con los dedos. Volteó los ojos y regresó a sus mapas. De pronto reinó un silencio incómodo, extraño. Jenks voló hasta su champiñón y me lo trajo, incluyendo la tierra. Estaba vestido con ropa ancha e informal. La seda era del color del musgo húmedo y el corte lo hacía ver como un jeque del desierto. Su pelo rubio estaba peinado hacia atrás y me pareció sentir olor a jabón. Nunca había visto a un duende en ropa casera. Se le veía muy bien.

"Ten," me dijo dejando el champiñón junto a mí. "Lo encontré en el jardín. Pensé que tal vez podrías usarlo para tu pizza."

"Gracias Jenks," le dije limpiando la tierra.

"Escucha" dijo, dando unos pasos hacia atrás. Sus alas se movían y luego se detenían intermitentemente. "Lo siento Raquel. Se supone que debí guardarte la espalda, pero en cambio me dejé atrapar."

Qué vergüenza, pensé, que un ser tan pequeño como una libélula me pidiera disculpas por no haberme protegido. "Vaya...eh...pues los dos metimos la pata," repuse amargamente, deseando que Ivy no estuviera presenciando esto. Ignorando su leve resoplido, lavé el champiñón y lo tajé. Jenks parecía satisfecho. Se fue a volar por encima de Ivy, describiendo molestos círculos alrededor de su cabeza hasta que ella empezó a manotearlo.

La dejó y regresó donde yo estaba. "Voy averiguar a qué huele Kalamack, así me cueste la vida," dijo Jenks mientras yo le agregaba su contribución a mi pizza. "Es una cuestión personal."

Bien, pensé, *¿por qué no?* Respiré profundo. "Volveré mañana por la noche," dije, recordando mi sentencia de muerte. Tarde o temprano, cometería un error; pero, a diferencia de Ivy, yo no podía regresar de la muerte. "¿Quieres acompañarme Jenks...no como asistente sino como socio?"

Jenks se levantó. Sus alas se tornaron moradas. "¡Seguro que sí! ¡Por mis barbas!"

"Raquel ¿qué crees que estás haciendo?"

Abrí el paquete de mozzarella y se lo agregué a la pizza. "Estoy ascendiendo a Jenks a socio. ¿Tienes alguna objeción? Ha estado trabajando tiempo extra y no merece nada menos."

"No," repuso mirándome desde el otro extremo de la cocina. "¡Me refiero a regresar donde Kalamack!"

Jenks voló a mi lado para formar un frente común. "Cierra la boca, Tamwood. Ella necesita uno de esos discos para demostrar que Kalamack trafica con drogas biológicas."

"No me queda otra alternativa," dije, haciendo tanta fuerza sobre el queso que se salió de la pizza.

Ivy se reclinó en su asiento con una lentitud exagerada. "Se que quieres atraparlo, pero piénsalo bien Raquel. Trent puede acusarte de todo, desde intrusión en propiedad privada hasta hacerte pasar por personal de la S.E. o de mirar mal a sus caballos. Si te atrapa, estás frita."

"Si lo acuso sin pruebas sólidas, se librará del proceso judicial de alguna manera." No podía mirarla a la cara. "Necesito pruebas rápidas y contundentes. Algo que la prensa pueda usar para profundizar en el asunto." Mis movimientos fueron algo torpes alzando el queso caído y poniéndolo otra vez en la pizza. "Necesito uno de esos discos y lo haré mañana."

Ivy hizo un leve sonido de incredulidad. "No puedo creer que de nuevo estés improvisando. Sin planear. Sin preparar. Nada. Ya probaste y te atraparon."

Me puse que ardía. "Sólo porque no planifico mis viajes al baño no significa que no sea buena agente," respondí secamente.

Apretó los dientes. "Nunca he dicho que no seas buena agente. Lo único que quiero decirte es que algo de planificación puede ahorrarte algunos errores vergonzosos, como el de hoy."

"¡Errores!," exclamé. "Escucha Ivy, ¡yo soy una agente de los mil demonios!"

Levantó las cejas. "No has hecho ni una sola captura completa en los últimos seis meses."

"Eso no es mi culpa. ¡Fue Denon! Inclusive lo admitió; además, si mis destrezas no te impresionan, ¿para que me rogaste que trabajáramos juntas?"

"No lo hice," dijo Ivy. Entrecerró los ojos y le comenzaron a salir manchas negras de ira en las mejillas.

No quería discutir con ella. Me di la vuelta para meter la pizza en el horno. La oleada de aire caliente me calentó la cara y se me metió el pelo en los ojos. "Sí, lo hiciste," masscullé, sabiendo que me oiría, y luego dije más fuerte, "Se exactamente lo que haré."

"¿Sí?," repuso justo detrás de mí. Reprimí un grito y giré velozmente. Jenks estaba sentado en la ventana al lado de Don Pez, lívido. "Pues, veamos... cuéntame," dijo con su voz fluida y sarcástica, "¿Cuál es tu *plan perfecto?*"

No queriendo que notara mi temor, pasé rozando junto a ella, dándole deliberadamente la espalda mientras limpiaba la harina de la mesa con un gran cuchillo. Se me pararon los pelos de la nuca y giré para verla exactamente donde la había dejado, pero ahora tenía los brazos cruzados y una sombra negra volaba detrás de sus ojos. Mi pulso se aceleró. Yo sabía que no debería discutir con ella.

Jenks voló como una flecha poniéndose en medio de nosotras. "¿Cómo vamos a entrar Raquel?," preguntó, poniéndose a mi lado junto a la mesa.

Me sentía más segura cuando Jenks estaba vigilando a Ivy y le di la espalda a propósito. "Voy a entrar como visón." Ivy hizo un ruido de incredulidad y luego se puso seria. Terminé de limpiar la harina regada poniéndola en mi mano y la tiré a la basura. "Aunque me vean, no sabrán que soy yo. Será un sencillo toma y corre." Las palabras de Trent acerca de mis actividades regresaron a mi mente y me quedé pensando.

"Robar la oficina de un concejal no es un sencillo toma y corre," dijo Ivy tensa. "Es un gran robo."

"Con Jenks estaré dentro y fuera de su oficina en dos minutos; y fuera del edificio en diez."

"Y enterrada en el sótano de la S.E. en una hora," agregó Ivy. "Están locos. Los dos están totalmente locos. ¡Esa oficina es una fortaleza en medio del maldito bosque! Además, eso no es un plan. Eso es una idea. Los planes se escriben en papel."

Habló con desdén. Estiré los hombros. "Si planificara estaría tres veces muerta," dije. "No necesito un plan. Simplemente aprendes todo lo que puedes, y luego lo haces. ¡Los planes no tienen en cuenta las sorpresas!"

"Si tuvieras un plan, no tendrías sorpresas."

Ivy se quedó mirándome y yo tragué saliva. Bastaba con una mínima traza de negro en sus ojos para que mi estómago se me revolviera.

"Conozco un camino más placentero, si lo que quieres es suicidarte," concluyó.

Jenks aterrizó en mi arete y de inmediato le quité la mirada a Ivy.

"Es la primera cosa inteligente que ha hecho en toda la semana," dijo. "Así es que quítate de en medio, Tamwood."

Ivy entrecerró los ojos y yo di un paso rápido hacia atrás notándola distraída. "Eres tan tonto como ella, duende," repuso, mostrando los dientes. Los dientes de los vampiros son como las pistolas: no se muestran a menos que se vayan a usar.

"¡Déjala hacer su trabajo!," gritó Jenks.

Ivy se puso tensa como un alambre. El viento frío producido por el aleteo de Jenks me golpeó en la nuca. "¡Ya basta!" grité, antes de que me abandonara. Lo necesitaba ahí donde estaba. "Ivy, si tienes una idea mejor, dímela. Si no, cállate."

Jenks y yo nos quedamos mirándola como unos estúpidos, pensando que juntos éramos más poderosos que solos. Sus ojos se volvieron negros y mi boca se secó. No parpadeaban. Estaban vivos. Su promesa se me hacía apenas una insinuación lejana. El cosquilleo en mi estómago subió hasta hacerme un nudo en la garganta. No podía saber si era temor o ansiedad. Me miró fijamente sin respirar. *No me mires el cuello*, pensé aterrada. *¡Oh Dios, no me mires el cuello!* "Púdrete y muérete," susurró Jenks.

Pero se estremeció, dio la vuelta y se inclinó en el fregadero. Yo sudaba y podría jurar que escuché a Jenks suspirar de alivio. Esto pudo haber terminado muy mal.

Ivy habló con voz de muerta. "Bien," dijo mirando el fregadero. "Háganse matar. Los dos." Comenzó a moverse y yo salté. Salió de la cocina encorvada y adolorida. Muy pronto sentimos el fuerte golpe de la puerta de la iglesia que se cerraba. Después, nada.

Alguien va resultar lastimado esta noche, pensé.

Jenks saltó de mi arete posándose en la ventana.

"¿Qué le pasa a esa?" preguntó beligerante en el repentino silencio. "Uno hasta pensaría que le importamos."

Dieciséis

Desperté de un sueño profundo alertada por el ruido distante de vidrios rotos. Olía a incienso y mis ojos se abrieron instintivamente.

Ivy estaba inclinada sobre mí, su cara apenas a unos centímetros de la mía. "¡No!" grité, lanzando un puño en la oscuridad. El golpe la alcanzó en el estómago. Ivy se agarró el abdomen y cayó al suelo luchando por respirar. Yo asumí mi posición de combate encima de la cama. Mis ojos saltaron de la ventana gris a la puerta. Mi corazón parecía estallar y me invadió el frío de una ráfaga de adrenalina al ver que ella estaba en el camino hacia la única salida que había.

"Espera," jadeó, la manga de su bata cayendo y dejando al descubierto un hombro tratando de agarrarme con la mano.

"Maldito vampiro traicionero chupa sangre," dije entre dientes.

De repente, me sorprendí al ver a Jenks...no, era Jax que entró por la ventana y voló sobre mí. "Srta. Raquel," dijo, distraído y preocupado. "¡Nos atacan! ¡Son hadas!" casi escupiendo la última palabra.

Hadas, pensé llena de temor mirando mi bolso. No podía luchar contra las hadas con mis hechizos. Eran demasiado veloces. Lo mejor que podía hacer era tratar de destripar una. Oh Dios, jamás había matado en mi vida, ni siquiera accidentalmente. Maldita sea, yo era agente. La idea era atrapar con vida...pero ¿hadas?

Mis ojos saltaron hacia Ivy y me sonrojé cuando entendí por qué estaba en mi habitación. Bajé de mi cama con la poca elegancia que me quedaba y le tendí la mano para ayudarla a pararse. "Perdóname," susurré.

Inclinó la cabeza y me miró entre la cortina que formaba su pelo. El dolor apenas ocultaba su rabia. De pronto una mano blanca me lanzó al suelo. Caí al suelo, aterrada de nuevo, mientras que ella me tapó la boca. "¡Cállate!," me dijo casi sin aliento. "¿Quieres que nos maten? Ya están adentro."

Con los ojos bien abiertos susurré entre sus dientes. "No van a entrar. Es una iglesia."

"Las hadas no respetan el suelo sagrado. Les importa un bledo."

Estaban adentro. Viendo mi preocupación, Ivy me quitó la mano de la boca. Dirigí la mirada hacia la rejilla de la calefacción. Con la mano estirada traté de cerrarla haciendo una mueca por el chirrido.

Jax se posó encima de mi rodilla con pijama. "Invadieron nuestro jardín," dijo. Su actitud asustada no concordaba con su cara infantil. "Lo pagarán, pero estoy aquí sentado cuidándolas a ustedes dos...grandulonas." Voló hasta la ventana.

De pronto sonó un golpe en la cocina pero Ivy me impidió alzarme. "Jenks se hará cargo de ellas."

"Pero..." me tragué mis reclamos cuando Ivy se dio vuelta para mirarme con sus ojos negros en la pálida luz de la mañana. ¿Qué podía hacer Jenks contra hadas asesinas? Estaba entrenado como asistente, pero no para luchar en una guerra de guerrillas. "Escucha, lo lamento," susurré, "me refiero al golpe."

Ivy no se movió. La transparencia de la emoción brilló en sus ojos y sentí que se me iba el aire. "Si quisiera poseerte, brujita, no podrías detenerme."

Temblando, tragué fuerte. Parecía una promesa.

"Algo ha cambiado," dijo fijando su atención en la puerta cerrada. "No esperaba que esto sucediera antes de tres días."

Las náuseas me invadieron. La S.E. había cambiado de táctica. Todo esto es por mi culpa. "Francis," dije. "Es mi culpa. La S.E. ya sabe que puedo escabullirme de su vigilancia." Apreté las yemas de los dedos contra las sienes. Keasley, el viejo de enfrente, me lo advirtió.

Ahora sonó un tercer golpe, más duro aun. Ivy y yo miramos hacia la puerta y yo podía oír los latidos de mi corazón; y me pregunté si ella también los oía. Luego de un momento que pareció una eternidad, alguien golpeó en la puerta suavemente. La tensión se apoderó de mí y sentí cómo Ivy tomaba una lenta bocanada de aire alistándose.

"¿Papá?" preguntó Jax. Un gemido provino del otro lado de la puerta y Jax voló junto a ella. "¡Papá!" gritó. Salté poniéndome en pie encendiendo la luz, entreabriendo los ojos por el destello de luz para ver la hora en el reloj que me regaló Ivy. Las cinco y media. Apenas había dormido una hora.

Ivy se levantó con una velocidad asombrosa. Abrió la puerta y saltó afuera. Su bata se agitó en el aire y yo me estremecí viéndola partir. No quise lastimarla. Bueno... eso no era cierto. Si quise. Pero yo pensé que me había tomado por desayuno.

Jenks entró y por poco se estrella contra la ventana tratando de aterrizar.

"¿Jenks?," pregunté, decidiendo que las disculpas para Ivy podían esperar. "¿Estás bien?"

"Esteeeee," dijo arrastrando la voz como si estuviera ebrio. "No tendremos que preocuparnos de hadas durante algún tiempo." Asombrada, abrí bien los ojos al observar la espada de hierro que llevaba en una mano. Tenía un mango de madera y era tan larga como un palito para ensartar aceitunas. Tambaleándose, se sentó duro doblando accidentalmente su par de alas inferiores.

Jax ayudó a su padre a levantarse. "¿Papá?," dijo preocupado. Jenks estaba hecho un desastre. Una de sus alas superiores estaba hecha jirones. Sangraba por varias cortadas, una de ellas justo debajo del ojo derecho. El otro lo tenía cerrado por la hinchazón y se recostó pesadamente sobre Jax que trataba de mantenerlo derecho.

"Ven," le dije poniendo mi mano debajo y detrás de Jenks, haciéndolo sentarse en mi palma. "Vamos a llevarte a la cocina. Hay más luz que aquí. Tal vez podamos pegarte el ala."

"Allá no hay luz," dijo con la voz entrecortada. "Las rompí." Parpadeó tratando de recomponer su visión. "Lo siento."

Preocupada, formé una cavidad sobre Jenks con mis manos ignorando sus protestas. "Jax, llama a tu madre." Jax agarró la espada de su padre y salió raudo volando a ras del techo. "¿Ivy?" la llamé, mientras caminaba a oscuras contra la pared del pasillo. "¿Qué tanto sabes sobre duendes?"

"Aparentemente no lo suficiente," respondió justo detrás mío haciéndome saltar. Golpeé el interruptor de la luz de la cocina con el codo. Nada. Las luces estaban dañadas.

"Aguarda," dijo. "Hay vidrios por todo el piso."

"¿Cómo puedes saberlo?" le pregunté incrédula, pero dudé seguir adelante con los pies descalzos en la oscuridad. Ivy pasó a mi lado rozándome y la brisa de su movimiento me produjo escalofríos. Estaba como un vampiro. Oí el ruido del vidrio triturado y se encendió la luz fluorescente del horno, iluminando la cocina con un incómodo resplandor.

Los pedazos de vidrio fluorecentes brillaban en el suelo, y un olor cáustico llenaba el aire. Alcé las cejas al darme cuenta que se trataba de polvillo de hadas, me irritó la garganta. Inmediatamente dejé a Jenks sobre el mostrador para no dejarlo caer accidentalmente por mis estornudos.

Contuve la respiración y me acerqué hasta la ventana para abrirla mejor. Don Pez yacía tendido inerte en el piso, su pecera destruida. Lo levanté cuidadosamente de los vidrios rotos y lo metí en una taza de plástico llena de agua. Don Pez se estremeció y cayó pesadamente al fondo. Lentamente, sus agallas se movieron otra vez. Estaba bien.

"¿Jenks?" lo llamé, girando para encontrarlo parado donde lo había dejado. "¿Qué sucedió?"

"Las vencimos," dijo, su voz a duras penas audible y reclinándose de lado.

Ivy tomó la escoba y comenzó a barrer los vidrios haciendolos un montón.

"Ellas pensaron que yo no sabía que estaban allí," prosiguió Jenks mientras que yo buscaba algo de cinta adhesiva, asombrada de encontrarme un ala de hada rota que más parecía de polilla que de libélula. Sus escamas se caían al frotarlas con mis dedos manchándolos de verde y morado. Dejé el ala a un lado. Hay varios hechizos complicados que requieren polvo de hada.

Diablos, pensé, dándome media vuelta. Esto me hacía enfermar. Alguien murió y yo estaba pensando usar parte de su cuerpo para fabricar un hechizo.

"La pequeña Jacey las detectó primero," dijo Jenks con una extraña cadencia en la voz. "Estaban al fondo del cementerio humano. Sus rosadas alas contrastaban contra el fondo de la luna descendente, a medida que la tierra entraba en su luminosidad de plata. Alcanzaron nuestras murallas. Nuestro frente presto. Lo que está escrito se cumplirá."

Desconcertada, miré a Ivy, ahí parada en silencio, inmóvil con la escoba. Lo miraba fijamente. Esto era muy extraño: Jenks no maldecía. Hablaba poéticamente, y aun faltaba más:

"La primera cayó junto al roble, muerta por el sabor al acero en su sangre. La segunda sobre el sagrado suelo descansó, acompañada de gemidos por su absurda temeridad. La tercera fracasó en el polvoriento y duro campo de batalla. Mirando a su a su jefe en una silenciosa advertencia." Jenks alzó la mirada pero no me veía. "Este suelo es nuestro. Así lo atestiguan nuestras maltrechas alas, nuestra sangre envenenada, nuestros muertos sin enterrar."

Ivy y yo nos miramos a través de la luz inquietante. "¿Qué demonios?" suspiró Ivy. Los ojos de Jenks se tornaron blancos. Giró la cabeza hacia nosotros, se llevó la mano a la frente en señal de saludo y se desplomó lentamente.

"¡Jenks!" gritamos Ivy y yo al mismo tiempo, saltando.

Ivy llegó primero. Alzó a Jenks con las manos y me miró aterrada. "¿¡Qué hago!?" gritó.

"¿Cómo voy a saberlo?" respondí. "¿Está respirando?"

Hubo un sonido de campanillas y la esposa de Jenks entró rauda a la habitación seguida de una fila de unos doce niños duendecillos. "El salón está limpio," dijo bruscamente, su manto de seda gris inflándose a su alrededor cuando se detuvo. "No hay hechizos. Llévenlo allí. Jhem, enciende la luz allá para que la Srta. Ivy pueda ver. Luego ayuda a Jinni a traerme mi equipo. Jax, lleva a los demás a revisar cuidadosamente toda la iglesia. Comiencen por el campanario. No dejen ranura sin revisar. Las paredes, las tuberías, los cables de la luz y el teléfono. Cuidado con los búhos. Además, te recomiendo revisar bien ese escondrijo del sacerdote. Si detectan el más mínimo olor de hechizos o de hadas, avísenme, ¿entendido? Ahora ¡a trabajar!"

Los niños duendes se desparramaron. Ivy, obediente, siguió las instrucciones de la diminuta mujer rápidamente y corrió al salón. Si no fuera porque Jenks yacía inmóvil en sus manos, no creería lo que estaba presenciando. Cojeando, los seguí.

"No querida," dijo la mujercita cuando Ivy quiso poner a Jenks sobre un mullido cojín. "En la mesa del fondo, por favor. Necesito una superficie dura para cortar."

¿Cortar? pensé mientras quitaba las revistas de Ivy de la mesa poniéndolas en el piso para abrirle espacio. Me senté en la silla más próxima y le di vuelta a la caperuza de la lámpara. La adrenalina comenzaba a abandonarme y sentí frío apenas cubierta con mi pijama de franela. ¿Qué pasaría si Jenks realmente estaba herido? Estaba horrorizada de que realmente hubiera matado a dos hadas. *Las mató.* Yo había mandado gente al hospital, sí . . . pero, ¿matar? Pensé en mis temores arrimándome en la oscuridad junto a un vampiro tenso y reflexioné si acaso yo sería capaz de hacer lo mismo.

Ivy depositó a Jenks como si se tratara de un papel fino y se retiró hasta la puerta. Estaba agachada y nerviosa, algo totalmente fuera de lugar en ella. "Voy a revisar afuera," dijo.

La Sra. Jenks sonrió cálidamente. "No querida," dijo. "Ahora estamos seguros. Pasará todo un día antes de que la S.E. logre hallar otro clan de hadas dispuestas a atravesar nuestras líneas. Además, cuesta muchísimo dinero convencer a unas hadas para que invadan el jardín de unos duendes, lo cual demuestra que no son otra cosa que primitivas salvajes. Pero, si quieres, puedes ir a cerciorarte. Hasta el niño más pequeñito podría bailar esta mañana entre las flores sin temor."

Ivy movió los labios como para protestar, pero cayó en la cuenta de que la Sra. Jenks hablaba en serio. Bajó la cabeza y se escabulló por la puerta trasera.

"¿Dijo Jenks algo antes de perder el sentido?" me preguntó la Sra. Jenks mientras le desplegaba las alas en una posición bastante extraña. Parecía un insecto clavado con alfileres en una exhibición y sentí náuseas.

"No," respondí, curiosa por su actitud tan calmada. Yo estaba frenética. "En realidad, habló como si estuviera recitando un soneto o algo así." Me subí el pijama hasta el cuello acurrucándome. "¿Va a estar bien?"

Se arrodilló junto a él y se vio más tranquila al pasarle un dedo debajo del ojo hinchado. "Está bien. Si maldecía o recitaba es porque está bien. Si me hubieras dicho que estaba cantando, me preocuparía." El movimiento de sus manos encima de su cuerpo se volvió más lento y su mirada distante. "La única vez que regresó a casa cantando casi lo perdemos." Sus ojos regresaron a la normalidad. Sonrió tristemente y abrió la bolsa que le trajeron los niños.

De pronto me invadió un sentimiento de culpa. "No sabe cuánto lo siento, Sra. Jenks," le dije. "De no ser por mí, esto jamás habría ocurrido. Si Jenks quiere terminar el contrato, está bien."

"¿¡Terminar su contrato!?" dijo la Sra. Jenks fijándome la mirada intensamente. "Por todos los cielos, hija mía, ¡no por algo tan insignificante como esto!"

"Pero Jenks no tenía por qué pelear," continué. "Pudieron matarlo."

"Apenas eran tres," respondió, extendiendo una sábana blanca junto a Jenks con un equipo que parecía de cirugía, con curas, bálsamos, inclusive algo que tenía el aspecto de membranas artificiales para alas. "Ellas sabían en qué se estaban metiendo. Vieron las advertencias. Las muertes fueron legítimas." Ella sonrió y entendí por qué Jenks usó su deseo para conservar a su esposa. Parecía un ángel, inclusive con ese cuchillo en la mano.

"Pero, no venían por ustedes venían por mí."

Agitó la cabeza haciendo mover su pelo ralo. "Eso no importa," dijo con voz lírica. "De todas formas se habrían metido al jardín. Yo creo que lo hicieron por *dinero*." Casi escupe la última palabra. "A la S.E. debió costarle mucho dinero convencerlas de medirse con Jenks," suspiró, mientras cortaba pequeños retazos de membrana según los agujeros que Jenks tenía en las alas, con la seguridad de quien remienda un par de medias.

"No se preocupe" dijo. "Ellas creyeron que como nosotros apenas tomamos posesión del lugar, iban a tomarnos con la guarda baja." Entonces me miró con suficiencia: "Pero se equivocaron, ¿no le parece?"

No supe que decirle. La animadversión entre duendes y hadas iba más allá de lo que podía imaginar. Concientes del hecho de que nadie podía ser el dueño de la Tierra, duendes y hadas rechazaban el concepto de títulos de propiedad y más bien esgrimían el dicho "el poder da derechos." Y, puesto que no estaban compitiendo con nadie más sino entre ellos, las cortes se hacían las ciegas en sus asuntos y los dejaban libres para ventilar sus diferencias, incluyendo matarse. Pensé qué habría sucedido con la persona que tenía el jardín antes de que Ivy arrendara la iglesia.

"Jenks te quiere mucho," dijo la mujercita, enrollando y guardando la membrana de alas. "La llama su amiga. Yo le daré a usted el mismo título para honrarlo a él."

"Gracias," tartamudeé.

"Pero no confío en usted," continuó. Yo parpadeé. Era tan directa como su marido, e igualmente "diplomática." "¿Es verdad que usted lo nombró su socio? ¿Es verdad o tan sólo una broma cruel?"

Asentí, más seria de lo que lo había estado en toda la semana. "Sí, señora. Él lo merece."

La Sra. Jenks tomó un par de tijeras en sus manos. Parecían más una reliquia que una herramienta funcional, con manijas de madera labradas con la figura de un ave. La punta era de metal. Abrí los ojos viendo cómo tomaba el frío metal y se arrodillaba delante de Jenks. "Por favor amor, sigue durmiendo," oí que susurraba. Observé asombrada cómo cortaba cuidadosamente los bordes pelados de las alas de Jenks. El olor de sangre cauterizada llenó el ambiente del cuarto cerrado.

Ivy apareció en el umbral de la puerta como por encanto. "Estás sangrando," dijo.

Moví la cabeza. "Es el ala de Jenks."

"No. Tú estás sangrando. Tu pie."

Me enderecé, angustiada. Cortando la mirada de Ivy, levanté el pie para mirar la planta. Una mancha roja me cubría el talón. Había estado demasiado concentrada en Jenks para notarlo.

"Te limpiaré," dijo Ivy. Dejé caer el pie y me encogí hacia atrás. "El *piso*," dijo Ivy molesta. "Dejaste huellas de sangre por todo el *piso*." Dirigí la mirada hacia donde señalaba en el pasillo. Mis huellas eran evidentes frente a la luz de la mañana que despuntaba. "No pensaba tocarte el pie," dijo Ivy entre dientes mientras salía otra vez.

Me sonrojé. Había despertado con Ivy respirando encima de mi cuello...

Sentí el golpe de las puertas del aparador y un chorro de agua en la cocina. Estaba molesta conmigo. Tal vez debería disculparme, pero ¿de qué? Ya le pedí disculpas por haberla golpeado.

"¿Está segura de que Jenks va a estar bien?" pregunté, tratando de eludir el tema de Ivy.

La mujer duende suspiró. "Si logro ponerle los parches antes de que despierte, sí." Se sentó sobre sus talones, cerró los ojos y rezó. Se frotó las manos en la falda y tomó una cuchilla sin brillo con mango de madera. Colocó un parche en su lugar y pasó la cara plana de la cuchilla por los bordes fundiendo la membrana contra las alas. Jenks se estremeció, pero no despertó. Cuando terminó, sus manos temblaban y polvo de duende salía de su cuerpo haciéndola brillar. Ciertamente, un ángel.

"¿Niños?" llamó. Aparecieron de todos lados. "Traigan a su papá. Josie ¿puedes asegurarte de que la puerta esté abierta?"

Observé cómo los niños descendían sobre él, levantándolo y sacándolo por el extractor de humo. La Sra. Jenks se levantó pesadamente mientras su hija mayor empacaba todo de nuevo en la bolsa. "Mi Jenks," dijo, "trata de alcanzar a veces más de lo que debería soñar un duende. No haga que mi marido muera en sus locuras, Srta. Morgan."

"Trataré," repuse, y los ví desaparecer por la chimenea. Me sentí culpable, como si estuviera manipulando a Jenks intencionalmente para protegerme. De pronto escuché los vidrios en el bote de la basura y me levanté a mirar por la ventana. Había salido el sol y hacía brillar las hierbas del jardín. Ya había pasado mi hora de dormir pero no creo que pudiera dormirme de nuevo.

Cansada y descontrolada, caminé hasta la cocina arrastrando los pies. Ivy estaba arrodillada con su bata negra lavando mis huellas. "Lo siento," le dije parada en medio de la cocina con los brazos cruzados.

Ivy alzó la mirada representando muy bien el papel de mártir. "¿De qué?," repuso queriendo arrastrarme hacia el trillado proceso de disculpas.

"Por…eh…golpearte. Estaba dormida," mentí. "No sabía que eras tú."

"Ya te disculpaste por eso," dijo, frotando de nuevo el piso.

"¿Por limpiar mis huellas?," probé de nuevo.

"Ofrecí hacerlo."

Moví la cabeza. Sí, se había ofrecido. No quería ahondar en los posibles motivos para aquello. Simplemente interpretaría su ofrecimiento como amabilidad. Pero había algo más que la molestaba. No tenía idea de qué podría ser. "Eh... está bien... dame una mano Ivy," dije finalmente.

Se levantó dirigiéndose hacia el fregadero, enjuagando metódicamente el trapo que dejó colgando sobre el grifo para secarlo. Se dio la vuelta recostándose contra el mesón. "¿Qué tal un poco de confianza? Te dije que no te mordería, y no lo haré."

Quedé con la boca abierta. ¿Confianza? ¿Ivy estaba molesta por la desconfianza? "¿Quieres que confíe en ti?" exclamé, cayendo además en la cuenta de que necesitaba estar molesta para hablar sobre este tema con Ivy. "Entonces, qué tal si te controlas un poco más. ¡Basta con contradecirte y te pones vampiro conmigo!"

"No es cierto," repuso abriendo los ojos.

"Vaya si es cierto," repuse gesticulando. "Como la primera semana que trabajamos juntas y discutíamos cuál es la mejor manera de atrapar a un ladrón en un centro comercial. Sólo porque no estoy de acuerdo contigo no significa que esté equivocada. Al menos escúchame antes de que decidas que lo estoy."

Respiró profundo y dejó escapar el aire lentamente. "Es verdad. Tienes razón."

Sus palabras me hicieron trastabillar. ¿Dijo que yo tenía razón? "Y algo más," agregué más calmada. "Ya deja de desaparecer en medio de las discusiones. Saliste de aquí esta noche como si fueras a cortarle la cabeza a alguien; y después me despierto contigo inclinándote sobre mí? Siento haberte golpeado, pero tienes que admitir que te lo merecías."

Una leve sonrisa se asomó en sus labios y desapareció. "Sí. Supongo que sí." Arregló el trapo en el grifo. Giró cruzando los brazos. "Está bien. No me iré en medio de una discusión, pero tú no te alteres tanto. Me sacudes de tal forma que no sé dónde estoy parada."

Vaya. ¿Quiso decir alterada como en asustada, molesta o ambas? "¿Cómo dices?"

"Y…¿tal vez deberías comprar otro perfume?," agregó un poco apenada.

"Pero si…si…recién compré perfume," dije sorprendida. "Jenks dijo que tapaba todo."

Repentinamente la mirada de Ivy se tornó de angustia. "Raquel, aun puedo olerme intensamente en ti. Eres como una gigantesca galleta de chocolate en un plato esperando a que alguien se la coma. Y cuando te agitas, es como si acabaras de salir del horno: toda calientita y blanda. Hace tres años que no pruebo una galleta. ¿Podrías calmarte para que no huelas tan provocativamente?"

"Oh, Dios." Helada, me hundí en el asiento. No me gustaba que me compararan con comida; y nunca más podría comer otra galleta de chocolate. "Volví a lavar mi ropa," le dije en un tono de voz muy leve. "Ya no uso ni tus sábanas ni tu jabón."

Ivy miraba al piso cuando di la vuelta. "Lo sé," respondió. "Te lo agradezco. Ayuda. No es tu culpa. El olor de un vampiro se prende a quienes viven con el. Es un rasgo de supervivencia que extiende la vida del compañero del vampiro advirtiéndoles a otros vampiros que se retiren. No pensé que lo notaría puesto que estamos compartiendo el espacio donde vivimos y no la sangre."

Sentí escalofrío al recordar mi clase de fundamentos de latín, cuando me enseñaron que la palabra compañero viene de comida. "Yo no te pertenezco," le dije.

"Lo sé." Respiró lentamente sin mirarme. "La lavanda ayuda. Tal vez si cuelgas más en tu armario bastaría. Y trata de no ponerte tan emotiva, sobre todo cuando estamos discutiendo acciones alternativas."

"Está bien," le dije suavemente, entendiendo lo compleja que iba a ser esta convivencia.

"¿Todavía piensas entrar donde Kalamack mañana?" preguntó Ivy.

Asentí, aliviada por el cambio de tema. "No quiero ir sin Jenks, pero no creo que pueda esperar a que esté en condiciones de volar."

Ivy guardó silencio un tiempo largo. "Te conduciré hasta allá, por lo menos hasta donde creas que sea seguro."

Quedé atónita. "¿Por qué?...disculpa, quise decir...¿en serio?"

"Porque tienes razón. Si no logras hacer esto rápido, no durarás una semana más."

Diecisiete

"**N**o vas a ir, amor," dijo la Sra. Jenks con firmeza.

Desocupé el último resto de café en el fregadero y miré hacia el jardín que brillaba con el sol de la tarde. Me sentía incómoda. Preferiría estar en cualquier otro sitio.

"¡Por mil demonios...voy a ir!," dijo Jenks entre dientes. Me di vuelta, cansada de la mañana sin sueño y sin ganas de ver cómo dominaban al pobre Jenks. Estaba parado en una mesa de acero inoxidable, furioso, con las manos en la cintura. Detrás estaba Ivy, agachada sobre su mesa de madera, planeando tres rutas hacia los terrenos de Kalamack. La Sra. Jenks estaba a su lado. Su posición inalterable hablaba por sí sola. Ella no quería que él fuera. Y, viendo su aspecto, yo no estaba dispuesta a contradecirla.

"Dije que no irás," repitió, esta vez con voz de hierro.

"¡Cuida tus palabras, mujer!" replicó; pero su aparente aspecto de tipo difícil tenía ciertos visos de súplica.

"Yo las cuidaré," continuó con tono severo. "Aún estás herido. Lo que yo digo se cumple. Es nuestra ley."

Jenks hizo un gesto lastimero. "Estoy bien. Puedo volar. Puedo pelear. Voy a ir."

"No lo estás. No puedes. No lo harás. Y mientras yo lo quiera, te quedarás de jardinero, no de agente."

"¡Puedo volar!" exclamó, y sus alas comenzaron a agitarse. Se alzó apenas un dedo del mostrador y descendió de nuevo. "Lo que pasa es que no quieres que yo vaya."

Se puso seria. "No voy a permitir que se diga que te mataron por mi culpa. Mi responsabilidad es mantenerte con vida, ¡y yo digo que *estás herido!*"

Alimenté a Don Pez con un trocito de hojuela de maíz. Esto era vergonzoso. Si por mi fuera lo dejaría ir, volara o no volara. Jenks se estaba recuperando más rápido de lo que se puede imaginar. Aun así, apenas habían transcurrido unas diez horas desde que recitaba sus poemas. Miré a la señora Jenks en interrogación arqueando mis cejas. La hermosa mujer duende agitó la cabeza. Nada que hacer.

"Lo siento Jenks," dije. "Estarás en el jardín hasta que tengas luz verde."

Dio tres pasos hasta el borde de la mesa con los puños cerrados.

Fui hacia Ivy que estaba en la otra mesa. "¿Entonces?" dije torpemente. "¿Cuál es tu idea para hacerme entrar?"

Ivy sacó el extremo del estilógrafo que sostenía entre los dientes. "Esta mañana hice algunas búsquedas en la red..."

"Quieres decir ¿luego de que me fui a dormir?" interrumpí.

"Sí." Volteándose para el otro lado, rebuscó entre sus mapas y sacó un folleto de colores. "Mira. Imprimí esto."

Lo tomé en las manos y me senté. No solamente lo había impreso sino que lo había doblado igual que un folleto. El panfleto anunciaba visitas guiadas de los jardines botánicos Kalamack: "'Venga a caminar en los espectaculares jardines privados del concejal Trenton Kalamack,'" leí en voz alta. "'Llame con anticipación para averiguar el horario y cuanto cuesta la entrada. Cerrado en luna llena por mantenimiento.'" Había más información, pero ya tenía mi sistema de entrada.

"Tengo otro para los establos," dijo Ivy. "Tienen visitas guiadas todo el año, menos en la primavera cuando nacen los potros."

"Qué considerados." Pasé el dedo sobre el dibujo de la

propiedad. No tenía idea de que a Trent le interesaran los jardines. A lo mejor *es* un brujo. Se escuchó un gemido duro y obvio y Jenks voló una distancia corta hasta la mesa. Apenas podía volar.

"Esto es maravilloso," dije, ignorando al beligerante duende que caminaba sobre el papel para detenerse directamente en mi campo de visión. "Pensé que tal vez podrías dejarme en algún lugar del bosque y desde allí buscar la manera de entrar, pero esto es maravilloso. Gracias."

Ivy me mostró una gran sonrisa. "Un poco de investigación ahorra tiempo."

Yo contuve un suspiro. Si Ivy se salía con la suya, tendríamos un plan en seis etapas colgando encima del retrete explicando qué hacer en caso de que el plan original no funcione.

"Creo que podría caber en una cartera grande."

"En una cartera para un trasero grande," complementó Jenks.

"Alguien me debe un favor," dijo Ivy. "Si ella compra el boleto, mi nombre no estará en la lista y podría usar un disfraz." Ivy sonrió ligeramente apenas dejando ver sus dientes. Yo le devolví una leve sonrisa. Se veía humana en la luz brillante del atardecer.

"Escuchen," dijo Jenks mirando a su esposa. "Yo también quepo en una cartera."

Ivy golpeó sus dientes con el estilógrafo. "Yo tomo la visita guiada y perderé desprevenidamente la cartera en algún lugar."

Jenks estaba parado encima del folleto agitando las alas torpemente. "Yo también voy."

Tiré del folleto debajo de Jenks y tropezó hacia atrás. "Nos vemos mañana más allá de la reja principal, en el bosque. Puedes recogerme justo donde nadie nos puede ver."

"Yo también voy," dijo Jenks más fuerte, pero lo ignoramos.

Ivy se reclinó en el asiento con aire de satisfacción. *"Eso sí es un plan."*

Todo esto era extraño. Anoche, Ivy por poco me arranca la cabeza cuando sugerí casi la misma cosa. Todo lo que necesitaba era algo de motivación. Satisfecha de haber descubierto este detalle sobre Ivy, me levanté y abrí mi armario de hechizos. "Trent ya sabe de ti," le dije mientras miraba todos mis conjuros. "Sólo Dios sabe cómo. Definitivamente necesitas un disfraz. Veamos... puedo hacer que te veas vieja."

"¿Es que nadie me escucha?" gritó Jenks con sus alas rojas de ira. "Voy a ir. Raquel, dile a mi esposa que estoy bien."

"Espera, espera," dijo Ivy. No quiero hechizos. Tengo mi propio disfraz."

Sorprendida, me di vuelta. "¿No quieres uno de los míos? No duele. Sólo es una ilusión. No es un hechizo de transformación."

No quiso mirarme a los ojos. "Ya tengo algo en mente."

"Dije que ¡voy a ir!," gritó Jenks.

Ivy se frotó los ojos con las manos.

"Jenks," comencé a hablar.

"Dile," pidió Jenks lanzándole una mirada a su esposa. "Si tú le dices que estoy bien, me dejará ir. Para entonces ya podré volar."

"Escucha," le dije. "Habrá otras oportunidades..."

"¿Para irrumpir en la hacienda Kalamack?" gritó. "No creo. Es ahora o nunca. Es mi única oportunidad de averiguar a qué huele Kalamack. Ningún duende ni hada ha podido descifrar qué es; y ni tú ni nadie van a impedir que aproveche esta oportunidad." Su voz sonaba desesperada. "Ninguna de ustedes dos puede."

Miré a la Sra. Jenks con ojos suplicantes. Él tenía razón. No habría otra oportunidad. Inclusive era arriesgado poner en juego mi vida, que de todas maneras ya estaba adentro de la batidora esperando a que alguien oprimiera el botón. La hermosa duende cerró los ojos y cruzó los brazos. Asintió con preocupación. "Está bien," dije mirando a Jenks. "Puedes venir."

"¿Qué?," aulló Ivy. Yo me encogí de hombros impotente.

"Ella dijo que está bien," repuse dirigiendo la mirada a la Sra. Jenks. "Pero solamente si promete salir tan pronto yo lo ordene. No voy a arriesgarlo más de lo que puede volar."

Las alas de Jenks se tornaron moradas de emoción. "Saldré cuando yo lo decida."

"Absolutamente NO." Estiré los brazos sobre la mesa poniendo un puño a cada lado de Jenks. "Vamos a entrar allá según mi criterio y saldremos de allá según mi criterio. Esta es una brujocracia... no una democracia... ¿entendido?"

Jenks se puso tenso y abrió la boca para protestar; pero entonces sus ojos saltaron de mí a su esposa. Su diminuto pie daba golpecitos en el piso.

"Está bien" dijo humildemente. "Pero sólo por esta vez."

Aprobé y crucé los brazos. "¿Concuerda esto con tu *plan,* Ivy?"

"Me da igual." Su silla raspó contra el suelo cuando se levantó. "Voy a llamar a lo del boleto. Tenemos que salir con tiempo para llegar hasta la casa de mi amiga y de la estación del autobús antes de las cuatro. Las visitas guiadas salen de allí." Su ritmo comenzó a tornarse vampiro cuando salió de la cocina.

"Jenks querido," dijo suavemente la pequeña mujer. "Estaré en el jardín por si acaso me..." Sus últimas palabras se le atoraron en la garganta y salió volando por la ventana.

Jenks reaccionó un segundo tarde. "Matalina, espera," gritó, sus alas agitándose velozmente, pero estaba prendido a la mesa. No pudo seguirle el paso. "¡Maldito Giro! Es mi única oportunidad," gritó.

Oí la voz apagada de Ivy en el salón que discutía con alguien por teléfono. "No me importa si son las dos de la tarde. Me debes." Hubo un corto silencio. "Yo puedo ir allá y retirarlo de tu escondite, Carmen. No tengo nada que hacer esta noche." Jenks y yo saltamos al oír un golpe seco contra la pared. Creo que fue el teléfono. Parece que todos disfrutábamos de una tarde apacible.

"¡Todo arreglado!" gritó con evidente alegría forzada.

"Podemos retirar el boleto dentro de media hora. El tiempo justo para cambiarnos."

"Excelente," dije suspirando, dirigiéndome a sacar una poción de visón. No creía que la simple ropa ofreciera un buen disfraz para un vampiro. "Oye, Jenks," dije en voz baja mientras escarbaba entre los cubiertos buscando un punzón de sangre. "¿A qué huele Ivy?"

"¿Qué?" gruñó, claramente alterado por lo de su esposa.

Pasé la mirada por el pasillo desocupado. "Ivy," le dije aun más bajo asegurándome de que ella no pudiera oírme. "Antes del ataque de las hadas salió de aquí furiosa. Parecía que fuera a sacarle el corazón a alguien. Yo no me voy a meter en su cartera a menos que esté segura que..." dudé un instante y luego susurré, "no está activa de nuevo."

Jenks se puso serio. "No." Se estiró y voló hacia mí. "Mandé a Jax a vigilarla, solo para asegurarnos de que nadie haya pasado un hechizo de contrabando dirigido a ti." Jenks resopló con aire paternal. "Le fue bien en su primera misión. Nadie lo vio. Igual que su viejo."

Me acerqué un poco más. "Entonces...¿dónde estaba?"

"En un bar de vampiros, cerca del río. Se sentó en una esquina, gruñéndole a todos los que trataban de acercarse. Y tomó jugo de naranja toda la noche," Jenks agitó suavemente la cabeza. "Si quieres que te de mi opinión, eso sí que me pareció extraño."

Sentimos un leve sonido cerca de la puerta. Jenks y yo nos pusimos derechos, tratando de ocultar cierta culpabilidad. Alcé la mirada parpadeando asombrada. "¿Ivy?," tartamudeé.

Sonrió sonrojándose un poco. "¿Qué te parece?"

"¡Oh! ¡Muy bien!," dije. "Te ves fantástica. Jamás te habría reconocido." Era verdad.

Ivy estaba vestida con un apretado vestido amarillo. Los dos delgados tirantes que lo sostenían sobresalían contra su piel blanca. Su cabello negro era una ola de ébano. El único color que tenía en la cara era el pintalabios rojo que la hacía verse más exótica de lo normal. Tenía puestos unos lentes de sol y un sobrero amarillo de alas que hacía juego con sus tacones altos. En el hombro cargaba una cartera tan grande como para meter a un potro.

Giró en círculo lentamente, como modelo profesional en pasarela. Sus tacones producían un agudo clic-clac y yo no pude menos que admirarla. Mirándola así pensé para mis adentros: no más chocolates, Raquel. Se detuvo y se quitó los lentes. "Creo que estará bien."

Moví la cabeza incrédula. "Sí, sí…eh…¿de verdad te vistes así a veces?"

"Antes sí. Además, tiene la ventaja de no activar los amuletos de detección de hechizos."

Jenks hizo una mueca parado en el umbral. "A pesar de lo mucho que estoy disfrutando de esta increíble emanación de estrógeno, creo que debo despedirme de mi esposa. Avísenme cuando estén listas. Estaré en el jardín, a lo mejor cerca de la hierba apestosa." Alzó el vuelo bamboleándose y salió por la ventana. De nuevo volví la mirada hacia Ivy. Era impresionante.

"Estoy asombrada de que aún me quede bien," dijo Ivy mirándose. "Era de mi madre. Lo heredé cuando murió." Me lanzó una mirada grave con el ceño fruncido. "Y si alguna vez se aparece en nuestra puerta, no le digas que me lo puse."

"Seguro," repuse débilmente.

Ivy lanzó su bolso sobre la mesa y se sentó con las piernas cruzadas. "Ella cree que mi tía abuela se lo robó. Si se entera de que yo lo tengo, me hará devolverlo. Como si ella pudiera usarlo. Un vestido amarillo después de ponerse el sol es de muy mal gusto."

Me regaló una gran sonrisa y yo contuve el temblor. Parecía humana. Una humana rica y apetecible. Caí en la cuenta de que ese vestido era un vestido de cacería.

Ivy se quedó quieta al ver mi cara de susto. Sus ojos se dilataron y eso me aceleró el pulso. El terrible negro pasó sobre sus ojos y empezó a juguetear con sus instintos. De pronto perdí conciencia de estar en la cocina Aunque ella estaba del otro lado del recinto, a mi me pareció que estaba a mi lado. Sentí calor y después frío. ¡Ella estaba arrastrándome el aura en plena tarde!

"Raquel," dijo respirando profundo. Su voz tentadora me produjo escalofrío. "Deja de temer."

Mi respiración se tornó rápida y corta. Atemorizada, me esforcé por darle la espalda. *¡Maldición, maldición, maldición!* Esta vez no era culpa mía. ¡Yo no hice nada! Parecía tan normal, pero ¿ahora esto? Vi cómo Ivy se quedaba quieta, luchando por controlarse. Si llegaba a moverse, yo me tiraba por la ventana.

Pero no se movió. Poco a poco, mi respiración volvió a la normalidad, mi pulso bajó y su tensión disminuyó. Me quité el cabello de la cara y fingí lavarme las manos. Ella se tiró en el asiento junto a la mesa. El temor era un afrodisíaco para su apetito y sin quererlo yo la estaba alimentando.

"No debí ponerme esto," dijo en voz baja y tensa. "Te espero en el jardín mientras que tú invocas tu hechizo." Asentí y ella se dirigió a la puerta, tratando de caminar normalmente. No caí en la cuenta en qué momento se levantó, pero ahí estaba ella, caminando por el pasillo. "Ah, Raquel," dijo suavemente parada en el umbral. "Si algún día vuelvo a la actividad, tú serás la primera en saberlo."

Dieciocho

"Creo que jamás podré librar mi nariz del hedor de ese costal." Jenks tomó una profunda bocanada del fresco aire de la noche.

"Bolsa," dije, oyendo que la palabra salió de mi boca como leve chillido. No podía articular otra cosa. Reconocí de inmediato el olor de la bolsa de la madre de Ivy, y de solo pensar que había pasado casi todo el día allí metida se me ponían los pelos de punta.

"¿Alguna vez habías sentido un olor así?" dijo Jenks risueño.

"Ya cállate Jenks"—chillido, chillido. En realidad, no es que me importara demasiado lo que lleva un vampiro cuando sale de cacería. Además, traté de no acordarme de la Tabla 6.1.

"No-o-o-o," dijo arrastrando las letras. "Más bien era un olor metálico almizclado como...eh..."

Pero el aire de la noche era agradable. Ya casi eran las diez y el jardín de Trent emitía el olor de la exuberante vegetación húmeda. La luna era un pequeño disco de plata perdido entre los árboles. Jenks y yo estábamos escondidos entre los matorrales detrás de un banco de piedra. Hacía ya horas que Ivy no estaba.

Esa tarde había dejado la cartera debajo del banco fingiendo estar mareada. Luego de echarle la culpa de su debilidad a una baja de azúcar en la sangre, la mitad de los hombres en el tour se ofrecieron para traerle una galleta del pabellón. Yo estuve a punto de echar a perder todo nuestro plan muriéndome de risa con la permanente y exagerada parodia de Jenks de lo que estaba ocurriendo afuera de la bolsa. Ivy había desaparecido en medio de un torbellino de hombres preocupados por ella. Yo no sabía si preocuparme o admirarme con la facilidad con la cual los dominó.

"Esto me huele tan mal como el viejo tío vampiro cuidando una fiesta de quinceañeras" dijo Jenks mientras salía de las sombras para dirigirse hacia el sendero. "No he oído ni un sólo pájaro en toda la tarde. Tampoco hay hadas ni duendes." Miró hacia la negra bóveda celeste.

"Vamos," chillé, mirando el sendero desolado. Lo veía todo en tonos grises y aun no lograba acostumbrarme a ello.

"No creo que haya duendes ni hadas," siguió Jenks. "Un jardín de este tamaño es capaz de mantener por lo menos a cuatro clanes. ¿Quién cuida las plantas?"

"¿A lo mejor es por aquel lado?" dije, tal vez ante la necesidad de hablar, pues él ni siquiera podía entenderme.

"Sí, sí..." continuó Jenks hablando solo. Grandulones. Brutos torpes de dedos gruesos que arrancan una planta enferma en lugar de darle una dosis de potasa.

No confiaba en la seguridad que Jenks tenía acerca de los duendes y las hadas. Yo estaba esperando que nos atacaran en cualquier momento. Después de ver el resultado de un enfrentamiento entre ambos, francamente no tenía apuro para experimentarlo de nuevo, especialmente ahora que era del tamaño de una ardilla.

Jenks estiró el cuello y escudriñó entre las ramas ajustando su sombrero. Me había dicho que era de color rojo fuego y que era el único color que protegía a un duende que osara entrar en el jardín de otro clan. Era un símbolo de buena voluntad y retiro rápido. Su constante cantaleta con el sombrero en el bolso de Ivy casi termina por enloquecerme. Además, haber permanecido detrás de ese banco toda la tarde no había sido propiamente divertido. Jenks se había pasado casi todo el día durmiendo, estirándose al despertar cuando el sol estaba por esconderse en el horizonte.

De pronto sentí una ráfaga de emoción que me abandonó tan rápido como había llegado. Chillé para llamar la atención de Jenks y mi dirigí siguiendo el olor de una alfombra. El tiempo que permanecimos en el bolso de Ivy detrás de ese banco le sentaron bien a Jenks. Pero, aun así, venía rezagado. Preocupada que tal vez el leve ruido de sus alas heridas pudieran alertar a alguien, me detuve y le indiqué que se subiera sobre mi lomo.

"¿Qué pasa Raque?," dijo Jenks ajustándose el sombrero. "¿Tienes piquiña?"

Le mostré los dientes, agaché la grupa y le señalé mis hombros.

"Ni por el infierno," refunfuñó. Miró luego hacia los árboles. "No voy a dejar que me lleven en cochecito como un bebé."

No tengo tiempo para perder en tonterías, pensé. Esta vez me paré y señalé al cielo. Era la señal que habíamos acordado dándole la orden de regresar a casa. Jenks bajó la mirada y yo saqué los dientes. Sorprendido, dio un paso hacia atrás.

"Está bien, está bien," se quejó. "Pero si le dices a Ivy, te voy a duendear todas las noches durante una semana, ¿comprendes?" Sentí su cuerpo liviano sobre mis hombros y se aferró a mi pelaje. Era una sensación extraña que no me gustó. "No vayas demasiado rápido," rezongó, sintiéndose también incómodo.

Aparte de su agarre mortal en mi piel, no podía sentirlo. Caminé tan rápido como pude. No me gustaba la idea de que hubieran ojos enemigos vigilándonos con el acero de las hadas, así que decidí salirme del sendero. Cuanto antes entráramos, mejor. Mis oídos y mi nariz trabajaban sin cesar. Podía olerlo todo, pero no era tan agradable como creía.

Las hojas se movían con cada brisa haciéndome parar o

meterme en la espesura. Jenks cantaba una monótona canción entre dientes. Algo acerca de sangre y margaritas.

Tejí mi paso a través de una barrera de zarzas y piedras caídas reduciendo la velocidad. Había algo diferente. "Las plantas han cambiado," dijo Jenks. Yo moví la cabeza. Los árboles por donde pasamos a medida que descendíamos por la loma eran más viejos. Además, olía a muérdago. La tierra vieja bien conservada tenía plantas crecidas. El aroma era más importante que la belleza visual. El estrecho pasadizo que encontré era de tierra prensada, no de ladrillo. El sendero estaba lleno de helechos hasta el punto de que una sola persona podía pasar. Se sentía el rumor del agua corriendo. Con más cautela aún, proseguimos hasta detenernos ante un olor muy conocido: Té Earl Gray.

Bajo la sombra de un lirio, me quedé quieta e intenté percibir el olor a humano. Todo estaba en silencio, excepto los insectos nocturnos. "Allá," me dijo Jenks. "Hay una taza en el banco." Se deslizó de mi espalda y desapareció en las sombras.

Me moví hacia adelante moviendo los bigotes y afinando el oído. El bosquecillo estaba desierto. Con un movimiento ágil subí al banco. Quedaba un trago de té en el fondo de la taza. El borde estaba cubierto de rocío. Su presencia decía tanto como el cambio de la vegetación. Sin saberlo, habíamos abandonado el parque público y estábamos en el jardín de Trent.

Jenks se encaramó en el asa, las manos en la cintura y el ceño fruncido. "Nada," dijo quejándose. "No puedo oler al hombre en la taza de té. Necesito entrar."

Salté del banco tratando de aterrizar bien. El hedor a área habitada era más fuerte hacia la izquierda y seguimos el sendero de tierra en medio de helechos. Muy pronto, el olor de muebles, alfombras y equipos electrónicos se hizo penetrante. No nos llamó la atención cuando hallamos la terraza al aire libre. Miré hacia arriba y pude ver un techo. Una enredadera nocturna florecía encima y su fragancia luchaba por sobresalir más que el hedor humano.

"¡Espera Raquel!," exclamó Jenks tirándome de una oreja cuando estaba a punto de pisar las tablas cubiertas de musgo. Algo rozó mis bigotes y retrocedí tocándolos con mis patas. Era pegajoso y accidentalmente pegué mis orejas sobre los ojos. Sentí pánico y me senté en las ancas. ¡Estaba pegada!

"No te frotes," me dijo Jenks con urgencia. "Quédate quieta."

No podía ver y mi pulso empezó a acelerar. Traté de chillar pero tenía la boca pegada. El olor a éter me invadió la garganta. Desesperada, traté de desprenderla con las manos, pero solo logré oír un zumbido apagado. ¡A duras penas podía respirar! ¿Qué demonios era esta cosa?

"Ya cálmate Morgan," dijo Jenks. "Deja de lanzarme golpes. Te voy a quitar esto."

Controlé mis instintos y me senté. Mi respiración era lenta y trabajosa. Una de mis patas estaba pegada a mis bigotes y me dolía. Si no me sentaba iba a caer por tierra.

"Está bien." Sentí la brisa que producían las alas de Jenks. "Voy a tocar tu ojo."

Mis manos temblaban a medida que Jenks limpiaba esa cosa de uno de mis párpados. Sus dedos eran suaves y diestros; pero el dolor me hacía sentir como si me estuviera arrancando el párpado. De pronto pude ver de nuevo. Con un solo ojo, ví como Jenks frotaba una bolita entre sus manos. Le salía polvillo de duende que lo hacía brillar. "¿Mejor?" preguntó mirándome.

"¡Claro que sí!" chillé, aun cuando sonó más sordo que de costumbre pues todavía tenía la boca pegada.

Jenks botó la bolita. Era esa cosa pegajosa mezclada con polvillo. "Quédate quieta y te quitaré el resto más rápido de lo que Ivy puede arrastrar un aura." Tiró de mi piel formando bolitas con la cosa pegajosa. "Lo siento," dijo, cuando me tiró la oreja. "No te advertí a tiempo."

"¿Cómo?," chillé mientras jalaba mis pelos. "Así fue como me atraparon ayer," dijo molesto. "Trent tiene el techo de su vestíbulo cubierto de seda pegajosa, justo arriba de la altura normal de los humanos. Es un material muy caro. Me llama la atención que también lo use en cualquier otro lugar." Jenks voló hacia mi otro costado. "Es un disuasivo contra hadas y duendes. Te lo puedes quitar, pero te demoras. Casi podría asegurar que todo el parque está cubierto. Por eso no hay nada que vuela."

Moví la cola para mostrarle que entendí. Había oído sobre la seda pegajosa pero nunca se me ocurrió pensar que la experimentaría en persona. Se sentía como telarañas.

Finalmente terminó y otra vez sentí mi nariz. Pensé si tendría la misma forma. Jenks se quitó el sombrero y lo lanzó debajo de una piedra. "Debí traer mi espada," dijo. La confrontación territorial entre hadas y duendes era de tal magnitud que cuando Jenks dejó su sombrero me convencí totalmente de que el jardín estaba libre de ambos. Su actitud sumisa de toda la tarde desapareció. Desde su punto de vista, seguramente todo el jardín le pertenecía, pues no había nadie que dijera otra cosa. Se paró a mi lado con las manos en la cintura, mirando detenidamente la terraza de Trent.

"Mira esto," dijo, sacudiendo polvillo de su cuerpo. Sus alas parecían una nube mientras soplaban el polvillo hacia la terraza con su brisa. La suave bruma parecía suspendida en el aire. Como por arte de magia, el polvillo se prendió a la seda marcando un trozo de malla. Jenks hizo una mueca de satisfacción con los labios. "Afortunadamente traje las tijeras de Matalina," dijo, sacando el par de tijeras con mango de madera de su bolsillo. Luego se acercó tranquilamente a la malla y cortó un agujero del tamaño de un visón. "Después de ti." Hizo una gran venia y yo me trepé a la terraza.

Mi corazón latió emocionado antes de regresar a un ritmo deliberadamente lento. Se trata tan sólo de una misión más, me dije a mí misma. Pero la emoción era un lujo que no podía darme ahora. Tenía que hacer de cuenta que mi vida no estaba de por medio. Mi nariz se movió buscando Entremundos o humanos. Nada.

"Me parece que es una oficina secundaria," dijo Jenks. "Mira. Ahí hay un escritorio."

¿*Oficina?*, pensé. Mis cejas peludas se alzaron. Era una terraza ¿no es así? Jenks se sacudía entusiasmado como un murciélago rabioso. Yo andaba a un paso más pausado. Después de recorrer unos cuatro metros las tablas cubiertas de musgo se convirtieron en una alfombra moteada encerrada por tres paredes. En todas partes había macetas con plantas muy bien cuidadas. El pequeño escritorio que había en la pared del fondo parecía con poco uso. También había un sofá grande y varias sillas alrededor de un bar. El cuarto era un lugar muy cómodo para descansar o para realizar trabajo ligero. Era una oficina que se extendía al exterior por la terraza y se convertía en jardín.

"¡Mira lo que encontré!," dijo Jenks emocionado.

Giré desde donde estaba junto a las orquídeas para ver a Jenks flotando encima de un grupo de equipos electrónicos. "Están ocultos tras la pared," explicó. "Fíjate en esto." Voló con los pies adelante hacia un botón adherido a la pared. El reproductor de CD y los discos se ocultaron en la pared. Satisfecho, Jenks oprimió de nuevo el botón y el equipo salió de nuevo. "¿Qué hará ese otro botón?," dijo, y voló como un destello atraído por la curiosidad de hallar nuevos juguetes.

Pensé que Trent tenía más discos de música que una residencia universitaria: pop, clásica, jazz, nueva era, hasta metálica. No tenía de música disco. Ganó un par de puntos conmigo.

Pasé nostálgicamente una de mis patitas sobre *El mar,* de Takata. De repente, el disco desapareció y entró en el reproductor. Yo di un salto hacia atrás. Alarmada, salté para oprimir el botón con las patas y todo se metió de nuevo en la pared.

"Aquí no hay nada, Raque. Vamos." Jenks miró decididamente hacia la puerta y se posó sobre la manija. Pero solamente giró cuando yo salté para sumar mi peso. Caí al suelo torpemente haciendo ruido. Jenks y yo nos quedamos sin respiración por un momento.

Mi pulso se aceleró. Empujé la puerta con la nariz

abriendo apenas lo suficiente para que Jenks lograra escurrirse. En un instante estaba de regreso. "Es un pasillo," dijo. "Puedes salir. Ya arreglé las cámaras."

De nuevo desapareció por la puerta mientras que yo tuve que usar toda mi fuerza para cerrarla. El sonido de la perilla fue duro y me acobardé, rezando para que nadie lo hubiese oído. Podía escuchar agua corriendo y el susurro de animales nocturnos que salía de una bocina invisible. Inmediatamente reconocí el pasillo como aquél que había atravesado ayer. Seguramente los sonidos estuvieron siempre allí pero eran tan subliminales que tan sólo podía escucharlos el oído de un roedor. Moví la cabeza para indicar que sabía dónde estábamos. Jenks y yo habíamos encontrado la oficina secundaria donde Trent entretenía a sus huéspedes "especiales."

"¿Hacia dónde?" susurró Jenks volando a mi lado. O bien sus alas funcionaban a la perfección o no quería que lo vieran montado en un visón. Segura, seguí caminando por el pasillo. En cada cruce decidí tomar el camino menos tentador y más desolado. Jenks trabajaba en la vanguardia ajustando cada cámara durante un lapso de quince minutos en los que no podíamos ser vistos. Afortunadamente, Trent operaba según el horario humano (por lo menos en público) y por eso el edificio estaba desocupado. O al menos eso creíamos.

"Mierda," dijo Jenks al mismo tiempo que quedé inmóvil. Sentimos voces en el vestíbulo. Mi pulsó comenzó a golpearme. "¡Corre!" dijo Jenks con urgencia. "¡No! Hacia la derecha. Esa silla y la planta en la maceta."

Me tiré hacia la maceta. El aroma de cítrico y terracota emanaba de la planta. Yo me acurruqué detrás de la maceta de barro y unos pasos suaves cruzaron por el piso. Jenks voló a esconderse entre las ramas.

"¿Tanto?" Reconocí claramente la voz de Trent que llegaba a mis sensibles oídos mientras que le daba la vuelta a la esquina con otra persona. "Averigua qué está haciendo

Hodgkin para incrementar la productividad. Si es algo que tú piensas que podría aplicarse en otros sitios, quiero un informe."

Contuve la respiración mientras Trent y Jonathan pasaron frente a nosotros.

"Sí, Sa'han." Jonathan garabateó en una libreta electrónica. "Ya terminé la revisión de antecedentes de las candidatas para nueva secretaria. Sería relativamente sencillo abrir espacio en su agenda de mañana en la mañana. ¿A cuántas quisiera entrevistar?"

"Pues...digamos que sólo a tres que te parezcan las más adecuadas y una que no. ¿Alguna que ya conozca?"

"No. Esta vez tuve que buscar por fuera del estado."

"Jon...¿hoy era tu día libre?"

Hubo un silencio. "Decidí trabajar, puesto que no tiene usted seretaria."

"Ah," repuso Trent con una sonrisa de satisfacción mientras giraban por la esquina.

"He ahí la razón de tu afán por terminar las entrevistas."

La negativa de Jon fue apenas un mero rumor mientras se alejaban.

"Jenks," chillé. No respondió. "¡Jenks!" chillé de nuevo, pensando si acaso habría hecho algo estúpido, como por ejemplo seguirlos.

"Aquí estoy," refunfuñó. Sentí alivio. La planta tembló mientras se deslizaba por el tronco. Se sentó en el borde de la maceta colgando los pies. "Lo olí bien" dijo. Yo me senté en las ancas esperando con ansiedad.

"No sé lo que es." Las alas de Jenks se tornaron azules a medida que su circulación se hacía más lenta y su estado de ánimo se apagaba. "Huele a pradera, pero no como brujo. No tiene trazas de hierro, por consiguiente no es vampiro." Los ojos de Jenks ondulaban confundidos. "Olí cómo su ritmo corporal disminuía, lo que significa que duerme toda la noche. Eso descarta a los lobos o cualquier otro Entremundo nocturno. ¡Duendes y relámpagos, Raque! No huele a nada que pueda reconocer. Pero...¿sabes qué es lo más extraño? Ese tipo que lo acompaña. Huele lo mismo que Trent. Tiene que ser un hechizo."

Mis bigotes temblaron. Extraño no era la palabra. Chillé.

"Así es." Se alzó lentamente, como una libélula, hasta la mitad del pasillo. "Deberíamos terminar ya la misión y largarnos de aquí."

Me estremecí de repente. *Largarnos de aquí,* pensé, dejando la seguridad de la planta. Podía apostar que no saldríamos por el mismo lugar por el que entramos. Pero de eso me preocuparía después de irrumpir en la oficina de Trent. Ya habíamos logrado lo imposible. Salir no era problema.

"Por acá," chillé, caminando por un pasillo ya conocido antes de llegar al vestíbulo. Podía oler la sal del tanque de peces en la oficina de Trent. Las puertas de vidrios esmerilados estaban a oscuras. Nadie trabajaba a esta hora y seguramente la puerta de madera de Trent estaría cerrada.

Veloz, Jenks se puso a trabajar. El seguro era electrónico y pasados unos momentos de jugueteo con la consola que estaba atornillada a la puerta, el seguro sonó y la puerta se abrió. "Estándard," dijo Jenks. "Hasta Jax podría abrirla."

El suave borboteo de la fuente en el escritorio salió por el pasillo. Jenks entró primero ajustando la cámara antes de que yo lo siguiera.

"No, espera," chillé, al ver que se lanzaba con los pies adelante hacia el interruptor de la luz. La habitación estaba bañada de un resplandor lúgubre. "¡Eh!" exclamé, tapándome la cara con las manos.

"Lo siento." Apagó la luz.

"Enciende la luz encima del acuario," chillé, tratando de ver algo con mis ojos ahora deslumbrados. "El acuario," repetí inútilmente, sentada en mis ancas y señalando con las manos.

"Raquel, no seas estúpida. No tienes tiempo de ponerte a comer." Entonces pensó un instante, bajó un poco y dijo: "¡Ah!, la luz. Buena idea."

La luz titiló y se encendió iluminando la oficina de Trent con un suave resplandor verde. Salté a su asiento giratorio y de allí al escritorio, moviendo torpemente las hojas de su agenda un par de meses. Finalmente arranqué una hoja. Mi pulso se aceleró. La dejé caer al piso y la recogí.

Abrí el cajón del escritorio y encontré los discos. No creí que Trent habría movido todo. *Tal vez,* me dije orgullosamente, *no pensó que yo fuera una amenaza importante.* Tomé el disco rotulado ALZHEIMER, tomé impulso sobre la alfombra y recargué todo mi peso contra el cajón para cerrarlo. Su escritorio estaba hecho de hermosa madera de cerezo. Lejanamente pensé en el triste contraste que habría entre mis muebles de madera prensada y los de Ivy.

Sentada en mis ancas, le indiqué a Jenks la cuerda. Jenks había doblado la hoja de manera que la pudiera sujetar y tan pronto me amarrara el disco, nos largaríamos de allí.

"Cuerda, ¿verdad?" Jenks hurgó en sus bolsillos.

De repente la luz del techo se encendió y yo quedé petrificada. Me agaché bajo el escritorio mirando hacia la puerta y vi dos pares de zapatos: un par de pantuflas suaves y un par de cuero duro. La luz se derramó por el pasillo.

"Trent," dijo Jenks con los labios sin hablar mientras aterrizaba a mi lado con el papel doblado.

Jonathan sonaba muy disgustado. "Ya se fueron, Sa'han. Voy a dar la alerta."

Se sintió un suspiro forzado. "Sí, anda. Veré que se llevaron."

El corazón me latía muy fuerte y me apretujé bajo el escritorio. Los zapatos de cuero dieron la vuelta dirigiéndose al pasillo. La adrenalina me invadió y pensé salir corriendo, pero no podía hacerlo con el disco entre las manos y tampoco pensaba dejarlo.

La puerta se cerró y maldije mi vacilación. Me acerqué a la tapa trasera del escritorio. Jenks y yo intercambiamos miradas. Yo le di la señal de irse a casa pero el agitó la cabeza enfáticamente. De nuevo nos agazapamos. Trent volvió y se detuvo frente al acuario.

"Hola, Sófocles," bufó Trent. "Si tan sólo pudieras decirme quién era."

Había dejado su saco de trabajo, lo cual lo hacía ver más informal. No me sorprendió la clara línea de sus hombros que se contorneaban contra su camisa al más mínimo movimiento. Suspirando, se sentó en su asiento. Su mano se dirigió al cajón de los discos y sentí que me flaqueaban las patas. Pasé saliva al darme cuenta de que estaba cantando la primera canción de *El mar, de Takata. Doble maldición. Le di todas las pistas.*

"Por eso lloran los recién nacidos; la elección fue real pero la oportunidad una mentira," susurró Trent. Era la letra de la canción.

Se quedó inmóvil con los dedos sobre los discos. Lentamente cerró el cajón con el pie. Sonó clic y me hizo saltar. Se acomodó aun más cerca del escritorio y escuché el sonido de la agenda que movió sobre la mesa. Estaba tan cerca que podía olerlo por fuera. "Oh," dijo sorprendido. "Imaginemos que..."

"¡Quen!" gritó.

Confundida, miré a Jenks. Una voz masculina que venía de un altoparalante llenó la oficina. "¿Sa'han?"

"¡Suelta a los perros!" dijo Trent. Su poderosa voz reverberó y temblé.

"Pero ¿acaso no..."

"¡Suelta a los perros, Quen!" repitió Trent con el mismo tono de voz, pero con rabia. Movía un pie rítmicamente debajo del escritorio.

"Sí, Sa'han."

Ahora su pie estaba quieto. "Espera." Oí que respiraba profundamente, como si degustara el aire.

"¿Señor?" dijo la voz.

Trent olió de nuevo. Lentamente, retiró el asiento del escritorio. Sentí que mi corazón estallaba y contuve el aire. Jenks se elevó para esconderse detrás de un cajón. Yo estaba paralizada, pues Trent se movió hacia atrás, se levantó y se agachó. No tenía dónde ir. Los ojos de Trent me encontraron y sonrió. El temor no me permitió moverme.

"Olvida esa orden," dijo suavemente.

"Bien, Sa'han." La voz quedó en silencio.

Miré a Trent sintiendo que iba a estallar.

"¿Srta. Morgan?" dijo Trent inclinando la cabeza con cortesía. Temblé. "Me gustaría decir que es un gusto." Aun así sonrió, moviéndose hacia adelante. Mostré mis dientes y chillé. Él retiró la mano frunciendo el entrecejo. "Salga de ahí. Usted tiene algo que me pertenece."

Sentí el disco junto a mí. Me habían atrapado y pasé de gran ladrón a idiota de pueblo en un segundo. ¿Cómo pude pensar que podía salirme con la mía? Ivy tenía razón.

"Venga, Srta. Morgan," me dijo estirando la mano debajo del escritorio.

Salté como un resorte hacia los espacios vacíos tratando de escapar, pero Trent lanzaba la mano dondequiera que yo estaba. De pronto chillé al sentir una mano fuerte que me atrapó por la cola. Mis garras se aferraban a la alfombra mientras que él tiraba. Giré aterrada hundiéndole mis dientes en la parte más gruesa de la mano.

"¡Maldita!" gritó y me sacó de un jalón. Todo daba vueltas y al mismo tiempo sacudió la mano violentamente golpeándome contra el escritorio. Vi millones de estrellas y sentí el sabor acanelado de su sangre. El dolor de cabeza me aflojó la mandíbula. Giraba por la cola de donde me tenía agarrada.

"¡Suéltela!" gritó Jenks.

El mundo giraba velozmente. "Trajo a su insecto," dijo Trent, golpeando un botón en su escritorio con la palma de la mano. Entonces sentí un ligero olor a éter.

"¡Véte Jenks!" chillé, al reconocer el olor de la malla pegajosa.

Jonathan abrió la puerta intempestivamente. Se quedó parado bajo el umbral con los ojos abiertos. "¡Sa'han!"

"¡Cierra la puerta!" gritó Trent.

Yo me retorcía desesperadamente tratando de escapar y Jenks salió como una flecha justo cuando logré clavarle de nuevo los dientes a Trent en el dedo pulgar. "¡Maldita bruja!" gritó, lanzándome contra la pared. De nuevo vi millones de estrellas que ahora se convertían en sombras negras. Las sombras crecieron más y más. Atontada, observé como la oscuridad crecía en mis ojos hasta que ya no veía nada más. Sentía calor. No podía moverme.

Estaba muriendo.

Tenía que ser.

Diecinueve

"Entonces, Srta. Sara Jane, ¿el horario dividido no es problema?"

"No señor. No me importa trabajar hasta las siete si puedo usar la tarde para hacer mis diligencias y cosas por el estilo."

"Le agradezco su flexibilidad. Las tardes las dedico a la contemplación. Trabajo mejor por la mañana y por la noche. Después de las cinco queda poco personal y sin distracciones puedo concentrarme mejor."

La suave voz de relaciones públicas de Trent me despertó haciéndome volver a mi estado de conciencia. Abrí los ojos sin saber por qué todo brillaba en gris y blanco. Entonces recordé. Era un visón. Pero estaba viva. Por pura suerte.

Las voces de Sara Jane y Trent continuaron mientras que me levanté temblorosa sobre mis cuatro patas. Estaba en una jaula. Mi estómago se tensó y sentí náuseas. Me acosté haciendo un esfuerzo por no vomitar. "Estoy destruída," susurré, a la vez que Trent me miraba por encima de sus lentes metálicos mientras que hablaba con una mujer delgada vestida de color pálido para la entrevista.

Me dolía la cabeza. Si no tenía una contusión, entonces era algo parecido. El hombro derecho, el que golpeó el escritorio, me dolía y también me dolía respirar. Puse mi pata delantera cerca para no moverme. Miré a Trent y traté de averiguar qué estaba sucediendo. Jenks no estaba en ninguna parte. *Ah, es verdad,* recordé con alivio. Logró escapar y estaría en casa con Ivy. Pero no podían hacer nada por mí.

En mi jaula había una botella de agua, un plato con bolitas de comida, una chozita de hurón lo suficientemente grande para meterme y una rueda de ejercicios. *Como si quisiera usarla,* pensé agriamente.

Estaba sobre una mesa en la parte de atrás de la oficina de Trent. Según la falsa luz solar de la ventana, apenas habían transcurrido unas pocas horas desde el amanecer. Demasiado temprano para mí. Pero, aun cuando me doliera en el orgullo, me iba a meter en esa choza a dormir. No me importaba lo que pensara Trent. Respiré profundo y me paré. "¡Ay! ¡Ay!" chillé, estremeciéndome de dolor.

"Oh, tiene un hurón de mascota," dijo suavemente Sara Jane.

Cerré los ojos en desgracia. No era un hurón. Era un visón. *Fíjate bien niña.*

Oí que Trent se levantaba de su escritorio y sentí, más que vi, que ambos se acercaron un poco más. Aparentemente la entrevista había terminado. Hora de comerse con los ojos al visón mascota. La luz se oscureció y abrí los ojos. Los dos estaban parados ahí, mirándome.

Sara Jane se veía muy profesional en su elegante vestido para la entrevista, su cabello largo y sencillo bajando hasta cierta distancia de los codos. La pequeña mujer era bonita. Pensé que a lo mejor nadie le prestaba mucha atención con esa nariz respingada, su vocecita de niña chiquita y su baja estatura. Sin embargo, pude ver en sus grandes ojos que estaba acostumbrada a trabajar en el mundo masculino y que sabía como hacer las cosas. También pensé que si la juzgaban mal sabría utilizar eso a su favor.

Su perfume era fuerte y me hizo estornudar. Me estremecí de dolor.

"Esta es....Ángela," dijo Trent. "Es un visón." Su sarcasmo fue sutil pero duro en mis oídos. Su mano izquierda masajeaba su derecha. La tenía vendada. *Tres vivas por el visón*, pensé.

"Se ve enferma." Las uñas cuidadosamente pintadas de Sara Jane estaban pulidas hasta la carne y sus manos se veían inusualmente fuertes, casi como las de un obrero.

"¿Le molestan los roedores, Sara Jane?"

Se enderezó y yo cerré los ojos mientras la luz los iluminaba. "Los desprecio, Sr. Kalamack. Vengo de una granja donde las alimañas se matan de inmediato. Pero no voy a perder un empleo por culpa de un animal." Tomó aire. "Necesito este empleo. Mi familia hizo grandes esfuerzos para pagar mis estudios y sacarme del campo. Tengo que pagarles lo que hicieron por mí. Tengo una hermana menor. Es demasiado inteligente para pasarse toda la vida cosechando remolachas. Quiere ser bruja. Obtener su título; pero no puedo ayudarla a menos que obtenga un buen empleo. *Necesito* este trabajo. Por favor, Sr. Kalamack. Yo sé que no tengo experiencia, pero soy inteligente y trabajo muy duro."

Entreabrí los párpados. Trent estaba serio. Pensaba. Su pelo lacio y su figura sobresalían con su elegante traje de negocios. Él y Sara Jane hacían bonita pareja, aun cuando ella era un poco baja. "Dicho en palabras simples, Sara Jane," dijo Trent con una sonrisa, "lo que más admiro en mis empleados es la honestidad. ¿Cuándo puede comenzar?"

"De inmediato" dijo con voz trémula. Sentí que enfermaba. Pobre mujer.

"Excelente," dijo complacido. "Jon le pedirá firmar algunos papeles. Luego le indicará sus responsabilidades. Será su sombra durante la primera semana. Puede preguntarle todo a él. Ha trabajado conmigo durante años y me conoce mejor que yo mismo."

"Gracias, Sr. Kalamack" repuso, alzando emocionada sus pequeños hombros.

"Es un gusto para mí." Trent la tomó del codo y la acompañó hasta la puerta. *La tocó*, pensé. *¿Por qué no me tocó a mí? ¿Acaso temió que pudiera averiguar lo que es?*

"¿Ya tiene un sitio donde vivir?," le preguntó. "No olvide preguntarle a Jon acerca de los alojamientos que tenemos fuera de la hacienda para empleados."

"Gracias, Sr. Kalamack. No, aún no tengo apartamento."

"Muy bien. Tómese el tiempo necesario para instalarse. Si lo desea, podemos depositar parte de su sueldo en un fondo libre de impuestos para su hermana."

"Sí, por favor." La sensación de alivio en la voz de Sara Jane era obvia, inclusive desde el pasillo. Estaba atrapada. Trent era una especie de dios para ella, un príncipe que llegó a su rescate y el de su familia. ¿Qué mal podía causarle?

Mi estómago dio vueltas. La habitación estaba vacía y yo me arrastré en la choza. Giré una vez para meter la cola y dejar la nariz apuntando hacia afuera. De pronto sentí que la puerta de la oficina se cerraba y de nuevo salté. Todo me dolió.

"Buenos días, Sr. Morgan," dijo Trent. La brisa llegó hasta mi jaula cuando pasó frente a ella. Se sentó en el escritorio y empezó a organizar sus papeles. "Pensaba dejarla aquí sólo hasta recibir una segunda opinión sobre usted. Pero no sé. Ahora es usted *motivo* de conversación."

"Vete al demonio," dije mostrándole los dientes. Todo soltaba chillidos.

"No me diga. No creo que eso haya sido un cumplido."

Un golpe en la puerta hizo que me pusiera alerta. Era Jonathan. Trent se veía ocupado. "¿Dime Jon?," le dijo, con la atención fija en el calendario.

El hombre alto se detuvo a una distancia respetuosa. "Sa'han, ¿la Srta. Sara Jane?"

"Posee justamente las cualidades que necesito." Trent dejó el lápiz. Se recostó en el asiento y se quitó las lentes mordiendo despreocupadamente una pata de la armadura hasta que cayó en la cuenta de la silenciosa mirada de desacuerdo de Jonathan. Trent las lanzó sobre el escritorio con una mirada molesta. "La hermana menor de Sara Jane necesita salir de la granja para estudiar brujería," le dijo. "Debemos apoyar la excelencia siempre que podamos."

"Ah... comprendo," dijo Jon un poco más relajado.

"Hazme el favor de averiguar el precio de venta de la granja de Sara Jane. Me gustaría jugar un poco en la industria del azúcar. Algo así como probar su dulce. Conserva a los trabajadores y traslada a Hodgkin como capataz durante seis meses para que entrene al capataz actual en sus métodos. Pídele que vigile a la hermana de Sara Jane. Si tiene algo de cerebro, pídele que la traslade donde tenga algunas responsabilidades."

Asomé la cabeza por la puerta, preocupada. Jonathan me miró con desprecio. "¿De nuevo con nosotros, Morgan?" dijo burlándose. "Si por mí fuera, la habría metido al triturador de desperdicios en el cuarto de descanso de los trabajadores y hubiera oprimido el interruptor."

"Bastardo," chillé, y le di la espalda para que entendiera.

Las arrugas de Jonathan se hicieron más profundas al fruncir el ceño y golpeó mi jaula con la carpeta que llevaba en la mano. Olvidando mi dolor me lancé contra los barrotes mostrándole los dientes.

Cayó hacia atrás asustado. Rojo de ira, el hombre tomó de nuevo impulso con la mano.

"Jon," dijo Trent suavemente, su voz apenas un susurro pero, aun así, el hombre quedó inmóvil. Yo permanecí aferrada a los barrotes con el corazón latiendo rápido. "Olvidas tu lugar. Deja en paz a la Srta. Morgan. Si tú la juzgas mal y ella se defiende, no es culpa suya. Es culpa tuya. Ya has cometido este error antes. Repetidamente."

Brava, bajé de nuevo al piso de la jaula y gruñí. No sabía que gruñía, pero lo hacía. Lentamente, Jonathan aflojó la mano. "Mi lugar es protegerlo a usted."

Trent alzó las cejas. "La Srta. Morgan no está en situación de lastimar a nadie. Ya basta."

Mis ojos saltaban de un hombre al otro. El más viejo aceptó la reprimenda de Trent sin reclamar. Jamás lo hubiera imaginado. Los dos tenían una relación muy extraña. Trent claramente tenía el control; pero recordé la cara de molestia de Trent cuando Jonathan había hecho manifiesto su desacuerdo cuando Trent mordía la pata de sus lentes. A lo mejor esa relación no siempre fue así. Pensé si acaso Jonathan se había encargado de la educación de Trent por un breve tiempo, cuando murió su madre y después su padre.

"Acepte mis disculpas, Sa'han," dijo Jonathan inclinando la cabeza.

Trent no respondió y regresó a sus papeles. Jonathan siguió allí parado aun cuando era obvio que ya podía retirarse. Trent alzó la cabeza. "¿Alguna otra cosa?" preguntó Trent.

"Su cita de las ocho treinta llegó temprano. ¿Traigo al Sr. Percy?"

"¡Percy!" chillé. Trent me miró. *¡No puede ser Francis Percy!*

"Sí," dijo Trent suavemente. "Por favor."

Demonios, pensé, mientras Jonathan regresaba al pasillo y cerraba lentamente la puerta al salir. La entrevista interrumpida de Francis. Caminé neviosamente alrededor de mi jaula. Mis músculos se estaban aflojando y el movimiento dolía pero se sentía bien. Me detuve al caer en la cuenta que Trent no me había quitado los ojos de encima. Entonces me metí de nuevo en mi choza, un poco avergonzada de su mirada.

Aun así, Trent seguía mirándome mientras enroscaba mi cola en la nariz para mantenerla caliente. "No se disguste con Jon," dijo suavemente. "El asume su trabajo con seriedad, como debe ser. Si lo presiona demasiado, la matará. Esperemos que usted no tenga que aprender esa lección."

Levanté el labio mostrando los dientes, pues no me gustaba que me diera lecciones de viejo sabio.

Un gemido hizo que los dos dirigiéramos nuestra atención hacia el pasillo. Francis. Le había dicho que podía convertirme en visón. Si conectaba bien los cables, era como estar muerta. Bueno…más muerta de lo que ya lo estaba. No quería que me viera. Y, aparentemente, Trent tampoco.

"Ummm…sí" dijo, poniéndose de pie a toda prisa, moviendo una de sus plantas grandes para esconder mi jaula. Ahora estaba tranquila y además podía ver a través de las hojas permaneciendo oculta. Golpearon en la puerta. "Adelante," dijo Trent.

"No, en serio..." decía Francis, pero Jonathan por poco lo hace entrar a empujones.

Pude ver cómo Francis miraba a Trent y tragaba saliva con dificultad. "Eh...hola, Sr. Kalamack," tartamudeó, quedándose quieto en una posición algo extraña. Estaba más desarreglado que de costumbre. Uno de sus cordones se asomaba debajo de los pantalones y su barba había crecido y se veía fea. Su pelo negro estaba alisado y sus pequeños ojos se veían cansados y con ojeras. Parecía que Francis no hubiera dormido y hubiese venido a la entrevista a conveniencia de Trent y no de la S.E.

Trent no dijo nada. Estaba sentado en su escritorio con la tranquilidad y la atención de un depredador junto a un pozo de agua.

Francis miró a Jonathan con los hombros encogidos. Francis se subió las mangas de poliéster de su chaqueta pero, acto seguido, las volvió a bajar. Quitándose el pelo de la cara, Francis se dirigió al asiento y se sentó en el borde. La tensión le resaltaba las facciones triangulares de la cara, especialmente cuando Jonathan cerró la puerta y se paró detrás de él con los brazos cruzados y las piernas abiertas. Dirigí toda mi atención hacia ellos. ¿Qué estaría sucediendo?

"¿Podría usted explicarme lo de ayer?" preguntó Trent con toda tranquilidad.

Yo estaba totalmente confundida, pero quedé boquiabierta cuando entendí. ¿Francis trabajaba para Trent? Eso explicaría su rápido ascenso y la forma en que un principiante como él llegó de repente a ser brujo. Me recorrió un escalofrío. Este acuerdo no tenía la bendición de la S.E. La institución no tenía ni idea. Francis era un espía. ¡El nene consentido era un cochino espía!

Miré a Trent entre las anchas hojas. Movió un poco los

hombros, como si estuviera de acuerdo con mis pensamientos. De nuevo sentí náuseas. Francis no era lo suficientemente bueno para meterse en algo tan resbaladizo. Sólo iba a lograr que lo mataran.

"Eh…uh…" tartamudeó Francis.

"Mi jefe de seguridad lo encontró hechizado en la cajuela de su propio auto," dijo Trent tranquilamente, apenas con una pequeña insinuación de amenaza. "La Srta. Morgan y yo tuvimos una conversación interesante."

"Ella…eh…ella dijo que me convertiría en un animal," interrumpió Francis.

Trent respiró profundo. "¿Y por qué habría de hacer eso?," preguntó como cansado de tener paciencia.

"Ella no me tiene estima."

Trent no respondió. Francis se encogió, tal vez al darse cuenta de lo infantil de su respuesta.

"Hábleme de Raquel Morgan," le ordenó Trent.

"Es…eh…es una piedra en un zapato," dijo, lanzándole una mirada nerviosa a Jonathan.

Trent tomó un lapicero entre los dedos y comenzó a darle vueltas. "Eso ya lo sé. Dígame algo más."

"¿Algo que usted aún no sabe?" soltó Francis. Sus ojos estaban fijos en el lapicero de Trent. "Seguramente usted le ha tenido puesta la mano más tiempo que a mí. ¿Le prestó dinero para pagar sus estudios?," dijo casi con celos, "¿o le susurró al oído a la persona que la entrevistó en la S.E.?"

Me puse seria. ¿Cómo se atrevía a sugerir semejante cosa? *Trabajé* para pagar mis estudios y el puesto lo conseguí *yo sola*. Miré a Trent odiándolos a todos. No le debía nada a nadie.

"No. No lo hice," dijo Trent dejando el lapicero. "La Srta. Morgan fue una sorpresa. Claro que le ofrecí trabajo," continuó, y Francis pareció hundirse en sí mismo. Su boca se movía pero no le salían palabras. Podía olerle el miedo, agrio y cortante.

"No el suyo," siguió Trent obviamente disgustado. "Dígame, ¿a qué le teme ella? ¿Qué le molesta? ¿Qué es lo que más valora en el mundo?"

Francis volvió a respirar con alivio. Se movió queriendo cruzar las piernas pero arrepintiéndose en el último movimiento. "No lo sé. ¿El centro comercial? Trato de mantenerme lejos de ella."

"Naturalmente," dijo Trent con su voz fluida. "Hablemos de eso un momento. Después de revisar sus actividades en los últimos días, uno podría poner sus lealtades en tela de juicio, Sr. Percy."

Francis cruzó los brazos. Se movió intranquilo en la silla y su respiración se aceleró. Jonathan dio un paso amenazante más cerca y Francis se quitó de nuevo el pelo de la cara.

Trent se puso terriblemente serio. "¿Sabe usted lo que me ha costado callar los rumores cuando salió corriendo de la bóveda de los archivos de la S.E.?"

Francis se lamió los labios. "Raquel me dijo que corriera, porque si no iban a pensar que la estaba ayudando."

"Y usted corrió, por supuesto."

"Ella dijo..."

"¿Y ayer?," interrumpió Trent. "Usted la condujo hasta mí."

La rabia de su voz me hizo salir de mi choza. Trent se inclinó hacia adelante y podría jurar que oí como se congelaba la sangre de Francis. El aura de hombre de negocios abandonó a Trent. Ahora era sólo poder. Puro y absoluto poder.

Me quedé observando ese cambio. Su semblante no era como el aura de poder de un vampiro. Era como chocolate sin endulzar: fuerte, amargo y aceitoso que deja un mal sabor al final. Los vampiros se hacían respetar con el miedo. Trent sencillamente exigía que lo respetaran. Y, por lo que pude ver, jamás le pasó por la mente que alguien se negara a hacerlo.

"Ella lo utilizó a usted para llegar a mí," susurró sin parpadear. "Eso es imperdonable."

Francis se acobardó en el asiento, su cara lívida y los ojos

Trent se frotó los dedos en la frente. "No," dijo finalmente. "Prefiero conservarlo hasta conseguir un reemplazo. Tal vez tenga otros planes para el Sr. Percy."

"Como usted prefiera, Sa'han," dijo Jonathan y cerró suavemente la puerta.

Veinte

"Ten Ángela," dijo persuasivamente Sara Jane. Una zanahoria se movía entre los barrotes de mi jaula. Me estiré para alcanzarla antes de que la dejara caer.

"Gracias," chirrié, a sabiendas de que no me entendía, pero de todas formas necesitaba decir algo. La mujer sonrió y metió los dedos cautelosamente en mi jaula. Rocé mis bigotes contra ellos. Sabía que eso le gustaría.

"¿Sara Jane?" llamó Trent desde su escritorio y la chica bonita giró velozmente sintiéndose culpable. "La contraté para que administre asuntos de mi oficina, no para que sea guardián de zoológico."

"Lo siento señor. Sólo trataba de deshacerme de mi irracional temor a los animales." Se pasó la mano por su falda de algodón que llevaba a la altura de las rodillas. No era tan elegante o profesional como el vestido para la entrevista, pero era nueva. Justo lo que pensé que vestiría una niña del campo en su primer día de trabajo.

Mordí desaforadamente la zanahoria del almuerzo de Sara Jane. Estaba muerta de hambre, pues me negué a comer esas bolitas rancias. *¿Qué pasa Trent?* pensé entre mordisco y mordisco. *¿Estás celoso?*

Trent se acomodó los lentes y volvió su atención hacia sus papeles. "Cuando haya terminado de liberarse de sus temores irracionales, me gustaría que bajara a la biblioteca."

"Sí, señor."

"El bibliotecario ha organizado alguna información que necesito; pero quiero que usted la seleccione. Tráigame lo que usted considera más importante."

"¿Señor?"

Trent dejó su bolígrafo. "Es información acerca de la industria de azúcar de remolacha." Sonrió con auténtica simpatía. Pensé si tendría su sonrisa patentada. "Tal vez decida experimentar en ese campo y necesito aprender más para tomar buenas decisiones."

Sara Jane salió como una flecha acomodando su bonito pelo detrás de una oreja, complacida pero a la vez apenada. Era obvio que adivinó la intención de Trent de comprar la hacienda donde servía su familia. *Eres una mujer inteligente,* pensé para mis adentros. *Piensa bien. Trent será el dueño de tu familia. Tú serás su propiedad, en cuerpo y alma.*

Volvió hacia mi jaula y dejó caer un último tallo de apio. Su sonrisa desapareció y la preocupación le hizo fruncir el ceño. Habría parecido atractiva en sus facciones de niña, sólo que su familia peligraba de verdad. Tomó aire para decir algo, pero cerró la boca. "Sí señor," dijo, su mirada distante. "Ya mismo le traeré la información."

Sara Jane salió y cerró la puerta. Sus pasos sonaban suaves en el pasillo.

Trent miró su puerta con sospecha mientras tomaba su taza de té: Earl Gray, sin leche y sin azúcar. Si seguía el mismo patrón de ayer, hablaría por teléfono y trabajaría con sus papeles de tres a siete, cuando la gente que trabajaba hasta tarde se iba a casa. Naturalmente, era más fácil traficar drogas ilegales desde la oficina cuando no había nadie alrededor mirando.

Trent había regresado esa tarde de su almuerzo de tres horas con su pelo recién peinado y oliendo a productos naturales. Estaba decididamente fresco. Mi teoría es que había pasado el mediodía durmiendo en su segunda oficina.

¿Por qué no? pensé, estirándome en la hamaca que había en mi celda. Él era lo suficientemente rico para decidir sus horas de trabajo.

Bostecé y mis ojos se cerraron. Era mi segundo día de cautiverio y estaba segura que no sería el último. Había pasado toda la noche anterior revisando minuciosamente mi jaula sólo para convencerme de que era a prueba de Raquel. Estaba diseñada para hurones. Era una jaula de dos niveles sorprendentemente segura. Las horas que pasé tratando de abrir las junturas fueron agotadoras. No hacer nada era un placer, pero mis esperanzas de que Jenks y Ivy hicieran algo para rescatarme eran casi nulas. Dependía de mí misma y llevaría tiempo transmitirle a Sara Jane que yo era una persona y que me dejara escapar de allí.

Abrí un párpado al sentir que Trent se levantaba de su asiento para dirigirse hacia sus discos de música que estaban en una repisa empotrada junto al equipo electrónico. Tenía una figura atractiva ahí parado junto a su música. Estaba tan absorto pensando en qué disco escuchar que no se dio cuenta de que yo estaba calificando su físico: 9.5 de 10. Le quité .5 porque casi todo su cuerpo estaba oculto bajo ese traje de negocios que a lo mejor costaba más que un auto.

Anoche también había tenido la oportunidad de echarle una provocadora mirada cuando se quitó el saco y no quedaba nadie en la oficina. El hombre tenía una espalda fuerte. Era un misterio y un pecado que la ocultara debajo de ese saco. Su abdomen liso se veía aun mejor. Tenía que hacer ejercicio, pero no sé en qué momento hallaba el tiempo para hacerlo. Daría lo que fuera por verlo en traje de baño—por lo menos. Sus piernas deberían ser musculosas, pues se decía que era un jinete experto. Tan vez sueno como una ninfómana hambrienta de sexo, pero no tenía nada más que hacer que mirarlo.

Trent había trabajado ayer hasta muy tarde después de ponerse el sol, aparentemente solo en el callado edificio. La única luz provenía de aquella ventana falsa. Lentamente, la luz palidecía a medida que caía el sol, imitando la luz natural hasta que encendía su lámpara. Varias veces caí en la cuenta de que me estaba quedando dormida pero me despertaba cuando él pasaba una página o sonaba alguna impresora. No paró de trabajar hasta que Jonathan entró para recordarle que comiera algo. Así se ganaba el sueldo, como me lo ganaba yo antes. La diferencia era que él tenía dos puestos: respetable hombre de negocios y capo de las drogas ilegales. Suficiente trabajo para ocuparlo todo el día.

Mi hamaca se mecía mientras observaba como Trent seleccionaba un disco. Giró y empezó a sonar una suave música de tambores. Me miró y se arregló el traje de lino gris y el pelo ralo como retándome a hablarle. Yo le devolví dos soñolientos dedos de aprobación y frunció el ceño. No era exactamente mi tipo de música, pero estaba bien. Era vieja, con cierta nostalgia que revolvía el alma. No era del todo mala.

Podré acostumbrarme a esto, musité mientras estiraba mi cuerpo que empezaba a sanar. No había dormido tan bien desde que abandoné la S.E. Era irónico estar a salvo de mi condena de muerte aquí, metida en una jaula en la oficina de un capo de las drogas.

Trent se acomodó de nuevo para trabajar. De vez en cuando acompañaba a los tambores con su bolígrafo deteniéndose a pensar. Obviamente, esta música era una de sus preferidas. Yo dormía y me despertaba a medida que transcurría la tarde, aplacada por el rumor de los tambores y el susurro de la música. Las ocasionales llamadas telefónicas hacían acentuar y bajar la melodiosa voz de Trent. Ahora yo esperaba la siguiente llamada con ansiedad sólo para oírle la voz.

De repente me despertó una conmoción en el pasillo. "Yo sé dónde queda su oficina," retumbó una voz segura que me hizo recordar a uno de mis profesores. Se oyó una leve reprimenda de Sara Jane. Trent y yo nos miramos con curiosidad.

"Maldita sea," musitó. Cerró sus ojos expresivos como tratando de controlar su reacción. "Le pedí que mandara a uno de sus asistentes." Escarbó en uno de sus cajones con inusitada prisa y el ruido me despertó del todo. Parpadeé para abrir bien los ojos y él apuntó el control remoto hacia el tocadiscos. Las flautas y los tambores cesaron. Luego tiró el control remoto en el cajón con aire de resignación. Podría asegurar que a Trent le gustaría compartir el día con alguien—alguien con quien no tuviera que fingir ser otra cosa de lo que realmente era—*lo que sea* que él fuera. La rabia que demostró con Francis hizo que mi termómetro escalofriante sobrepasara el límite máximo.

Sara Jane golpeó y entró. "Sr. Kalamack, el Sr. Faris quiere verlo."

Trent tomó aire. "Hágalo entrar."

"Sí, señor." Dejó la puerta abierta y sentí como se alejaba el sonido de sus tacones. Pero pronto sonaron de nuevo. Acompañaba a un hombre grande y pesado que vestía una bata gris de laboratorio. El hombre se veía gigantesco parado junto a la pequeña mujer. Sara Jane salió, pero su mirada reflejaba preocupación.

"No puedo decir que me gusta su secretaria," refunfuñó Faris mientras cerraba la puerta. "Sara…¿ese es su nombre?"

Trent se puso de pie y le extendió la mano, el desagrado oculto detrás de su aparente sonrisa. "Gracias por venir con tan poco tiempo de aviso, Faris. Se trata de algo muy sencillo. Uno de sus asistentes habría bastado. Espero no haber interrumpido seriamente sus investigaciones."

"Para nada. Siempre estoy dispuesto a madrugar," resolló sin aliento.

Faris apretó la mano con los mordiscos que le había propinado a Trent ayer y desapareció su sonrisa. El pesado hombre se acomodó trabajosamente en el asiento frente al escritorio de Trent como si fuera el dueño. Cruzo una pierna dejando ver sus pantalones de vestir y zapatos brillantes. Tenía una mancha oscura en la solapa y emanaba olor a desinfectante, casi ocultando su olor a secoya. Tenía las mejillas y las manos cubiertas de viejas marcas de viruela.

Trent regresó detrás de su escritorio y se reclinó hacia atrás, ocultando su mano vendada debajo de la otra. Hubo un momento de silencio.

"Bueno ¿para qué me necesita?" preguntó Faris en un tono fuerte, casi dándole una orden.

Me pareció notar un destello de molestia en Trent. "Directo como siempre," comentó Trent. "¿Qué puede decirme de esto?"

Me estaba señalando y contuve la respiración. De inmediato me escondí en mi refugio. Faris se levantó rezongando y su fuerte olor a secoya me golpeó a medida que se acercaba. "Vaya vaya," dijo. "Pero si es la pobre estúpida."

Disgustada, lo miré a los ojos casi perdidos entre los dobleces de su piel. Trent se había colocado al frente de su escritorio, apoyándose en él. "¿La reconoce?" le preguntó.

"No personalmente." Golpeó suavemente los barrotes de mi jaula con uno de sus dedos gruesos.

"¡Escucha!," grité desde mi choza. "¡Ya me estoy cansando de esto!"

"Cállate," repuso con desprecio. "Es una bruja," siguió Faris, descartándome como si yo no fuera nada. "Sólo manténgala lejos de su acuario y así no podrá transformarse. Tiene un poderoso hechizo. Seguramente la apoya una organización importante, pues es costoso. Además, es estúpida."

Eso iba dirigido a mí, pero resistí la tentación de lanzarle bolitas.

"¿Podría explicármelo?" Trent hurgó en su cajón del fondo y sacó dos vasos de cristal para servir dos tragos del whiskey añejo de 40 años.

"La transformación es un arte difícil. Se usan pociones en lugar de amuletos. Eso significa que se prepara una poción para una sola ocasión." Lo que sobra se bota. Es muy costosa. Puede pagar el sueldo de su bibliotecólogo asistente y montar un negocio para que el seguro la venda con lo que cuesta ese brebaje.

"¿Dice que es difícil?" dijo Trent dándole un vaso a Faris. "¿Podría usted preparar un hechizo así?"

"Si tuviera la receta," repuso, inflando el pecho al sentir su orgullo en entredicho. "Es un hechizo antiguo ¿tal vez preindustrial? No puedo identificar quién diseñó este hechizo." Se acercó un poco más respirando profundamente. "Afortunadamente para él, de lo contrario me iría a reemplazar al brujo de su biblioteca."

Esta conversación se pone interesante, pensé.

"Entonces, ¿usted no cree que ella misma preparó la poción?," preguntó Trent. Estaba de nuevo sentado en su escritorio y se veía increíblemente delgado y musculoso comparado con Faris. El pesado hombre agitó la cabeza y se sentó de nuevo. No se podía ver el vaso en su mano gruesa. "Podría apostar mi vida. No puede ser tan inteligente para preparar esta poción y al mismo tiempo ser tan bruta de dejarse atrapar. No tiene sentido."

"A lo mejor estaba impaciente," dijo Trent. Faris estalló en carcajadas. Yo salté tapándome los oídos con las manos.

"Sí, claro," repuso Faris entre risotadas. "Estaba impaciente. Está buena esa."

Vi que la compostura usual de Trent empezaba a resquebrajarse mientras se acercaba de nuevo a su escritorio y dejaba de lado su vaso aun sin probar.

"Entonces ¿quién es?" preguntó Faris, inclinándose hacia adelante con aire mordaz. "¿Una periodista audaz buscando el reportaje de su vida?"

"¿Existe algún hechizo que me ayude a entenderla?," preguntó Trent, ignorando la observación de Faris. "Todo lo que habla son chillidos."

Faris gruñó inclinándose para dejar su vaso desocupado sobre el escritorio, pidiendo otro trago sin hablar. "No. Los roedores no tienen cuerdas vocales. ¿Piensa quedarse con ella más tiempo?"

Trent giró el vaso en la mano. Se quedó en silencio y me alarmó.

Faris sonrió siniestramente. "¿Qué está tramando en esa mente malvada, Trent?"

El crujido del asiento de Trent sonó duro al inclinarse hacia adelante. "Faris, si no necesitara tanto de su talento lo haría azotar en su propio laboratorio."

El hombre hizo una mueca y cambió de semblante. "Lo sé."

Trent guardó la botella. "Tal vez la haga participar en el torneo del viernes."

Faris parpadeó. "¿El torneo de la ciudad?," dijo en voz baja. "Una vez presencié uno pero los combates no terminan hasta que alguno muere."

"Eso he oído decir."

El miedo me hizo lanzarme contra la malla metálica. "Eh, un momento," chillé. "¿Qué quieren decir con que alguno muere? ¡Oigan! ¿¡Podría alguien hablar con el visón!?"

Le lancé una bolita a Trent pero cayó apenas medio metro más allá. Probé de nuevo, pero la pateé en lugar de lanzarla con la mano. Esta vez golpeó la parte de atrás del escritorio. "¡El Giro te arrastre, Trent!" grité. "¡Háblame!"

Trent me miró alzando las cejas. "Naturalmente, esta rata pelea."

Mi corazón saltaba. Aterrada, me senté en las ancas. Combates de ratas. Son ilegales. Anónimas. A muerte. Me iban a llevar a un cuadrilátero en una lucha a muerte contra una rata.

Estaba confundida. Posé mis largas patas de pelo blanco contra la malla de mi jaula. Me sentía traicionada. Faris pareció enfermar. "No hablará en serio," susurró, su cara pálida. "¿De verdad piensa apostarla? ¡No puede hacer eso!"

"¿Por qué demonios no puedo?"

Faris luchaba por emitir las palabras. "¡Es una persona!," exclamó. "No durará tres minutos. La van hacer jirones."

Trent se alzó de hombros con una indiferencia que no fue fingida. "Sobrevivir es problema suyo, no mío." Se puso sus lentes de alambre y concentró la mirada en sus papeles. "Buenas tardes, Faris."

"Kalamack, vas demasiado lejos. Ni siquiera tú estás por encima de la ley." Tan pronto terminó esa frase, tanto Faris como yo sabíamos que fue un error. Trent alzó la mirada. Observó a Faris en silencio por encima de los lentes y apoyó un codo encima de sus papeles. Aguardé sin poder respirar y la tensión me hizo erizar la piel. "¿Cómo está su hija menor, Faris?" preguntó Trent con su hermosa voz pero incapaz de ocultar la suciedad de su pregunta.

El hombre cambió de color. "Está bien" susurró. Su arrogante seguridad se había desvanecido. Ahora sólo era un hombre asustado.

"¿Cuántos años tiene...quince?" Trent se recostó en su asiento, puso sus lentes junto a la caja de documentos y cerró el puño. "Hermosa edad. Quiere ser oceanógrafa, ¿no es cierto? ¿hablar con los delfines?"

"Sí," a duras penas se escuchó su respuesta.

"No sabe usted lo satisfecho que estoy de ver que el tratamiento contra el cáncer de los huesos haya funcionado."

Observé la parte posterior del cajón de Trent donde guardaba los comprometedores discos. Luego miré a Faris, pero esta vez interpreté su bata de laboratorio desde otro punto de vista. Se me heló la sangre y volví la mirada hacia Trent. No solamente traficaba con drogas biológicas sino que las producía. Yo no sabía qué me horrorizaba más: si el hecho de que Trent estaba jugando con la misma tecnología que borró del mapa a la mitad de la población del mundo o el hecho de que estaba chantajeando con ella a la gente, amenazando a sus seres queridos. ¡Era tan agradable, tan encantador, tan desgraciadamente simpático con esa personalidad y tan seguro de sí mismo! ¿Cómo podía algo tan oscuro convivir junto con algo tan atractivo?

Trent sonrió. "Ha estado en remisión por cinco años. No es fácil hallar buenos médicos que estén dispuestos a explorar técnicas ilegales. Además, cuestan mucho."

"Sí, señor," repuso Faris.

Trent lo miró inquisitivamente. "Buenas tardes, Faris."

"¡Basura!," dije. "¡Eres una basura, Trent! ¡Eres la porquería que se le pega a mis botas!"

Faris se dirigió tembloroso hacia la puerta. Me tensé cuando olí cierta actitud desafiante. Trent lo tenía arrinconado y el pobre hombre ya no tenía nada que perder.

Trent también lo presintió. "Va a tratar de escapar, ¿cierto Faris?" le dijo cuando él abría la puerta y se filtraba el sonido externo de la oficina. "Usted sabe que eso no puedo permitírselo."

Faris se dio vuelta con una mirada desesperada. Estupefacta, vi cómo Trent desatornillaba la tapa de su bolígrafo e introducía un pequeño proyectil en el tubo vacío. Con un pequeño soplido de aire le disparó a Faris.

El pobre hombre abrió los ojos y dio un paso adelante hacia Trent agarrándose la garganta. Emitió un ruido áspero y su cara empezó a hincharse. Estaba demasiado impactada para sentir miedo y ví cómo Faris caía de rodillas. El hombre metió una mano en el bolsillo de la camisa. Sus dedos buscaban a tientas y una jeringa cayó al piso. Trató de alcanzarla estirando el brazo pero rodó por el suelo. Trent se puso de pie. Su cara era inexpresiva y pateó la jeringa de la mano de Faris.

"¿Qué le hiciste?" chillé, observando cómo atornillaba su bolígrafo de nuevo. Faris se puso morado. Emitió un último sonido carrasposo. Luego quedó en silencio.

Trent guardó su bolígrafo en un bolsillo y pasó por encima de Faris para llegar hasta la puerta abierta. "¡Sara Jane!" gritó. "Llama a los paramédicos. El Sr. Faris está mal."

"¡Se está muriendo!," chillé, "¡eso es lo que sucede! ¡Tú lo mataste, maldito!"

El rumor de los comentarios aumentó a medida que todos salían de sus oficinas. Reconocí los pasos veloces de Jonathan que se detuvieron en seco bajo el umbral de la puerta mientras observaba el cuerpo de Faris tirado en el suelo. Luego le hizo una mueca de desacuerdo a Trent.

Trent estaba en cuclillas junto a Faris tomándole el pulso.

Se encogió de hombros mirando a Jonathan y luego inyectó a Faris con la jeringa a través de los pantalones. Yo sabía que ya era demasiado tarde. Faris no respondía. Estaba muerto y Trent lo sabía.

"Ya vienen los paramédicos," dijo Sara Jane desde el pasillo mientras sus pasos se acercaban. "Puedo traer..." Se detuvo detrás de Jonathan y puso su mano sobre la boca mirando a Faris.

Trent se puso de pie dejando caer la jeringa al suelo con algo de dramatismo. "Oh, Sara Jane," le dijo suavemente mientras la hacía regresar al pasillo. "Lo siento. No mire. Es demasiado tarde. Creo que fue una picadura de abeja. Faris es alérgico a las abejas. Traté de aplicarle su antitoxina pero no hizo efecto con suficiente rapidez. Seguramente trajo una abeja consigo sin darse cuenta. Se dio una palmada en la pierna justo antes de caer."

"Pero él..." tartamudeó ella mirando una vez más hacia atrás mientras Trent la alejaba.

Jonathan se agachó y arrancó un pelo de la pierna derecha de Faris que guardó en el bolsillo. El hombre me miró con ojos sarcásticos.

"Lo siento mucho," dijo Trent en el pasillo. "¿Jon?" llamó, y Jonathan se puso de pie. "Por favor, asegúrate de que todos salgan temprano. Desocupa el edificio."

"Sí, señor."

"Esto es terrible, espantoso," continuó Trent como si realmente lo sintiera. "Vete a casa, Sara Jane. Trata de no pensar en ello."

Escuché que trataba de contener un sollozo y sus pasos se alejaron.

Hacía apenas unos minutos Faris estaba ahí parado. Horrorizada observé cómo Trent pasaba por encima de su brazo. Tranquilo como si nada se dirigió a su escritorio y oprimió el intercomunicador. "¿Quen? Lamento molestarte. ¿Podrías venir a mi oficina? Hay un equipo de paramédicos en camino a la hacienda y seguramente alguien de la S.E. vendrá luego."

Hubo un momento de duda pero al final sonó la voz de Quen por el altoparlante. "¿Sr. Kalamack? Voy enseguida."

Miré a Faris hinchado y tirado en el piso. "Lo mataste," dije acusándolo. "Dios me ayude. ¡Lo mataste en tu propia oficina delante de todos!"

"Jon," dijo Trent suavemente, rebuscando indiferentemente en uno de sus cajones. "Asegúrate de que su familia reciba los mejores beneficios. Quiero que su hija menor estudie en la universidad que quiera. Que todo quede anónimo. Preséntalo como una beca."

"Sí, Sa'han." Su voz era informal, como si los cadáveres fueran cosa de todos los días.

"Qué generoso eres, Trent," chillé. "Pero creo que preferiría tener a su papá."

Trent me miró. Había una línea de sudor sobre su frente. "Quiero hablar con el asistente de Faris antes de que termine el día," dijo suavemente. "¿Cómo se llama, Darby?"

"Darby Donnelley, Sa'han."

Trent asintió, frotándose la frente como si estuviera preocupado. Cuando bajó la mano ya no sudaba. "Sí, eso es. Donnelley. No quiero que esto retrase mi agenda."

"¿Qué quiere usted que le diga?"

"La verdad. Faris era alérgico a las picadas de abejas. Todos sus empleados lo saben."

Jonathan empujó a Faris con el pie y salió. Sus pasos sonaron fuerte ahora que no había ruido de fondo. La oficina se había desocupado muy rápido y me pregunté cuántas veces sucedería esto.

"¿Le gustaría reconsiderar mi oferta inicial?" me preguntó Trent. Sostenía su vaso de whiskey intacto en la mano. No podría asegurarlo, pero creo que le temblaba. Por un instante pensó tomarse un trago, pero luego lo dejó de lado. Colocó el vaso suavemente. "Olvídese de la isla. Es más prudente tenerla más cerca. La forma en que usted se infiltró en mi propiedad es impresionante. Creo que podría convencer a Quen para contratarla. Por poco se muere de risa viendo cómo usted inutilizó al Sr. Percy con cinta adhesiva en la cajuela, y después estuvo a punto de asesinarla cuando le dije que usted se había metido a mi oficina principal."

Estaba tan aterrorizada que mi mente quedó en blanco. No pude responder. *Faris estaba muerto en el piso* y Trent me estaba ofreciendo trabajar para él.

"Faris estaba muy impresionado con su poción," continuó. "Decodificar técnicas de cambios genéticos anteriores al Giro no será más difícil que preparar una poción complicada. Si usted no está interesada en explorar sus fronteras en el mundo físico podría probar con el mundo mental. ¡Usted tiene una gran combinación de destrezas, Srta. Morgan! Eso la hace excepcionalmente valiosa."

Me senté en ancas sin palabras.

"Verá, Srta. Morgan," continuó diciendo. "Yo no soy mala persona. A todos mis empleados les ofrezco condiciones justas de trabajo, la posibilidad para mejorar y oportunidades para que alcancen su potencial máximo."

"¿Oportunidades? ¿Posibilidades de mejorar?" farfullé a pesar de que él no podía entenderme. "¿Quién te crees que eres, Dios? Puedes irte al mismísimo infierno."

"Creo que entendí la idea general de eso," dijo, y sonrió fugazmente. "Por lo menos le he enseñado a ser honesta." Acercó el asiento al escritorio. "Voy a amansarla, Morgan, hasta que esté dispuesta a hacer cualquier cosa con tal de salir de esa jaula. Jon se demoró quince años, no como una rata, pero sí como un esclavo. Da igual. Creo que usted saldrá mucho antes."

"Eres un maldito, Trent" dije llena de cólera.

"No sea burda." Trent tomó su bolígrafo. "Estoy seguro de que su moral es tan fuerte, ó más fuerte aún, que la de Jon. Claro que él no tuvo que enfrentarse con ratas que trataban de destrozarlo. Con él me di el lujo de tomarme mi tiempo. Lo hice mucho más lento, y eso que en ese entonces no era tan bueno como ahora." Su mirada se perdió en el vacío, pensando. "Aún así, jamás se dio cuenta de que lo estaba amansando. La mayoría no se dan cuenta. Él aún no se da cuenta. Y si por si acaso usted llegara a sugerírselo, la mataría."

Trent reaccionó de nuevo con la mirada. "Me gusta tener todas las cartas destapadas sobre la mesa. Resulta más satis-factorio. ¿No le parece? Es mejor no ser tan diplomático so-bre las cosas. Los dos sabemos lo que está sucediendo, pero si usted no sobrevive, no será una gran pérdida. No he inver-tido tanto en usted. Una jaula de alambre, unas cuantas boli-tas de comida y algo de aserrín."

De repente, la idea de hallarme encerrada en una jaula me abrumó. Atrapada. "¡Déjame salir," grité, jalando la malla de mi celda. "¡Sácame de aquí, Trent!"

Golpearon la puerta y yo giré. Jonathan entró pisando junto a Faris. "El equipo de médicos está estacionando la ambulancia. Ellos pueden ocuparse de Faris. La S.E. sola-mente solicita una declaración. Nada más." Luego me diri-gió una mirada de desprecio. "¿Qué le ocurre a tu bruja?"

"¡Déjame salir Trent!" chillé cada vez más frenética. "¡Déjame salir!" Corrí hasta la parte baja de la jaula. Con el corazón martillándome, subí de nuevo al segundo nivel. Me lancé contra los barrotes tratando de voltear la jaula. ¡Tenía que salir de allí!

Trent sonrió, su mirada tranquila y controlada. "La Srta. Morgan acaba de darse cuenta de lo convincente que soy. ¡Golpea su jaula!"

Jonathan dudó, confundido. "Pensé que usted no quería que la atormentara."

"En realidad, lo que te dije fue que no reacciones con ra-bia cuando has juzgado mal cómo puede reaccionar una per-sona. Ahora no estoy reaccionando con rabia. Le enseño a la Srta. Morgan su nuevo lugar en la vida. Ella está dentro de una jaula y yo puedo hacer lo que quiera con ella." Sus fríos ojos se fijaron en los míos. "¡Pégale-a-su-jaula!"

Jonathan hizo una mueca. Con la carpeta que tenía en la mano, lanzó el brazo contra la malla de alambre. El duro golpe me asustó, a pesar de que ya sabía que venía. La jaula se estremeció y yo me aferré a la malla con mis cuatro patas.

"Cállate, bruja," agregó Jonathan con una dulce satisfacción. Corrí a esconderme en mi choza. Trent acababa de darle permiso para atormentarme cuanto quisiera. Si no me mataban las ratas, lo haría Jonathan.

Veintiuno

"**V**amos Morgan, haz algo," bufaba Jonathan clavándome un palo y empujándome. Yo temblaba tratando de no reaccionar.

"Sé que sientes rabia," continuó, cambiando de posición para clavarme el palo en el otro costado. El piso de mi jaula estaba lleno de lápices, todos masticados hasta la mitad. Jonathan me había atormentado intermitentemente toda la mañana. Luego de muchas horas de chillarle y embestirlo, caí en la cuenta de que mis esfuerzos no sólo conseguían agotarme sino alimentar el entusiasmo de ese maldito sádico. Ignorarlo no resultaba tan satisfactorio como atacarlo para quitarle los lápices de la mano y mordisquearlos hasta la mitad, aunque guardaba la esperanza de que se aburriera y se largara.

Trent había salido para su almuerzo-siesta hacía una media hora. Pero Jonathan no mostraba señales de querer irse. Estaba contento de quedarse para acosarme entre bocado y bocado de pasta. Ni siquiera estaba a salvo en medio de la jaula. Simplemente metía un palo más largo y me habían quitado la choza.

"Bruja maldita. Reacciona." Jonathan giró el palo para golpearme en la cabeza. Me golpeó una, dos, tres veces en medio de las orejas. Mis bigotes temblaban. Sentía como mi pulso se aceleraba y me dolía la cabeza por el esfuerzo para no reaccionar. Al quinto golpe no aguanté más. Me moví en reverso y agarré el palo partiéndolo en dos.

"¡Eres hombre muerto!," chillé, lanzándome contra la malla de alambre. "¿Escuchaste? ¡Cuando salga de aquí serás hombre muerto!"

Se enderezó y se pasó las manos por el pelo. "Sabía que lograría hacerte mover."

"Haz la prueba cuando esté fuera de esta jaula," dije, temblando de ira.

Oí el sonido de tacones altos que se acercaban en el pasillo y sentí alivio. Reconocí los pasos y aparentemente también Jonathan. Se puso serio y dio un paso atrás. Esta vez Sara Jane entró a la oficina sin golpear. "¡Oh!," exclamó llevándose la mano a la solapa de su nuevo traje de oficina que había comprado el día anterior. Trent les pagaba a sus empleados por adelantado. "Lo siento, Jon. No pensé que aún había alguien aquí." Hubo un extraño silencio. "Venía a darle a Ángela lo que sobró de mi almuerzo antes de salir a mis vueltas."

Jonathan la miró directamente. "Yo lo haré por ti."

Oh, no, por favor, pensé. A lo mejor empaparía primero la comida en tinta, y ni siquiera así me la daría. Las sobras de Sara Jane era lo único que tenía para comer y ya estaba medio muerta de hambre.

"Gracias, pero no" dijo. Me acurruqué aliviada. "Yo cerraré la oficina del señor Kalamack si usted quiere irse."

Sí, vete, pensé con el pulso latiéndome rápido. *Lárgate para que yo pueda decirle a Sara Jane que soy una persona.* Lo había intentado todo el día, pero la primera vez Trent estaba observando y Jonathan golpeó mi jaula tan fuerte que la hizo caer.

"Estoy esperando al Sr. Kalamack," dijo Jonathan. "¿Estás segura de que no quieres que la alimente?" dijo con actitud petulante, colocándose justo detrás del escritorio de Trent fingiendo ordenarlo. Mis esperanzas de que se largara se desvanecieron. Sabía lo que estaba haciendo.

Sara Jane se agachó para que sus ojos quedaran al nivel de

los míos. Creo que eran azules, pero no estaba segura. "No. No me demoraré. ¿Trabajará el Sr. Kalamack durante el amuerzo?" le preguntó.

"No. Sólo me pidió esperarlo."

Me moví hacia adelante oliendo la zanahoria. "Ven Ángela," dijo la mujer. Su voz suave era tranquilizante. Abrió una servilleta de papel. "Hoy sólo hay zanahoria. Ya no quedaba apio."

Miré sospechosamente a Jonathan. Chequeaba detenidamente la punta de los lápices en el escritorio de Trent así es que tomé una zanahoria con mucha cautela. De pronto sentí un golpe fuerte y salté. Dejó ver una sonrisita en los labios. Había dejado caer un archivo sobre el escritorio. La mirada iracunda de Sara Jane era suficiente para cuajar leche. "Ya basta," le dijo indignada. "La has acosado todo el día." Frunció los labios y empujó las zanahorias a través de la malla. "Aquí tienes cariño," dijo calmándome. "Come tus zanahorias. ¿No te gustan tus bolitas?" Soltó las zanahorias y dejó sus dedos entre la malla.

Los olí dejando que me acariciara la cabeza con sus uñas gastadas y maltrechas. Confiaba en Sara Jane y yo no confiaba en la gente así nomás. Tal vez era porque las dos estábamos atrapadas y ambas lo sabíamos. No pensé que ella supiera acerca del tráfico de drogas biológicas de Trent; pero era demasiado inteligente para no estar preocupada por la forma como murió su predecesora. Trent la usaría tal como usó a Yolin Bates dejando su cadáver tirado en algún callejón.

Sentí una presión en el pecho como si fuera a llorar. Percibí un leve olor de secoya en ella casi opacado del todo por su perfume. Sintiéndome miserable, jalé las zanahorias y me las comí lo más rápido posible. Olían a vinagre y me puse a pensar en la preferencia de aliño para ensaladas de Sara Jane. Me había dado tres. Yo hubiera podido comer el doble.

"Yo pensé que ustedes los granjeros odiaban a los asesinos de gallinas" dijo Jonathan fingiendo ser indiferente pero observándome para asegurarse de que no demostrara algún comportamiento diferente al de los visones.

Las mejillas de Sara Jane enrojecieron y se enderezó inmediatamente de su posición agachada. Antes de pronunciar palabra alguna estiró el brazo tembloroso y se aferró a mi jaula. "Oooh" dijo, fijando los ojos en la distancia. "Me levanté demasiado rápido."

"¿Estás bien?" preguntó indiferente, como si no le importara.

Ella se llevó las manos a los ojos. "Sí, sí... estoy bien."

Dejé de masticar al oír pasos suaves en el pasillo. Trent entró a la oficina. Se había quitado el saco. Su ropa era lo que lo hacía ver como ejecutivo en lugar de un salvavidas. "Sara Jane, ¿no es tu hora de almuerzo?" preguntó amablemente.

"Ya me iba, Sr. Kalamack," respondió. Nos miró a Jonathan y a mí con preocupación antes de salir. Sus tacones sonaron levemente en el pasillo y desapareció. Sentí algo de alivio. Si Trent estaba aquí tal vez Jonathan me dejaría en paz y yo podría comer.

El altanero Jon se sentó en el asiento frente al escritorio de Trent. "¿Cuánto tiempo?," preguntó, cruzando la pierna y fijándome la mirada.

"Depende." Trent alimentó a sus peces de una bolsa. El pez amarillo llegó a la superficie produciendo sonidos leves.

"Debe ser muy fuerte," dijo Jonathan. "No pensé que le hiciera efecto."

Paré de masticar. *¿Ella? ¿Sara Jane?*

"Yo pensé que sí," repuso Trent. "Estará bien." Volteó la cabeza pensando. "En el futuro tendré que ser más directo en mis negociaciones con ella. Toda la información que me trajo sobre la industria del azúcar de remolacha estaba recargada. Toda indicaba que es un mal negocio."

Jonathan aclaró la garganta sonando condescendiente. Trent cerró la bolsa y la guardó en el cajón debajo del acuario. Se paró detrás de su escritorio con la cabeza inclinada mientras organizaba unos papeles.

"¿Y por qué no un hechizo, Sa'han?" Jonathan se estiró y se puso de pie, arreglándose las arrugas del pantalón. "Yo diría que así estaríamos más seguros."

"Es contra las reglas hechizar a los animales en la competencia." Escribió una nota en su agenda.

Jonathan sonrió con malicia. "Pero las drogas no. Es una perversión que tiene sentido."

Mastiqué más lento. Hablaban de mí. El sabor de vinagre estaba más fuerte en esta última zanahoria y sentía un hormigueo en la lengua. Dejé caer la zanahoria y toqué mis encías. Estaban entumecidas. *Maldición. Era viernes.*

"¡Bastardo!" grité lanzándole la zanahoria a Trent, sólo para ver cómo rebotaba contra la malla. "¡Me drogaste y drogaste a Sara Jane para que me drogara!" Iracunda me lancé contra la puerta sacando una pata para tratar de alcanzar la perilla. Sentí náuseas y mareo.

Los dos hombres se acercaron a mí, mirándome. La expresión dominante de Trent me heló. Aterrada, corrí hasta el segundo nivel, luego bajé al primero. La luz me lastimaba los ojos. Tenía la boca entumecida y me tambaleé perdiendo el equilibrio. *¡Me había drogado!*

En medio del pánico, caí en la cuenta de que la portezuela se abriría. Esta podía ser mi única oportunidad. Me quedé inmóvil en medio de la jaula, jadeando. Lentamente, me di vuelta. *Por favor,* pensé desesperada. Por favor, abran la portezuela antes de que pierda el conocimiento del todo. Mi corazón latía veloz y mis pulmones se hincharon. No sabía si era por la droga o por mi esfuerzo.

Los dos estaban callados. Jonathan me pinchó con un lápiz. Hice vibrar mi pata como si fuera incapaz de moverla. "Creo que está dormida" dijo emocionado.

"Dale tiempo." La luz me golpeó en los ojos cuando Trent se alejó y los entreabrí.

Sin embargo, Jonathan estaba impaciente. "Voy por el maletín."

La jaula tembló mientras abría la portezuela. Mi pulso se aceleró cuando Jonathan enroscó sus dedos alrededor de mi cuerpo. ¡Pero yo volví de nuevo a la vida y le clavé los dientes en un dedo!

"¡Maldita asquerosa!," maldijo Jonathan sacando la mano y jalándome también a mí hasta afuera. Me solté cayendo pesadamente al suelo. Nada me dolía. Estaba totalmente entumecida. Salté hacia la puerta, despatarrada, pues mis patas no respondían.

"¡Jon! ¡La puerta!," gritó Trent.

El piso tembló y sentí el duro golpe de la puerta que se cerraba. Dudé, incapaz de pensar. Tenía que correr. ¿Dónde diablos estaba la puerta?

La sombra de Jonathan se acercó. Le mostré los dientes y retrocedió, acobardado por mis diminutos incisivos. Emanaba el agudo hedor de miedo. Estaba asustado, el valentón. De pronto se lanzó hacia adelante agarrándome por el pescuezo. Yo me retorcí clavándole mis dientes en el pulgar. Gritó de dolor y me soltó. De nuevo caí al piso. "¡Maldita bruja!," gritó. Me tambaleé, incapaz de correr. Sentía la sangre de Jon en la lengua. Sabía a canela y vino.

"Tócame de nuevo y te arrancaré todo el dedo," chillé.

Jonathan retrocedió asustado. Fue Trent quien me alzó. Estaba bajo el efecto profundo de la droga y no podía hacer nada. Sentí como una bendición sus manos frías que me acunaban. Me depositó suavemente en el maletín y cerró la portezuela. La jaula trepidó.

Sentía la boca seca y el estómago retorcido. Alguien alzó el maletín poniéndolo sobre el escritorio. "Aun tenemos unos minutos antes de partir. Veamos si Sara Jane tiene crema antibiótica en su escritorio para esas mordidas."

La voz de Trent era tan borrosa como mi mente. La oscuridad se volvió total y quedé inconsciente. Maldije mi estupidez.

Veintidós

Alguien hablaba. Eso podía entenderlo. En realidad eran dos voces y ahora que recuperaba mi capacidad de pensar, caí en la cuenta que habían estado conversando durante algún tiempo. Una de las voces era la de Trent. Su extraordinaria elocuencia me hizo reaccionar otra vez. Al fondo se oía el agudo chillido de ratas.

"Ay, ¡maldición!," susurré, pero con un chillido débil. Tenía los ojos abiertos pero me esforcé por cerrarlos. Los sentía tan secos como papel de lija. Unos cuantos dolorosos parpadeos más y comenzaron a fluir las lágrimas. Lentamente logré enfocar de nuevo las paredes grises del maletín.

"¡Sr. Kalamack!," dijo una voz dándole la bienvenida y el mundo dio vueltas cuando giraron el maletín. "Me dijeron en la segunda planta que usted estaba aquí. Es un gusto." La voz se acercó más. "¡Y además trajo un contrincante! Espere usted a verlo, sólo espere" dijo el hombre, desbordado de emoción agitando para arriba y para abajo la mano que le había ofrecido Trent. "Un nuevo contrincante hace que el concurso sea mucho más emocionante."

"Buenas tardes Jim," repuso Trent cálidamente. "Disculpe que haya llegado así no más sin avisar."

La sosegada voz de Trent fue un bálsamo que hizo desaparecer mi dolor de cabeza. La amaba y la odiaba a la vez. ¿Cómo podía algo tan hermoso pertenecerle a alguien tan funesto?

"Usted siempre es bienvenido, Sr. Kalamack." El tipo olía a aserrín. Yo me acurruqué en un rincón. "¿Ya se registró? ¿Le han asignado un puesto para el primer asalto?"

"¿Acaso habrá más de una pelea?" interrumpió Jonathan.

"Sí señor, así es," repuso Jim animadamente al tiempo que giró el maletín para quedar de frente a la portezuela. "Uno apuesta su rata hasta que muere, o la retira. ¡Oh!" exclamó al verme. "Un visón. Vaya...es usted muy elegante. Naturalmente, eso hará que sus posibilidades cambien. Pero no se preocupe. En el pasado hemos tenido tejones y serpientes. Apreciamos la diversidad y a todos les encanta cuando un contrincante nuevo es devorado."

Empecé a respirar aceleradamente. Tenía que salir de allí.

"¿Está seguro de que su animal luchará?" preguntó Jim. "Las ratas que tenemos aquí han sido criadas para atacar; claro que ahora tenemos a una rata callejera que ha dado espectáculo los últimos tres meses."

"Tuve que drogarlo para meterlo en el maletín," dijo Trent con voz seria.

"Ah, un batallador. Veamos..." dijo Jim solícito, arrebatándole un cuaderno de registro a un trabajador que pasaba por ahí. "Permítame cambiar el primer asalto que le correspondía por uno de los últimos. Así tendrá más tiempo de eliminar el sedante. Además, a nadie le gustan los primeros turnos. No hay suficiente tiempo para que los animales se recuperen antes del siguiente asalto."

Me acerqué impotente a la parte delantera del maletín. Jim parecía un buen tipo con mejillas redondas y panza grande. Con un pequeño hechizo podría convertirse en el San Nicolás del centro comercial. ¿Qué estaba haciendo en los antros de Cincinnati?

La mirada amable de Jim pasó por encima del hombro de Trent y agitó el brazo saludando a alguien. "Por favor, conserve siempre a su animal con usted," dijo fijando la mirada en la persona que acababa de llegar. "Tiene cinco minutos para meter a su animal en la arena una vez que lo llamen. De lo contrario queda eliminado."

La arena... qué divertido, pensé.

"Ahora sólo necesito saber el nombre de su animal," dijo Jim.

"Ángela," repuso Trent con sinceridad burlona, pero Jim lo anotó sin dudarlo ni un instante.

"Ángela," repitió Jim. Adiestrado y propiedad de Trent Kalamack.

"¡No te pertenezco!" chillé, y Jonathan le dio un golpe al maletín.

"Vamos arriba, Jon," dijo Trent dándole la mano a Jim. "El ruido de estas ratas me está atravesando la cabeza."

Me paré en mis cuatro patas para equilibrarme ante la oscilación del maletín al ponernos en movimiento. "No voy a pelear Trent," chillé con fuerza. "No puedes ignorarme así."

"Quédese quieta, Srta. Morgan," dijo Trent mientras subíamos. "No me dirá que no está entrenada para esto. Todos los agentes saben cómo matar. Bien sea que trabaje para mí o para ellos ¿cuál es la diferencia? Es sólo una rata."

"¡Nunca he matado a nadie en la vida!" grité golpeando la portezuela, "y no lo haré por ti." Pero pensé que no tenía opción. No podía razonar con una rata, decirle que todo era un grave error ¡y que por qué no arreglábamos las cosas amigablemente!

El ruido de las ratas fue opacado por las conversaciones en voz alta en la parte superior de las escaleras. Trent hizo un pausa para acomodarse al ambiente. "Mira," dijo. "Ahí está Randolph."

"¿Randolph Mirick?" preguntó Jonathan. "¿No ha tratado usted de organizar una reunión con él para incrementar sus derechos sobre el agua?"

"Sí." Trent pareció saborear la palabra. "Desde hace siete semanas. Aparentemente es un hombre muy ocupado. Y mira más allá. ¿Ves a la mujer que sostiene a ese asqueroso perrito? Es la Jefe Ejecutiva de la compañía de vidrios con la que hemos hecho negocios. Me gustaría hablar con ella sobre la posibilidad de obtener un buen descuento por volumen. No pensé que esta sería una oportunidad para hacer contactos."

Empezamos a movernos entre la multitud. Trent mantenía conversaciones ligeras y amigables, exhibiéndome como si fuera una mula premiada. Me agazapé al fondo de la jaula ignorando los gestos que me hacían las señoras. Sentía la boca como una secadora de pelo y podía oler sangre vieja, orines y ratas.

También podía oírlas chillando en tonos tan agudos que la gente no escuchaba. Ya habían comenzado los enfrentamientos aun cuando ninguna persona parada lo sabía. Barrotes y plásticos gruesos separaban a los combatientes, pero ya emitían sus violentas amenazas.

Trent encontró un asiento al lado de la miserable alcaldesa de la ciudad y luego de acomodarme en medio de sus pies empezó a hablarle sobre los beneficios globales de zonificar nuevamente su propiedad como propiedad industrial y no comercial. Argumentaba que la mayor parte de su terreno se empleaba de una u otra manera en ganancias industriales. Ella no parecía escucharlo hasta que Trent sugirió que tal vez tendría que trasladar a sus industrias más afectadas hacia otros lugares más... amigables.

Pasé una hora de pesadilla. Los chillidos ultrasónicos atravesaban los sonidos más graves, pero la multitud humana no los sentía. Jonathan hacía comentarios complejos que no redundaban en beneficio mío, pues adornaba las monstruosidades que tenían lugar en la arena. Ninguno de los asaltos duró mucho—diez minutos por mucho. El repentino silencio seguido de la explosiva gritería de los espectadores era una barbarie. Pronto pude oler la sangre de la que Jonathan parecía obtener inspiración. Yo saltaba con cada movimiento de pies de Trent.

El público aplaudió educadamente el resultado oficial del último asalto. Evidentemente hubo un ganador. Gracias a Jonathan me enteré de que la rata ganadora le había abierto el vientre a su oponente antes de que el perdedor pudiera rendirse, y que todavía le clavaba los dientes en una de sus patas.

"¡Ángela!" llamó Jim con voz profunda y espectacular que retumbó por los altoparlantes. "Adiestrado por Kalamack y propiedad de Kalamack."

Invadida de adrenalina, mis patas comenzaron a temblar. *Tengo que superar a una rata,* pensé, mientras sentía cómo el público vitoreaba a mi oponente en la arena, El Barón Sanguinario. No me dejaría matar por una rata.

Sentí un nudo en el estómago cuando Trent pasó junto al banco vacío junto a la arena. El olor era cien veces peor. Sabía que él también sentía el olor por la expresión de malestar que puso. Jonathan le seguía los pasos entusiasmado. A pesar de ser un mojigato elegante de cuello planchado y medias almidonadas, al hombre le gustaban los deportes sangrientos. Ahora casi no podía oír los chillidos de las ratas. La mitad estaban muertas y la otra mitad se lamían las heridas.

Hubo un momento de intercambio de cumplidos entre los propietarios seguido de una dramática emoción orquestada por Jim. Yo no escuchaba su palabrería de maestro de ceremonias. Estaba más concentrada en echarle una primera mirada a la arena.

El círculo era del tamaño de una piscina para niños rodeado de paredes de un metro de altura. El piso era de aserrín. Tenía manchas oscuras que indicaban ser de sangre. El hedor a orina y miedo era penetrante, tanto que me asombré de no poder verlo. Alguien con humor negro había colocado animales de juguete en la arena.

"¿Caballeros?" dijo Jim teatralmente, llamando la atención. "Pongan a sus combatientes."

Trent acercó la cara a la jaula. "He cambiado de opinión, Morgan," murmuró. "Ya no te necesito como agente. Para mí vales más matando ratas que matando a mis competidores. Los contactos que puedo hacer aquí son asombrosos."

"Muérete," gruñí.

Ante mi osco chillido abrió la portezuela y me tiró al ruedo.

Caí suavemente en el aserrín. La sombra de un movimiento del otro lado del ruedo me anunció la llegada del Barón Sanguinario. El público emitió un "¡Oh! de asombro al verme y yo salté rápidamente escondiéndome detrás de una pelota. Yo era mucho más atractiva que una rata."

Era espantoso tener la nariz metida en el aserrín: sangre, orina, muerte. Sólo pensaba en escapar. Mis ojos buscaron a los de Trent y sonrió. Él pensaba que podía torcerme el brazo y yo lo odiaba.

El público gritaba y me di vuelta para ver cómo el sanguinario venía hacia mí. No era tan largo como yo pero sí más fornido. Tal vez pesábamos lo mismo. Chillaba sin cesar en su carrera. Me paralicé sin saber qué hacer. En el último instante decidí saltar para quitarme del camino, dándole una patada al pasar. Era una fórmula de ataque que usé cientos de veces cuando era agente. Fue una reacción instintiva, aun cuando para un visón no tenía mayor gracia y no era muy efectiva. Terminé la patada girando y cayendo de cuclillas viendo cómo la rata resbalaba hasta detenerse.

El Barón dudó un instante examinando con su hocico el flanco donde lo había golpeado. Quedó en silencio.

Me atacó de nuevo y el público lo animaba. Esta vez apunté mejor acertándole en la cara al tiempo que yo saltaba hacia un lado. Aterricé de cuclillas y mis manos asumieron automáticamente la posición de combate, como si estuviera peleando contra una persona. La rata resbaló de nuevo hasta detenerse, chillando y agitando la cabeza como tratando de enfocar. El campo de visión de una rata debe ser muy limitado. Podía usar eso a mi favor.

Chillando con ira, El Barón se abalanzó contra mí por tercera vez. Me concentré en la idea de saltar directamente hacia arriba, caer sobre sus espaldas y ahogarlo hasta que perdiera el sentido. Sentía náuseas. No mataría por Trent. Ni siquiera a una rata. Si sacrificaba mis principios o mi ética, me poseería en cuerpo y alma. Si le daba mi brazo a torcer con ratas, mañana sería con gente.

La muchedumbre gritaba a más no poder y El Barón embistió de nuevo. Salté. "¡Mierda!" chillé al ver que se detuvo debajo de mí. ¡Le caería encima! Caí suavemente y chillé cuando me clavó los dientes en la nariz. Aterrada, traté de zafarme pero se aferró con fuerza, no permitiéndome liberarme. Me retorcí, lo golpeé en la boca con las manos y le propiné un par de patadas en la panza. Chilló con los golpes y aflojó su agarre. Finalmente me soltó y pude escabullirme.

Retrocedí un poco frotándome la nariz. No sé por qué no me la arrancó de la cara.

El Barón se puso de pie. Se tocó el costado donde lo había golpeado primero, luego la cara y finalmente la panza donde habían aterrizado mis patadas. Estaba haciendo un inventario de mis golpes. Su pata derecha se alzó para frotarse la nariz y me pareció entender que me estaba imitando. ¡El Barón era una persona!

"¡Demonios!" chillé. El Barón movió la cabeza una vez. Respiraba muy rápido y pasé la mirada por las paredes del ruedo y la gente que se abarrotaba contra ellas. Juntos podíamos escapar pero solos no teníamos ninguna opción. El Barón me hizo unos sonidos suaves. El público quedó en silencio. No iba a dejar escapar esta oportunidad. Torció los bigotes y yo lo embestí. Rodamos por el suelo en una lucha inofensiva. Todo lo que necesitaba era idear la manera de salir de allí y decírselo a El Barón sin que Trent se diera cuenta.

Nos trenzamos en una serie de vueltas y luego nos separamos. Me puse de pie y giré para buscarlo. Nada. "¡Barón!," grité. ¡Se había ido! Di vueltas y vueltas pensando si acaso lo habrían sacado del ruedo. De pronto sentí unos rasguños rítmicos detrás de una torre de bloques de madera. Luché contra la urgencia de darme vuelta pero finalmente sentí alivio. Ahí estaba. Ahora tenía una idea.

El único momento en que las manos se metían al ruedo

era cuando terminaba el combate. Uno de los dos tendría que fingir que moría.

"¡Escucha!" grité al tiempo que El Barón se lanzaba sobre mí. Sus afilados dientes se clavaron en mi oreja rasgándola. Mis ojos se llenaron de sangre cegándome. Furiosa, lo lancé por encima del hombro. "¿Qué demonios te pasa?" chillé mientras él caía pesadamente. El público estalló de la emoción, olvidando de inmediato nuestro comportamiento no roedor de segundos atrás.

El Barón hizo una serie larga de chillidos, sin duda tratando de explicarme lo que pensaba. Yo lo embestí agarrándolo por la tráquea haciéndolo callar. Me aporreó con las patas traseras a medida que le cortaba el suministro de aire. Se retorció agarrándome de la nariz con las uñas. Yo aflojé mi agarre al sentir los alfileres de sus garras dejándolo respirar.

Rengueó. "Se supone que no tienes que morirte todavía" dije chillando trabajosamente pues tenía su piel en mi boca. Lo atenacé hasta que lo sentí quejarse y patalear. El público empezó a murmurar pensando que Ángela se anotaría la primera victoria de la noche. Miré a Trent pero el instinto me hizo recapacitar al reconocer que sospechaba algo. Esto no iba a funcionar. Tal vez El Barón podía escapar. Yo no. Sería yo quien tendría que morir, no él.

"Ven, pelea" chillé, sabiendo que no me entendía. Aflojé mi agarre. Pero él no entendió. Se quedó inmóvil. Entonces le lancé una patada en la entrepierna.

Gritó de dolor y se zafó de mí. Yo me alejé rodando. "Atácame, mátame," chillé. Movió la cabeza tratando de recuperar su enfoque. Yo le hice una señal moviendo mi cabeza hacia el público. Él parpadeó como si hubiera entendido y me atacó. Su mandíbula fue directa a mi tráquea dejándome sin aire. Me sacudí con fuerza y los dos nos fuimos contra las paredes. Escuché los gritos de emoción de la gente y la presión de la sangre me reventaba en la cabeza.

Me tenía agarrada muy duro, demasiado duro para poder respirar. *Ahora, en cualquier momento,* pensé desesperada.

Puedes dejarme respirar en cualquier momento. Nos fuimos contra una pelota pero aún no me soltaba. El pánico me invadió. ¿Acaso no era una persona? ¿Había dejado que una rata me agarrara con un mordisco mortal?

Comencé a luchar por zafarme pero me mordió más fuerte. Sentí que mi cabeza iba a estallar. La sangre me latía. Me retorcí y pataleé clavándole una garra en el ojo hasta que le salieron lágrimas; pero aun así no me soltaba. Logré hacer una voltereta que nos lanzó contra las paredes. Entonces logré atraparlo por el cuello. Me soltó de inmediato y por fin pude respirar.

Lo mordí furiosa y sentí el sabor de su sangre en mis dientes. Me devolvió el mordisco y chillé de dolor. Aflojé mi agarre y él hizo lo mismo. Los gritos del público presionaban tanto como el calor de las lámparas. Estábamos tirados en el piso sobre el aserrín tratando de disminuir el ritmo de la respiración para que pareciera que nos estábamos asfixiando el uno al otro. Finalmente comprendí. Su dueño también sabía que él era una persona. Los dos teníamos que morir.

La gente gritaba. Querían saber quién era el ganador o si los dos estábamos muertos. Miré con los ojos entreabiertos y vi a Trent. No estaba contento. Entendí que nuestro teatro apenas tenía éxito parcialmente. El Barón se quedó muy quieto. Emitió un pequeño chillido y yo le respondí muy bajo. Sentí de repente un nuevo ánimo.

"¡Señoras y señores!" sonó finalmente la voz profesional de Jim acallando el ruido. "Parece que tenemos un empate. ¿Podrían los propietarios retirar a sus animales por favor?" El público quedó en silencio. "Haremos una breve pausa para determinar si alguno de los combatientes está vivo."

Mi corazón comenzó a martillar al percibir que se aproximaban sombras. El Barón emitió tres chillidos breves y de repente saltó. Yo reaccioné un poco tarde agarrando la primera mano que encontré.

"¡Cuidado!" gritó alguien. Volé por el aire cuando la mano me soltó intempestivamente. Me arqueé con mi cola formando círculos frenéticamente. Pude ver una cara sorprendida y aterricé sobre el pecho de un hombre. Gritó como una niñita tratando de quitarme de encima y caí duro al piso. Tomé aire y me arrastré debajo de su silla.

El ruido era ensordecedor. Uno diría que se había escapado un león y no dos roedores. La gente se dispersó. El sonido de pasos que pasaban junto a la silla parecía irreal. Alguien que olía a aserrín trató de agarrarme pero lo amenacé con los dientes y retrocedió.

"Tengo al visón," gritó un empleado en medio del escándalo. "¡Tráiganme una red!" Apenas volteó la mirada salí corriendo. Mi pulso latía tan rápido que sonaba como un zumbido. Esquivé piernas y asientos casi estrellándome de cabeza contra la pared del fondo. La sangre que me chorreaba de la oreja caía en mis ojos nublándome la vista. ¿Cómo saldría de allí?

"Todo el mundo tranquilo," sonó la voz de Jim por los altavoces. "Por favor, diríjanse al vestíbulo a disfrutar de un refrigerio mientras continuamos la búsqueda. Les pedimos que mantengan cerradas las puertas exteriores hasta que hayamos atrapado a los combatientes." Hubo una pausa. "¡Y saquen a ese perro de aquí!" concluyó molesto.

¿Puertas? pensé, mirando aquel manicomio. Yo no necesito puertas. Necesito a Jenks.

"¡Raquel!" dijo una voz arriba de mí. Chirrié al tiempo que Jenks aterrizaba sobre mis hombros con un leve golpe. "Estás hecha una mierda," gritó en mi oído herido. "Pensé que esa rata te había matado; ¡pero cuando saltaste y agarraste la mano de Jonathan estuve a punto de orinarme en los pantalones!"

"¿¡Dónde está la puerta!?" traté de preguntarle. Cómo logró encontrarme es una historia que tendríamos que dejar para más tarde.

"No sé," dijo. "Me fui tal como lo ordenaste. Apenas regresé hoy. Tan pronto Trent salió con esa caja para gatos supe que tú estabas adentro. Yo me escondí en el parachoques. Te apuesto a que no sabías que así viajan los duendes por la ciudad ¿lo sabías? Más vale que saques tu trasero peludo de aquí antes de que alguien te encuentre."

"¿¡Hacia dónde!?" chillé. "¿¡Para qué lado!?"

"Por atrás. Hay una ruta de escape. Hice un reconocimiento durante el primer combate. Oye…estas ratas salvajes. ¿Viste como esa le arrancó la pierna a la otra? Sigue esta pared por unos seis metros y luego bajas tres escalones hasta llegar a un pasillo."

Empecé a moverme y sentí que Jenks se aferraba a mi piel.

"Huy…tu oreja esta hecha trizas" dijo Jenks mientras descendíamos los tres escalones. "Muy bien. Ahora continúa por el pasillo a la derecha. Hay una abertura…¡No! ¡No te metas ahí!" gritó Jenks cuando ya empezaba a hacerlo. "Es la cocina."

Di media vuelta y me quedé paralizada al oír un ruido de pasos. Mi pulso se aceleró. No me dejaría atrapar. ¡Eso jamás!

"El fregadero," susurró Jenks. "La puerta del armario no está con llave. ¡Corre!"

Lo vi. Correteé por el piso, mis garras raspando suavemente. Me escurrí adentro mientras Jenks voló junto a la puerta para espiar. Retrocedí para esconderme detrás de un balde y escuché en silencio.

"No están en la cocina," gritó una voz apagada. Sentí un poco de alivio. Había dicho "están." El Barón seguía libre.

Jenks regresó aleteando sin parar y se paró en el armario. "Demonios, no sabes cuánto me alegra verte. Ivy no hace otra cosa que estudiar un plano que encontró de la propiedad de Trent," susurró. "Se pasa la noche rezongando y escribiendo papeles. Después arruga y tira cada hoja en una esquina. Mis hijos gozan de lo lindo jugando en la montaña que formó. No creo que ella sepa que estoy aquí. Sólo piensa en ese mapa y en tomar jugo de naranja."

Sentí olor a tierra. Mientras Jenks cacareaba como un adicto al azufre que necesita su dosis, exploré el oloroso armario y descubrí que la tubería del fregadero pasaba debajo del piso de madera de la casa. El espacio entre el metal y el piso era apenas suficiente para mis hombros. Comencé a masticar.

"Dije que sacaran a ese perro de aquí," ordenó una voz apagada.

"No, espera. ¿Puedes darle una pista? Tal vez pueda encontrarlos."

Jenks se acercó. "Claro, el piso. ¡Es buena idea! Te ayudaré." Se puso junto a mí.

"Busca a El Barón," chillé.

"¿Quién dice que no puedo ayudar?" dijo Jenks orgulloso. Arrancó un palito de madera del tamaño de un palillo cerca del agujero.

"La rata," chillé. "No puede ver." Frustrada dejé caer un recipiente de detergente. El polvo se derramó y el olor a pino me invadió. Le arrebaté el palillo a Jenks y con él escribí: "Busca a la rata."

Jenks se elevó y tapándose la nariz con una mano preguntó. "¿Por qué?"

"Hombre" escribí. "No ve."

Jenks gruñó. "¿Encontraste un amigo? Espera a que Ivy se entere."

Mostré los dientes señalando la puerta con el palillo. Aún así dudó. "¿Te quedarás aquí agrandando ese agujero?"

Desesperada le lancé el palo. Jenks retrocedió un poco. "¡Está bien, está bien! No te vuelvas loca."

Su risa retumbó por todas partes libremente cuando pasó por la ranura de la puerta. Yo seguí mordisqueando la madera. Tenía un sabor horrible, una mezcla pútrida de jabón, grasa y moho. Sentí que enfermaba. Mi cuerpo se tensó. Cada golpe que escuchaba me sobresaltaba. Estaba esperando a escuchar el grito triunfal de la captura. Afortunadamente, el perro no entendió que diablos esperaban de él. Sólo quería jugar y a todos se les estaba agotando la paciencia.

Me dolía la mandíbula pero contuve mis lamentos. Un poco de jabón había entrado en la herida que tenía en la oreja y me ardía como el mismísimo infierno. Traté de meter la cabeza en el agujero para llegar al espacio por donde podría arrastrarme. Si lograba meter la cabeza, de seguro pasaría también mi cuerpo. Pero aún no era lo suficientemente grande.

"¡Miren!" gritó alguien. "Está funcionando. Parece que ya detectó el olor."

Saqué la cabeza del agujero con desesperación. Me raspé la oreja y empezó a sangrar de nuevo. De repente oí un rasguño en el pasillo y redoblé mi esfuerzo. Sentí la voz de Jenks. "Es la cocina. Raquel está debajo del fregadero. No. Es el siguiente armario. ¡Rápido! Creo que te vieron."

De pronto entró un destello de luz acompañado por aire. Me senté escupiendo madera.

"¡Hola! ¡Ya regresamos! Aquí está tu rata, Raquel."

El Barón me miró. Sus ojos brillaban e inmediatamente formamos un equipo. Metió la cabeza en el agujero y comenzó a roer. No había suficiente espacio para acomodar sus anchas espaldas. Yo continué agrandando el agujero arriba. Ahora escuchábamos los ladridos del perro en el pasillo. Por un instante se nos heló el corazón pero seguimos mordiendo. Sentí un nudo en el estómago.

"¿Suficientemente grande?" gritó Jenks. "¡Váyanse rápido!"

Metí la cabeza en el agujero junto a El Barón mordisqueando frenéticamente. De repente oímos rasguños en la puerta del armario. La luz invadió el mueble al abrirse la puerta. "¡Aquí!" gritó una voz. "¡Encontró a uno aquí!"

Estaba perdiendo las esperanzas. Alcé la cabeza y me dolía la mandíbula. El detergente de pino me cubría la piel y me hacía arder los ojos. Giré la cabeza y pude ver las patas que nos buscaban. Pensé que el agujero aún no era lo suficientemente grande. De pronto sentí un chillido agudo. El Barón estaba acurrucado señalando hacia abajo. "No es lo suficientemente grande para ti," le dije.

Se abalanzó sobre mí jalándome y metiéndome en el agujero. El ruido del perro se hizo más fuerte y yo caí en el aire.

Estiré las patas tratando de engancharme a la tubería. Con una de mis patas delanteras logré fijarme a unos tubos soldados y me detuve. Arriba el perro ladraba sin cesar. Los rasguños de sus patas sonaban en el piso de madera y entonces sentí un chillido. Terminé mi caída y toqué fondo. Me quedé ahí escuchando el gemido de muerte de El Barón.

Debí quedarme, pensé desesperada. *Nunca debí dejar que me metiera por este hueco.* Sabía que él no cabía.

De repente sentí un golpe seco y que raspaban la tierra a mi lado.

"¡Lo lograste!" chillé al ver cómo El Barón se revolcaba en la tierra a mi lado.

También llegó Jenks brillando con su tenue luz. Traía un bigote de perro en una mano. "¡Debiste verlo, Raque!" me dijo emocionado. "Le propinó un mordisco a ese perro en la nariz ¡yahoo! ¡pum! ¡bam-bam! ¡esto es para ti grandulón!"

El duende siguió volando en círculos a nuestro alrededor, demasiado excitado para quedarse quieto. Sin embargo, El Barón estaba tiritando. Se enroscó como una bola de peluche y se veía enfermo. Me acerqué para agradecerle. Le toqué los hombros y saltó, mirándome con sus ojos negros bien abiertos.

"¡Saquen a ese perro de aquí!," dijo una voz furiosa arriba en el piso. Alzamos la mirada para ver una tenue luz. Los ladridos cesaron y mi pulso comenzó a normalizarse. "Así es," dijo Jim. "Son mordiscos frescos. Uno se escapó por aquí."

"¿Cómo llegamos allá abajo?" Era Trent. Me llené de pánico acurrucándome contra la tierra.

"Hay una escotilla en el pasillo pero el espacio tiene acceso a la calle por cualquiera de los respiraderos." Sus voces se alejaron. "Lo siento mucho, Sr. Kalamack. Es la primera vez que tenemos una fuga," continuó Jim. "Haré que alguien baje allá inmediatamente."

"No. Ya escapó." Sonó frustrado y yo sentí un aire de victoria. Jonathan no iba a tener un viaje de regreso nada agradable. Me estiré un poco y suspiré cansada. Me ardían los oídos y los ojos. Quería regresar a casa.

El Barón chilló para llamar mi atención y señaló la tierra. Había escrito algo: "Gracias."

No pude contener una sonrisa. Me acurruqué junto a él y escribí: "Por nada." Mis letras se veían desordenadas junto a las suyas.

"Vaya, que *ternura*" se burló Jenks. "¿Ahora podemos largarnos de aquí?"

El Barón saltó hacia la malla que tapaba el respiradero aferrándose con las cuatro patas y empezó a morder cuidadosamente las soldaduras.

Veintitrés

Raspé con la cuchara el fondo del recipiente plástico de requesón formando un montoncito con lo que quedaba. Sentía frío en las rodillas y las cubrí con mi bata azul de felpa. Me arreglé la cara mientras que El Barón se transformaba en hombre y se duchaba en el segundo baño, el que Ivy y yo habíamos decidido que sería el mío. Me moría de ganas de ver cómo era. Las dos estuvimos de acuerdo en que si había sobrevivido a las peleas de ratas tanto tiempo tenía que ser un monumento de hombre. Era valiente, caballeroso y no le molestaban los vampiros—esto último era lo más asombroso pues, según Jenks, El Barón es un humano.

Jenks había llamado a Ivy por cobrar desde el primer teléfono que vimos. El ruido de su motocicleta—recién retirada del taller luego de que se metió bajo un camión la semana anterior—nos pareció una bella canción. Por poco me hace llorar cuando saltó de su silla vestida de cuero negro de pies a cabeza, apenas me vio. Por lo menos había alguien que se preocupaba si yo vivía o estaba muerta, así fuese un vampiro cuyos motivos aún no lograba descifrar.

Ni El Barón ni yo quisimos meternos en la cajita que había traído para transportarnos. Después de discutir cinco minutos—ella protestando y nosotros chillando—decidió botar la cajita en el callejón refunfuñando frustrada y nos dejó subir adelante. No estaba de muy buen humor cuando salió del callejón con un visón y una rata subidos en el tanque de gasolina con las patitas encima del velocímetro. Finalmente logramos salir del tráfico del viernes en la tarde y tomar velocidad. ¡Al fin entendí por qué a los perros les gusta sacar la cabeza por las ventanillas!

Montar en moto siempre me pareció emocionante, pero ahora como roedor sentía un torrente de excitación. Estaba feliz de regresar a casa con el aire que me doblaba los bigotes y me hacía tener los ojos semiabiertos. No me importaba que la gente mirara a Ivy con extrañeza y que sonaran la bocina. Sentí que tendría un orgasmo cerebral por la sobrecarga emocional. Hasta sentí tristeza cuando Ivy finalmente giró para tomar nuestra calle.

Empujé con el dedo el último poco de queso en la cuchara sin prestarle atención a los ruidos de marrano que emitía Jenks parado en el cucharón que colgaba de la mesa en medio de la cocina. No había parado de comer desde que me transformé de nuevo, pero como sólo había probado zanahorias durante los últimos tres días y medio, tenía derecho a una comilona.

Puse el recipiente desocupado junto al plato sucio que tenía al frente. Pensé si duele más transformarse siendo humano. Según el quejido masculino de dolor que se escuchó en el baño antes de prenderse la ducha, diría que duele igual.

A pesar de haberme jabonado dos veces, sentía aun el olor de visón bajo mi perfume. Mi oreja herida palpitaba, mi cuello tenía perforaciones con manchas rojas donde El Barón me había mordido y mi pierna izquierda me dolía por la caída que tuve de la rueda de ejercicios. Pero qué bien se sentía ser de nuevo una persona. Observé a Ivy lavando los platos. Tal vez debí taparme la oreja.

Aún no les había contado a Ivy y a Jenks todo lo sucedido durante los últimos días. Sólo les había contado de mi cautiverio pero no de todas las cosas que aprendí. Ivy no había dicho nada pero presentí que se moría de ganas de decirme lo idiota que fui por no tener un plan alterno de escape.

Cerró la llave tan pronto terminó de enjuagar el último

vaso. Lo dejó escurriendo y se dio vuelta para secarse las manos con la toalla de los platos. Ver a un vampiro delgado vestido de cuero lavando platos era una escena que solamente podía suceder en mi vida de locos. "Veamos. Explícame bien las cosas" dijo Ivy reclinándose en la mesa. "Trent te atrapó con las manos en la masa; pero en vez de entregarte te metió a las peleas de ratas de la ciudad para que dieras tu brazo a torcer y trabajaras para él."

"Ajá." Me estiré para alcanzar el paquete de galletas que tenía Ivy junto a su computadora.

"Tiene sentido." Se movió y tomó mi plato vacío. Lo lavó y lo puso a escurrir junto a los vasos. Además de mis platos, no vi más platos, cubiertos ni tazas. Sólo veinte vasos con una gota de jugo de naranja en el fondo.

"La próxima vez que te enfrentes a alguien como Trent ¿podríamos tener por lo menos un plan si te atrapan?," dijo dándome la espalda.

Alcé la cabeza del paquete de galletas fastidiada. Tomé aire para decirle que podía hacer papel higiénico con sus planes, pero dudé. Sus hombros estaban tensos y la cara seria. Recordé que Jenks me dijo lo preocupada que estaba y también cómo yo despertaba sus instintos. Dejé escapar el aire lentamente. "Sí, claro," repuse con algo de duda. "Podemos tener un plan libre de errores para cuando yo meta la pata, siempre y cuando también tengamos uno para ti."

Jenks dejó escapar una risilla e Ivy lo miró. "No necesitamos uno para mí," dijo.

"No olvides escribir eso y pegarlo junto al teléfono," repuse indiferentemente. "Yo haré lo mismo." Le estaba tomando el pelo, pero luego pensé que a lo mejor era capaz de hacerlo puesto que tomaba todo tan en serio.

Sin decir más, Ivy decidió empezar a secar los platos y los vasos que había dejado escurriendo. Mastiqué las galletas de jengibre observando cómo sus hombros se relajaban y sus movimientos se volvían más lentos. "Tenías razón," dije, pues pensé que al menos le debía eso, "nunca he contado con nadie antes, no estoy acostumbrada."

Ivy dio media vuelta y me sorprendió su actitud relajada. "Oye, no hay problema."

"¡Oh! ¡Ayuda!" dijo Jenks desde el organizador de cubiertos. "Creo que voy a vomitar."

Ivy le dio un golpe con la toalla con una sonrisa irónica. La observé detenidamente mientras seguía secando los platos. Las cosas eran distintas cuando lograba calmarse y acomodarse al momento. Ahora que lo pensaba, el año que logramos trabajar juntas fue justamente porque logramos acomodarnos a las circunstancias. Sin embargo, para mí era más difícil acomodarme estando rodeada de todas sus cosas pero ninguna mía. Me había sentido vulnerable y al borde del precipicio.

"Debiste verla, Raquel," dijo Jenks susurrando en voz alta para que ella lo oyera. "Se pasó todos los días sentada con sus mapas buscando una manera para rescatarte de Trent. Le dije que solo podíamos estar atentos y ayudarte cuando se presentara la oportunidad."

"¡Cierra la boca, Jenks!" dijo Ivy intempestivamente con voz grave de advertencia. Comí la última galleta y me levanté para botar el paquete.

"Si vieras. Tenía este plan maravilloso" continuó Jenks, "pero lo botó cuando te estabas duchando. Iba a llamar a todos los que le deben favores. Hasta habló con su madre."

"Voy a conseguir un gato," dijo Ivy seriamente. "Un gato grande y negro."

Saqué un paquete de pan y la miel de la alacena donde la había escondido de Jenks. Llevé las cosas a la mesa y las puse en orden.

"Afortunadamente, escapaste en ese momento," dijo Jenks haciendo oscilar el cucharón que llenó la cocina de destellos. "Ivy estaba a punto de gastar lo poco que aún le queda para salvarte, de nuevo."

"Voy a llamar a mi gato Polvo de Duende. Lo dejaré en el jardín y no le daré de comer."

Pasé la mirada de la boca cerrada de Jenks a Ivy. Habíamos tenido una conversación cálida y punzante sin que ella se pusiera vampiro ni yo me asustara. ¿Por qué Jenks tenía que arruinarlo todo? "Jenks," le dije suspirando "¿No tienes nada que hacer?"

"No." Saltó y metió una mano en el chorro de miel que estaba sirviendo en el pan. Se agachó un poco y luego se levantó. "Entonces ¿se quedarán con él?"

Miré a Jenks inquisitivamente y se rió.

"Tu nuevo n-o-o-o-vio," dijo arrastrando las letras.

Mis labios se movieron instantáneamente al ver el asombro de Ivy. "No es mi novio."

Jenks se quedó estático en el aire encima del frasco sacando miel con los dedos para llevársela a la boca. "Yo los vi juntos en la moto," dijo. "Ummm... esto está bueno." Tomó más y ahora sus alas sonaron más fuerte. "Se estaban tocando las colas" agregó burlonamente.

Enfadada lo palmoteé pero voló fuera de mi alcance y luego regresó. "Debiste verlos, Ivy. Se revolcaron por el suelo mordiéndose." Jenks estalló en una aguda risa tonta. Yo incliné levemente la cabeza cuando aterrizó a mi lado izquierdo. "Fue amor al primer mordisco."

Ivy dio media vuelta. "¿Te mordió en el cuello?" dijo con seriedad de muerte, excepto por sus ojos. "Entonces debe ser amor. A *mí* no me deja morderle el cuello."

¿Y todo esto? ¿Noche de emprenderla contra Raquel? No me parece divertido. Saqué otra tajada de pan para terminar mi emparedado y ahuyenté a Jenks de la miel que salió dando tumbos. Trataba de conservar el equilibrio en vuelo pues el aumento de azúcar lo emborrachó.

"Oye, Ivy," dijo Jenks volando de medio lado y lamiéndose los dedos. "¿Has oído lo que dicen acerca del tamaño de la cola de las ratas? Cuanto más larga tienen la cola más largo tienen el..."

"¡Ya cierra la boca!" grité. En ese momento apagaron la ducha y contuve el aire. Una oleada de ansiedad hizo que me sentara derecho en mi silla. Miré a Jenks que reía borracho de miel. "Jenks," dije. "Vete." No quería que El Barón tuviera que aguantarse a un duende borracho.

"N-o-o-o-o" respondió, tomando más miel con una mano. Molesta, cerré de nuevo el frasco y Jenks emitió un leve sonido de desagrado. Con la mano lo ahuyenté hasta los utensilios que colgaban. Con suerte permanecería allí hasta pasar la borrachera, es decir, unos cuatro minutos como mucho.

Ivy salió musitando algo sobre vasos que había en la sala. El cuello de mi bata se había mojado con el pelo. Me limpié la miel de los dedos y me movía nerviosamente como si se tratara de una primera cita. Que tontería. Ya nos habíamos conocido. Inclusive, tuvimos una versión roedora de primera cita: un resonante combate en el gimnasio, una carrera escapando de la gente y los perros y un paseo por el parque en moto. ¿Pero qué le dices a un tipo que no conoces y que te salvó la vida?

Oí que la puerta del baño chirriaba abriéndose. Ivy frenó en seco en el pasillo con dos tazas colgándole de los dedos. Yo me cubrí las piernas con la bata y no supe si ponerme de pie. La voz de El Barón viajó suavemente por el aire y llegó a la cocina. "Tú eres Ivy ¿verdad?"

"Uhh" dudó Ivy. "Tú tienes puesta mi bata," dijo y sonrió. Grandioso. El Barón ya estaba impregnado con el olor de Ivy. Buen comienzo.

"Oh, lo lamento," dijo con voz agradable y sonora. No podía aguantar más las ganas de verlo. Ivy parecía no hallar palabras. El Barón respiró ruidosamente. "La encontré en el tendedero y no había nada más que ponerse. Mejor busco una toalla."

Ivy dudó un poco. "Eh…no," repuso con inusual voz de asombro. "¿Estás bien? Ayudaste a Raquel a escapar."

"Sí. ¿Está en la cocina?" preguntó.

"Entra." Ivy volteó los ojos. Ella venía adelante. "Es un nerdo" me dijo con los labios pero sin hablar. Quedé paralizada. *¿Un nerdo me salvó la vida?*

"Eh, hola," dijo, torpemente parado bajo el umbral de la puerta.

"Hola," respondí desconcertada sin hallar otras palabras, mirándolo de arriba abajo. No era propiamente justo decir que era un geek, pero comparado con los tipos a los que estaba acostumbrada Ivy, tal vez.

El Barón era tan alto como Ivy pero sus músculos eran tan escasos que parecía más alto. Sus brazos pálidos que se transparentaban detrás de la bata negra de Ivy mostraban algunas cicatrices leves, seguramente de anteriores peleas de ratas. Tenía las mejillas rasuradas—tendría que ir a comprar una cuchilla nueva pues la que me prestó Ivy ya estaría dañada. Los lóbulos y los arcos de las orejas tenían rasguños. Dos agujeros sobresalían en su cuello. Se veían rojos e irritados. Eran como los míos y sentí verguenza.

A pesar de su figura angosta—o tal vez debido a ella—se veía bien. Tenía el pelo largo y oscuro y la forma como se lo quitaba permanentemente de los ojos me hizo pensar que normalmente lo llevaba más corto. La bata lo hacía verse cómodo y tranquilo; pero la forma en que la seda negra caía encima de sus músculos flacos hizo que mis ojos vagaran. Ivy había exagerado su crítica. Tenía demasiados músculos para ser un nerdo.

"Tienes el pelo rojo" dijo, y comenzó a moverse. "Yo pensé que era castaño."

"Y yo pensé que...eh...que eras más bajo." Me levanté a medida que se aproximaba y, luego de una extraña pausa, me tendió la mano desde el otro lado de la mesa. Está bien. No era precisamente Arnold Schwarzenegger pero me había salvado la vida. Digamos que estaba entre un bajito y joven Jeff Goldblum y un descuidado Buckaroo Banzai.

"Mi nombre es Nick" dijo mientras me daba la mano. "Bueno, en realidad es Nicolás. Gracias por ayudarme a escapar de ese nido de ratas."

"Yo soy Raquel." Tenía una mano agradable al tacto. Lo suficiente para saludar con firmeza sin tratar de demostrar lo fuerte que era. Hice un ademán indicando las sillas de la cocina y nos sentamos. "No hay de qué. En realidad, nos ayudamos mutuamente. Dirás que no es asunto mío, pero ¿cómo diablos terminaste como rata de pelea?"

Nick se frotó una oreja con la mano mirando el techo. "Yo

...eh...estaba organizando la colección privada de libros de un vampiro. Hallé algo interesante y cometí el error de llevarlo a casa." Me miró a los ojos, avergonzado. "No pensaba quedármelo."

Ivy y yo intercambiamos miradas. *S-ó-o-o-l-o- lo tomó prestado*...claro. Si había trabajado con vampiros antes, eso explicaba su calma frente a Ivy.

"Al enterarse, me transformó en rata," continuó Nick. "Luego me regaló a uno de sus socios comerciales. Fue él quien me inscribió en las peleas pues sabía que yo tenía la ventaja mental de un ser humano. Ganó mucho dinero conmigo. ¿Y tú? ¿Cómo llegaste allá?"

"Eh...preparé una poción para convertirme en visón y terminé en las peleas por equivocación." No le estaba mintiendo. No lo tenía en mis planes, de manera que fue un accidente. Es la verdad.

"¿Eres bruja?" preguntó con una sonrisa grande. "Qué bien. No estaba seguro."

Yo también sonreí. Me había topado varias veces con humanos como Nick que pensaban que los Entremundos eran tan sólo el otro lado de la moneda humana. Siempre fueron sorpresas agradables.

"¿Qué son esas peleas?" preguntó Ivy. "¿Una especie de forma para deshacerse de la gente sin mancharse las manos de sangre?"

Nick agitó la cabeza. "No creo. Raquel es la primera persona con quien me topé y estuve allí tres meses."

"¡Tres meses!" exclamé espantada. "¿Fuiste una rata durante tres meses?"

Se acomodó en la silla y anudó bien la bata. "Sí. Imagino que han vendido todas mis cosas para pagar mis pagos atrasados de arriendo. Pero...ahora tengo manos de nuevo." Las alzó y observé que, aun cuando eran delgadas, tenían muchos callos.

Hice un gesto de dolor en señal de compasión. En Los Hollows la práctica corriente era vender los bienes del inquilino en caso de que desapareciera y la gente desaparecía con demasiada frecuencia. Tampoco tenía empleo pues obviamente lo habían "despedido" del anterior.

"¿De verdad viven en una iglesia?" preguntó.

Mi mirada siguió a la suya que se paseaba por nuestra cocina institucional. "Así es. Ivy y yo nos mudamos hace un par de días. No nos molestan los cuerpos enterrados en el jardín de atrás."

Sonrió forzadamente. Dios me perdone, pero eso lo hizo parecer un niño perdido. Ivy, quien de nuevo estaba en el fregadero, rió entre dientes.

"Miel." Sentí la voz de Jenks que se quejaba y alcé la vista para verlo. Nos miraba aferrado al cucharón y agitando sus alas velozmente. Voló inestable y por poco cae sobre la mesa. Me encogí avergonzada pero Nick sonrió. "Jenks ¿verdad?" preguntó Nick.

"Barón," repuso Jenks dando tumbos mientras se esforzaba por hacer su pose de Peter Pan. "Me alegro que puedas hacer algo diferente a chillar. Eso me produce dolor de cabeza. Chillidos, chillidos, chillidos. Ese ruido ultrasónico me perfora la cabeza."

"Nick. Nick Sparagmos."

"Escucha Nick, Raquel quiere saber qué se siente tener pelotas tan grandes como tu cabeza que se arrastran por el suelo."

"¡Jenks!" grité. *Oh Dios, por favor.* Agité la cabeza negándolo y miré a Nick. Él, sin embargo, pareció tomarlo con calma. Sus ojos brillaron e hizo una larga mueca.

Jenks tomó aire apresuradamente y salió disparado cuando traté de atraparlo. Estaba recuperando rápidamente el equilibrio. "Vaya cicatriz que tienes en la muñeca," dijo. "Mi esposa—es una chica dulce—me remienda. Hace maravillas con sus puntadas."

"¿Quieres algo para el cuello?" le pregunté, tratando de cambiar el tema.

"No. Estoy bien" dijo Nick. Se estiró lentamente como si estuviera entumecido y saltó poniéndose derecho cuando me rozó suavemente uno de mis pies. Traté de no ser demasiado obvia al mirarlo. Jenks fue menos diplomático.

"Nick," dijo Jenks aterrizando a su lado en la mesa. "¿Alguna vez has visto una cicatriz como esta?" Jenks se arremangó la camisa para exhibir un arrugado zigzag desde la muñeca hasta el codo. Siempre vestía camisa de seda de mangas largas. No sabía que tuviera cicatrices.

Nick silbó con asombro y eso le dio cuerda a Jenks. "Me la hizo un hada," dijo. "Estaba ocultando al objetivo que mi agente estaba persiguiendo. Bastaron un par de segundos de lucha en el techo y se perdió."

"Vaya vaya," dijo Nick impresionado y se inclinó hacia adelante. Olía bien: masculino sin caer en lobo y ni rastros de sangre. Sus ojos eran pardos. Bonitos. Me gustaban los ojos humanos porque los ves y sólo encuentras lo que esperas encontrar.

"¿Y esa otra?" preguntó Nick señalando una cicatriz redonda en la clavícula.

"Picada de abeja," repuso Jenks. "Me mandó a la cama tres días con escalofríos y sacudidas; pero hicimos respetar nuestro territorio alrededor de las macetas con flores. ¿Y esa que tienes ahí?" preguntó Jenks elevándose y apuntando hacia una cicatriz con ribetes que tenía Nick en la muñeca.

Nick me miró y luego se fijó en su cictraiz. "Me la hizo una rata grande llamada Hugo."

"Por poco te arranca la mano."

"Trató."

"Mira esta otra" dijo Jenks quitándose una de sus botas dejando ver un pie casi deforme detrás de su media transparente. "Un vampiro casi me hace papilla cuando no me quité de en medio a tiempo."

Nick hizo una mueca y yo sentí enfermar. Debe ser difícil medir diez centímetros en un mundo de uno ochenta. Abrió la parte superior de la bata para mostrar su hombro y algunos músculos. Yo me incliné hacia adelante para ver mejor. El tejido de cicatrices parecían boquetes producidos por clavos y quise averiguar qué tanto bajaban. Llegué a la conclusión de que Ivy estaba equivocada. No era un nerdo. Los nerdo no tienen abdominales como una tabla. "Éstas me las hizo una rata llamada Pan el Terrible" explicó Nick.

"¿Y qué tal esto?" Jenks dejó caer su camisa hasta la cintura. Yo estaba asombrada de ver cómo el cuerpo de Jenks estaba tan lastimado y lleno de cicatrices. "¿Ves eso?" dijo señalando una cicatriz cóncava y circular. "Mira, atraviesa hasta el otro lado." Giró para mostrar una cicatriz más pequeña abajo en su espalda. "Fue una espada de hada. Pudo haberme matado, pero acababa de casarme con Matalina. Ella me mantuvo con vida hasta que las toxinas fueron eliminadas de mi cuerpo."

Nick agitó la cabeza despacio. "Tu ganas," dijo. "Eso no puedo igualarlo."

Jenks se elevó varios centímetros sintiéndose orgulloso. Yo no supe qué decir. Mi estómago hacía ruidos y finalmente se me ocurrió decir: "Nick, ¿te gustaría comer un sándwich o algo?"

Nuestros ojos se encontraron. "Si no es mucha molestia."

Me levanté y caminé con mis peludas pantuflas rosadas hasta el refrigerador. "Ninguna molestia. De todas formas pensaba preparar algo para mí."

Ivy terminó de guardar el último vaso y comenzó a lavar el fregadero con polvo blanqueador. Inmediatamente le hice una mirada cortante. El fregadero no necesitaba una lavada. Simplemente estaba metiendo las narices. Tan pronto abrí el refrigerador repasé cuidadosamente las bolsas de comida de cuatro restaurantes diferentes. Aparentemente Ivy había pedido todo eso. Escarbando un poco encontré algo de mortadela y una lechuga que comenzaba a marchitarse. Mis ojos se posaron en el tomate que había en la repisa de la ventana. Me mordí los labios con la esperanza de que Nick no lo hubiera visto. No quería ofenderlo, pues casi ningún humano se atrevía a probar los tomates. Me interpuse entre Nick y el tomate y lo escondí detrás de la tostadora.

"¿Comiendo todavía?" murmuró Ivy entre dientes.

"Tengo hambre" rezongué. "Además, esta noche necesito todas mis fuerzas." Volví a meter la cabeza en el refrigerador para buscar la mayonesa. "Podría hacer buen uso de tu ayuda, si tienes tiempo."

"¿Ayuda para qué?" preguntó Jenks. "¿Para meterte a la camita?"

Me di vuelta con las manos llenas de cosas para preparar sándwiches y cerré la puerta del refrigerador con el hombro. "Necesito tu ayuda para atrapar a Trent y sólo tenemos hasta la medianoche para hacerlo."

Jenks saltó en el aire. "¿Qué?" preguntó secamente. Su buen humor desapareció.

Miré con preocupación a Ivy pues sabía que esto no le iba a gustar. A decir verdad, quería que Nick estuviera presente pues tal vez con un testigo Ivy no armaría una escena.

"¿Esta noche?" dijo Ivy, poniendo sus manos sobre los muslos y clavándome la mirada. "¿Quieres tratar de atraparlo esta noche?" Sus ojos se fijaron en Nick y luego en mí. Lanzó su trapo en el fregadero y se secó las manos con una servilleta de papel, "Raquel, ¿podemos hablar en el pasillo?"

Fruncí el ceño ante su implicación de que no podíamos confiar en Nick. Entonces dejé escapar un suspiro de exasperación y dejé caer en la mesa todo lo que tenía en los brazos. "Disculpa," le dije a Nick con una sonrisa.

Fastidiada, la seguí. Me detuve abruptamente al verla ahí parada en medio del pasillo en dirección a nuestras habitaciones. Su silueta cáustica la hacía verse peligrosa en la oscuridad del pasillo. Me tensé además por el penetrante olor a incienso. "¿Qué?" pregunté a secas.

"No creo que sea buena idea que Nick sepa tu pequeño problema" dijo.

"Ha sido una rata durante tres meses," repuse retrocediendo. "¿Cómo diablos podría ser un asesino de la S.E.? El pobre hombre ni siquiera tiene ropa y tú te preocupas de que pueda matarme?"

"No," protestó moviéndose más cerca poniéndome de

espaldas contra la pared. "Pero cuanto menos sepa de ti, más seguros estarán *ambos*."

"Oh." Me puse lívida. Ivy estaba demasiado cerca y eso no era buen síntoma.

"¿Y de qué piensas acusar a Trent?" preguntó. "¿De dejarte como visón? ¿De meterte a las peleas de ratas de la ciudad? Si piensas presentarte gimiendo a la S.E. con esa historia, estás muerta."

Sus palabras se habían tornado lentas y sofocantes. Tenía que salir de ese pasillo. "Después de tres días con él, tengo mucho más que eso."

La voz de Nick se escuchó en la cocina. "¿La S.E.?" habló fuerte. "¿Fueron ellos quienes te metieron en las peleas de ratas, Raquel? No serás una bruja negra ¿verdad?"

Ivy se sobresaltó. Sus ojos se tornaron pardos instantáneamente. Desconcertada, retrocedió. "Lo siento," dijo en voz baja. Claramente disgustada, Ivy regresó a la cocina. Yo la seguí aliviada para encontrarme a Jenks parado sobre el hombro de Nick. No sabía si Nick tenía un oído tan agudo o si Jenks le había transmitido todo, pero podría apostar que era lo segundo. Lo inquietante fue su pregunta tan informal acerca de la magia negra.

"No-o-o-o," repuso Jenks con petulancia. "La magia de Raquel es tan blanca como su trasero. Abandonó a la S.E. y se llevó consigo a Ivy. Ella era lo mejor que tenían y por eso Denon, su jefe, le puso precio a la cabeza de Raquel."

"Vaya, *eras* agente de la S.E." comentó Nick. "Ya entiendo. Pero, ¿cómo terminaste en las peleas de ratas?"

Aún a la defensiva, observé a Ivy que seguía fregando el fregadero encogiéndose de hombros. Bien. Hasta aquí llegaron los secretos para el chico rata. Regresé a la mesa arrastrando los pies y saqué seis tajadas de pan. "El Sr. Kalamack me atrapó en su oficina buscando pruebas de su participación en el tráfico de drogas biológicas," expliqué. "Pensó que sería más divertido meterme a las peleas de ratas que entregarme."

"¿Kalamack?" exclamó Nick asombrado. "¿Te refieres a

Trent Kalamack, el concejal? ¿Traficante de drogas biológicas?" La bata de Nick se abrió a la altura de sus rodillas y yo quería que se moviera tan sólo un p-o-o-qui-i-i-t-o más.

Con aire de suficiencia puse dos capas de mortadela en tres tajadas de pan. "Así es, pero mientras estuve enjaulada donde Trent aprendí que no solamente las trafica. También las *produce*," concluí teatralmente.

Ivy se dio vuelta. Se quedó mirándome desde el otro lado de la cocina con el trapo colgando de la mano. Podía escuchar a los niños que jugaban en la casa vecina. Así fue el silencio. Quité las partes marchitas de la lechuga disfrutando la reacción de Ivy.

La cara de Nick se puso pálida. Era apenas normal pues a los humanos les aterraba la manipulación genética por razones obvias. Pero que Trent Kalamack estuviera jugando con ellas... eso era preocupante, sobre todo cuando no se sabía a qué lado del campo pertenecía: humano o Entremundos. "No puede ser el mismo Sr. Kalamack," dijo Nick consternado. "Yo voté por él ambas veces. ¿Estás segura?"

Ivy también se veía preocupada. "¿Es bioingeniero?"

"Al menos los financia," dije. *Y los asesina y los deja morir en el piso de su oficina.* "Esta noche enviará un cargamento al Suroeste. Si logramos interceptarlo e incriminarlo, podría pagar mi contrato. Jenks, ¿tienes esa hoja de papel de su agenda?"

El duende asintió. "La tengo bien oculta entre las piernas."

Por un instante iba a protestar, pero me di cuenta que no era tan mal escondite. El cuchillo hizo bastante ruido mientras untaba los panes con mayonesa y terminaba los sándwiches. Nick alzó la cabeza de las manos. Su cara estaba larga y pálida. "¿Ingeniería genética? ¿Trent Kalamack tiene un laboratorio biológico? ¿El concejal?"

"Y la segunda parte te va a encantar," continué. "Francis trabaja para él encubriéndolo en la S.E."

Jenks saltó hasta el techo y cayó de nuevo. "¿Francis? ¿Estás segura de que no te golpearon en la cabeza Raque?"

"Es tan cierto que trabaja con Trent como que llevo cuatro

días comiendo zanahorias. Yo lo vi. ¿Recuerdan esos decomisos de azufre que hizo Francis? ¿Su ascenso? *¿Ese auto?*" Terminé ahí mi explicación dejando que Jenks y Ivy descifraran el resto.

"¡Hijo de perra!," exclamó Jenks. "¡Los decomisos son para distraer la atención!"

"Exacto." Corté los sándwiches por la mitad. Satisfecha, puse uno para mí en un plato y dos para Nick en otro: estaba flaco. "Trent mantiene ocupadas a la AFE y la S.E. con azufre mientras que lo que produce el dinero de verdad sale por el otro lado de la ciudad."

Ivy se movió lentamente, pensando, mientras se enjuagó las manos de nuevo. "Francis no es tan inteligente," dijo, secándose los dedos dejando a un lado el trapo de los platos.

"No. No lo es. Lo van a hacer trocitos y empacar."

Jenks aterrizó a mi lado. "Denon se va a orinar en los pantalones cuando se entere," dijo.

"Esperen un momento" dijo Ivy concentrándose. El círculo de sus ojos pardos comenzó a disminuir por la agitación, no por el apetito. "¿Quién dice que Denon no está en la nómina de pagos de Trent? Necesitarás obtener pruebas antes de ir a la S.E. Te matarían antes de ayudarte a atraparlo. Y para atraparlo no bastará con nosotras dos y una tarde de planificar."

Apreté la frente preocupada. "Esta es mi única oportunidad, Ivy," protesté. "No importa lo alto que sea el riesgo."

"Umm." La mano temblorosa de Nick tomó un sándwich. "¿Por qué no van a la AFE?"

Ivy y yo nos miramos en silencio mientras Nick mordía y tragaba. "La AFE iría a medianoche a cualquier tugurio de Los Hollows tratándose de pistas sobre drogas biológicas, especialmente si el Sr. Kalamack está implicado. Si consiguen cualquier tipo de pruebas, ellos le echarán una mirada."

Ivy y yo nos miramos incrédulas. ¿La AFE?

Me tranquilicé un poco y sonreí. Nick tenía razón. La sola rivalidad que existía entre la AFE y la S.E. sería suficiente para que se interesaran. "Trent quedará frito, pagaré mi contrato y la S.E. quedará como una estúpida. Me gusta." Mordí mi sándwich limpiándome la mayonesa del extremo de la boca. Nick y yo nos miramos.

"Raquel," dijo Ivy preocupada. "¿Puedo hablar contigo un momento?"

Miré a Nick y de nuevo empecé a sentir ira. ¿Ahora qué? Ya había salido. "Disculpa," dije poniéndome de pie y amarrando nerviosamente el nudo de mi bata. "La princesa paranoia quiere hablarme." Ivy se veía bien. No habría problema.

Nick se limpió impasible algunas migas de los labios. "¿Te importa si preparo café? Me muero por una taza desde hace tres meses."

"Seguro. Como quieras" repuse, contenta de que no se sintiera ofendido por la desconfianza de Ivy. Yo sí lo estaba. Él propuso un buen plan pero a Ivy no le gustó porque ella no fue quien lo pensó primero. "El café está en el refrigerador," le dije, mientras seguí a Ivy hacia el pasillo.

"¿Cuál es tu problema?" le dije antes de estar cerca de ella. "Es tan sólo un tipo común y corriente y tiene razón. Convencer a la AFE para que persiga a Trent es mucho más seguro que convencer a la S.E. de que me ayude a mí."

No podía ver el color de los ojos de Ivy en la luz tenue y afuera estaba oscureciendo. El pasillo era de un negro inquietante con ella ahí. "Raquel, esta no es una redada en un nido de vampiros," me dijo. "Se trata de hacer caer a uno de los ciudadanos más poderosos de la ciudad. Una sola palabra equivocada de Nick y estarás muerta."

Se me formó un nudo en el estómago al recordarlo. Respiré profundo y entonces respondí lentamente. "Continúa."

"Yo se que Nick quiere ayudar. No sería humano si no quisiera pagarte de alguna manera por ayudarlo a escapar. Pero se hará daño."

No dije nada pues entendí que tenía razón. Nosotros éramos profesionales pero él no. Tendría que sacarlo del camino de alguna forma. "¿Qué sugieres?" pregunté y ella se tranquilizó.

"¿Por qué no lo llevas al campanario para que se pruebe ropa mientras que yo reservo un cupo en ese vuelo?" preguntó. "¿Qué vuelo dijiste que era?"

Me acomodé un mechón de pelo detrás de la oreja "¿Por qué? Solo necesitamos saber a qué hora sale."

"Tal vez necesitemos más tiempo. Como están las cosas, ya vamos atrasadas. Casi todas las compañías retrasan un vuelo si les dices que tienes restricciones diurnas. Le echan la culpa al mal tiempo o cualquier cuestión de mantenimiento. Y no despegan hasta que el sol no se vea a 12.000 metros de altura."

¿Restricciones diurnas? Eso lo explicaba todo. "Último vuelo a Los Ángeles antes de la medianoche" contesté.

La actitud de Ivy era resuelta. Entró en lo que yo llamaba "modalidad de planificación." "Jenks y yo iremos a la AFE a explicarlo todo" dijo preocupada. "Luego nos reuniremos contigo en el momento de atraparlo."

"Este…espera un minuto. Yo iré a la AFE. Este es mi caso."

Su molestia fue obvia, inclusive en la oscuridad del pasillo. Yo retrocedí, incómoda. "Es la AFE, Raquel. Puede que estés un poco más segura, pero podrían atraparte por el prestigio de atrapar a alguien que se le ha escurrido a la S.E. Algunos de esos tipos darían lo que fuera por matar a una bruja y tú lo sabes."

Sentí que enfermaba. "Está bien," dije lentamente mientras que mi boca se me hacía agua al oler el aroma de café. "Tienes razón. Me mantendré al margen hasta que le informes a la AFE lo que estamos haciendo."

La mirada decidida de Ivy se tornó de pronto en mirada de asombro. "¿Tú crees que yo tengo razón?"

El olor a café me arrastró hacia la cocina. Ivy me siguió en silencio. Cruzé los brazos al entrar al cuarto iluminado. El recuerdo de ocultarme en la oscuridad durante el ataque de las hadas asesinas sofocó cualquier sentimiento de emoción ante la posibilidad de atrapar a Trent. Tenía que preparar otros hechizos. Unos fuertes. Diferentes. Realmente diferentes, tal vez negros. Sentí que iba a enfermar.

Nick y Jenks estaban muy cerca. Jenks estaba convenciéndolo para que abriera el frasco de miel. Pero por las muecas y negativas que hacía, entendí que Nick conocía algo sobre duendes y vampiros. Me dirigí hacia la cafetera a esperar a que terminara. Ivy abrió el armario y me pasó tres tazas. En sus ojos leí que no entendía por qué yo estaba tan preocupada. Ella era un vampiro. Leía el lenguaje corporal mejor que la Dra. Ruth.

"La S.E. todavía me busca" dije en voz baja. "Cada vez que la AFE hace una jugada importante, la S.E. busca la manera de involucrarse. Si voy a aparecer en público, necesitaré algo para protegerme de ellos. Algo poderoso. Puedo prepararlo mientras que ustedes van a la AFE. Luego nos vemos en el aeropuerto" concluí.

Ivy estaba junto al fregadero con los brazos cruzados. Tenía sospechas. "Suena como una buena idea" dijo. "Algo de trabajo preliminar. Está bien."

La tensión me invadió el cuerpo. La magia negra siempre involucraba matar algo antes de agregárselo a la mezcla, especialmente las pociones fuertes. Estaba a punto de averiguar si sería capaz de hacerlo. Bajé la mirada y puse las tazas en fila. "¿Jenks? ¿Cómo están organizados mis perseguidores?"

La brisa de sus alas movió mi pelo mientras aterrizaba en mi mano. "Es leve. Ya son cuatro días desde la última vez que te vieron. Sólo están las hadas. Dales cinco minutos a mis hijos para que puedas escabullirte, si necesitas."

"Perfecto. Voy a salir a buscar nuevos hechizos tan pronto termine de vestirme."

"¿Para qué?" preguntó Ivy preocupada. "Ya tienes suficientes libros de magia."

Sentí que el sudor me empapaba el cuello y no me gustaba que Ivy se diera cuenta. "Necesito algo más poderoso." Me di vuelta y me llamó la atención la cara flácida de Ivy. Sentí pavor. Respiré profundo y bajé la mirada. "Necesito algo para atacar," dije con voz trémula, agarrándome la clavícula con una mano y tomándome el codo con la otra.

"Huy...Raque," empezó a decir Jenks mientras volaba justo frente a mis ojos. Sus diminutas facciones reflejaban preocupación, lo cual no me hacía sentir precisamente mejor. "Eso suena a magia negra ¿no es así?"

El corazón me martillaba el pecho y ni siquiera había empezado. "¿Te suena? ¡Pues nada!" repuse. Miré a Ivy. Su aspecto parecía normal, igual Nick. No parecía trastornado al levantarse por el tan anhelado café. Pensé en Nick como practicante de magia negra. Los humanos podían penetrar las líneas ley. En los círculos de Entremundos se consideraba que ese tipo de brujos y brujasnos eran más que una broma.

"La luna está creciendo," dije, "y eso está de mi lado. No voy a preparar hechizos para lastimar a alguien en particular..." El silencio fue incómodo.

La respuesta suave de Ivy fue desconcertante. "¿Estás segura Raquel?" dijo, y apenas pude percibir una leve advertencia en su voz.

"Voy a estar bien" repuse sin mirarla. "No lo hago por maldad sino para salvar mi vida. Hay una diferencia." *Eso espero. Dios, protege mi alma si me equivoco.*

Las alas de Jenks se agitaron y aterrizó en el cucharón. "Quemaron todos los libros de magia negra."

Nick sacó la cafetera y comenzó a servirse café. "La biblioteca de la universidad tiene algunos" dijo. La base metálica caliente sonó al gotear algo de café.

Todos nos volteamos a mirarlo y se encogió de hombros. "Los guardan en el armario de los libros antiguos."

Sentí una pizca de temor. *No debería hacer esto,* pensé. "Y tú tienes la llave ¿verdad?" dije sarcásticamente, pero me retracté cuando asintió.

Ivy exhaló incrédula. "Tienes la llave" se burló. "Hace una hora eras una rata pero tienes la llave de la biblioteca de la universidad."

De repente me pareció más peligroso ahí parado tranquilamente en la cocina, vestido con la bata de Ivy que le caía encima de su cuerpo delgado. "Trabajaba ahí al mismo tiempo que estudiaba."

"¿Fuiste a la universidad?" le pregunté sirviéndome una taza de café después que él.

Tomó un sorbo y cerró los ojos, como agradeciendo un milagro. "Tenía una beca completa. Estudié adquisición de datos, organización y distribución."

"Eres bibliotecario," comenté aliviada. Así fue como se enteró de los libros de magia negra.

"Lo fui. Puedo ayudarte a entrar y salir. No hay ningún problema. La señora que estaba a cargo de nosotros, los que trabajábamos y estudiábamos, escondía las llaves de los cuartos cerrados cerca de las puertas para que no la molestáramos." Tomó otro sorbo y sus ojos parecieron cristalizarse con la cafeína.

Ahora Ivy parecía preocupada de verdad y sus ojos pardos se redujeron.

"¿Raquel, puedo hablarte?"

"No," repuse suavemente. No quería volver a ese pasillo. Estaba nerviosa. El que mi corazón estuviera latiendo con fuerza por el temor a la magia negra y no por ella, daba lo mismo para sus instintos. Ir con Nick a la biblioteca era menos peligroso que fabricar un hechizo negro—lo cual aparentemente no le importaba. "¿Qué quieres?"

Ivy nos miró a Nick y a mí. "Sólo te iba a sugerir que llevaras a Nick al campanario. Tenemos ropas que podrían servirle."

Me retiré de la mesa con la taza de café sin probar en la mano. *Mentirosa,* pensé. "Dame un minuto para vestirme, Nick. Te acompañaré arriba. Espero que no te importe vestirte con ropa heredada de un antiguo sacerdote."

Nick pareció sorprenderse. "No. Está bien."

"Muy bien" repuse, pero mi cabeza estaba por estallar. "Cuando te hayas vestido iremos a la biblioteca y me mostrarás todos los libros de magia negra."

Miré a Ivy y Jenks al salir. Jenks estaba pálido. Era obvio que no le gustaba lo que yo estaba haciendo. Ivy estaba preocupada; pero lo que más me preocupaba a mí era la tranquilidad de Nick con todo lo relativo a Entremundos. Y ahora, con la magia negra. No sería un practicante ¿o sí?

Veinticuatro

Esperaba en el andén a que Nick bajara del taxi contando el dinero que tenía en mi billetera antes de guardarla de nuevo. Mi último pago se reducía. Si no tenía más cuidado, tendría que pedirle a Ivy que me sacara dinero del banco. Estaba gastando más rápido que de costumbre y no entendía por qué pues ahora mis gastos eran menores. *Deben ser los taxis,* pensé y prometí movilizarme más en autobús.

Nick había encontrado un par de viejos jeans de trabajo en el campanario que le quedaban grandes. Los llevaba ajustados con una de mis correas más conservadoras. Parecía que el viejo sacerdote había sido un hombre grande. El suéter con el escudo de la Universidad de Cincinnati le quedaba igualmente grande y ni para qué hablar de las botas de jardinero. Con todo, Nick caminaba como un personaje de una mala película de Frankenstein. De alguna manera su altura y buena cara hacían que se viera atractivo sin importar su aspecto descuidado. Yo en cambio parecía un desastre.

El sol no se había puesto aún pero las luces de la calle estaban encendidas puesto que el día estaba nublado. Nos habíamos demorado más llevando la ropa del sacerdote a la lavandería que viniendo hasta acá. Cerré con las manos el cuello de mi abrigo de invierno para protegerme del aire frío mientras observaba la calle iluminada. Nick hablaba unas últimas palabras con el conductor. Las noches podían ser frías los últimos días de primavera, pero de todas formas me hubiera puesto este abrigo largo para cubrir el vestido de cuadros escoceses que llevaba puesto. Tenía que continuar con mi disfraz de señora anciana. Lo había usado sólo una vez cuando no se por qué terminé metida en uno de esos banquetes para madres e hijas.

Nick salió del taxi. Cerró la puerta y le dio un golpecito al techo. El conductor lo saludó con un saludo y se alejó. Había autos por todas partes. La ciudad tenía mucho movimiento al atardecer, cuando tanto humanos como Entremundos estaban muy activos.

"Oye," me dijo Nick mirándome bajo la luz tenue. "¿Qué pasó con tus pecas?"

"Eh…" musité llevándome un dedo frente a los labios "yo no tengo pecas."

Nick tomó aire para decir algo pero luego cambió de opinión. "¿Dónde está Jenks?" preguntó finalmente.

Señalé nerviosamente hacia las escalinatas de la biblioteca. "Va adelante para revisar que todo esté bien." Observé a las pocas personas que entraban y salían de la biblioteca. ¡Gente que estudia los viernes en la noche! Hay personas que tienen el insaciable deseo de arruinarles a los demás la normalidad. Nick me tomó del codo pero yo me zafé. "Gracias. Puedo cruzar la calle yo sola."

"Se supone que eres una anciana. Ya deja de agitar los brazos y camina más lento."

Suspiré y traté de caminar más despacio mientras Nick cruzaba en la mitad de la calle. Sonaron bocinas pero Nick no les prestó atención. Estábamos en territorio estudiantil. Si hubiéramos cruzado en la intersección habríamos llamado la atención. Tuve la tentación de hacerles un par de señas a los conductores con los dedos, pero pensé que echaría a perder mi imagen de anciana.

"¿Estás seguro que nadie te reconocerá?" pregunté mientras subíamos por las escalinatas y llegábamos a las puertas de vidrio. Demonios, con razón los viejos mueren. Les toma el doble hacer cualquier cosa.

"Seguro." Me abrió la puerta y entré con mi andar cansado. "No he trabajado aquí desde hace cinco años y los únicos que están aquí los viernes son los estudiantes de primer año. Ahora encórvate y trata de no atacar a nadie." Le hice una sonrisa sarcástica y agregué: "Así está mejor."

Cinco años significa que él no era mucho mayor que yo. Era más o menos lo que yo había pensado, aun cuando era difícil asegurarlo con todas esas cicatrices que le hicieron las ratas.

Me detuve en la entrada para orientarme. Me gustan las bibliotecas. Huelen bien y hay silencio. La luz fluorescente de la entrada era muy débil pero la complementaba la luz natural que entraba por los grandes ventanales de dos pisos de alto, pero a esta hora la penumbra de la tarde oscurecía todo.

De pronto volví la mirada hacia algo borroso que caía del techo. ¡Venía directo hacia mí! Me agaché y Nick me tomó del brazo. Perdí el equilibrio y mis zapatos de tacón resbalaron dejándome despatarrada. Me sonrojé de rabia al ver a Jenks volando a mi alrededor riendo. "¡Maldita sea, vete al demonio!" grité. "¡Cuidado con lo que haces!"

Hubo un grito ahogado colectivo y todos se voltearon a mirarme. Jenks se ocultó en mi pelo, su risita haciéndome enfurecer aun más. Nick se agachó y me tomó del codo. "Lo siento abuela," dijo en voz alta, mirando a todos avergonzado. "La abuela no oye bien," prosiguió con su discurso que buscaba comprensión, "pobre vieja murciélago." Se volvió hacia mí serio, pero los ojos le brillaban. "¡Ya estamos en la biblioteca!" habló fuerte. "¡Tienes que guardar silencio!"

Estaba tan caliente como un horno. Rezongué un par de palabras y dejé que me ayudara a levantarme. La gente hizo comentarios de asombro pero pronto regresó a sus deberes.

Un chico con la cara llena de granos corrió hasta nosotros preocupado seguramente por una demanda. Haciendo más escándalo de lo necesario, nos acompañó hasta las oficinas de atrás parloteando sobre lo resbalosos que estaban los pisos pues los terminaban de encerar. Hablaría inmediatamente con el encargado de la limpieza.

Yo me apoyé en el brazo de Nick lamentándome de mi cintura y actuando como una ancianita. El asustado chico nos llevó zumbando por un área semi restringida. Preocupado por mí, me ayudó a sentar en un asiento ayudándome a subir los pies en una silla giratoria. Pero se detuvo un momento al ver el cuchillo de plata que llevaba aferrado a mi tobillo. Yo susurré algo sobre agua y él voló a traerla. Le tomó tres intentos pasar por la puerta con alarma; pero finalmente hubo silencio cuando se cerró tras él. Le hice una mueca sarcástica a Nick. Esta no era precisamente la manera como lo habíamos planeado, pero al fin de cuentas, aquí estábamos.

Jenks salió de su escondite. "Somos más resbalosos que un moco en la perilla de la puerta," dijo mientras volaba a examinar las cámaras. "¡Ajá!" exclamó. "Son falsas." Nick me tomó de las manos y me ayudó a ponerme de pie. "Iba a llevarte por la puerta del cuarto de descanso de los empleados, pero creo que esto va a funcionar." Lo miré sin musitar palabra y él continuó: "El sótano es por ahí."

Sonreí al tiempo que observaba el candado. "¿Jenks?"

"Aquí estoy" dijo saltando y empezó a hurgarlo. Lo abrió en tres segundos. "Ya está." Nick murmuró mientras giraba la perilla. La puerta se abrió y vimos unas escaleras en la oscuridad. Encendió las luces y esperamos. "No hay alarmas" dijo.

Saqué un amuleto de detección invocándolo rápidamente. Permaneció verde y cálido en mi mano. "Tampoco hay alarmas silenciosas" dije, colgándolo del cuello.

"Oigan" refunfuñó Jenks. "Esto es de primer año."

Comenzamos a descender. El aire en las escaleras estrechas era frío y no sentíamos el reconfortante olor a libros. Cada dos metros había una pálida bombilla que lanzaba rayos amarillentos y dejaba ver el polvo al abrigo de los escalones. Una franja de mugre de 15 centímetros de grueso cubría las paredes de lado y lado. También había un pasamanos pero no quise usarlo.

Los escalones terminaban en un pasillo oscuro donde se escuchaba todo. Nick me miró y yo revisé el amuleto. "Vamos bien" susurré. Él encendió las luces que iluminaron un pasillo de techo bajo y paredes de piedra. Rejas de alambre del techo al piso recorrían todo el pasillo dejando ver los libros que había detrás.

Jenks salió disparado delante de nosotros. Seguí a Nick taconeando hasta una de las rejas con seguro. Era la sección de libros antiguos. Jenks entraba y salía pasando por los agujeros en forma de diamante y yo pasé los dedos por la malla parada en las puntas de los pies con todos mis sentidos alertas. Fruncí el ceño. Tal vez era mi imaginación, pero podría jurar que sentía la magia flotando de las repisas llenas de libros y arremolinándose alrededor de mis tobillos. La sensación de la magia antigua era tan diferente del olor que había sentido arriba como lo es un chocolate cualquiera de una tableta de fino chocolate Belga: embriagador, intenso y dañino.

"¿Y la llave?" pregunté, segura de que Jenks no podía abrir las clavijas de los antiguos y pesados candados mecánicos. A veces los seguros viejos son mejores.

Nick pasó los dedos debajo de una repisa cercana. Sus ojos parecían recordar las frustraciones del pasado y de repente detuvo su mano. "Demasiado jóvenes para entrar al depósito de libros ¿verdad?" murmuró entre dientes al tiempo que sacaba una llave pegajosa. Miró fijamente unos segundos la vieja llave que sostenía entre las manos antes de abrir la reja de malla.

Mi corazón comenzó a latir aceleradamente pero se tranquilizó tan pronto chirrió la puerta. Nick metió la llave en el bolsillo con un movimiento abrupto y decidido. "Después de ti," dijo, encendiendo las luces fluorescentes.

Dudé un instante. "¿Hay alguna otra salida?" pregunté, pero Nick lo negó con la cabeza. Me di vuelta buscando a

Jenks. "Quédate aquí. Cúbreme la espalda" Me mordí los labios. "¿Me cubrirás la espalda Jenks?" repetí con un nudo en el estómago.

El duendecillo debió percibir el leve temblor de mi voz pues aterrizó en la mano que le ofrecía. Asintió con los ojos. Su camisa de seda negra comenzó a brillar iluminándolo más aún que el destello de sus alas en movimiento. "No te preocupes Raque" me dijo solemnemente. "Nada pasará por aquí sin que tú lo sepas, lo prometo."

Respiré nerviosamente. Nick estaba confundido. Todos en la S.E. sabían cómo había muerto papá. Le agradecí a Jenks el no mencionarlo y que tan sólo me dijera que estaría allí para ayudarme.

"Muy bien" dije, y me quité el amuleto de detección colgándolo donde Jenks pudiera verlo. Seguí a Nick ignorando la escalofriante sensación de mi piel. Bien fuera que enseñaran magia negra o blanca, eran tan sólo libros. El poder venía de usarlos.

La reja se cerró con un chirrido y Nick me indicó que lo siguiera. Me quité el amuleto de disfraz y lo metí en la bolsa. Luego me deshice el moño del pelo y lo solté. Ahora me sentía medio siglo más joven.

Observé los títulos mientras caminaba lentamente a medida que el pasillo se convertía en un salón más amplio escondido detrás de estantes y estantes de libros. Había una mesa y tres sillas giratorias diferentes que ni siquiera servirían para estudiantes.

Nick caminó seguro hacia el gabinete con puertas de vidrio del otro lado del salón. "Aquí, Raquel," dijo abriéndolas. "Busca aquí a ver si encuentras lo que necesitas." Se dio vuelta quitándose el pelo negro de los ojos. Parpadeó y observé en él una mirada pícara.

"Gracias. Esto es maravilloso. De verdad te lo agradezco." Dejé mi bolso en la mesa y me paré a su lado. Sentí preocupación y empujé el bolso un poco. Si el hehizo era demasiado repugnante, sencillamente no lo haría.

Saqué con cuidado el libro que parecía más viejo. El

empaste del lomo estaba roto y tuve que usar ambas manos para sostener el pesado tomo. Lo puse en una esquina de la mesa y acerqué una de las sillas. Aquí abajo hacía tanto frío como en una cueva y me alegré de tener mi abrigo. El aire seco olía a papas fritas. Sofoqué mis nervios y abrí el libro. Le habían arrancado la página del título. Usar un hechizo de un libro sin título era preocupante. El índice estaba intacto, pero me impresionó. *¿Un hechizo para hablar con fantasmas?* Qué bien.

"Tú no eres como los demás humanos que conozco," le dije mientras le daba un vistazo al índice.

"Mi madre estaba sola," dijo. "No podía pagar nada en los suburbios y prefería dejarme jugar con brujas y vampiros que con los hijos de adictos a la heroína. Los Hollows eran el menos grave de los dos males." Nick tenía las manos en los bolsillos de atrás y leía los títulos de las filas de libros. "Crecí aquí y estudié en Emerson."

Lo observé con curiosidad. El que hubiera crecido en Los Hollows explicaba por qué sabía tanto sobre Entremundos. Tenía que saberlo para sobrevivir. "¿Estudiaste en la Secundaria Entremundos de Los Hollows?" pregunté.

Sacudió la puerta cerrada de un armario grande. La madera se veía roja bajo el brillo de las luces fluorescentes. ¿Qué habría de peligroso allí para que estuviera en un armario con llave en una bóveda con llave detrás de una puerta con llave en el sótano de un edificio oficial?

Nick se encogió de hombros hurgando el candado. "No era mala. El rector pasó las reglas por alto después de que me causaron una conmoción cerebral. Me dejaron portar una daga de plata para alejar a los lobos y podía lavarme el pelo con agua bendita para evitar a los vampiros. Eso no los detenía, pero al menos el mal olor que sentían en mí los mantenía alejados."

"¿Agua bendita? Uumm." Al oírlo decidí que conservaría mi perfume de lilas en lugar de tener un olor corporal que sólo los vampiros podían sentir.

"Los problemas surgieron con las brujas y los brujos"

dijo, dándose por vencido con el candado. Se sentó entonces en una de las sillas y estiró sus largas piernas. Sonreí levemente. Ya imaginaba por qué las brujas lo molestaban. "Pero las bromas terminaron cuando me hice amigo del brujo más grande, malo y feo de la escuela." Dejó escapar una leve sonrisa. "Turco. Le hice las tareas durante cuatro años. Tenía que haberse graduado años atrás. Los maestros se hacían los de la vista gorda con tal de que se fuera de la escuela. Yo no iba gimiendo a la oficina del rector todos los días como los otros humanos que asistían a esa escuela. Era lo suficientemente fresco para meterme con los Entremundos. Mis amigos me defendían y así aprendí cosas que de otra forma no hubiera aprendido."

"Como por ejemplo que no se le debe temer a los vampiros," agregué, dándome cuenta de lo extraño que era que un humano supiera más de vampiros que yo.

"Por lo menos no al mediodía. Pero me sentiré mucho mejor tan pronto pueda ducharme para eliminar el olor de Ivy. No sabía que esa era su bata." Se acercó un poco. "¿Qué estás buscando?"

"No estoy segura" respondí nerviosa al ver que estaba mirando por encima de mi hombro. Tenía que haber algo que pudiera usar que no me mandara hasta el otro lado de la "Fuerza." De repente me invadió un preocupante destello de asombro. *¡Tú no eres mi padre, Darth. Jamás me uniré a tí!*

Los ojos de Nick se aguaron ante el penetrante olor de mi perfume y retrocedió. Las ventanillas del taxi estaban abiertas y ahora comprendí por qué él no había dicho nada al respecto.

"¿No has vivido con Ivy mucho tiempo, verdad?"

Levanté la mirada del índice sorprendida y su expresión se volvió tímida. "Eh . . . bueno, sólo me pareció que tú y ella no son. . . ."

Me sonrojé y bajé la mirada de nuevo. "No, no lo somos," dije, "no si podemos evitarlo. Sólo somos compañeras de casa. Yo estoy del lado derecho del pasillo y ella del izquierdo."

Nick dudó un instante. "Entonces ¿te molestaría si te doy un consejo?"

Lo miré perpleja y él se sentó en una esquina de la mesa. "Prueba un perfume cítrico en lugar de uno de flores."

Abrí los ojos asombrada. Esto no lo esperaba y moví lentamente la mano hacia el cuello donde me había salpicado ese detestable perfume. "Jenks me ayudó a escogerlo" expliqué. "Me dijo que cubría muy bien el olor de Ivy."

"Estoy seguro que así es," sonrió Nick queriendo disculparse. "Pero tiene que ser demasiado fuerte para que funcione. Los perfumes cítricos no sólo tapan el olor a vampiro: lo neutralizan."

"Oh" suspiré, recordando el gusto de Ivy por el jugo de naranja.

"El olfato de los duendes es bueno, pero el de los vampiros es especializado. La próxima vez sal de compras con Ivy. Te ayudará a escoger algo que funcione."

"Lo haré" respondí, dándome cuenta de que pude evitar ofender a todo el mundo si hubiera pedido ayuda la primera vez. Cerré el libro sin título sintiéndome estúpida y me paré a escoger otro.

Saqué el siguiente libro de la repisa y me di cuenta que era más pesado de lo que pensé. Golpeó la mesa con fuerza y Nick se encogió. "Disculpa," dije acomodando la tapa tratando de ocultar que había roto el empaste podrido. Me senté y lo abrí.

Mi corazón dio un vuelco y quedé petrificada sintiendo cómo se me paraban los pelos de la nuca. No lo estaba imaginando. Con preocupación alcé la mirada hacia Nick para ver si él también lo había notado. Estaba mirando hacia uno de los pasillos que formaban los gabinetes de libros. La sensación fantasmagórica no provenía del libro. Provenía detrás de mí. *Maldición.*

"¡Raquel!" llamó una vocecilla desde el pasillo. "Tu amuleto cambió a rojo . . . ¡pero aquí no hay nadie!"

Cerré el libro y me puse de pie. Sentía algo en el aire. Mi corazón saltó de nuevo cuando algunos libros en el pasillo se movieron hacia el fondo de la repisa. "Eh...¿Nick? ¿Sabes si hay fantasmas en la biblioteca?"

"No que yo sepa."

Doble maldición. "Entonces ¿qué demonios es eso?"

Se veía dubitativo. "No lo se."

Jenks entró volando. "No hay nada en el pasillo Raque. ¿Estás segura de que el hechizo que me diste funciona?" preguntó mientras señalaba la alteración en el pasillo.

"¡Mierda!" exclamó, volando en medio de nosotros a medida que en el aire se iba formando una figura. De repente, todos los libros se movieron hacia adelante al mismo tiempo. Eso fue aun más aterrador.

La bruma se volvió amarilla y luego sólida. Silbé. Era un perro, un perro tan grande como un pony y con colmillos tan grandes como mi mano y cuernos que le salían de la cabeza...¿un perro? "Por favor, díganme que este es el sistema de seguridad de la biblioteca" susurré.

"No se que será" dijo Nick pálido y aterrado. El perro estaba entre nosotros y la puerta. Tenía saliva cayéndole de la mandíbula y podría jurar que escuchaba un siseo cuando tocaba el piso y producía humo amarillo. Olía a azufre. "¿Qué era esta cosa?"

"¿Tienes algo en tu bolso contra esto?" susurró Nick, quedándose inmóvil al ver que las orejas del perro se levantaban en alerta.

"¿Algo para detener a un perro amarillo del infierno? ¡No!"

"Si no le demostramos miedo tal vez no nos ataque."

El perro abrió la boca y dijo: "¿Quién de ustedes es Raquel Mariana Morgan?"

Veinticinco

Estaba jadeando y mi corazón parecía estallar. El perro abrió la boca bostezando con un pequeño gemido al final. "Debes ser tú" dijo. Sus pelos se pararon y se abalanzó hacia nosotros.

"¡Cuidado!" gritó Nick empujándome. El perro babeante aterrizó sobre la mesa.

Caí al suelo y asumí mi posición de defensa. Nick gritó de dolor. La mesa resbaló y se estrelló contra los estantes y se deslizó más cuando el perro saltó de nuevo. El plástico se rompió.

"¡Nick!" grité al verlo atrapado debajo de una pila de libros. El monstruoso perro estaba sobre él hurgándolo con el hocico. Había sangre en el piso. "¡Quítate de encima!" le grité al perro. Jenks estaba impotente en el techo.

El perro se volteó hacia mí. Contuve el aire. Sus iris eran rojos rodeados de un enfermizo halo anaranjado. Las pupilas eran sesgadas, como las de una cabra. Retrocedí sin quitarle la mirada de encima ni un segundo. Titubeando, saqué mi daga de plata del tobillo. Podría jurar que lo vi hacer una sonrisa de canino salvaje apenas me quité el abrigo y me deshice de mis tacones de anciana.

Nick se movió quejándose. Estaba vivo y sentí alivio. Jenks estaba parado sobre su hombro gritándole al oído que se levantara.

"Raquel Mariana Morgan," habló el perro con voz lúgubre pero suave. Yo me quedé esperando sintiendo escalofríos en el aire frío del sótano. "Uno de ustedes le teme a los perros" siguió diciendo asombrado. "No creo que seas tú."

"Ven y lo averiguas," le repuse audazmente. El corazón me latía aceleradamente, y empuñé mi cuchillo. Empecé a temblar. Los perros no hablan. No hablan.

Di un paso hacia adelante boquiabierta al ver cómo sus patas delanteras se estiraban y se paraba derecho para caminar. Adelgazó y asumió forma humana. Estaba vestido: jeans rasgados, chaqueta de cuero negro y una cadena que iba desde la cintura hasta la billetera. Tenía el pelo en punta y teñido de color rojo. No podía verle los ojos pues llevaba puesto lentes oscuros. No podía moverme del asombro viendo cómo aparecía ahora este muchacho fanfarrón.

"Me mandaron a matarte," me dijo hablando con sórdido acento londinense a medida que terminaba de transformarse en pandillero de callejón. "Me pidieron que me asegurara de hacerte morir asustada, nena. No me dieron mayor información, así que a lo mejor me tomará un buen rato."

Retrocedí intempestivamente al darme cuenta de que estaba casi encima de mí. Con un movimiento demasiado veloz para notarlo, me lanzó un golpe con el puño pegándome sin que me diera cuenta de que se había movido. El dolor que sentí en la mejilla fue intenso y luego sentí que se entumecía. Un segundo golpe en el hombro me alzó del piso. Me doblé y me fui de espaldas contra un anaquel de libros.

Caí al suelo y encima cayeron los libros. Me levanté tratando de despejar la vista. Nick se había metido en medio de dos anaqueles de libros. Sangraba en la cabeza y el cuello y su mirada era de espanto y asombro. Se tocó la cabeza mirando la sangre como si le dijera algo. Nuestras miradas se encontraron. La cosa estaba en medio de los dos.

De pronto se lanzó de nuevo contra mí. Caí de rodillas atravesándolo con el cuchillo dando tumbos. Aterrada, logré zafarme pero siguió atacándome. Ahora su cara era nebulosa y comenzó a transformarse cuando le clavé el cuchillo. *¿Qué demonios era esto?*

"Raquel Mariana Morgan," rió sarcásticamente. "¡He venido por ti!"

Me levanté y comencé a correr pero una mano gruesa me tomó por el hombro y me giró de regreso. La cosa me tenía agarrada y me paralicé viendo cómo su otra mano se convertía en un puño asesino. Sonrió mostrando sus dientes perfectamente blancos y tomó impulso con el brazo. Iba a pegarme en el estómago.

A duras penas logré bajar mi brazo para bloquear el golpe pero el puño me golpeó en el brazo. El dolor me dejó sin aire y caí de rodillas. Grité de dolor tomándome el brazo mientras caía. La cosa también me siguió y rodé por el piso tratando de alejarme. Me cayó encima. Sentía cómo me aplastaba. Sentía su aliento en la cara y sus largos dedos me apretaron los hombros haciéndome gritar. Metió su otra mano debajo de mi vestido pasándola sobre mis muslos, buscando. Abrí los ojos asombrada. *¿Qué demonios?*

Tenía su cara a centímetros de la mía y podía ver mi expresión de terror reflejada en sus lentes. Sacó la lengua caliente y repugnante y recorrió mi cara con ella desde el mentón hasta la oreja. Con las uñas buscó mi ropa interior tirando y enterrándomela salvajemente.

Reaccioné de nuevo tumbándole los lentes enterrándole las uñas en sus iris anaranjados.

Su sorpresivo gemido me dio un rápido respiro. Aproveché su instante de confusión para rodar y alejarme de él. Sin embargo me pateó un riñón con sus botas oliendo a ceniza. Jadeando, me doblé en posición fetal escondiendo mi cuchillo con el cuerpo. Esa vez lo tenía. La cosa se distrajo y no comenzó a transformarse. Si sentía dolor entonces también podía morir.

"¿No te asusta que te viole, nena?" me dijo con placer. "Eres una maldita ramera luchadora."

Me agarró por un hombro y traté de defenderme, indefensa frente a los dedos largos que me levantaban a trancazos. Miré a Nick alertada por el ruido de unos golpes fuertes. Estaba golpeando el candado de uno de los gabinetes de madera con una pata de la mesa. Su sangre estaba en todas partes. Jenks estaba encima de su hombro con sus alas rojas de susto.

Todo era borroso frente mí. Quedé pasmada al ver que esa cosa se transformaba de nuevo. Ahora, la mano que me tomaba del hombro era suave. Traté de recuperar el aliento y ví que era un hombre joven, alto, elegante y con levita. Tenía unos lentes opacos sobre su nariz delgada. Estaba segura de haberlo golpeado pero no tenía heridas en los ojos ¿Era un vampiro? ¿Un vampiro realmente viejo?

"¿Tal vez le temes al dolor?," dijo esa visión de hombre elegante, hablando con tanta propiedad como el mismo profesor Henry Higgins.

Me alejé de un salto cayendo contra un gabinete de libros pero me siguió haciendo una mueca espantosa. Me levantó lanzándome contra Nick que seguía golpeando el mueble al otro lado de la habitación.

Mi espalda lo golpeó con tanta fuerza que perdí el aire y mi cuchillo sonó al caer al suelo. Me deslicé por el gabinete roto luchando por respirar. Terminé sentada a medias sobre una repisa detrás de las puertas destrozadas. Estaba impotente frente a la cosa que me levantó por el vestido.

"¿Qué eres?," dije carraspeando.

Sonrió mostrando sus dientes blancos. "¿Qué te asusta, Raquel Mariana Morgan?" preguntó. "No es el dolor. No es la violación. Tampoco los monstruos."

"¡Nada!" dije jadeante y le escupí en la cara.

Mi saliva siseó al caer en su cara y temblé al recordar la saliva de Ivy en mi cuello.

La cosa pareció disfrutarlo. "Le temes a las sombras sin alma," susurró con placer. "Temes morir en los amorosos brazos de una sombra sin alma. Tu muerte será un placer para ambos, Raquel Mariana Morgan. Qué forma tan contradictoria de morir—con placer. Habría sido mejor para tu alma temerle a los perros."

Lancé mis manos de nuevo dejándole cuatro heridas en la cara con mis uñas. No se inmutó. La sangre salió densa y roja. Me retorció los dos brazos en la espalda agarrándome las dos muñecas con una mano. Sentí nauseas. Me tiró del brazo y el hombro aplastándome contra la pared, pero logré zafar una mano para lanzarle un golpe.

Me bloqueó antes de que pudiera pegarle. Lo miré a los ojos y sentí que mis rodillas flaqueaban. La levita de caballero se había convertido en chaqueta y pantalones negros de cuero. Su tez rojiza se transformó en una carita un tanto cachetona con cabello rubio. Le brillaban dos aretes. Entonces ví que Kisten me sonreía mostrándome su lengua roja. "¿Te gustan los vampiros, brujita?" susurró.

Me retorcí tratando de zafarme. "No estés tan seguro" murmuré. Seguí luchando y ahora se transformaba de nuevo. Se volvió más pequeño, apenas una cabeza más alto que yo. El cabello le creció largo, lacio y negro. El rubio desapareció y su cara se volvió la de un fantasma. La mandíbula cuadrada de Kisten se hizo más suave y ovalada.

"Ivy" susurré paralizada de terror.

"Me diste un nombre," dijo con voz suave y femenina. "¿Quieres esto?"

Quise tragar y no podía moverme. "No me asustas," murmuré.

Sus ojos centellaron. "Pero Ivy sí."

Reuní fuerzas tratando de zafarme a medida que me acercaba más por la muñeca. "¡No!" grité en el instante en que abrió la boca mostrándome los colmillos. Mordió profundo y grité. Fuego corrió por mi brazo entrando en mi cuerpo. Me mordió la muñeca como un perro mientras yo me contorsionaba tratando de escapar.

Sentí que me destrozaba la piel al retorcerme. Levanté la rodilla, lo empujé y me solté. Caí de espaldas jadeando petrificada. Era como si Ivy estuviera ahí en frente con mi sangre goteándole de la boca. Alzó una mano quitándose el pelo de los ojos dejando una mancha roja sobre su frente.

No podía, no podía enfrentarme a esto. Tomé difícilmente una bocanada de aire y corrí hacia la puerta.

La cosa estrechó un brazo como una serpiente con la velocidad de un vampiro y me jaló hacia atrás. Sentí un dolor intenso al estrellarme contra la pared de cemento. La mano pálida de Ivy me atrapó. "Deja que te muestre lo que hacen los vampiros a puerta cerrada, Raquel Mariana Morgan."

Comprendí que moriría en el sótano de la biblioteca universitaria.

Esa cosa que se transformó en Ivy se inclinó más cerca. Sentía que el pulso me empujaba la piel y un cosquilleo caliente en la muñeca. La cara de Ivy estaba a centímetros de mi cara y me pareció que sacaba las imágenes de mi cabeza. Llevaba un crucifijo colgado alrededor del cuello y olía a jugo de naranja. Sus ojos se veían ahumados lanzando una mirada de apetito sofocante. "No," suspiré, "No, por favor."

"Puedo poseerte cuando me de la gana, brujita" susurró con una voz que imitaba la de Ivy.

Entré en pánico luchando inútilmente. La cosa que se parecía Ivy sonrió mostrando sus dientes. "Tienes tanto miedo" susurró cariñosamente, ladeando la cabeza para que su cabello negro rozara mi hombro. "No tengas miedo. Te gustará. ¿No te lo dije antes?"

Me sacudí al sentir que algo me tocaba el cuello. Dejé escapar un gemido al caer en la cuenta de que era una lengua que se movía veloz. "Te va a encantar" dijo con el mismo susurro gutural de Ivy. "Palabra de explorador."

Por mi mente pasó la imagen de Ivy cuando me sujetó en el asiento. La cosa gemía de placer apretándome contra la pared. De pronto empujó mi cabeza de lado y yo pegué un alarido aterrorizada.

"Oh, por favor" suspiraba la cosa mientras que yo ya sentía el filo helado de sus dientes en mi cuello. "Oh por favor. Ahora..."

"¡No!" grité, pero me clavó los dientes. Penetró tres veces con movimientos rápidos. Yo me aferré a sus puños y así, aferrados, caímos al piso. Me aplastó contra el cemento frío. Mi cuello ardía como fuego. La misma sensación subió por mi muñeca hasta la cabeza. Temblé de escalofrío. Podía sentir cómo me chupaba rítmicamente tratando de tomar más de lo que mi cuerpo podía dar.

Jadeante, sentí que me invadía una sensación agria. No podía distinguir dolor de placer. Era…era…

"¡Quítate de encima!" gritó Nick.

Oí un golpe y sentí una sacudida. La cosa se levantó.

Yo no podía moverme. No quería moverme. Estaba tirada en el piso, paralizada y entumecida bajo el letargo inducido por el vampiro. Jenks voló sobre mí y la brisa de sus alas sobre mi cuello me producía vibraciones.

Nick estaba de pie con los ojos cubiertos de sangre. Tenía un libro tan grande en las manos que le costaba trabajo sostenerlo. Murmuraba entre jadeos, pálido y asustado. Sus ojos pasaron del libro a la cosa que estaba a mi lado.

De nuevo se transformó en perro. Gruñendo, lo atacó.

"Nick" susurré al tiempo que Jenks me cubría el cuello con polvo de duende. "¡Cuidado!"

"¡Laqueo!," gritó Nick, haciendo malabares con el libro sobre su rodilla levantada lanzando una mano al aire.

El perro se estrelló contra algo y luego cayó. Yo observaba tirada en el piso. Se levantó de nuevo aturdido agitando la cabeza. Gruñó otra vez y lo atacó de nuevo, pero cayó por segunda vez. "¡Me encerraste!" rabió, cambiando de una forma a otra en un grotesco caleidoscopio de formas. Miró el piso y el círculo que Nick había formado con su propia sangre. "¡Tú no tienes los conocimientos para llamarme desde el más allá!," gritó.

Agachado sobre el libro, Nick se pasó la lengua por los labios. "No. Pero puedo encerrarte en un círculo una vez que estás aquí," repuso algo dudoso, como si no estuviera del todo seguro.

Jenks esparcía polvo de duende sobre mi muñeca parado en la palma de mi mano mientras que la cosa se estrellaba contra la barrera invisible. Del piso salía humo donde sus pies tocaban el cemento. "¡No de nuevo!," se lamentaba. "¡Sácame de aquí!"

Nick pasó saliva y pasó junto a la sangre y los libros caídos dirigiéndose hacia mí. "Dios mío, Raquel" dijo, dejando caer el libro al suelo con el ruido de páginas rotas. Jenks secaba la sangre de mi cara cantando una canción de cuna sobre rocío y rayos de luna.

Miré el libro roto en el piso y luego a Nick. "¿Nick?" llamé con voz trémula mirando su silueta contra la lúgubre luz fluorescente. "No puedo moverme. ¡No puedo moverme Nick! ¡Creo que me paralizó!" le dije agobiada por el pánico.

"No, no," repuso mirando al perro. Se puso detrás de mí y me alzó sentándome desplomada encima de él. "Es la saliva del vampiro. El efecto desaparecerá."

Acunada en sus brazos y muslos, sentí que comenzaba a enfriarme. Entumecida, lo miré. Sus ojos pardos estaban medio cerrados. Tenía la mandíbula tensa de la preocupación. La sangre le manaba de la cabeza formando un pequeño riachuelo que le empapaba la camisa. Tenía las manos rojas y pegajosas pero sus brazos eran cálidos. Comencé a temblar.

"¿Nick?" dije. Los dos miramos a la cosa. De nuevo era un perro. Ahí estaba mirándonos, goteando saliva. Le temblaban los músculos. "¿Es un vampiro?"

"No," repuso lacónicamente. "Es un demonio, pero tiene mucho poder. Posee las destrezas de cualquier forma que toma. Pronto podrás moverte." Su cara era de angustia mirando la sangre esparcida por el cuarto. "Vas a estar bien." Aún acunándome en sus muslos, usó mi cuchillo de plata para cortar la parte inferior de su camisa. "Estarás bien" susurró, mientras amarraba el trapo alrededor de mi muñeca poniéndola luego suavemente sobre mi muslo. Gemí ante el inesperado movimiento de mi muñeca.

"¿Nick?" Veía destellos negros frente a las luces. Me fascinaron. "No hay más demonios. No han habido más ataques demoníacos desde el Giro."

"Estudié tres años de demonología como segunda lengua para perfeccionar mi latín," dijo mientras se estiraba para alcanzar mi bolso que Jenks rescató de abajo de la mesa destrozada. "Esa cosa es un demonio." Tenía mi cabeza recostada en sus muslos mientras él hurgaba en mi bolso. "¿Tienes algo aquí contra el dolor?"

"No. Me gusta el dolor." Nick me miró primero y luego a Jenks. "Nadie estudia demonología," le dije asombrada tratando de sonreír. "Es...cómo podría decirlo, lo más inútil del mundo." Dirigí la mirada hacia el gabinete. Las puertas seguían cerradas pero las láminas estaban rotas por los golpes que le propinó Nick y por las veces que me estrellé contra el mueble. Detrás de la madera astillada había un espacio vacío del tamaño del libro que estaba en el piso junto a mí. *De manera que esto es lo que esconden en un armario con llave en un cuarto con llave detrás de una puerta con llave en el sótano de un edificio oficial.* Miré incrédula a Nick. "¿Tú sabes parar demonios?," le pregunté. Dios me perdone, pero ahora me sentía bien, liviana como una pluma. "Eres un practicante de magia negro. Yo arresto a gente como tú" le dije, pasándole un dedo por la mandíbula.

"No precisamente," respondió Nick tomando mi mano y bajándola de nuevo. Agitó un poco el puño de su suéter para limpiarme la sangre de la cara. "No trates de hablar Raquel. Perdiste mucha sangre." Se volvió hacia Jenks. "¡No puedo llevarla así en el autobús!"

Jenks puso cara de tragedia. "Iré por Ivy." Voló hasta mi hombro y susurró: "Aguanta Raque. Ya vuelvo." Luego se dirigió hacia Nick refrescándome con la brisa de sus alas. Cerré los ojos esperando que nunca se terminara.

"Si la dejas morir aquí yo mismo te mataré," amenazó Jenks y Nick asintió con la cabeza. Salió volando con el zumbido de mil abejas y el sonido retumbó en mi cabeza inclusive cuando ya Jenks no estaba.

"¿Puede escapar?" pregunté abriendo los ojos. Mis emociones pasaban de un extremo al otro y finalmente las lágrimas formaron lagunas en mis ojos.

Nick metió el gran libro de hechizos demoníacos en mi bolso. Sus huellas sangrientas estaban sobre ambos. "No. Y

cuando salga el sol, ¡puff! desaparecerá y estarás a salvo."
Metió mi cuchillo en el bolso y alcanzó mi abrigo.

"Pero estamos en el sótano. Aquí no hace sol," argumenté.

Nick rasgó el forro de mi abrigo y lo presionó sobre mi
cuello. Gemí al sentir el éxtasis por el efecto de la saliva de
vampiro que aún permanecía activa. La hemorragia había
disminuido y pensé si acaso se debería al polvo de duende
de Jenks. Aparentemente servía para otras cosas, además de
producirle rasquiña a la gente.

"No es la luz del sol la que hace que un demonio regrese
al más allá," dijo Nick pensando que me lastimaba. "Tiene
algo que ver con rayos gamma o protones, diablos Raquel.
Ya deja de hacer tantas preguntas. Enseñaban demonología
como ayuda para entender el desarrollo del lenguaje, pero
no para aprender a controlar demonios."

El demonio se había transformado de nuevo en Ivy y yo
temblé al ver que se relamía los labios con la lengua manchada de sangre, provocándome. "¿Qué nota sacaste, Nick?
Por favor, dime que sacaste una A."

"Umm" tartamudeó Nick cubriéndome con mi abrigo.
Estaba muy preocupado. Me tomó en sus brazos, casi arru-
llándome. Yo sentía los latidos de mi muñeca al mismo
ritmo de los latidos del cuello. "Despacio," murmuró. "Todo
saldrá bien."

"¿Estás seguro?" se escuchó una voz que provenía de una
esquina.

Nick levantó la mirada y juntos miramos al demonio. De
nuevo tenía el aspecto de un caballero vestido de levita.
"Déjame salir. Yo puedo ayudarte," dijo con toda simpatía.

Nick tuvo un momento de duda. "¿Nick?" dije súbitamente invadida por el miedo. "¡No lo escuches! ¡No!"

El demonio sonrió y miró por encima de sus lentes opacos. Tenía los dientes blancos y parejos. "Rompe el círculo y
la llevaré donde su Ivy. De lo contrario…" Frunció el ceño,
como si estuviera preocupado. "Parece que tuviera más sangre afuera que adentro."

Nick pasó la mirada por la sangre esparcida en los libros y paredes y sentí que me agarraba más fuerte. "Trataste de matarla," dijo con voz entrecortada.

El demonio se encogió de hombros. "Me obligaron a hacerlo. Ahora que me encerraste en el círculo eliminaste a quien me convocó y con ello desapareció mi obligación de obedecerle. Ahora soy todo tuyo, pequeño brujo." Sonrió y mi respiración se volvió rápida y jadeante.

"Nicky" susurré, ahora que el letargo producido por la pérdida de sangre empezaba a desaparecer lentamente. Estaba mal, muy mal. Recordé aterrorizada su ataque salvaje y mi corazón comenzó a latir aceleradamente.

"¿Puedes llevarnos de vuelta a la iglesia?" preguntó Nick.

"¿La que está junto a la línea ley pequeña?" La silueta del demonio tembló un instante con cara de asombro. "Alguien cerró un círculo ahí hace seis noches. La onda expansiva que envió hasta el más allá me hizo temblar las entrañas." Luego inclinó la cabeza cuestionando. "¿Fuiste tú?"

"No," repuso Nick débilmente.

Sentí enfermar. Puse mucha sal. Dios me acompañe. No sabía que los demonios podían sentir cuando uno arrastra una línea ley. Si salía de esto con vida no lo haría nunca más.

El demonio me fijó la mirada. "Yo puedo llevarlos allá," dijo, "pero a cambio no quiero que me impongan la obligación de regresar al más allá."

Nick me apretó fuerte. "¿Quieres que te deje libre en Cincinnati toda la noche?"

El demonio sonrió como demostrando su poder. Exhaló lentamente y escuché cómo sonaban las articulaciones de sus hombros. "Quiero matar a quien me convocó. Luego me iré. Aquí hay demasiado hedor." Su mirada me hizo estremecer. "Tú no vas a llamarme ¿no es cierto, pequeño brujo? Yo podría enseñarte las cosas que tú quieres saber."

El temor y el dolor luchaban dentro de mí durante el tiempo que Nick estuvo dudando. Finalmente movió la cabeza.

"No vas a lastimarnos mental, física ni emocionalmente. Tomarás el camino más directo y no harás nada que nos lastime después", dijo.

"Nick, Nicky" repuso el demonio con asombro. "¿No confías en mí? Yo podría llevarlos por una línea ley antes de que Ivy salga de allá. Pero tienes que apurarte. Raquel Mariana Morgan parece desvanecerse rápidamente."

¿Por el más allá? ¡No! Eso fue lo que mató a papá.

Nick tragó saliva, preocupado. "¡No!" traté de gritar contorsionándome para zafarme de sus brazos. El estupor que me producía la saliva de esa cosa ya casi desaparecía del todo y con cada movimiento sentía mucho dolor. Pero prefería el dolor sabiendo que el placer había sido un espejismo. Nick estaba pálido. Se esforzaba por no dejarme mover y me sostenía el cuello con el forro del abrigo.

"Raquel," susurró. "Ya has perdido mucha sangre. ¡No sé que hacer!"

Mi garganta estaba demasiado seca para tragar. "¡No! ¡No lo dejes salir!," insistí. "¡Por favor!" le rogué quitándole las manos de encima. "Estoy bien. Ya no estoy sangrando. Voy a estar bien. Déjame aquí y ve a llamar a Ivy. Ella vendrá a buscarnos. No quiero pasar por el más allá."

El demonio frunció el ceño, mostrándose preocupado. "Ummm" musitó suavemente jugando con el corbatín de seda. "Parece que está incoherente. Mala cosa. Tic-Tac, Nicky, tienes que decidir rápido."

Nick repiró profundo y reflexionó. Miró el pozo de sangre en el piso y luego me miró a mí. "Tengo que hacer algo," susurró. "Estás helada, Raquel."

"¡No, Nick!" grité. Me dejó en el suelo levantándose. Con un pie rompió el círculo de sangre.

Escuché un gemido aterrador y me tapé la boca al darme cuenta de que era yo misma. El terror me invadió completamente cuando vi cómo se sacudía el demonio. Lentamente, dio un paso sobre la línea. Luego pasó la mano sobre la pared manchada de sangre chupándose el dedo, con la mirada fija en mí.

"¡No dejes que me toque!" Estaba totalmente histérica.

"Raquel," dijo Nick tratando de calmarme arrodillado a mi lado. "Dijo que no va a lastimarte. Los demonios no mienten. Lo dicen todos los textos que estudié."

"Y tampoco dicen la verdad!" exclamé.

Los ojos del demonio centellaban de ira, pero después cambiaron de expresión como si estuviera preocupado por mí antes de que Nick pudiera darse cuenta. Se acercó a mí y yo traté de retroceder. "¡No dejes que me toque! ¡No me obligues a hacer esto!"

El temor de Nick era por mi actitud y no por el demonio. Él no entendía. Pensó que sabía lo que hacía. Pensó que sus libros tenían todas las respuestas. Pero no sabía lo que estaba haciendo. Yo sí.

Nick me tomó del hombro y le habló al demonio. "¿Puedes ayudarla?," le preguntó. "Se va a matar."

"¡No, Nick!" chillé mientras que el demonio se arrodilló y puso su cara sonriente junto a la mía.

"Duerme, Raquel Mariana Morgan," exhaló. No recuerdo nada más.

Veintiséis

"¿Qué pasó? ¿Dónde está Jenks?" dijo Ivy. Su voz seca y preocupada me sacó del aturdimiento. Sentí que me mecía hacia adelante. Había sentido calor pero ahora sentía frío. El olor a sangre era fuerte. El recuerdo de algo muy malo permanecía en mi memoria: carroña, sal y ámbar quemado. No podía abrir los ojos.

"La atacó un demonio." Era una voz suave y profunda. Nick.

Es verdad, pensé, y comencé a armar el rompecabezas. Estaba en sus brazos. De ahí venía el único olor agradable, masculino y dulce. Era su suéter manchado de sangre que frotaba mis ojos hinchados lastimándolos más aún. Comencé a temblar. ¿Por qué sentía frío?

"¿Podemos quitarnos de la calle?" preguntó Nick. "Ha perdido mucha sangre."

Sentí una mano cálida sobre la frente. "¿Un demonio hizo esto?" dijo Ivy. "No había ocurrido un ataque de demonios desde el Giro. Maldición. No debí dejar que saliera de la iglesia."

Los brazos que me sostenían se pusieron tensos y me moví hacia adelante y hacia atrás apenas se detuvo. "Raquel sabe lo que hacer," dijo Nick seriamente. "No es tu bebé, desde ningún punto de vista."

"¿A no?" dijo Ivy. "Pero actúa como si lo fuera. ¿Cómo permitiste que la atacaran así?"

"¿Yo? ¡Vampiro despiadado!" gritó Nick. "¿Tú crees que yo permití que esto sucediera?"

Se me formó un nudo en el estómago y sentí náuseas. Traté de ponerme el abrigo con mi mano sana. Entreabrí los ojos ante el brillo de las luces de la calle. ¿Podrían terminar de discutir después de meterme en la cama?

"Ivy," dijo Nick calmadamente. "No te tengo miedo, así es que ya deja la mierda del aura y no estorbes. Yo sé lo que buscas y no pienso permitir que lo hagas."

"¿A qué te refieres con eso?" tartamudeó Ivy.

Nick se inclinó hacia ella y yo quedé en medio de los dos. "Si no me equivoco, Raquel cree que tú y ella se mudaron el mismo día" dijo. "A lo mejor a ella le podría interesar saber que todas tus revistas llegan a la dirección de la iglesia." Escuché cómo Ivy respiraba asombrada mientras que él continuó amenazante. "¿Cuanto tiempo llevas viviendo aquí esperando a que Raquel renuncie? ¿Un mes? ¿Un año? ¿La estás cazando lentamente, Tamwood? ¿Quieres convertirla en tu lacayo cuando mueras? Estamos planificando por adelantado ¿verdad? ¿No es así?"

Me esforcé por retirar mi cabeza del pecho de Nick para poder oír mejor. Traté de pensar pero estaba muy confundida. ¿Acaso Ivy no se había mudado el mismo día que yo? Su computadora aun no estaba conectada a la red y tenía todas esas cajas en su habitación. Entonces, ¿por qué sus revistas llegaban a la iglesia? Mi mente pasó entonces al jardín perfecto para una bruja que había atrás y a los libros de hechizos en el ático. Dios me proteja. Soy una estúpida.

"No," repuso Ivy. "Las cosas no son como parecen. Por favor, no le digas eso. Puedo explicarlo todo."

Nick se puso en marcha ayudándome a subir las escalinatas de piedra. Estaba recuperando la memoria. Nick había hecho un trato con el demonio. Lo había dejado libre. El demonio me durmió y me hizo viajar por las líneas ley. Maldición. El portazo del santuario me hizo saltar y gemí de dolor.

"Está volviendo en sí," dijo Ivy lacónicamente. Su voz sonó en eco. "Déjala en la sala."

No en el sofá, pensé. Ahora me embriagaba la sensación de paz del santuario. No quería dejar mi sangre en el sofá de Ivy, aun cuando de todas formas había tenido sangre en el pasado.

Sentí un vacío en el estómago tan pronto Nick se agachó y por fin sentí la suavidad de los mullidos cojines bajo mi cuerpo. Escuché el clic de la lámpara de mesa y arrugué la cara ante el cálido y repentino brillo que percibía a través de mis párpados cerrados.

"¿Raquel?"

Sentía a alguien cerca que me acariciaba suavemente la cara.

"Raquel." El cuarto estaba en silencio. Sólo desperté con los susurros. Entreabrí los ojos y vi a Nick arrodillado junto a mí. Aún le chorreaba sangre de la frente y un riachuelo seco se le había formado entre la mandíbula y el cuello. Tenía mal aspecto y el cabello desordenado y alborotado. Estaba hecho un desastre. Ivy estaba detrás de él, preocupada.

"Eres tú," susurré, sintiéndome mareada y desubicada. Nick se reclinó hacia atrás con un respiro de alivio. "¿Puedo beber agua? No me siento bien" carraspeé.

Ivy se inclinó obstruyendo la luz. Me examinó con un profesionalismo que cesó apenas levantó el borde del vendaje improvisado que me puso Nick alrededor del cuello. Sus ojos se abrieron con asombro. "Prácticamente ha dejado de sangrar."

"Amor, confianza y polvo de duende" dije arrastrando las palabras. Ivy asintió.

Nick se puso de pie. "Llamaré a una ambulancia."

"¡No!" exclamé. Intenté sentarme pero la fatiga y las manos de Nick me lo impidieron. "Me atraparán. La S.E. sabe que estoy viva." Me recosté jadeando. Las heridas que me hizo el demonio en la cara latían rítmicamente con mi corazón. En mi brazo sentía la misma pulsación. Estaba mareada y el hombro me dolía al respirar. Cuando exhalaba lo veía todo oscuro.

"Jenks la cubrió con polvo," dijo Ivy, como si eso lo explicara todo. "Mientras que no vuelva a sangrar, no creo que empeore. Voy por una manta." Se puso de pie con esa velocidad graciosa e inquietante suya. Estaba entrando en la onda vampiro y yo no me hallaba en condición de defenderme.

Miré a Nick que salía. Parecía enfermo. El demonio lo había engañado. Estábamos en casa como lo había prometido; pero ahora había un demonio suelto en Cincinnati cuando todo lo que Nick tenía que hacer era esperar a que llegaran Jenks e Ivy.

"¿Nick?" musité.

"¿Qué? ¿Qué podía hacer?" Su voz suave y preocupada dejaba entrever sentimiento de culpa.

"Eres un imbécil. Ayúdame a sentar."

Haciendo un gesto me tendió las manos con cuidado para ayudarme hasta que mi espalda estuvo contra el brazo del sofá. Me senté mirando al techo mientras que los puntos negros que bailaban ante mis ojos desaparecían. Respiré profundo y me miré. Mi vestido estaba manchado de sangre y mi abrigo me servía de manta. Un delgado hilillo de sangre había hecho que mis medias se me pegaran a los pies. El brazo mordido tenía un color grisáceo y lleno de manchas de sangre seca. La manga de la camisa de Nick aún estaba amarrada alrededor de mi muñeca y la sangre seguía chorreando con la velocidad de una llave goteando: plop, plop, plop. A lo mejor a Jenks se le agotó el polvo. Tenía hinchado el otro brazo y sentí que tenía roto el hombro. Sentía el cuarto caliente y luego frío. Miré a Nick sintiéndome lejana y fuera de la realidad.

"Mierda," musitó mirando hacia el pasillo. "Vas a perder el sentido de nuevo." Me tomó por los tobillos suavemente y me hizo recostar de nuevo hasta que mi cabeza quedó sobre el brazo del sofá. "¡Ivy!," gritó. "¿Dónde está esa manta?"

Miré al techo hasta que dejó de dar vueltas. Nick estaba acurrucado en una esquina dándome la espalda. Tenía una mano sobre el vientre y con la otra se tomaba la cabeza. "Gracias," susurré. Él se dio vuelta.

"¿De qué?" respondió con amargura, deshecho, con la cara manchada de sangre. Sus manos estaban negras de sangre y le sobresalían líneas blancas.

"Por hacer lo que creíste que era mejor." Sentí escalofríos.

Se veía enfermo pero sonrió. Se veía preocupado. "Había tanta sangre que sentí pánico. Lo siento." Su mirada se fijó en el pasillo. No me extrañé al ver entrar a Ivy con una manta colgando de un brazo, varias toallas rosadas debajo del otro y un recipiente de agua en las manos.

El malestar que sentí fue más fuerte que el dolor. Aún sangraba; y ahí venía Ivy. Me estremecí.

"¿Qué?" dijo de repente mientras dejaba las toallas y el agua sobre la mesa de centro y me envolvía con la manta como si fuera un niño.

Tragué saliva y traté de mirarla directamente a los ojos. "Nada," repuse humildemente mientras que ella se enderezaba de nuevo y retrocedía. Aparte de verse más pálida que de costumbre, estaba bien. Pensé que no podría aguantar si se ponía vampiro. Estaba totalmente indefensa.

Sentí más calor con la manta que me cubría la quijada y por la luz de la lámpara. Temblé cuando se sentó en la mesa y acercó el cuenco de agua. Pensé en el color de las toallas y recordé que en el rosado no se notan las manchas viejas de sangre.

"¿Ivy?" dije asustada mientras que ella acercó las manos al trapo que tenía alrededor de mi cuello.

Retiró la mano y su expresión antes perfecta ahora se veía insultada y molesta. "No seas estúpida, Raquel. Déjame revisarte el cuello."

De nuevo acercó la mano pero yo me encogí. "¡No!" grité alejándome. Vi ante mí la imagen del demonio que se transformaba en Ivy. No pude luchar contra él y estuvo a punto de matarme. El terror me invadió completamente y reuní fuerzas para sentarme. El dolor del cuello parecía dar alaridos queriendo escapar a cambio de aquella exquisita mezcla de dolor y apetito que suministraba la saliva del vampiro. Me sacudía y me horrorizaba. Los ojos de Ivy se agrandaron hasta tornarse negros.

Nick se paró en medio de ambas cubierto de sangre seca y oliendo a miedo. "¡Atrás, Tamwood!" amenazó. "No vas a tocarla si le quieres arrastrar el aura."

"Tranquilízate niño rata," exclamó Ivy. "No estoy arrastrando auras. Estoy furiosa. Además no mordería a Raquel ahora ni aunque me lo rogara: apesta a infección."

Eso era más de lo que me interesaba oír. Sus ojos se habían tornado pardos otra vez. Fluctuaba entre la rabia y la necesidad de ser comprendida. De pronto me sentí culpable. Ivy no me había apretado contra la pared para morderme. Tampoco me había aterrorizado clavándome los dientes. No me había chupado el cuello gimiendo de placer aferrándome con fuerza mientras me contorsionaba. Maldición. No-fue-ella.

Nick seguía en medio de ambas. "Nick, está bien," le dije con voz trémula. Él sabía por qué yo tenía tanto miedo. "Todo está bien." Miré a Ivy. "Disculpa. Por favor, mira mi cuello."

Ivy se relajó de inmediato. Se acercó más sintiendo el derecho de hacerlo mientras que Nick se quitaba de en medio. Dejé escapar lentamente el aire que retenía mientras que ella me quitaba la tela empapada. "Muy bien," advirtió. "Esto va doler un poco."

"¡Ay!" grité. Mi reacción fue jalar cuando ella levantó la tela. Me mordí los labios para no hacerlo de nuevo. Ivy dejó el trapo sucio en la mesa y sentí que se me retorcía el estómago. Estaba negro de sangre húmeda y podría jurar que tenía pegados trocitos de piel. Temblé por el frío que sentí en el cuello pues tuve la sensación de sangre fresca que fluía.

Ivy me miró a la cara. "Llévate eso de aquí," ordenó Ivy. Nick salió con el trapo empapado.

Sin expresión en la cara, Ivy puso una toalla de manos sobre mi hombro para atrapar el nuevo flujo. Miré fijamente a la televisión apagada mientras ella empapaba una toallita y la escurría encima del cuenco de agua. Sus movimientos eran suaves, limpiando desde los bordes de las heridas hacia el centro. Aun así, yo no podía contener el dolor. El amenazante anillo negro que me cubría la visión comenzó a crecer.

"¿Raquel?" dijo suavemente. Inmediatamente volví la atención hacia ella sin saber con qué me encontraría. Sin embargo, su expresión era neutra y sus ojos y manos examinaban mis heridas en el cuello. "¿Qué sucedió?" preguntó. "Nick mencionó algo acerca de un demonio, pero esto parece..."

"Parece un mordisco de vampiro" terminé de manera insulsa. "Se transformó en vampiro y me hizo esto." Tomé aire temblando. "Se transformó en tu figura, Ivy. Discúlpame si estoy demasiado sensible ahora. Yo se que no eras tú. Sólo dame tiempo para convencer a mi subconsciente de que tú no trataste de matarme. ¿Está bien?"

Nuestras miradas se encontraron y las dos sentimos temor cuando un relámpago de claridad cruzó por su mente. Yo había sido atacada por un vampiro. Había sido iniciada a un club del cual Ivy trataba de alejarse. Ahora éramos dos. Luego recordé lo que dijo Nick respecto a que Ivy quería convertirme en su lacayo. No sabía qué pensar.

"Raquel, yo..."

"Después," dije. Nick regresó. Me sentía muy mal y de nuevo empecé a ver todo borroso. Matalina venía con él y con dos de sus niños. Traían una bolsa tamaño duende. Nick se arrodilló a mi lado. Sosteniendo el vuelo en el aire en medio de la habitación, Matalina evaluó la situación y tomó la bolsa que llevaban los niños. Luego los hizo salir por la ventana. "Vayan, vayan" oí que susurraba. "Ya sé que les había dicho otra cosa pero cambié de opinión. Váyanse a casa." Protestaron y se retiraron aterrados. ¡Cómo estaría de mal!

"¿Raquel?" dijo Matalina volando frente a mí de un lado a otro, tratando de determinar hacia dónde miraban mis ojos. La sala había quedado bajo un preocupante silencio y sentí escalofríos. Matalina era realmente hermosa. Con razón Jenks haría lo que fuera por ella. "Trata de no moverte, querida," me dijo.

De pronto, una brisa de aire proveniente de la ventana hizo que Matalina se elevara. "¡Jenks!," dijo aliviada la pequeñita mujer duende. "¿Dónde estabas?"

"¿Yo?," respondió volando frente a mis ojos. "¿Cómo llegaron aquí antes que yo?"

"Tomamos el autobús expreso" repuso Nick sarcásticamente.

Jenks estaba muy preocupado. Tenía los hombros caídos pero por fin pude sonreír. "¿Está muy cansado de trabajar este buen mozo hombrecito duende?" Respiré profundo y Jenks se acercó tanto que tuve que entrecerrar los párpados.

"Ivy, tienes que hacer algo" dijo. "Le cubrí las heridas con polvillo para disminuir la hemorragia, pero jamás he visto a alguien tan pálido que siga vivo aún."

"Eso es lo que estoy tratando de hacer," gruñó. "¡Quítense de mi camino!"

Sentí cómo cambiaba la brisa. Ivy y Matalina se acercaron a mí. Era reconfortante saber que un vampiro y un duende me estaban examinando el cuello; y puesto que una infección era motivo para bajar el apetito, debería encontrarme a salvo. Ivy podría determinar si mis heridas eran o no mortales . Y Nick...sentí deseos de reír, Nick me rescataría si Ivy perdía el control.

Ivy me tocó el cuello con los dedos y grité. Ivy también se sobresaltó y Matalina se elevó en el aire. "Raquel," dijo Ivy preocupada. "Yo no puedo arreglar esto. El polvillo de duende te ayudará sólo durante cierto tiempo, pero necesitas que te cosan. Tenemos que llevarte a emergencias."

"Nada de hospitales," dije suspirando. Ya no temblaba y sentía mi estómago extraño. "Allá los agentes entran pero nunca salen." Me permití una sonrisa.

"¿Prefieres morir en mi sofá?" dijo Ivy y Nick comenzó a seguirla.

"¿Qué le pasa a esa?" dijo Jenks en voz alta.

Ivy se puso de pie y cruzó los brazos. Se veía seria y molesta. Un vampiro molesto. Vaya, qué gracioso. Eso ameritaba una risa y reí de nuevo.

"Es la pérdida de sangre," dijo Ivy impaciente. "Será como un yo-yo entre la lucidez y la irracionalidad hasta que se equilibre o se muera. Odio esta parte."

Mi mano buena se arrastró hacia mi cuello pero Nick me obligó a meterla bajo la manta.

"¡No puedo arreglarlo, Raquel!" exclamó Ivy frustrada. "Te hicieron demasiado daño."

"Yo haré algo," dije con firmeza. "Soy una bruja." Me incliné para rodar del sofá y levantarme. Tenía que ir a la cocina. Tenía que cocinar la cena para Ivy.

"¡Raquel!" gritó Nick, tratando de agarrarme. Ivy saltó tomándome y haciéndome regresar al sofá. Sentí perder hasta el último aliento. La sala me daba vueltas. Miré el techo con los ojos totalmente abiertos haciendo un gran esfuerzo por no perder el sentido. Si eso sucedía, Ivy me llevaría a emergencias.

Matalina voló siguiendo mi mirada. "Ángel," susurré, "Eres un ángel hermoso."

"¡Ivy!" gritó Jenks. "¡Está delirando!"

El duende ángel me hizo una sonrisa que me pareció una bendición. "Alguien debe ir a buscar a Keasley," dijo.

"El viejo grandulón...eh...brujo del otro lado de la calle?"

Matalina asintió. "Dile que Raquel necesita ayuda médica."

Ivy también se mostró asombrada. "¿Crees que él puede hacer algo?" preguntó con temor patente en su voz. Ivy temía por mí. Tal vez yo también debería estar asustada.

Matalina se ruborizó. "El otro día pidió permiso para tomar unas ramitas del jardín. No hay nada de malo con eso." La hermosa duende zumbaba con la mirada baja. "Todas eran plantas con propiedades fuertes: milenrama, verbena, cosas por el estilo. Pensé que si las quería es porque sabe qué hacer con ellas."

"Mujer," repuso Jenks advirtiéndole.

"Estuve todo el tiempo a su lado," dijo con ojos desafiantes. "Sólo tocó lo que le permití. Fue muy educado y preguntó por el bienestar de todos."

"Matalina, este no es nuestro jardín," dijo Jenks, y el ángel se molestó.

"Si tú no vas por él, iré yo," dijo decididamente y salió como un rayo por la ventana. Yo apenas pude parpadear mirando hacia el sitio donde había estado.

"¡Matalina!" gritó Jenks. "No vueles dejándome así. Este no es nuestro jardín y no puedes hacer de cuenta que lo es," repuso volando frente a mi campo de visión. "Lo lamento," dijo Jenks evidentemente avergonzado y molesto. "No volverá hacerlo." Se puso muy serio y salió volando tras ella. "¡Matalina!"

"S'tá bien..." susurré, aun cuando ninguno de los dos estaba allí. "Digo que está bien. El ángel puede invitar al jardín a quien le plazca." Cerré los ojos. Nick puso la mano en mi frente y sonreí. "Hola Nick," dije suavemente abriendo los ojos. "¿Aún estás aquí?"

"Sí, aún estoy aquí."

"Muy bien," repuse, "porque tan pronto pueda ponerme de pie te voy a dar un beso m-u-u-u-y grande."

Nick me soltó la mano y retrocedió un paso.

Ivy hizo una mueca. "Odio esta parte," murmuró. "La odio. La odio."

Arrastré la mano hacia mi cuello pero Nick me la quitó. De nuevo oí el goteo en la alfombra: plop, plop, plop. La sala daba vueltas extraordinarias y yo observaba fascinada. Era gracioso y traté de reír.

Ivy hizo un sonido de frustración. "Si ríe es porque va a estar bien. ¿Por qué no te bañas?"

"Yo estoy bien. Voy a esperar hasta estar seguro."

Ivy se quedó en silencio por un segundo. "Nick," dijo Ivy. "Raquel apesta a infección. Tu apestas a sangre y miedo. Ve a bañarte."

"Oh." Un largo momento de duda. "Lo siento."

Le sonreí a Nick que estaba parado en la puerta. "Ve a bañarte Nick, Nicky," le dije. "No hagas que Ivy se ponga oscura y aterradora. Demórate todo lo que quieras. Hay jabón y…" dudé por un instante tratando de recordar qué quería decir, "toallas en el cajón," concluí satisfecha de mi logro.

Me tocó el hombro mirándome a mí y a Ivy. "Vas a estar bien."

Ivy cruzó los brazos impaciente esperando a que se fuera. Luego escuché la ducha. Eso me produjo mucha sed. Sentía mi brazo estallar y las costillas inflamadas. Mi hombro y cuello eran un sólo dolor. Giré para ver fascinada cómo se movía la cortina con la brisa.

De repente sentí un golpe fuerte al frente de la iglesia que acaparó toda mi atención hacia el pasillo oscuro. "Hola" sonó la voz distante de Keasley. "¿Srta. Morgan? Matalina me dijo que entrara."

"Quédate aquí" dijo Ivy inclinándose sobre mí hasta que no tuve otra opción que mirarla. "Y no te levantes hasta que yo regrese, ¿bien? ¿Raquel? ¿Me escuchas? *No te levantes*."

"Sí, sí." De nuevo miré hacia las cortinas. Si entreabría los ojos a-p-e-e-e-n-a-s lo suficiente, el gris se convertía en negro. "Quédate aquí."

Mirándome una última vez recogió sus revistas y salió. El sonido de la ducha me atrajo. Me lamí los labios y pensé: ¿si me esfuerzo de verdad puedo llegar hasta el fregadero de la cocina?

Veintisiete

En el pasillo se escuchó el chasquido de una bolsa de papel y yo levanté un poco la cabeza del brazo del asiento. Esta vez no sentí que la sala daba vueltas y la visión nublada se tornó clara. Entonces entró un encorvado Keasley seguido de cerca por Ivy. "Qué bien," susurré casi sin aire. "Compañía."

Ivy pasó muy cerca de Keasley y fue a sentarse en la silla más cercana. "Te vez mejor," dijo. "¿Ya volviste en sí o todavía estás en la tierra de la fantasía?"

"¿Qué?"

Movió la cabeza y yo le sonreí a Keasley lánguidamente. "Disculpe que no le ofrezca un chocolate."

"Srta. Morgan," dijo, fijando la mirada en mi cuello. "¿Discutió con su compañera de vivienda?" dijo secamente pasándose la mano por su negro pelo crespo.

"No," repuse de inmediato. Ivy se puso seria.

Arqueó las cejas con incredulidad y puso su bolsa de papel sobre la mesita. "Matalina no me dijo lo que necesitaría, así es que traje un poco de todo." Miró la lámpara de la mesa con los ojos entreabiertos. "¿Tiene una luz más brillante?"

"Tengo una lamparita fluorescente." Ivy salió hacia el pasillo pero se detuvo. "No deje que se mueva. Se pondrá incoherente de nuevo."

Abrí la boca para decir algo pero desapareció y la reemplazaron Matalina y Jenks. Jenks parecía estar molesto, pero

Matalina no parecía estar arrepentida. Los dos estaban suspendidos en el aire en una esquina pero hablaban tan rápido y en una tono tan agudo que no pude entender lo que decían. Finalmente Jenks se fue. Estaba tan furioso que parecía que mataría lo primero que se le cruzara por enfrente. Matalina se acomodó su hermoso vestido blanco y voló hasta el brazo del asiento donde estaba mi cabeza.

Keasley se sentó en la mesita emitiendo un suspiro de preocupación. Su barba de tres días se estaba tornando blanca, lo que lo hacía verse muy descuidado. Las rodillas de sus overoles estaban manchadas de tierra húmeda y pude oler su exterior. Sus oscuras manos toscas se veían lastimadas obviamente de trabajar. Entonces sacó un periódico de la bolsa y lo extendió como un mantel. "¿Y quién está en la ducha? ¿Su madre?"

Resoplé sintiendo la hinchazón en mi ojo hinchado. "Se llama Nick," dije en el momento en que regresó Ivy. "Es un amigo."

Ivy hizo ruido poniendo una pequeña luz a un lado de la lámpara de mesa y la conectó. Yo cerré los ojos al sentir el calor y la intensidad de la luz.

"¿Nick?" comentó Keasley hurgando en su bolsa y sacando amuletos, paquetes envueltos en papel de aluminio y botellas que iba poniendo encima del periódico. "¿Es un vampiro?"

"No. Es humano," respondí. Keasley miró a Ivy con desconfianza.

Ivy no lo vio y se acercó un poco más. "El cuello es lo peor. Ha perdido una cantidad peligrosa de sangre."

"Eso ya lo sé," repuso el hombre mirando a Ivy agresivamente hasta que retrocedió un poco. "Necesito más toallas. ¿Por qué no le trae a Raquel algo de tomar? Necesita estar hidratada."

"Lo se" dijo Ivy, dando un paso en falso hacia atrás antes de dirigirse a la cocina. Se escuchó el sonido de vasos y el glorioso sonido del líquido. Matalina abrió su equipo de herramientas y comparó sus agujas con las de Keasley.

"Algo tibio" recalcó Keasley en voz alta. Ivy tiró la puerta del refrigerador. "Vamos a ver," dijo mientras me apuntaba con la luz. Él y Matalina estuvieron en silencio durante un buen tiempo. Luego se recostó hacia atrás dejando escapar un poco de aire. "Primero algo para calmar el dolor" dijo suavemente tomando un amuleto.

Ivy apareció en la entrada. "¿Dónde obtuvo esos hechizos?" preguntó sospechosa.

"Tranquilícese," repuso mientras inspeccionaba cuidadosamente cada paquete. "Los compré hace varios meses. Más bien sea útil y ponga a hervir una olla de agua."

Ivy refunfuñó y dio media vuelta regresando furiosa a la cocina. Escuché varios ruidos y después el sonido del gas que prendía. Abrió las llaves de agua al máximo para llenar la olla y de mi baño provino un pequeño gruñido de sorpresa.

Keasley había untado su dedo en sangre y había invocado el hechizo antes de que yo cayera en la cuenta. Colocó el amuleto alrededor de mi cuello y luego de mirarme fijo a los ojos para comprobar su eficacia, concentró toda su atención en mi cuello. "De verdad le agradezco esto" le dije al sentir que sus dedos aliviaban mi cuerpo. Mis hombros se encorvaron. Salvación.

"Yo usted, aguardaría a dar las gracias después de que reciba mi cuenta," murmuró Keasley. Alcé las cejas por el viejo chiste y él sonrió. Se acomodó de nuevo y me pinchó la piel. El dolor fue más fuerte que el hechizo y tuve que respirar profundo. "¿Aún duele?" preguntó innecesariamente.

"¿Por qué no la duerme?" preguntó Ivy.

Me sobresalté. No la había oído entrar. "No" dije a secas. No quería que lo convenciera de llevarme a emergencias.

"Así no sentirías dolor" siguió diciendo, parada desafiante y vestida de cuero y seda. "¿Por qué tienes que hacer las cosas de la forma más difícil?"

"No las hago difíciles. Simplemente no quiero que me duerman," reclamé. Mi visión se oscureció y me concentré en respirar para no perder el sentido.

"Señoras," dijo Keasley. "Estoy de acuerdo que sedar a Raquel sería más fácil para ella, pero yo no la voy a obligar."

"Gracias" dije lánguidamente.

"Ivy, ¿más ollas de agua por favor? ¿y las toallas?"

El microondas sonó e Ivy regresó a la cocina. ¿Y ahora qué mosco la picó? Me quedé pensativa.

Keasley invocó un segundo amuleto y lo puso junto al primero. Era otro hechizo para el dolor. Yo agradecí el alivio y cerré los ojos. Pero pronto los abrí cuando Ivy puso una taza de chocolate caliente sobre la mesa seguida de más toallas rosadas. Frustrada, regresó a la cocina haciendo ruido en un gabinete.

Lentamente saqué de debajo de la manta el brazo que me mordió el demonio. La inflamación había bajado un poco y me tranquilicé al notar que no estaba roto. Moví los dedos y Keasley puso el chocolate caliente en mi mano. El calor de la taza era reconfortante y tomé con placer la bebida. Sentí que me protegía.

Keasley me ponía toallas alrededor del hombro derecho mientras tomaba mi bebida. Lavó las últimas manchas de sangre del cuello empapando las toallas con el líquido de una botellita que sacó de la bolsa. Luego comenzó a examinar mi piel. "¡Ay!" grité casi derramando mi chocolate del salto. "¿Realmente necesita hacer eso?"

Keasley refunfuñó y me puso un tercer amuleto alrededor del cuello. "¿Mejor?" preguntó. La potencia del hechizo hizo que mi visión se volviera borrosa. ¿Dónde habría obtenido un hechizo tan fuerte? Pero luego recordé que él sufría de artritis. Se necesitaba un hechizo muy poderoso para aliviar ese dolor y me sentí culpable de que estuviera gastando sus hechizos medicinales en mí. Esta vez solamente sentí una leve presión mientras pinchaba y jalaba. Yo asentí. "¿Hace cuánto tiempo la mordieron?"

"Eh…" murmuré tratando de luchar contra la somnolencia que me producía el amuleto. "¿a la puesta del sol?"

"¿Y qué hora es? ¿Las nueve?" dijo mirando el reloj en el reproductor de discos compactos. "Muy bien. Podemos coserte." Se acomodó con aire de maestro y le hizo señas a Matalina para que se acercara. "Mira," le dijo a la mujercita duende. "¿Ves cómo la piel ha sido rajada en lugar de rasgada? Prefiero coser mil veces una mordida de vampiro que una de lobo. No sólo es más clara sino que no hay que eliminar las enzimas."

Matalina se acercó más. "Las lanzas de espinas producen heridas como estas, pero nunca he encontrado algo que mantenga el músculo en su lugar mientras que los ligamentos se vuelven a insertar."

Palidecí y bebí mi chocolate caliente de un trago deseando que dejaran de hablar como si yo fuera un experimento científico o un trozo de carne para la parrilla.

"Yo utilizo suturas veterinarias" dijo Keasley.

"¿Suturas veterinarias?" pregunté asombrada.

"Nadie controla las clínicas veterinarias" dijo con indiferencia. "Pero he oído decir que la nervadura que recorre el pecíolo de la hoja de laurel es suficientemente resistente para duendes y hadas. Pero yo no usaría nada distinto a la tripa de gato para los músculos de las alas. ¿Quieres un poco?" Esculcó en su bolsa y puso varios sobres de papel sobre la mesa. "Has de cuenta que es en pago por esas ramitas que arranqué."

Las alitas de Matalina se tornaron color rosa. "Esas plantas no eran mías."

"Sí que lo eran," interrumpí. "A mí me descuentan cincuenta del alquiler por mantener el jardín. Eso lo hace mío, aun cuando ustedes lo cuidan. Y yo digo que eso lo hace de ustedes."

Keasley levantó la mirada y Matalina puso cara de asombro.

"Digamos que es el sueldo de Jenks," agregué. "Naturalmente, eso si él quiere que el jardín sea su sueldo."

Hubo un momento de silencio. "Creo que eso le va a gustar," susurró Matalina y metió los pequeños sobres en su bolsa. Los dejó allí y voló hacia la ventana y de vuelta, evidentemente confundida. Era obvio que estaba nerviosa con mi propuesta. Yo no sabía si había hecho algo mal y observé las cosas de Keasley sobre el periódico.

"¿Usted es médico?" le pregunté, poniendo mi taza sobre la mesa. Tenía que acordarme de pedirle la receta de este hechizo. No sentía nada en ninguna parte.

"No." Escurrió las toallas empapadas de agua y sangre y las tiró al piso.

"Entonces, ¿dónde consiguió todas estas cosas?" insistí.

"No me gustan los hospitales," dijo a secas. "Matalina, yo haré las suturas internas y tú las de la piel. Estoy seguro de que tu trabajo es más parejo que el mío," sonrió acongojado. "Apuesto a que Raquel preferirá una cicatriz más pequeña."

"Todo se facilita cuando se está a milímetros de la herida," dijo Matalina satisfecha de que le pidieran ayuda.

Keasley me lavó el cuello con una gelatina fría. Yo me quedé mirando el techo mientras que él tomó un par de tijeras. Pensé que sería para cortar los bordes rasgados. Luego seleccionó una de sus agujas e hilo. Sentí presión en el cuello y respiré profundo. Dirigí la mirada hacia Ivy que se acercó obstruyéndole la luz a Keasley.

"¿Y esa otra herida?" dijo apuntando. "¿No debería coser esa primero? Es la que más sangra."

"No" repuso suturando una más. "¿Por qué no me trae otra olla con agua hirviendo?"

"¿Cuatro ollas con agua hirviendo?" cuestionó Ivy.

"Si fuera tan amable," repuso. Keasley siguió cosiendo mientras yo contaba las suturas con la mirada fija en el reloj. El chocolate no me sentó tan bien como hubiera deseado. No me habían cosido puntos desde que mi mejor amiga se escondió en mi armario de la escuela pretendiendo ser un zorro. Al final del día nos habían expulsado a las dos.

Ivy dudó, pero finalmente recogió las toallas mojadas y las llevó a la cocina. Se escuchó el agua de las llaves y de nuevo escuchamos un reclamo desde la ducha. "¡Ya deja de abrir la llave!" sonó la voz molesta y no pude evitar sonreír. Pero Ivy ya estaba de regreso vigilando sobre el hombro de Keasley.

"Esa sutura no está bien" dijo.

Me sentí un poco incómoda al ver que Keasley fruncía el ceño. Me caía bien, pero Ivy estaba comportándose como una pesada. "Ivy," murmuró Keasley, "¿por qué no hace una revisión del terreno?"

"Jenks está afuera. Estamos a salvo."

Keasley apretó los dientes. Tiró del hilo verde concentrado en su trabajo. "Tal vez necesite ayuda," dijo.

Ivy se puso seria cruzando los brazos y la bruma negra comenzó a invadir sus ojos. "Lo dudo."

Matalina agitó las alas tanto que no se veían cuando vio que Ivy se acercaba tapándole la luz a Keasley.

"Vete," le dijo suavemente sin moverse. "Me estás rondando."

Ivy retrocedió asombrada. Me miró a los ojos y yo le sonreí como disculpándome pero señalándole que estaba de acuerdo con Keasley. Agitada, dio media vuelta. Sentí el taconear de sus botas en el pasillo de madera y el santuario. Luego oímos reverberar por toda la iglesia el golpe de la puerta principal.

"Lo siento" dije, sintiendo que alguien debía presentar excusas.

Keasley se estiró difícilmente. "Está preocupada por usted y no sabe cómo demostrarlo sin morderla. O bien es eso o no le gusta perder el control."

"No es la única. Yo también comienzo a sentir que soy una fracasada" dije.

"¿Fracasada? ¿Cómo es eso?"

"Míreme," repuse secamente. "Estoy hecha una ruina. He perdido tanta sangre que no puedo ponerme de pie. No he logrado nada yo sola desde que abandoné la S.E. aparte de dejarme atrapar por Trent y convertirme en comida para ratas." Ya no me sentía como un agente. *Papá estaría desilusionado*, pensé. Debí quedarme donde estaba segura aunque aburrida.

"Está viva," dijo. "Eso no es cualquier cosa cuando se está bajo una amenaza de muerte de la S.E." Acomodó la lámpara haciéndola brillar en mi cara. Cerré los ojos dando un respingo apenas me puso una toalla fría en el párpado hinchado. Matalina comenzó a coser mi cuello y yo apenas sentía sus diminutas puntadas. No nos prestó mucha atención concentrada en su trabajo.

"Estaría muerta dos veces de no ser por Nick," dije mirando hacia la ducha.

Keasley apuntó la lámpara hacia mi oreja. Salté cuando la frotó con algodón húmedo con el que limpió la sangre vieja. "Usted habría escapado de Kalamack tarde o temprano. Pero en cambio asumió el riesgo de ayudar a escapar a Nick," dijo. "No veo dónde está el fracaso."

Lo miré con el ojo bueno entreabierto. "¿Cómo se enteró de la pelea de ratas?"

"Me lo dijo Jenks cuando veníamos hacia acá."

Satisfecha, hice una mueca cuando frotó un líquido maloliente en mi oreja herida. Vibré debajo de los tres amuletos contra el dolor. "Es todo lo que puedo hacer. Lo lamento."

Matalina voló frente a mis ojos mirándonos. "Terminado," dijo con su dulce voz de muñeca de porcelana. "Si usted puede terminar lo que falta, me gustaría…eh…" Sus ojos encantadores estaban impacientes. Parecía un ángel portador de buenas noticias. "Hablarle a Jenks acerca de su oferta de subarrendar el jardín."

Keasley asintió. "Ve tranquila," repuso. "Ahora sólo falta la muñeca."

"Gracias, Matalina," le dije. No sentía nada.

"No hay de qué." La diminuta duende salió disparada hacia la ventana y luego regresó. "Gracias a usted" susurró antes de desaparecer en la oscuridad del jardín.

La sala estaba desocupada. Quedamos solos Keasley y yo. Hacía tanto silencio que podíamos oír las tapas de las ollas de agua hirviendo que saltaban en la cocina. Keasley tomó las tijeras y cortó el algodón empapado que tenía en la muñeca. Apenas cayó, sentí nauseas en el estómago. Mi muñeca estaba aún allí, pero nada estaba en su lugar. Con razón el polvillo de duende de Jenks no logró detener la hemorra-

gia. Pedazos de carne blanca se amontonaban y tenía pequeños agujeros llenos de sangre. Si así estaba mi muñeca,
¿cómo estaría mi cuello? Cerré los ojos y me concentré en
respirar. Iba a perder el sentido. Lo presentía.

"Ahora ya tiene una aliada muy fuerte," dijo Keasley.

"¿Matalina?" dije conteniendo la respiración esperando
no hiperventilarme. "No se por qué" continué. "He puesto
en riesgo permanente a su marido y su familia."

"Ummm." Puso la olla de agua de Ivy sobre las rodillas metiendo lentamente mi muñeca en ella. Gemí al sentir el ardor
pero luego logré tranquilizarme al ver que los amuletos alejaban el dolor. Mi pinchó la muñeca y yo grité tratando de zafarme. "¿Quiere que le de un consejo?," preguntó.

"No."

"Muy bien. Escuche de todas formas. Me da la sensación
de que usted se ha convertido en un líder aquí. Acéptelo.
Sepa que eso tiene un precio. La gente hará cosas por usted.
No sea egoísta. Déjelos."

"Les debo la vida a Nick y a Jenks" dije, pero no me
gustó. "¿Qué tiene eso de extraordinario?"

"No. No es así. Gracias a usted, Nick ya no tiene que matar ratas para seguir con vida y la esperanza de vida de Jenks
se ha duplicado."

Retiré la mano y esta vez me soltó. "¿Cómo sabe eso?"
pregunté con desconfianza.

Keasley puso a un lado la olla y el golpe sobre la mesa fue
claro y seco. Puso una toalla rosada debajo de mi muñeca y
yo hice el esfuerzo de mirarla. El tejido se veía mejor. Salió
un lento brote de sangre que ocultó las heridas y fluyó sobre
mi piel mojada hacia la toalla empapada.

"Usted hizo a Jenks su socio," continuó mientras abría
una almohadilla de gasa para limpiarme. "Ahora tiene más
que cuidar que un empleo: tiene un jardín; y esta noche usted acaba de dárselo indefinidamente. Nunca he sabido que
alguien le arriende propiedades a los duendes, pero apuesto
a que las cortes Entremundos lo aceptarían en caso de que
otro clan la desafiara. Usted le garantizó que *todos* sus hijos

tendrán un lugar donde vivir hasta que sean adultos, no sólo los primeros. Eso para él debe ser el equivalente a una tarde jugando a las escondidas en un cuarto lleno de gente grande."

Observé cómo ensartaba un hilo en una aguja y me esforcé por mirar al techo. Los punzones y pinchazos empezaban lentamente. Todo el mundo sabía que los duendes y las hadas competían entre sí por un pequeño pedazo de tierra pero nunca pensé que tuvieran motivos tan profundos. Pensé en lo que Jenks había dicho acerca de arriesgar la vida por una picada de abeja por un miserable par de macetas con flores. Ahora tenía un jardín. Con razón Matalina había sido tan realista respecto al ataque de las hadas.

Ahora Keasley trabajaba con un ritmo de dos puntadas y un frote. El sangrado no se detenía. Yo no quise mirar. Pasé la mirada por la habitación gris hasta detenerlos en la mesita del fondo donde Ivy tenía sus revistas antes. Tragué saliva y sentí náuseas. "Keasley, usted ha vivido aquí algún tiempo, ¿verdad?" le pregunté. "¿Cuándo se mudó Ivy?"

Levantó la mirada de los puntos con asombro en su cara oscura y arrugada. "El mismo día que usted. Las dos se retiraron el mismo día, ¿no es así?"

Quise asentir pero me detuve. "Puedo entender por qué Jenks arriesga la vida por mí, pero..." le eché un vistazo al pasillo. "¿Qué gana Ivy con todo esto?" susurré.

Keasley miró mi cuello con repugnancia. "¿Acaso no es obvio?" Ella se alimenta de usted y a cambio evita que la S.E. la asesine.

Yo estaba indignada. "¡Ya le dije que Ivy no me hizo esto!" exclamé esforzándome para alzar la voz. "¡Fue un demonio!"

No pareció sorprenderse como esperaba. Se quedó mirándome esperando más. "Salí de la iglesia para buscar una receta" dije suavemente. "La S.E. me mandó un demonio que se transformó en vampiro para matarme. Nick lo encerró en un círculo, de lo contrario lo habría logrado." Me desvanecí exhausta. Sentía mi pulso martillar. Estaba demasiado débil hasta para molestarme.

"¿La S.E.?" dijo Keasley liberando la aguja y mirándome con el ceño fruncido. "¿Está segura de que era un demonio? La S.E. no usa demonios."

"Los usan ahora" repuse agriamente. Le di un rápido vistazo a mi muñeca y alejé la mirada. Aún sangraba. La sangre se coagulaba entre los puntos de las suturas, pero por lo menos se había detenido en mi cuello. "El demonio sabía mis tres nombres, Keasley. Mi segundo nombre ni siquiera está en mi registro de nacimiento. ¿Cómo pudo averiguarlo la S.E.?"

Keasley se veía preocupado mientras me secaba la muñeca.

"Si se trataba de un demonio entonces no debe preocuparse de quedar enlazada con los vampiros debido a las mordidas, creo."

"Pequeños favores" dije amargamente.

De nuevo tomó mi muñeca y acercó la lámpara. Puso otra toalla debajo para recoger la sangre que aún goteaba. "¿Raquel?" murmuró.

De repente sonaron las campanas de sospecha en mi cabeza. Siempre me había llamado señorita Morgan. "¿Qué?"

"Sobre el demonio, ¿hizo algún trato con él?"

Observé que su mirada seguía fija en mi muñeca y sentí miedo.

"Nick," respondí de inmediato. "Acordó dejarlo salir del círculo si me traía aquí con vida. Nos trajo por las líneas ley."

"Oh," respondió. Sentí que me helaba al oír el tono seco de su voz. Él sabía algo que yo no sabía.

"¿Qué?" le exigí. "¿Qué sucede?"

Tomó una lenta bocanada de aire. "Esto no va a sanar por sí sólo," dijo suavemente poniendo la muñeca sobre mis muslos.

"¿Qué?" exclamé tomándome la muñeca y sintiendo que

se me revolvía el estómago con el chocolate amenazando con devolverse. La ducha se apagó y sentí un instante de pánico. ¿Qué hizo Nick conmigo?

Keasley abrió un vendaje medicinal y lo puso sobre mi ojo. "Los demonios no hacen nada gratis," dijo. "Usted le debe un favor."

"¡Yo no acordé nada con él!" repuse. "¡Fue Nick! ¡Le dije a Nick que no lo dejara salir!"

"No es nada que haya hecho Nick," dijo Keasley tomando mi brazo herido frotándolo hasta que empecé a jadear. "El demonio quiere un pago extra por haberla traído a través de las líneas ley. Pero tiene opciones. Puede pagar ese viaje dejando que su muñeca gotee sangre el resto de su vida o deberle un favor al demonio y sanará. Yo le sugeriría lo último."

Me desmoroné en los cojines. "Qué bien." Maldición. Le pedí a Nick que no lo hiciera.

Keasley acercó mi muñeca hacia él y comenzó a vendarla con un rollo de gasa. La sangre la empapó tan rápido como le daba vueltas. "No permita que ese demonio no le permita a usted poner también condiciones" dijo mientras terminaba de colocarme todo el rollo sujetándolo al final con cinta adhesiva. "Puede negociar su paso hasta que lleguen a un acuerdo. Hasta puede negociar durante años. Los demonios dan opciones y son pacientes."

"¡Vaya opción!" exclamé. "Deberle un favor o vivir marcada el resto de la vida."

Se encogió de hombros mientras envolvía sus agujas, hilo y tijeras en el periódico para doblarlo. "A mí me parece que le fue muy bien para ser la primera vez que se enfrenta a un demonio."

"¡Primer enfrentamiento!" exclamé jadeando. *¿Primero? Como si fuera a tener otro.* "¿Cómo sabe usted todas estas cosas?" susurré.

Metió su periódico en la bolsa y dobló el borde hacia abajo. "Se vive bastante, se aprende bastante."

"Grandioso" Alcé la mirada al ver que Keasley me quitaba del cuello el amuleto más poderoso contra el dolor. "Aguarde" reclamé apenas sentí que regresaba el dolor con fuerza. "Necesito ese amuleto."

"Estará bien con dos." Se puso de pie y guardó el tercero en su bolsillo. "Así no se lastimará por tratar de hacer alguna cosa. Deje esos puntos una semana. Matalina le dirá cuándo se los puede quitar. No más transformaciones por ahora." Luego sacó un cabrestillo. "Úselo. Tiene el brazo herido. No está roto" dijo. Arqueó las cejas. "Tuvo suerte."

"Keasley, espere" dije, haciendo un esfuerzo por respirar y poner mi cabeza en orden. "¿Qué puedo hacer por usted? Hace una hora pensé que estaba muriendo."

"Hace una hora usted estaba muriendo" rió entre dientes. Luego se puso serio. "Es importante que no le deba nada a nadie, ¿no es así?" Dudó un instante. "La envidio por sus amigos. Ya estoy muy viejo y no me da miedo decirlo, pero los amigos son un lujo que no disfruto desde hace mucho tiempo. Si me deja confiar en usted, estamos a mano."

"Pero eso no es nada" protesté. "¿Necesita más plantas del jardín? ¿O una poción de visón? Aún está buena para un par de días y yo no la necesitaré más."

"No esté tan segura" dijo mirando hacia el pasillo al oír que se abría la puerta del baño. "Además, confiar en usted puede resultar costoso. Algún día podría necesitar esconderme. ¿Está dispuesta a aceptar?"

"Claro que sí" repuse, pensando de qué podría estar huyendo un viejo como Keasley. No podía ser algo peor de lo que me perseguía a mí. La puerta del santuario se cerró. Ivy ya había terminado de refunfuñar y Nick salió de la ducha. Muy pronto estarían enfrentándose otra vez y yo estaba muy cansada para hacer de árbitro. Jenks entró volando por la ventana y yo cerré los ojos para acumular fuerzas. Los tres juntos podían acabar de matarme.

Con su bolsa en la mano, Keasley dio media vuelta para salir. "Por favor, no se vaya todavía" le rogué. "Nick podría necesitar algo. Tiene una cortada grave en la cabeza."

"Raque" empezó Jenks volando alrededor de Keasley

para saludarlo. "¿Qué demonios le dijiste a Matalina? Está volando por todo el jardín como si estuviera bajo el efecto de azufre, riendo y llorando al mismo tiempo. No logro que esa mujer diga una sola palabra coherente." Se detuvo en pleno vuelo, sosteniéndose en el aire, escuchando.

"Oh grandioso," murmuró. "De nuevo están en las mismas."

Keasley y yo intercambiamos miradas a medida que nos llegaba la conversación del pasillo. Ivy entró poniendo cara de satisfacción y Nick la seguía de cerca. Cambió el ceño fruncido por una sonrisa cuando me vio sentada y de mejor semblante. Se había vestido con una camiseta blanca de algodón demasiado grande y un par de jeans limpios recién sacados de la secadora. Claro que su encantadora sonrisa no funcionó conmigo. La razón por la cual sangraba mi muñeca era demasiado grave.

"Usted debe ser Keasley" dijo Nick extendiendo la mano sobre la mesa como si nada hubiera pasado. "Yo soy Nick."

Keasley aclaró la garganta y le dio la mano. "Mucho gusto" respondió, aun cuando sus palabras no coincidían con su cara de desaprobación. "Raquel quiere que te examine la frente."

"Estoy bien. Dejó de sangrar en la ducha."

"¿De verdad?" Entrecerró los ojos. "La muñeca de Raquel no deja de sangrar."

Nick se puso lívido. Me miró y abrió la boca, pero de nuevo la cerró. Lo miré desafiante. Al infierno con todo. Él sabía exactamente lo que eso significaba. "Eh…ummm…" susurró.

"¿Qué?" presionó Ivy. Jenks aterrizó sobre su hombro pero ella lo espantó.

Nick se pasó la mano por la quijada sin decir palabra. Nick y yo íbamos a hablar…íbamos a hablar muy pronto. Keasley empujó agresivamente su bolsa de papel contra el pecho de Nick. "Sostén esto mientras preparo el baño de Raquel. Quiero asegurarme de que su temperatura sea la correcta."

Nick apenas retrocedió. Ivy nos miró a todos con sospecha. "Un baño," dije animadamente para que no se diera cuenta de que algo estaba mal. Sería capaz de matar a Nick si llegase a enterarse de lo sucedido. "Suena magnífico." Empujé la manta y el abrigo y giré los pies para ponerlos en el piso. Pero de pronto todo se oscureció y sentí frío.

"Aguarda, despacio" dijo Keasley poniendo su mano oscura sobre mi hombro. "Espera a que esté listo."

Respiré hondo pues no quería descansar la cabeza entre las piernas. Era tan poco decoroso.

Nick se veía enfermo ahí en el rincón. "Eh…creo que tendrás que esperar para bañarte. Acabé con el agua caliente."

"Está bien. Eso fue lo que te pedí que hicieras." Pero por dentro estaba siendo mordaz.

Keasley interrumpió. "Para eso son las ollas de agua."

Ivy puso mala cara. "¿Por qué no lo dijo antes?" gruñó mientras salía. "Yo lo haré."

"Fíjese que el agua no esté demasiado caliente" le dijo Keasley.

"Yo se cómo tratar la pérdida de sangre" repuso beligerante.

"Eso no lo dudo, jovencita." Luego dio media vuelta y empujó a Nick contra la pared. "Tú ve a decirle a la Srta. Morgan a lo que tiene que atenerse con su muñeca," le dijo arrebatándole la bolsa.

Nick asintió una vez, sorprendido del brujo pequeño y aparentemente inofensivo.

"Raque," dijo Jenks zumbando cerca. "¿Qué sucede con tu muñeca?"

"Nada."

"¿Qué está sucediendo con tu muñeca, Candela?"

"¡Nada!" respondí alejándolo con la mano casi jadeando por el esfuerzo.

"¿Jenks?" llamó Ivy por encima del sonido del agua de la llave. "Tráeme esa bolsa negra que hay en mi armario, ¿quieres? Voy a ponerla en el baño de Raquel."

"¿La que apesta a verbena?" repuso volando encima de mí.

"¡Te metiste entre mis cosas!" exclamó y Jenks sonrió avergonzado. "¡Apúrate!" agregó. "Cuanto antes esté Raquel en la tina más pronto nos largaremos de aquí. Mientras que ella esté bien tenemos que terminar su misión."

La idea del envío de Trent me regresó a la memoria. Miré el reloj y suspiré. Aún teníamos tiempo de avisarle a la AFE para atraparlo. Pero yo no participaría de ello desde ningún punto de vista.

Maldición.

Veintiocho

Deberían vender las burbujas como medicamento para el bienestar. Suspiré y me alcé un poco para meter el cuello en el agua. Opacados por los dos amuletos y el agua caliente, los latidos de dolor comenzaron a hacerse más leves. Hasta sentía mejor mi muñeca que tenía alzada sobre el borde seco de la tina. Podía escuchar a través de las paredes a Nick que hablaba por teléfono con su madre contándole que tuvo muchísimo trabajo durante los últimos tres meses, disculpándose por no haberla llamado. Aparte de eso, la iglesia estaba en silencio. Jenks e Ivy no estaban. "Estaban haciendo mi trabajo" susurré con amargura.

"¿Cómo dijo, Srta. Raquel?" dijo Matalina. La mujercita estaba parada sobre un montón de toallas y parecía un ángel con su vestido de seda blanca bordando un hermoso chal con retoños de flores de cerezo para su hija mayor. Me acompañaba desde que me metí a la tina para asegurarse de que no perdiera el sentido y me ahogara.

"Nada" dije, alzando difícilmente mi brazo herido acercando más las burbujas. El agua empezaba a enfriarse y mi estómago hacía ruidos. El baño de Ivy tenía un aspecto misterioso como el de mi madre, con pequeños jabones en forma de conchas y cortinas de encajes en los vitrales de colores. Había un florero de violetas en la cómoda y me llamó la atención que un vampiro se interesara por esas cosas. La tina era negra haciendo contraste con las paredes color pastel decorado con botones de rosas.

Matalina dejó su encaje de lado y voló encima de la porcelana negra. "¿Está bien que sus amuletos se mojen?"

Miré los hechizos contra el dolor que colgaban de mi cuello y pensé que me veía como una prostituta borracha el día de Mardi Gras. "Están bien" suspiré. "El agua con jabón no los disuelve como el agua salada."

"La Srta. Tamwood no quiso decirme qué le puso al baño," dijo Matalina preocupada. "Podría contener sal."

Ivy tampoco me dijo nada, pero a decir verdad, no quería saberlo. "No tiene sal. Ya pregunté."

Matalina aterrizó sobre mi dedo gordo que sobresalía del agua. Sus alitas se veían borrosas y en el agua se formó un espacio libre de burbujas. Levantándose el vestido, se inclinó cuidadosamente hundiendo una mano y llevándose una gota hasta la nariz. Formó hondas diminutas en el agua.

"Verbena," dijo con voz aguda. "Mi Jenks tenía razón. Sanguinaria, Sello de Oro." Nuestros ojos se encontraron. "Se usan para cubrir cosas muy potentes. ¿Qué estará tratando de ocultar?"

Mire hacia el techo. Mientras me aliviara el dolor, no me importaba.

De repente se escucharon pasos en las tablas de madera del pasillo y me quedé quieta. "¿Nick?" pregunté, viendo que la toalla estaba lejos de mi alcance. "Aún estoy en la tina. ¡No entres!"

Se detuvo de inmediato junto al enchape de madera que nos separaba. "Eh...hola Raquel, sólo quería saber cómo estás." Hubo un instante de duda. "Eh...necesito hablar contigo."

Se me revolvió el estómago cuando miré hacia la muñeca. Aún sangraba empapando la gasa de dos centímetros de grosor. El hilillo de sangre encima de la tina parecía un ribete. Tal vez por eso Ivy tenía una tina negra. La sangre no contrastaba tanto en el negro como en el blanco.

"¿Raquel?" dijo de nuevo ante mi silencio.

"Estoy bien" repuse fuerte. Mi voz rebotó en las paredes rosadas. "Dame un minuto para salir de la tina, ¿de acuerdo? Yo también necesito hablar contigo, pequeño brujo."

Dije lo último con malicia y sentí que daba media vuelta. "No soy brujo," contestó en voz baja. "¿Tienes hambre? Puedo preparar algo de comer." En su voz presentía culpabilidad.

"Sí, gracias" repuse, con la esperanza de que se alejara de la puerta. Tenía un hambre canina. Tal vez mi apetito se debía a una galleta parecida a un pastellillo que Ivy me hizo comer antes de salir. Era tan fea como un panqueque de arroz y después de que logré tragarla Ivy me dijo que mejoraría mi metabolismo, especialmente la producción de sangre. Aún sentía el sabor en la garganta. Era una especie de mezcla entre almendras, bananos y cuero de zapatos.

Nick se alejó y yo traté de alcanzar la llave del agua caliente con el pie. Seguro que el agua del calentador ya estaba caliente.

"No querida, no la calientes" advirtió Matalina. "Ivy dijo que salieras una vez estuviera fría."

¡Qué molestia! Sabía lo que había dicho Ivy pero me abstuve de hacer cualquier comentario.

Me alcé lentamente para sentarme en el borde de la tina. Sentí que se oscurecía el cuarto y me envolví instintivamente con una toalla rosada en caso de que perdiera el conocimiento. Cuando desapareció el gris, tiré del tapón de la tina y me levanté con cuidado. Se desocupó ruidosamente y limpié el vapor del espejo. Me incliné sobre el lavamanos para mirarme.

Escuché un suspiro y giré el cuerpo. Matalina aterrizó sobre mis hombros mirándome con tristeza. Me veía como si hubiera caído de un camión. Tenía un lado de la cara con un verdugón morado que me llegaba hasta el ojo. La venda de Keasley se había caído dejando expuesta una herida que seguía el contorno de la ceja. Me veía terriblemente. Ni siquiera me acordaba de esa herida. Me acerqué más para verme mejor. Entonces reuní fuerzas para quitarme el pelo greñudo del cuello.

Dejé salir un suspiro de resignación. El demonio no había hecho perforaciones claras sino más bien tres grupos de rasgados que se unían entre sí como ríos y tributarios. Las puntadas de Matalina parecían diminutas líneas de tren recorriendo mi clavícula.

Sentí escalofríos al recordar al demonio. Estuve cerca de morir. El sólo recuerdo me aterrorizaba; pero lo que realmente me desvelaría todas las noches sería el hecho de que, a pesar del terror y el dolor, la saliva de vampiro que me inyectó en la sangre me hizo sentir bien. Verdadera o falsa, la sentí sorprendentemente maravillosa.

Me envolví más fuerte con la toalla y di media vuelta.

"Gracias Matalina," susurré. "No creo que las cicatrices se noten demasiado."

"No hay de qué, querida. Es lo menos que podía hacer. ¿Quiere que la acompañe a vestirse?"

"No." Escuché el sonido de la mezcladora en la cocina. Abrí la puerta y le eché un vistazo al pasillo. Olí el aroma de huevos. "Creo que puedo hacerlo sola."

La pequeña mujer asintió y salió volando con su encaje, sus alitas produciendo un suave zumbido. Me quedé escuchando un buen rato hasta cerciorarme de que Nick estaba bien ocupado. Llegué hasta mi habitación cojeando y respirando aliviada por haber llegado sin que me viera.

Me senté en el borde de la cama para recuperar las fuerzas y mi cabello aun goteaba agua. No me gustaba la idea de ponerme pantalones, pero tampoco podía vestirme con falda y medias. Al final me decidí por los jeans amplios y una camisa escocesa fácil de poner sin tener que pasar tanto dolor del brazo y el hombro. Jamás me verían vestida a sí en la calle, pero la verdad es que no estaba interesada en atraer a Nick.

El piso todavía me daba vueltas mientras que me vestía y las paredes parecían inclinarse si me movía muy rápido, pero al final lograba recuperarme gracias a mis dos húmedos amuletos que colgaban de mi cuello. Caminé por el pasillo con mis pantuflas arrastrando los pies. Tal vez debía cubrir mis heridas en la cara con un hechizo, pues el maquillaje corriente no haría el trabajo.

Nick salió corriendo de la cocina buscándome con un sándwich en la mano. "Ahí estás" dijo con los ojos bien abiertos mirándome de pies a cabeza. "¿Quieres un sándwich de huevo?"

"No, gracias" repuse. Mi estómago hacía ruidos. "Demasiado azufre." Recordé la imagen de Nick sosteniendo ese libro negro mientras lanzaba una mano para detener en seco a ese demonio: asustado, temeroso y poderoso. Jamás había visto a un humano poderoso. Fue sorprendente. "Más bien necesito ayuda para cambiar el vendaje de mi muñeca," concluí cáusticamente.

Entonces se encogió destruyendo la imagen que había formado en mi cabeza.

"Discúlpame Raquel"

Seguí de largo y entré a la cocina. Sus pasos me seguían ligeros. Yo me incliné sobre el fregadero para darle de comer a Don Pez. Afuera estaba completamente oscuro y podía ver los pequeños destellos de luz que emitía la familia de Jenks vigilando el jardín. Me llamó la atención ver el tomate de nuevo en la ventana. Sentí preocupación y maldije mentalmente a Ivy. Fruncí el ceño. ¿Qué me importa lo que piense Nick? Esta era mi casa. Yo era un Entremundos. Si no le gustaba, peor para él.

Nick estaba detrás de mí, en la mesa. "Raquel, de verdad lo lamento" siguió. Yo di media vuelta con los brazos cruzados. Si perdía el conocimiento, mi indignación no tendría ningún efecto. "No sabía que tú tendrías que pagar. Lo digo de verdad."

Molesta, alejé el pelo mojado de mis ojos y permanecí parada con los brazos cruzados. "Esto es una deuda con un demonio, Nick, un maldito y miserable demonio."

Nick dobló su desgarbado cuerpo sobre uno de los asientos. Con los codos sobre la mesa, puso la cabeza entre las manos. Con la vista fija en la mesa dijo: "La demonología es una disciplina muerta. Nunca pensé que tuviera que poner en práctica mis conocimientos. La estudié sólo para obtener fácilmente las clases requeridas para lenguas extranjeras."

Alzó la cabeza para mirarme. Su preocupación, su necesidad de que lo escuchara y comprendiera me hicieron controlar mi siguiente comentario.

"De verdad que lo lamento" dijo. "Si pudiera transferir tu deuda hacia mí lo haría. Yo pensé que morirías. No podía dejar que eso sucediera en el asiento trasero de un taxi."

Poco a poco mi rabia desapareció. Había estado dispuesto a aceptar una deuda con un demonio para salvarme, pero no estaba obligado a hacerlo. Era una estúpida.

Nick movió el cabello de su sien izquierda. "Mira. ¿Ves cómo ya no sangra?"

Miré su piel justo donde lo había golpeado el demonio. Tenía una dolorosa herida roja recientemente cicatrizada. En medio del círculo había una línea. ¡Maldición! Ahora yo tendría que vivir con una marca demoníaca. Las brujas negras de líneas ley tenían marcas demoníacas, pero no las brujas blancas terrestres. ¡Yo no!

Nick dejó caer su cabello otra vez. "Desaparecerá cuando pague el favor. No es permanente."

"¿Favor?" pregunté.

Entrecerró sus ojos pardos rogando comprensión. "Tal vez sea algo así como información. Al menos eso es lo que dicen los textos."

Alcé una mano pasando los dedos por la frente. En realidad no tenía opción. No era como si Kotex vendiera toallas para estas cosas. "Entonces ¿cómo le hago saber al demonio que estoy de acuerdo en deberle un favor?"

"¿Estás de acuerdo?"

"Sí."

"Acabas de hacerlo."

Sentí que enfermaba. No me gustaba estar atada a un demonio de tal manera que pudiera enterarse instantáneamente que estaba de acuerdo con sus términos. "¿Nada de documentos? ¿Nada de contratos?," pregunté. "No me gustan los acuerdos verbales."

"Si quieres que venga aquí para firmar papeles sólo tienes que pensarlo. Vendrá."

"No." Mis ojos se fijaron sobre la muñeca y sentí un cosquilleo. Me asombré cuando sentí que aumentaba hasta convertirse en una rasquiña que luego fue ardor. "¿Dónde están las tijeras?" pregunté muy seria. Nick miró alrededor pero ahora sentía como si mi muñeca estuviera en llamas. "¡Me quema!," grité. El dolor crecía mientras trataba frenéticamente de quitarme la gasa.

"¡Quítamela! ¡Quítamela!" grité. Girando, abrí toda la llave del agua y metí la muñeca debajo. El agua fría atravesó la gasa aliviando la sensación de fuego. Me incliné sobre el fregadero con el pulso palpitante mientras que el agua aliviaba mi dolor.

La brisa húmeda de la noche pasaba a través de las cortinas mientras miraba el jardín oscuro y el cementerio esperando a que desaparecieran los puntos oscuros. Sentía débiles las rodillas pues sólo la adrenalina me mantenía de pie. Luego sentí el sonido de las tijeras que Nick arrastró sobre la mesa.

Cerré la llave. "Gracias por la advertencia" le dije sarcásticamente.

"A mí no me dolió" repuso. Estaba preocupado, confundido y perplejo. Tomé la toalla de secar los platos y las tijeras y me dirigí hacia mi puesto en la mesa. Metí las tijeras entre la gasa empapada y comencé a cortar. Le lancé una mirada a Nick que estaba parado junto al fregadero con cara de culpa. Yo estaba en crisis.

"Discúlpame por rezongar tanto Nick," dije cambiando de opinión. Decidí desenvolver la gasa en lugar de cortarla. "De no ser por tí estaría muerta. Tuve suerte de que estuvieras allí para evitarlo. Te debo la vida y de verdad te agradezco lo que hiciste." Hubo un momento de silencio. "Esa cosa me aterró. Sólo quería olvidarla, pero ahora no puedo. No sé cómo reaccionar. Por eso me es fácil gritarte."

Nick dejó salir una tímida sonrisa y acercó una silla para sentarse a mi lado. "Déjame ayudarte," dijo, y me tomó la mano.

Al principio dudé, pero luego dejé que pusiera mi muñeca sobre sus muslos. Inclinó la cabeza sobre mi mano y sus rodillas casi tocaban las mías. Creo que le debía más que sólo gracias. "¿Nick? Lo digo en serio. Gracias. Me has salvado la vida dos veces. Esta cuestión estará bien. Lamento que ahora tengas una marca demoníaca por ayudarme."

Nick alzó la cabeza buscando mis ojos con su mirada. De pronto caí en la cuenta de lo cerca que estaba. Recordé cuando me tenía abrazada y me entró cargada a la iglesia. ¿Me habría tenido en sus brazos cuando cruzamos el más allá?

"Me alegro que estaba allí para ayudar" dijo suavemente. "En realidad, fue culpa mía."

"No. Me hubiera encontrado en cualquier sitio" repuse. Finalmente había quitado la última venda. Tragué saliva y miré mi muñeca. Estaba totalmente sana. Hasta los puntos verdes habían desaparecido. La cicatriz blanca parecía vieja. La mía era en forma de círculo con la misma línea que la cruzaba.

"Vaya," dijo Nick recostándose hacia atrás. "Creo que le gustas a ese demonio. A mi no me sanó del todo. Sólo detuvo la sangre."

"Ummm." Froté la marca que tenía en la muñeca. Me pareció mejor que la venda, eso creía. La gente no sabría de qué se trataba esa cicatriz pues nadie había visto demonios desde el Giro. "¿Ahora sólo tengo que esperar a que me pida algo?"

"Así es." Nick se levantó para dirigirse hacia la estufa.

Descansé los codos sobre la mesa y sentí cómo entraba el

aire a mis pulmones. Nick estaba frente a la estufa dándome la espalda pero el silencio creció volviéndose incómodo.

"¿Te gusta la comida de estudiantes?" preguntó súbitamente.

"¿Cómo dices?"

"Comida de estudiantes." Sus ojos se fijaron en el tomate de la ventana. "Lo que haya en el refrigerador mezclado con pasta."

Preocupada, me puse de pie y caminé hasta allá para ver qué había en la estufa. Había macarrones en una olla. Junto a ella había una cuchara de palo y levanté las cejas. "¿Usaste esa cuchara?" le pregunté.

Nick asintió. "Sí. ¿Por qué?"

Alcancé la sal y desocupé todo el recipiente en el agua.

"¡Oye!" exclamó Nick. "Ya le puse sal al agua. No se necesita tanta."

Sin prestarle atención, lancé la cuchara en mi vasija de disolución y saqué una de metal. "Hasta tanto no recupere mis cucharas de barro, el metal es para cocinar y la madera para conjurar. Enjuaga bien esos macarrones. Estarán bien."

Nick alzó las cejas. "Yo habría pensado que usabas cucharas metálicas para conjuros y de madera para cocinar puesto que los hechizos no se pegan al metal."

Me acerqué lentamente al refrigerador sintiendo que aumentaban los latidos de mi corazón inclusive por este mínimo esfuerzo. "¿Por qué crees que los hechizos no se pegan al metal? A menos que se trate de cobre, los metales echan todo a perder. Si no te importa, yo haré los hechizos y tú te dedicas a preparar la cena."

Sorprendentemente, Nick no se enfurruñó ni se puso a la defensiva. Sólo se sonrió.

De pronto sentí dolor a pesar de los amuletos cuando traté de abrir el refrigerador. "No puedo creer el hambre que tengo" dije mientras buscaba algo que no estuviera envuelto en papel o en plástico. "Creo que Ivy me dio algo sin darme cuenta."

Nick desocupó el agua para escurrir los macarrones. "¿En la galleta?"

Saqué la cabeza y le hice una seña con un ojo. ¿A él también? "Sí."

"Lo vi." Tenía los ojos puestos en el tomate mientras salía vapor del fregadero. "Cuando estaba escribiendo mi tesis de maestría tuve acceso a la bóveda de libros curiosos. Queda justo al lado del depósito de libros antiguos. El caso es que los diseños arquitectónicos de las catedrales preindustriales son aburridos y una noche encontré el diario de un sacerdote británico del siglo diecisiete. Lo habían juzgado y acusado de asesinar a tres de sus feligreses más bonitas."

Nick devolvió la pasta a la olla y abrió un frasco de salsa Alfredo. "Allí hablaba de esa sustancia. Decía que eso permitía que los vampiros tuvieran orgías de sangre y lujuria todas las noches. Desde el punto de vista científico deberías considerarte con suerte. Supongo que rara vez se lo dan a alguien que no pertenezca a su esfera y luego están obligados a mantener la boca cerrada."

Me sentí intranquila. ¿Qué demonios me dio Ivy?

Sin quitarle los ojos al tomate, Nick desocupó la salsa en la pasta. La cocina se llenó de un exquisito aroma y mi estómago comenzó a hacer ruido. Mientras revolvía, Nick miraba el tomate en la ventana. Se veía enfermo. Desesperada por la repulsión ilógica de los humanos por los tomates, cerré la refrigeradora y me acerqué a la ventana. "¿Cómo entró esto aquí?," musité. Lo metí en el agujero del duende tirándolo al jardín. Lo sentí caer.

"Gracias," dijo respirando tranquilo.

Yo regresé a mi asiento suspirando. Pensaba que Ivy y yo nos habíamos ganado a un cabezón, pero al menos era satisfactorio saber que al menos tenía un defecto humano.

Nick siguió cocinando agregándole champiñones, salsa de Worcestershire y salchichón a la mezcla. Sonreí al darme cuenta que se trataba de uno de los ingredientes de mi última pizza. Olía bien y apenas tomó el cucharón que colgaba de la mesa le pregunté: "¿Hay suficiente para dos?"

"Hay suficiente para todo un dormitorio." Nick me pasó un plato hondo y se sentó abrazando el suyo. "Comida de estudiantes" dijo con la boca llena. "Pruébala."

Miré el reloj encima del lavadero. Seguramente Ivy y Jenks estaban ahora en la AFE tratando de convencer al tipo de la portería de que no eran unos simples tontos. Y yo aquí, comiendo macarrones Alfredo con un humano. No era normal. Me refiero a la comida. Habría sido mejor con una salsa de tomates. Probé con algo de dudas. "Vaya," dije satisfecha. "Está muy buena."

"Te lo dije."

Por unos momento sólo se escucharon los sonidos de las cucharas y el canto de los grillos en el jardín. Nick comenzó a comer más lentamente y miró el reloj. "Eh...sabes..." dijo un poco dudoso. "Tengo que pedirte un gran favor."

Tragué y alcé la cabeza. Imaginaba lo que iba a decir. "Puedes quedarte aquí esta noche si quieres," le dije. "Pero no te garantizo que despiertes con todos tus líquidos completos o a lo mejor sin líquidos." La S.E. me tiene en la mira. Ahora apenas son esas hadas asesinas pero tan pronto corra la voz de que sigo con vida, es posible que quedemos a merced de ellos. Creo que estarías más seguro en un banco de un parque."

"Gracias" repuso. "Creo que me arriesgaré. Ya mañana te dejaré tranquila. Veré si aún haya algo que me pertenezca, iré donde mamá" Se veía muy preocupado, tanto como cuando pensó que moriría desangrada. "Le diré que lo perdí todo en un incendio. No será fácil."

Sentí un golpe de compasión. Yo sabía lo que era hallarse en la calle con una caja llena como única propiedad en la vida. "¿Estás seguro de que no quieres quedarte con ella esta noche? Es mucho más seguro."

Nick siguió comiendo. "Puedo cuidarme solo."

Sí, seguro, pensé, recordando ese libro sobre demonios que tomó de la biblioteca. Ya no estaba en mi bolso. Apenas quedaba una pequeña mancha de sangre para demostrar su existencia. Quería preguntarle si había hecho magia negra, pero si respondía que sí, entonces tendría que decidir qué hacer con él y no quería hacer eso en este momento. Me gustaba la confianza que Nick tenía en sí mismo y ver esa virtud en un humano era intrigante.

Una parte de mí rechazaba la idea de que me atraía por aquello del síndrome de la dama en apuros rescatada y en este momento yo necesitaba algo de seguridad en mi vida. Un humano que sabía magia y que podía mantener a los demonios a raya antes de que me rasgaran la garganta no estaba mal, sobre todo con un aspecto tan inofensivo con el suyo.

"Además," dijo Nick echándolo todo a perder, "Jenks me hechizaría si me voy antes de que regrese."

Exhalé desilusionada y molesta. Nick estaba haciendo de niñera.

De pronto sonó el teléfono. Miré a Nick sin moverme. Todo me dolía. Maldición.

Sonrió a medias y se puso de pie. "Yo contesto." Seguí comiendo mientras el desaparecía pensando que le diría que fuéramos de compras juntos tan pronto consiguiera algo de ropa nueva. Los jeans le quedaban demasiado anchos.

"¿Sí?" contestó Nick con voz sorprendentemente profesional. "Morgan, Tamwood y Jenks, servicio de agentes vampiros y brujos."

¿Servicio de agentes vampiros y brujos? pensé. Un poco de Ivy, un poco de mí. Estaba bien. Soplé la siguiente cucharada pensando que tampoco cocinaba nada mal.

"¿Jenks?" dijo Nick. Yo dudé y alcé la cabeza para ver a Nick que aparecía en el pasillo con el teléfono. "Está comiendo. ¿Ya están en el aeropuerto?"

Siguió una pausa larga y suspiré. La AFE era más abierta y estaba más interesada en ponerle el guante a Trent de lo que imaginé.

"¿La AFE?" dijo Nick ahora con tono preocupado. Me puse seria oyendo lo que siguió. "¿Ella hizo qué? ¿Hay algún muerto?"

Cerré los ojos lentamente por un instante dejando de lado

la cuchara. La comida de Nick me supo amarga y tragué con dificultad.

"Eh...sí, claro" dijo, entrecerrando los ojos. "Danos media hora." Colgó. Me miró a los ojos y dijo: "Tenemos problemas."

Veintinueve

Me incliné hacia la derecha del taxi mientras daba una curva cerrada. El dolor traspasaba mis amuletos y sólo atinaba a aferrarme a mi bolso sintiéndome muy mal. El chofer era humano y había dejado muy claro que no le gustaba manejar en Los Hollows después de oscurecer. No dejó de murmurar hasta que cruzó el río Ohio y sintió que estaba de nuevo donde permanecía la "gente decente." Para sus ojos, lo único que nos salvaba era que nos había recogido en una iglesia y que íbamos para la AFE: "Una institución decente del lado de la ley."

"Muy bien," dije a medida que Nick me ayudaba a sentarme derecha. "De modo que esa gente buena y decente de la AFE estaba acosando a Ivy y jugando al policía rudo. Alguien la tocó y…"

"Estalló" concluyó Nick. "Se necesitaron ocho policías para controlarla. Jenks dice que tres están en el hospital bajo observación. Otros cuatro fueron dados de alta."

"Idiotas," murmuré. "¿Y Jenks?"

Nick estiró un brazo al detenernos repentinamente frente a un gran edificio de vidrio. "Lo soltarán cuando llegue una persona responsable." Se veía un poco nervioso pero continuó. "Y en el caso de que no haya ninguna, entonces te lo darán a ti."

"Ja, ja" reí secamente. Miré a través del sucio vidrio del taxi y vi un letrero que decía: AGENCIA FEDERAL EN-

TREMUNDOS en las dos puertas. Nick salió primero y me ofreció la mano para ayudarme. Me bajé lentamente tratando de orientarme mientras que él le pagaba al taxista con el dinero que le di. Estaba claro bajo las luces de la calle y asombrosamente había poco tráfico para esa hora. Estábamos en el distrito humano de Cincinnati. Al ver el imponente edificio no pude menos que sentirme en minoría y muy nerviosa.

Escudriñé las ventanas oscuras a mi alrededor buscando señas de un posible ataque. Jax dijo que las hadas asesinas se fueron inmediatamente después de la llamada telefónica. *¿Para llamar refuerzos o tenderme una emboscada aquí?* No me gustaba la idea de hadas catapultas tomando impulso mientras que yo esperaba. Claro que ni siquiera un hada sería tan audaz de atacarme dentro del edificio de la AFE, pero en la acera era un blanco.

Por otra parte, era posible que las hubieran relevado de la misión puesto que ahora la S.E. estaba mandando demonios. Sentí un poco de satisfacción al pensar que ese demonio ya habría destrozado a quien lo invocó. No creía que fueran a mandar otro por el momento. La magia negra siempre regresa para atraparte. Siempre.

"Usted debería cuidar mejor a su hermana" dijo el taxista tomando el dinero. Nick y yo nos miramos asombrados. "De todas formas, yo creo que ustedes los Entremundos no se preocupan tanto por los demás como nosotros, la gente decente. Volvería papilla a cualquiera que se atreviera a tocar a mi hermana" agregó antes de arrancar.

Me quedé confundida mirando las luces del auto hasta que Nick dijo: "Cree que alguien te dio una paliza y que venimos a presentar una demanda."

Estaba demasiado nerviosa para reír y además me habría hecho perder el conocimiento, pero al menos sonreí apoyándome en su brazo para no caer. Alzando las cejas, Nick abrió la puerta de vidrio para mí como todo un caballero. De repente, me invadió la angustia tan pronto crucé la puerta. Me estaba poniendo en la posición de confiar en una institución manejada por humanos. Estaba caminando en arena movediza y no me gustaba.

El sonido de la gente hablando y el olor a café recalentado me eran familiares y me tranquilizaron un poco. Por todas partes sentía que estaba en una institución: piso de baldosas grises, gente hablando fuerte, sillas anaranjadas y padres preocupados por los jóvenes en dificultades que estaban sentados en ellas. Sentí que entraba a mi casa y mis hombros se aflojaron un poco.

"Ummm, allá" dijo Nick indicando el mostrador de la recepción. Mi brazo palpitaba en el cabestrillo y me dolía el hombro. O bien estaba disolviendo los amuletos con mi sudor o el exceso de esfuerzo los estaba anulando. Nick caminaba detrás de mí y eso me molestaba.

La secretaria de la recepción me miró con ojos de asombro. "Por Dios cariño, ¿qué te sucedió?" preguntó en voz baja.

"Eh…este…" hice una mueca poniendo los codos en el mostrador para pararme firme. El hechizo para la cara no era suficiente para ocultar mi ojo morado ni los puntos. ¿Qué se supone que debía a decirle? ¿Que había un demonio suelto en Cincinnati otra vez? Miré detrás de mí pero Nick no era de mucha ayuda. Estaba mirando hacia la puerta. "Eh…" tartamudeé. "Vengo a recoger a alguien."

"Espero que no sea el que te hizo eso."

No pude evitar sonreír por su preocupación. Le agradecí su compasión. "No."

La mujer se acomodó un mechón de pelo gris detrás de la oreja. "No quisiera tener que decirte esto, pero tienes que dirigirte a la oficina de la calle Hillman y esperar hasta mañana. No dejan salir a nadie después de las horas de oficina."

Suspiré. Detestaba el laberinto de la burocracia con toda el alma pero había descubierto que la mejor forma de lidiar con ella es sonreír y hacerse el estúpido. Así nadie se confunde. "Pero acabo de hablar con una persona hace menos de veinte minutos," insistí. "Me dijeron que viniera."

Se asombró y puso una expresión de asombro. "Ah," repuso mirándome de lado. "Tú vienes por…" dudó un instante, "¿duende?" Se frotó una pequeña ampolla detrás del cuello. La había hechizado un duende.

Nick aclaró la garganta. "Se llama Jenks" dijo secamente con la cabeza agachada. Se había dado cuenta de que por poco dijo "insecto."

"Sí," dijo despacio mientras bajaba la mano para rascarse el tobillo. "El señor Jenks. ¿Podrían tomar asiento allá?" nos dijo señalando con la mano. "Los atenderán tan pronto el capitán Edden esté disponible."

"El capitán Edden." Tomé a Nick del brazo. "Gracias." Me sentía vieja y cansada y me dirigí hacia las horribles sillas anaranjadas que estaban contra las paredes del vestíbulo. No me extrañó el cambio de actitud de la señora. En un instante pasé de ángel a ramera. A pesar de que había vivido con humanos durante cuarenta años me sentía tensa. Vivían asustados y tenían sus buenas razones para estarlo. No es fácil levantarse y saber que los vecinos son vampiros y que la maestra de cuarto grado en realidad es una bruja.

Nick escudriñó el vestíbulo con la mirada mientras me ayudaba a sentarme. Las sillas eran tan desagradables como lo había imaginado: duras e incómodas. Nick se sentó a mi lado en el borde de una de ellas. "¿Cómo te sientes?" me preguntó. Yo refunfuñaba tratando de acomodarme más cómodamente.

"Bien" repuse. "Muy bien." Hice una mueca siguiendo a dos guardias de uniforme con la mirada. Uno caminaba con muletas. El otro tenía un ojo negro que comenzaba a ponerse morado y se rascaba los hombros vigorosamente. *Mil gracias Jenks e Ivy.* Otra vez me sentí intranquila. ¿Ahora cómo convencería al capitán de la AFE para que me ayudara?

"¿Quieres comer algo?" dijo Nick atrayendo mi atención de nuevo. "Puedo ir al otro lado de la calle por algo. ¿Te gustan los helados de pacana?"

"No." Me salió más brusco de lo que pensé y sonreí para suavizar mi respuesta. "No, gracias" corregí. Sentía la preocupación en la boca del estómago.

"¿Qué tal algo de la máquina de dulces? ¿Sal y carbohidratos?" agregó. "Comida de campeones."

Agité la cabeza y puse mi bolso en medio de los pies. Traté de mantener calmada la respiración concentrándome en el rayado piso de baldosas. Si comía algo, iba a vomitar. Había comido otro plato de macarrones antes de que llegara el taxi por nosotros, pero ese no era el problema.

"¿Se acaba el poder de los amuletos?" adivinó Nick y yo lo confirmé.

De repente se detuvieron un par de zapatos pardos frente a mí. Nick se sentó bien con los brazos cruzados y yo alcé la cabeza.

Era un hombre fornido vestido con camisa blanca y caqui, esbelto y con apariencia de haber estado en la armada antes de pasar a la vida civil. Usaba lentes con aros plásticos pero demasiado pequeños para su cara redonda. Olía a jabón y su cabello corto estaba húmedo. Estaba parado como si fuera un bebé orangután. Pude intuir que lo habían hechizado pero tuvo la precaución de darse un baño antes de que le salieran ampollas. Llevaba la muñeca derecha vendada en un cabestrillo idéntico al mío. Cabello negro corto y bigote negro corto. Ojalá tuviera buen humor. "¿Srta. Morgan?" preguntó. Yo me enderecé con un suspiro. "Soy el capitán Edden."

Grandioso, pensé, esforzándome por ponerme de pie. Nick me ayudó. Caí en la cuenta de que podía mirar a Edden directamente a los ojos y que así disminuía un poco esa actitud tan oficial. Hasta me atrevería a decir que tenía algo de sangre de gnomo, si es que aquello era biológicamente posible. Mis ojos se fijaron en el arma que portaba alrededor de la cintura. Por un momento deseé tener otra vez mis esposas de la S.E. Entrecerró los ojos por la intensidad de mi perfume y me ofreció la mano izquierda en lugar de la derecha, puesto que ninguno de los dos podíamos utilizarla.

Mi pulso se aceleró mientras nos saludábamos. Era incómodo y habría preferido saludarlo de nuevo con la derecha. "Buenas tardes, capitán" dije tratando de ocultar mi nerviosismo. "Este es Nick Sparagmos. Me ayuda a mantenerme en pie."

Edden le hizo un gesto cortés a Nick, pero dudó un instante. "Sr. Sparagmos...¿nos hemos conocido anteriormente?"

"No. Creo que no."

Nick habló muy rápido y yo lo examiné con los ojos de pies a cabeza. Nick había estado antes aquí y estoy segura de que no fue para recoger los boletos de la cena anual de beneficencia de la AFE.

"¿Está seguro?" preguntó el hombre pasándose la mano por el pelo.

"Sí."

El capitán lo siguió mirando. "Sí," dijo abruptamente. "Creo que estoy pensando en otra persona."

Nick se relajó imperceptiblemente haciendo aumentar mi interés.

La mirada del capitán Edden se concentró en mi cuello. Tal vez debería cubrir mis heridas y puntos con una bufanda o algo por el estilo. "¿Tendrían la amabilidad de seguirme?" dijo el fornido hombre. "Quisiera hablar con usted antes de dejar al duende bajo su custodia."

Nick se puso serio. "Se llama Jenks" musitó, apenas perceptible por el ruido del vestíbulo.

"Sí. El Sr. Jenks." Edden hizo una pausa. "Vengan a mi oficina del fondo."

"¿Y qué hay de Ivy?" le pregunté. No quería abandonar el área pública del vestíbulo. Mi pulso comenzó a acelerarse. Apenas tenía energías para mantenerme de pie. Si caminaba rápido perdería el conocimiento.

"La Srta. Tamwood permanecerá donde está ahora. Será entregada a la S.E. en la mañana para que inicien un proceso judicial."

La rabia pudo más que la precaución. "Usted debió pensar antes de tocar a un vampiro furioso," le dije. Nick me apretó el brazo. De todas formas yo no podía zafarme de él.

Edden dejó escapar una leve sonrisa. "No importa. Atacó

al personal de la AFE. Tengo las manos atadas con respecto a Tamwood. Nosotros no estamos preparados para lidiar con Entremundos." Luego dudó. "¿Quiere venir a mi oficina? Podemos discutir sus opciones."

Mi preocupación creció aún más. Nada le agradaría más a Denon que encarcelar a Ivy. Nick me pasó mi bolso y moví la cabeza. Esto se veía mal. Parecía que Edden hubiera acosado a Ivy hasta hacerla perder el control para hacerme venir hasta acá con el sombrero en la mano. Seguí a Edden hasta una oficina con paredes de cristales en una esquina del vestíbulo. Al principio me pareció que quedaba alejada de todo, pero si recogía las persianas podía verlo todo. Ahora estaban cerradas para que su oficina no pareciera una pecera. Dejó la puerta abierta y se oían todos los ruidos de afuera.

"Tome asiento" dijo, señalando las dos sillas verdes frente a su escritorio. Me senté agradecida. Estas sillas eran un poco más cómodas que las sillas plásticas del vestíbulo. Le eché una miraba a la oficina de Edden mientras Nick se acomodaba en su silla. Observé el polvo acumulado sobre los trofeos de bolos y las montañas de carpetas. Una pared estaba tapada por archivadores y encima de ellos había álbumes de fotos casi hasta el techo. De su escritorio colgaba un reloj. Tenía una foto de él junto a mi antiguo jefe, Denon, dándose la mano frente a la Municipalidad. Edden se veía bajo y corriente al lado del vampiro de Denon. Los dos sonreían.

Regresé la atención hacia Edden. Estaba inclinado en su silla esperando a que yo terminara de explorar su oficina. Si me lo hubiera preguntado, le habría dicho que es un marrano; pero el ambiente de esa oficina indicaba que allí se trabajaba de verdad. Era tan diferente a la oficina esterilizada de Denon repleta de tonterías como lo era mi viejo escritorio del patio de una iglesia. Me gustaba. Si tenía que confiar en alguien prefería que fuera una persona tan desordenada como yo.

Edden se puso serio. "Debo admitir que mi conversación con Tamwood fue fascinante, Srta. Morgan. Como ex funcionaria de la S.E., usted entenderá lo que podría causarle a la imagen de la AFE el detener a Trent Kalamack bajo el cargo de lo que sea...más aún bajo el cargo de fabricar y distribuir productos biológicos ilegales."

Directo al grano. Vaya si me empezaba a caer bien este tipo. Sentí un nudo en el estómago pero no dije nada. Aún no había terminado.

Edden descansó un brazo sobre su escritorio y colocó el cabestrillo sobre los muslos detrás de la mesa. "Pero usted también debe entender que no puedo pedirle a mi gente que arresten al concejal Kalamack por sugerencia de una ex agente de la S.E. Usted está bajo amenaza de muerte, así sea ilegal."

Mi respiración se aceleró casi a la par de mi pensamiento. Yo tenía razón. Encerró a Ivy para hacerme venir hasta acá. Sentí pánico al pensar si acaso estaría haciendo tiempo conmigo mientras llegaba la S.E. para atraparme, pero deseché la idea. La S.E. y la AFE estaban trenzadas en una agria rivalidad. Si Edden quería reclamar el precio de mi vida lo haría el mismo. No necesitaba invitar a la S.E. a su edificio. Me había hecho venir para evaluarme. ¿Para qué? No podía imaginarlo y me preocupé aún más.

Decidí tomar el control de nuestra conversación y sonreí, entrecerrando los ojos pues mi párpado inflamado me molestaba. Lo miré de frente librándome de la tensión de mis hombros y concentrándola en el estómago donde él no pudiera verla. "Quisiera disculparme por el comportamiento de mis socios, capitán Edden." Miré su muñeca vendada. "¿Se la rompió ella?"

Apenas dejó ver una brizna de asombro. "Peor que rota. Está fracturada en cuatro partes. Mañana sabré si necesito un yeso o si basta esperar a que sane. Esa maldita enfermería no me deja tomar nada más fuerte que aspirina. La próxima semana es luna llena, Srta. Morgan. ¿Se imagina el retraso de trabajo si tengo que tomar un día libre?"

Con esta conversación no íbamos para ningún lado. El dolor empezó a regresar y tenía que averiguar qué quería Edden antes de que fuera demasiado tarde para movernos contra Kalamack. Había algo más aparte de Trent. Él sólo podía encargarse de Ivy si quisiera.

Me enderecé quitándome uno de mis amuletos y lo empujé hacia él. Mi bolso estaba lleno de hechizos pero ninguno contra el dolor. "Lo entiendo, capitán Edden. Estoy segura de que podemos llegar a un acuerdo que nos beneficie a los dos." Mis dedos soltaron el pequeño disco y traté de esforzarme para controlar la ola de dolor. Las náuseas me revolvieron el estómago y me sentí tres veces más débil. Ojalá no hubiera cometido un error dándoselo. Como lo vimos con la secretaria de la recepción, eran pocos los humanos que aceptaban a los Entremundos y menos aún su magia. Me pareció que valía la pena arriesgarse. Edden parecía inusualmente abierto. Tendríamos que ver cuánto.

Tomó el amuleto con curiosidad. "Usted sabe que no puedo aceptar esto" dijo. "Para un oficial de la AFE estos se considera..." Se puso serio mientras sus dedos se cerraban alrededor del amuleto disminuyendo el dolor. "Soborno," dijo en voz baja.

Sus ojos oscuros se fijaron en mi cara. Yo le sonreí a pesar del dolor. "Un cambio." Alcé las cejas ignorando la tensión que me producían las curas. "Aspirina por aspirina." Si era suficientemente astuto entendería que yo estaba probando las aguas. Pero si era un estúpido, daba igual. Yo estaría muerta este fin de semana. Claro que si no existiera una manera de "convencerlo," entonces yo no estaría ahí sentada en su oficina.

Por un momento Edden se quedó inmóvil, como temiendo moverse y romper el hechizo. Finalmente sonrió. Se inclinó hacia la puerta abierta y gritó por el pasillo. "¡Rosa! Tráigame unas cuantas aspirinas. Me estoy muriendo aquí." Se inclinó hacia atrás con una mueca colgándose el amuleto alrededor del cuello y escondiéndolo detrás de la camisa. Sintió alivio y entendí que teníamos un buen comienzo.

Sentí intranquilidad al ver que entraba apuradamente una mujer. Estaba asombrada de vernos en la oficina de Edden.

Sin mirarme, sacó dos vasos de papel mientras que Edden le indicaba dejarlos en el escritorio. La mujer frunció el ceño dejando las aspirinas junto a las manos del capitán y se retiró en silencio. Apenas salió, Edden estiró el pie y cerró la puerta. Esperó un momento acomodándose bien los lentes sobre la nariz antes de poner su brazo bueno sobre el herido.

Tomé uno de los vasos y miré las pastillas. Ahora era mi turno de confiar. Esas diminutas pastillas blancas podían contener cualquier cosa, pero ante todo necesitaba aliviar mi dolor.

Había oído hablar de pastillas. Tuve una compañera de habitación que las usaba siempre. Mantenía un frasquito junto al cepillo de dientes. Decía que funcionaban mejor que los amuletos y tampoco había necesidad de pincharse los dedos. Una vez la vi tomarse una. Hay que tragarlas enteras.

Nick se acercó. "Trágalas enteras" dijo y yo asentí con la cabeza. Volteé el vaso sintiendo el sabor amargo de corteza de sauce que pasé con un poco de agua tibia. Me esforcé por no toser sintiendo cómo bajaban las aspirinas, pero me tensé por el repentino dolor que sentí al moverme. ¿Se supone que esto me haría sentir mejor?

Nick me dio unos golpecitos consoladores en la espalda. Vi reír a Edden por mi ineptitud a través de mis ojos llorosos. Alejé a Nick con la mano y reuní mis fuerzas para sentarme derecha. Pasó un momento. Luego otro. Nada. La aspirina no surtía efecto. Con razón los humanos sospechaban tanto. Sus remedios no funcionaban.

"Puedo entregarle a Kalamack, capitán Edden" dije, observando el reloj que tenía detrás del escritorio. Eran las diez y cuarenta y cinco. "Puedo demostrar que está traficando con drogas ilegales: producción y distribución."

Se le iluminó la cara. "Déme las pruebas e iremos al aeropuerto."

No lograba entender esto. Ivy le había dicho todo, pero aún quería hablar conmigo. ¿Por qué no aceptó la información para cubrirse de gloria? Sólo Dios lo sabe. ¿Qué estaría tramando? "No las tengo" acepté. "Escuché cuando organizó todo. Si hallamos las drogas, será prueba más que suficiente."

Edden apretó los labios moviendo su bigote. "No voy a realizar una captura basándome en pruebas circunstanciales. Ya he hecho el papel de idiota ante la S.E."

Miré el reloj de nuevo. Diez y cuarenta y seis. Nuestros ojos se encontraron pero le dejé ver que estaba molesta. Ahora sabía que yo estaba contra el tiempo. "Capitán," dije, tratando de que mi voz no sonara implorante. "Penetré a la oficina de Trent Kalamack para obtener las pruebas pero me atraparon. Pasé los últimos tres días encerrada allá y presencié varias reuniones que confirman mis sospechas. Él es productor y distribuidor de drogas ilegales."

Tranquilo y sereno, Edden se recostó en su silla giratoria. "¿Usted estuvo tres días donde Kalamack y espera que le crea que dijo todas esas cosas delante de usted?"

"Yo me había transformado en visón" repuse secamente. "Se supone que iba a morir en las peleas de ratas de la ciudad. No que escaparía viva."

Nick se acomodó intranquilo en la silla pero Edden movió la cabeza, como si yo acabara de confirmarle alguna sospecha.

"Trent maneja una red de drogas biológicas casi semanalmente" continué tratando de no jugar con mi pelo. "Chantajea a quien puede y a quienes se encuentran en la desafortunada necesidad de adquirir esas drogas. Usted puede detectar sus ganancias secretas identificando los decomisos de zufre de la S.E. Los usa como…"

"Distracción" dijo Edden terminando mi frase. Le dio un golpe al archivador que tenía al lado hundiéndolo. Nick y yo saltamos. "¡Maldición! Por eso es que nunca hacemos decomisos."

Asentí. Era ahora o nunca. Ya no importaba si confiaba en él o no. Si no me ayudaba, estaba muerta. "Pero hay más," continué, rezando que estuviera haciendo lo correcto. "Trent tiene un agente de la S.E. en su nómina de pagos que ha estado a la cabeza de casi todos los decomisos de azufre."

Edden se puso más serio aún. "Fred Perry."

"Francis Perry" corregí, sintiendo un repentino destello de rabia.

Edden se acomodó en la silla entrecerrando los ojos. Era obvio que le molestaba la idea de un policía corrupto tanto como a mí. Tomé aire temblando. "Esta noche sale un cargamento de drogas biológicas. Con mi ayuda, usted puede atraparlos a los dos. La AFE recibe el crédito por el arresto, la S.E. queda mal y su departamento paga secretamente mi contrato." Sentí que me dolía la cabeza y sólo recé que no hubiera soltado mi única oportunidad por el escusado. "Digamos que son honorarios de asesoría. Aspirina por aspirina."

Con los dientes apretados, Edden miró hacia el techo de tablas. Lentamente se fue tranquilizando mientras que yo esperaba y jugaba con mis uñas al mismo ritmo que el tic-tac del reloj.

"Me siento tentado a dejar a un lado las reglas por usted, Srta. Morgan" dijo, haciendo saltar mi corazón. "Pero necesito más. Algo que los de arriba puedan anotar en su libro de ganancias y pérdidas y que mantenga su valor por mucho tiempo."

"¿Más?" preguntó Nick molesto.

La cabeza me palpitaba. *¿Quería más?* "No tengo más, capitán" dije con frustración.

Sonrió malévolamente. "Sí tiene."

Traté de alzar las cejas pero la cinta adhesiva me lo impidió.

Edden miró la puerta cerrada. "Si esto funciona... me refiero a atrapar a Kalamack" Se pasó sus manos gruesas por la frente. Cuando las bajó, el capitán de la AFE confiado, accesible y seguro de sí mismo ya no estaba. En cambio, vi a un hombre motivado e inteligente que me asombró. "He trabajado para la AFE desde que me retiré del servicio militar" dijo suavemente. Llegué arriba buscando las cosas que hacían falta y hallándolas.

"Yo no soy una mercancía, capitán" repuse ofuscada.

"Todo el mundo es una mercancía," dijo. "Mis departamentos en la AFE están en gran desventaja, Srta. Morgan. Los Entremundos han evolucionado y conocen las debilidades humanas. Demonios, ustedes tal vez son responsables de la mitad de nuestros complejos mentales. La triste realidad es que no podemos competir."

Edden quería que me volviera en contra de mis compatriotas Entremundos. Debería ser más astuto. "No hay nada que yo sepa que no se encuentre en una biblioteca," repuse aferrando mi bolso fuertemente. Quería levantarme y salir de allí, pero él me tenía justo donde quería tenerme y yo sólo podía verlo sonreír. Sus dientes planos eran totalmente humanos comparados con sus ojos depredadores.

"Estoy seguro de que eso no es del todo cierto," dijo. "Pero yo sólo le estoy pidiendo un consejo, no una traición." Edden se reclinó en su silla pensando. "A veces, por ejemplo esta noche con la Srta. Tamwood, algunos Entremundos vienen a nosotros con información o solicitando ayuda para algo que prefieren no llevar a la S.E. Para serle sincero, no sabemos qué hacer con ellos. Mi gente sospecha tanto que no logra hacer buen uso de esa información; y en las contadas ocasiones que logramos entender, no logramos capitalizar la información. El único motivo por el cual pudimos controlar a la Tamwood fue porque aceptó dejarse encarcelar como requisito para escucharla a usted. Hasta la fecha, les traspasamos a regañadientes estos casos a la S.E." Nuestras miradas se encontraron. "Nos hacen parecer unos tontos, Srta. Morgan."

Me estaba ofreciendo trabajo pero en lugar de tranquilizarme me preocupé más.

"Si quisiera tener un jefe, me habría quedado en la S.E. capitán."

"No," repuso de inmediato. Su asiento chirrió al sentarse recto. "Tenerla a usted aquí sería un error. Mis superiores no sólo pondrían mi cabeza en una estaca, sino que tenerla a usted en la nómina de pagos es contrario a los acuerdos de la

AFE/S.E." Ahora su sonrisa era realmente malévola. Esperé lo que vendría. "La quiero como asesora ocasional, según las necesidades."

Dejé salir el aire lentamente. Ya entendí lo que quería.

"¿Cómo dijo que se llama su empresa?" preguntó Edden.

"Agentes vampiros y brujos" dijo Nick.

Edden rió. "Suena como un servicio de parejas."

Hice una mueca, pero era tarde para cambiar el nombre. "Supongo que me pagarán por estos servicios *ocasionales*" dije mordiéndome el labio inferior. *A lo mejor funcionaría*.

"Naturalmente."

Ahora era mi turno de mirar hacia el techo. El pulso me latía al saber que había encontrado la manera de salir de esto. "Soy parte de un equipo, capitán Edden." Al decirlo pensé si acaso Ivy estaría pensando continuar aun en sociedad. "No puedo hablar por ellos."

"La Srta. Tamwood ya aceptó. Me parece que dijo: 'Si la brujita dice sí, yo también.' El Sr. Jenks expresó el mismo sentimiento, aun cuando sus palabras precisas fueron un tanto más... coloridas."

Miré a Nick quien se encogió de hombros incómodamente. No teníamos ninguna garantía de que al final Edden pagara mi contrato. Pero había algo en su humor sarcástico y reacciones auténticas que me convencieron de que sí lo haría. Además, esta noche ya había hecho un pacto con un demonio. Esto no podía ser peor.

"De acuerdo, capitán Edden" dije de repente. "Es el vuelo de las 11:45 de Southwest hacia Los Ángeles."

"¡Excelente!" Golpeó el escritorio con la mano buena y yo salté otra vez. "Sabía que aceptaría. ¡Rosa!," gritó con la puerta cerrada pero luego gruñó y se inclinó para abrirla. "Mande una escuadra con perros detectores de azufre a..." Se quedó mirándome. "¿Dónde será el decomiso?" me preguntó.

"¿Ivy no se lo dijo?" pregunté sorprendida.

"Tal vez sí. Quería asegurarme de que no mentía."

"La antigua estación de autobuses" respondí con el corazón martillándome en el pecho. *En realidad lo estábamos logrando. Íbamos a capturar a Trent y pagar mi contrato.*

"¡Rosa!" gritó de nuevo. "A la antigua estación de autobuses. ¿Quién trabaja esta noche que no esté en el hospital?"

Una vez femenina pero gruesa respondió en medio del ruido exterior. "Está Kaman, pero en este instante se está bañando tratando de quitarse ese polvo de insecto. Dillon, Ray…"

"Basta," dijo Edden. Se puso de pie saliendo de la oficina y nos indicó a Nick y a mí que lo siguiéramos. Respiré profundo y me levanté. Ahora el dolor se me había convertido en leves latidos. Seguimos a Edden por el pasillo. La agitación me hizo acelerar el paso. "Creo que la aspirina funciona al fin" le susurré a Nick mientras alcanzábamos al capitán. Estaba inclinado sobre un escritorio brillante como un cristal hablando con la misma mujer que había llevado las pastillas.

"Llame a Rubén y a Simón. Necesito alguien con la cabeza fría. Mándelos al aeropuerto y dígales que me esperen."

"¿A usted, señor?" Rosa nos miró a Nick y a mí por encima de los lentes. Su frente fruncida lo decía todo. No estaba contenta con dos Entremundos en el edificio, menos aún parados detrás de su jefe.

"Sí. Yo. Haga venir la camioneta sin distintivos. Esta noche estoy de misión." Se acomodó bien el cinturón en la cintura. "Sin errores. Esto tiene que hacerse bien."

Treinta

El piso de la camioneta de la AFE estaba limpio. Había un cierto olor a humo de pipa que me recordaba a papá. Adelante iban Edden y el conductor, Clayton. Nick, Jenks y yo íbamos sentados en el asiento del medio. Las ventanillas estaban abiertas para ventilar mi perfume. De haber sabido que no soltarían a Ivy hasta después de llegar a un acuerdo, a lo mejor no lo hubiera usado. Por ahora, apestaba.

Jenks estaba furioso. Su vocecilla me atolondraba el cerebro con la cantaleta y sólo lograba producirme más y más ansiedad. "Métete una media en la boca, Jenk" susurré mientras pasaba mi dedo por el fondo de la bolsita de maní para comerme la sal del fondo. Tan pronto la aspirina me controló el dolor sentí mucha hambre. Tal vez era mejor no tomar aspirinas si después me iba a morir de hambre.

"Vete al Giro" gruñó Jenks desde el soporte para vasos donde lo había puesto. "¡Me metieron en una maldita jarra de agua, como si estuviera en exposición! ¡Me rompieron los flecos de las alas! ¡Mira! Destrozaron la nervadura principal. Tengo la camisa con manchas de metal ¡arruinada! ¿Y mis botas? ¿Las viste? Jamás podré quitarles las manchas de café."

"Te pidieron disculpas" dije, aun cuando sabía que era un caso perdido. Estaba insoportable.

"Me tomará toda una semana para que me crezca esta ala. Matalina me va a matar. Todos huyen de mí cuando no puedo volar, ¿sabías? Inclusive mis hijos."

Hice de cuenta que Jenks no existía. La diatriba comenzó tan pronto lo soltaron y no paraba. Aun cuando a Jenks no lo habían acusado de nada a pesar de animar a Ivy desde el techo y llenar de polvillo a los policías de la AFE, sí empezó a meter la nariz donde no le correspondía hasta que lo atraparon y lo metieron en una jarra desocupada de agua.

Ahora empezaba a comprender aquello que había dicho Edden. Él y su gente no tenían ni la más remota idea de cómo manejar a los Entremundos. Pudieron atraparlo en un cajón o en un armario mientras curioseaba. Así sus alas no se habrían mojado y puesto tan frágiles como papel higiénico. Tampoco habría ocurrido la persecución de diez minutos con una red... ¡Y así no habría hechizado a medio piso de oficinas! Ivy y Jenks habían ido a la AFE a las buenas pero terminaron creando un caos. Era preocupante lo que podía llegar a hacer un Entremundos violento y poco colaborador.

"No tiene sentido," dijo Nick lo suficientemente fuerte para que Edden escuchara. "¿Por qué quiere Kalamack llenarse los bolsillos con ganancias ilegales? Ya es millonario."

Edden dio media vuelta en su asiento. Tenía puesta una gorra amarilla de la AFE. Era su único símbolo de autoridad. "A lo mejor estará financiando un proyecto que no quiere que se conozca. Es difícil rastrear el dinero cuando se adquiere ilegalmente y se gasta de la misma manera."

Me detuve a pensar qué podría ser. ¿Algo más en curso en el laboratorio de Faris?

El capitán puso la quijada sobre su brazo. Su cara estaba iluminada por los faros de los autos que venían detrás de nosotros. "Sr. Sparagmos," dijo. "¿Alguna vez ha tomado el paseo turístico en ferry por el río?"

Nick puso cara de asombro. "¿Disculpe?"

Edden agitó la cabeza. "Es muy extraño, estoy seguro que lo he visto antes."

"No," repuso Nick echándose para atrás. "No me gustan los botes."

El capitán emitió un sonido leve y giró de nuevo en su asiento. Jenks y yo cruzamos una mirada. El duende puso una mirada astuta y entendió antes que yo. Mi bolsa de maní desocupada crujía y la metí en mi bolso. No iba a lanzarla al piso limpio. Nick estaba en la sombra y sentado muy cerca. La luz lejana de los autos que venían en el otro sentido apenas dejaban ver su nariz respingada y su cara delgada. Me acerqué un poco más y susurré: "¿Qué hiciste?"

Su mirada siguió fija en la ventanilla y su pecho subía y bajaba lentamente al respirar. "Nada."

Miré la parte de atrás de su cabeza. *Sí. Te creo. Y yo soy la nena en los carteles de la S.E.* "Escucha. Lamento haberte metido en esto. Si quieres irte tan pronto lleguemos al aeropuerto, te entiendo." En el fondo yo no quería enterarme de lo que hizo.

Movió la cabeza sonriéndome. "Todo está bien" dijo. "Te acompañaré esta noche. Te lo debo por haberme sacado de ese nido de ratas. Una semana más y enloquecería."

Sentí un escalofrío de sólo pensarlo. Había penas peores que la de estar en la lista negra de la S.E. Toqué su hombro un instante y volví a recostarme en mi asiento mirándolo de reojo. Poco a poco se fue calmando y su respiración se normalizó. Cuanto más lo iba conociendo, más diferencias le encontraba con la mayoría de los humanos. Pero en lugar de preocuparme me hacía sentir más segura. Otra vez regresé a mi síndrome de la dama en peligro y el caballero. Tal vez había leído demasiados cuentos de hadas siendo niña pero también vivía en la realidad y no me molestaba ser rescatada de vez en cuando.

El silencio era incómodo y mi ansiedad aumentó. ¿Qué pasaría si llegábamos tarde? ¿Qué tal si Trent hubiera cambiado el vuelo? ¿Y si todo era una distracción bien montada? *Ayúdame, Dios mío,* pensé. Me estaba jugando el todo por el todo en las próximas horas. Si no salía bien, estaba perdida.

"¡Bruja!" gritó Jenks para llamar mi atención. Caí en la cuenta que estaba tratando de que le prestara atención durante los últimos minutos. "¡Álzame!" exigió. "No veo nada desde aquí."

Le ofrecí la mano para que trepara. "No se me ocurre por qué la gente se aleja de ti cuando no puedes volar" le dije secamente.

"Esto *no* habría sucedido si cierta persona no me hubiera roto la maldita *ala*," dijo en voz alta.

Lo puse sobre mi hombro desde donde podía ver el tráfico a medida que nos acercábamos al aeropuerto internacional de Cincinnati–Kentucky del Norte. Casi todo el mundo lo llamaba Hollows Internacional, o más fácil aún: el H.I. Los autos eran levemente iluminados por las escasas luces de la calle pero se hicieron más numerosas a medida que estábamos más cerca de la terminal. De repente me invadió la emoción y me enderecé en mi asiento. Todo saldría bien. Lo atraparía. No importaba lo que fuera Trent, iba a atraparlo. "¿Qué hora es?" pregunté.

"Las once y quince" murmuró Jenks.

"Las once y veinte" corrigió Edden señalando el reloj de la camioneta.

"Las once y quince," rebatió Jenks. "Yo sé mejor dónde está el sol que usted por qué orificio orinar."

"¡Jenks!" grité disgustada. Nick soltó los brazos que tenía cruzados.

Edden alzó la mano en señal de paz. "No se preocupe Srta. Morgan."

Clayton me miró por el retrovisor. Era un policía serio que aparentemente no confiaba en mí. "Señor, a decir verdad, nuestro reloj está adelantado cinco minutos" dijo a regañadientes.

"¿Se da cuenta?" dijo Jenks.

Edden levantó el teléfono del auto y encendió el altoparlante para que todos pudiéramos oír. "Vamos a asegurarnos de que ese avión se quede en tierra y que ocupen sus posiciones," dijo.

Llena de ansiedad, acomodé mi cabestrillo mientras Edden oprimía tres números del teléfono. "¡Rubén!" ladró en la bocina sosteniéndola como si se tratara de un micrófono. "Háblame."

Hubo un momento de silencio y de pronto se escuchó una voz masculina por el altoparlante. "Capitán, estamos en la puerta de embarque, pero el avión no está aquí."

"¿¡No está!?" grité al tiempo que me abalancé hacia el asiento delantero. "Ya deberían estar abordando."

"Nunca llegó hasta la rampa, señor" continuó Rubén. "Todos esperan en la terminal. Dicen que es una reparación menor que tomará sólo una hora. ¿Esto no es por orden suya?"

Miré a Edden. Casi podía ver cómo sus ideas daban vueltas alrededor de su cara llena de conjeturas. "No," repuso. "Quédense ahí." Luego cortó la comunicación.

"¿Qué está sucediendo?" le grité al oído. Él me devolvió una mirada molesta.

"Ponga el trasero en su asiento, Morgan" dijo el capitán. "Probablemente se trata de las restricciones de luz diurna de su amigo. La compañía no va a dejar a los pasajeros esperando en la pista cuando la terminal está desocupada."

Observé a Nick que tocaba nerviosamente un ritmo desconocido con los dedos. Nerviosa, me acomodé en el asiento. Podía ver la luz del faro del aeropuerto que brillaba bajo las nubes. Ya estábamos por llegar.

Edden marcó un número de memoria, sonriendo tranquilo al levantar la bocina. "Hola ¿Chris?" preguntó. Escuché la voz lejana de una mujer que contestaba. "Tengo una pregunta. Parece que hay un vuelo de Southwest detenido en la pista. El de las once y cuarenta y cinco para Los Ángeles. ¿Cuál es el problema?" Escuchó atentamente mientras yo me comía el pellejo de las uñas. "Gracias Chris," rió. "¿Qué tal el filete más grande de la ciudad?" Rió de nuevo y podría jurar que sus orejas se pusieron rojas.

Jenks se rió de algo que no pude oír. Miré a Nick pero me ignoraba.

"Chrisy," dijo Edden arrastrando las letras. "Tal vez mi esposa se moleste con eso." Jenks se rió al tiempo con Edden y me ponían nerviosa. "Hablamos luego" y colgó el teléfono.

"¿Entonces?" pregunté desde mi asiento.

Edden seguía sonriendo. "El avión está detenido en tierra. Parece que la S.E. tenía conocimiento de que transportaba una bolsa de azufre."

"Maldición," dije. El señuelo era la estación de autobuses, no el aeropuerto. ¿Qué hacía Trent?

Los ojos de Edden destellaron. "La S.E. está a quince minutos de aquí. Nosotros podríamos quitárselo en las narices."

Jenks empezó a maldecir en mi hombro.

"No vinimos aquí por azufre," protesté al ver que todo comenzaba a desbaratarse. "¡Vinimos por drogas biológicas!" Estaba echando humo pero cerré la boca mientras pasaba un ruidoso auto en sentido contrario.

"Ese si que está violando el código urbano," comentó Edden. "Clayton, trata de localizar su número."

La mente me daba vueltas. Esperé a que pasara antes de hablar de nuevo. El motor rugía y parecía que fuera a treinta millas por encima del límite de velocidad, pero el auto apenas se movía. Los cambios chillaron y reconocí un sonido familiar: *Francis,* pensé, y contuve el aire.

"¡Ese es Francis!" gritamos Jenks y yo al tiempo mientras me daba vuelta para ver la luz de parqueo rota. La visión se me nubló por el dolor que sentí con el movimiento al pasar casi gateando hacia la parte posterior del coche. Jenks seguía sobre mi hombro. "¡Es Francis!" grité con el corazón. "¡Deténganse, de media vuelta! ¡Es Francis!"

Edden golpeó el tablero con fuerza. "¡Maldición! ¡Llegamos demasiado tarde!"

"¡No!" grité. "¿No lo entiende? Trent está haciendo el cambio. Las drogas y el azufre. La S.E no ha llegado aún. ¡Francis está haciendo el cambio!"

Edden se quedó mirándome. Las luces y las sombras pasaban por su cara a intervalos y seguíamos camino al aeropuerto.

"Francis tiene las drogas ¡den media vuelta!" grité.

La camioneta se detuvo en una luz roja. "¿Capitán?" dijo el chofer.

"Morgan, usted está loca si piensa que voy a dejar pasar la oportunidad de hacer un decomiso de azufre en las narices de la S.E. Usted ni siquiera está segura si era él."

Jenks rió. "Era Francis. Raquel le quemó el embrague a ese auto. Sí señor."

Tensé la cara. "Francis tiene las drogas. Las mandará en autobús. Apostaría mi vida por ello."

Edden abrió bien los ojos y apretó los dientes. "Así es. Ya lo hizo" dijo a secas. "Clayton, da la vuelta."

Me hundí en mi asiento dejando salir el aire. No me había dado cuenta de que lo había guardado tanto.

"¿Capitán?"

"¡Ya me oíste!" dijo claramente. No estaba contento. "Da media vuelta. Haz lo que dice la bruja." Entonces se volteó a mirarme muy serio. "Más te vale que tengas la razón, Morgan" dijo bufando.

"La tengo" repuse sintiendo un nudo en el estómago. Me recosté y me aferré bien cuando viramos. *Más me valía tener razón,* pensé mirando a Nick.

Nos cruzamos con un camión de la S.E. que se dirigía al aeropuerto, silencioso, con las luces intermitentes encendidas. Edden golpeó el tablero tan duro que no entendí cómo no se activó la bolsa de aire. Tiró de la radio. "¡Rosa!" bramó. "¿Qué hallaron los perros en la estación de autobuses?"

"Nada, capitán. Ya vienen de regreso."

"¡Mándelos allá otra vez!" ordenó. "¿A quién tenemos en Los Hollows vestido de civil?"

"¿Señor?" dijo confundida.

"¡¿Quién hay en Los Hollows que no haya mandado al aeropuerto!" gritó.

"Briston está en el centro comercial de Newport." Entonces los interrumpió un lejano timbre de teléfono y el capitán gritó de nuevo: "¡Que alguien conteste ese teléfono!" Hubo un instante de silencio. "Gerry la está acompañando, pero está uniformado."

"Gerry," musitó Edden poco satisfecho. "Mándelos a la estación."

"Briston y Gerry a la estación," repitió lentamente.

"Dígales que lleven sus EAC," agregó Edden mirándome.

"¿EAC?" preguntó Nick."

"Equipo Anti Conjuros" le expliqué.

"Buscamos a un hombre blanco de unos treinta años. Brujo. El nombre es Francis Percy, agente de la S.E."

"No es ni siquiera un principiante," interrumpí, aferrándome cuando frenamos abruptamente en un semáforo.

"El sospechoso podría estar transportando hechizos" continuó Edden.

"Es inofensivo" musité.

"No lo confronten a menos que trate de largarse," concluyó el capitán.

"Sí," dije, y nos pusimos en movimiento de nuevo. "Es capaz de hacernos morir de aburrición."

Edden se volteó a mirarme. "¿Por qué no se calla la boca?"

Me encogí de hombros y luego me arrepentí, pues regresó el dolor.

"¿Me entendió Rosa?" dijo el capitán.

"Armado, peligroso, no confrontarlo a menos que trate de largarse. Entendido."

Edden refunfuñó. "Gracias, Rosa," y apagó la radio con un dedo.

Jenks se aferró de mi oreja y solté un grito.

"¡Ahí está!" gritó el duende. "Miren. Justo delante de nosotros."

Nick y yo nos inclinamos hacia adelante para ver. La luz rota era como un faro. Vimos a Francis hacer una señal para girar, haciendo chirriar las llantas para dirigirse a la estación de autobuses. De pronto sonó una bocina fuerte: por poco se estrella contra un autobús.

"Bien," dijo Edden mientras dábamos la vuelta para estacionar del otro lado del estacionamiento. "Tenemos cinco minutos mientras que llegan los perros, quince para Briston y Gerry. Francis tiene que registrar sus paquetes en la recepción. Será una bonita prueba de que son de su propiedad." Se quitó el cinturón de seguridad y giró en el asiento al tiempo que la camioneta se detenía. Parecía un vampiro ansioso con esa sonrisa mostrando los dientes. "Ni siquiera lo miren hasta que no hayan llegado todos. ¿Entendido?"

"Sí. Entendido" repuse alegremente. No me gustaba estar bajo las órdenes de otra persona, pero lo que dijo tenía sentido. Me deslicé nerviosamente en el asiento para apretar mi cara contra la ventanilla de Nick y ver cómo Francis luchaba con tres cajas planas.

"¿Es él?" preguntó Edden fríamente.

Asentí. Jenks bajó por mi brazo y se detuvo en el borde de la ventanilla tratando de conservar el equilibrio con sus alas. "Así es. Ese es nuestro pastelito."

De pronto caí en la cuenta de que estaba casi encima de los muslos de Nick. Rápidamente retrocedí hasta mi puesto. El efecto de la aspirina empezaba a desaparecer y aun cuando el amuleto aun servía un par de días más, el dolor me molestaba cada vez más. Pero lo que más me preocupaba era la fatiga. Mi corazón latía como si acabara de terminar una carrera. No creía que fuera solo por la emoción.

Francis cerró la puerta del auto de una patada y comenzó a moverse tambaleando. Se jactaba de su imagen de persona importante entrando a la terminal con su escandalosa camisa y el cuello volteado hacia arriba. Reí al verlo sonreírle a una mujer que salía, pero que no le prestó atención. Recordé de pronto su cara de temor ahí sentado en la oficina de Trent y mi desprecio se convirtió en lástima por ese hombre inseguro.

"Muy bien chicos y chicas," dijo Edden distrayendo mi

atención. "Clayton, quédate aquí. Dile a Briston que entre apenas llegue. No quiero a nadie en uniforme cerca de las ventanas." Se quedó observando a Francis mientras entraba por las puertas dobles. "Dile a Rosa que mande a todos los que están en el aeropuerto. Parece que la bruja, quise decir, la Srta. Morgan tenía razón."

"Sí, señor," dijo Clayton. Alcanzó el teléfono con desgano. Las puertas se abrieron y era obvio que no éramos el típico grupo que viene a tomar el autobús, pero Francis era demasiado estúpido para darse cuenta. Edden metió su gorra amarilla de la AFE en el bolsillo trasero del pantalón y Nick era un flaco don nadie. Él sí parecía pertenecer a ese lugar. Mis heridas y el cabestrillo llamaban más la atención que si llevara un letrero que dijera: "Trabajo a cambio de hechizos."

"¿Capitán Edden?" dije mientras descendía y esperaba de pie. "Un minuto."

Edden y Nick me miraron intrigados mientras buscaba algo en mi bolso. "Raquel," dijo Jenks parado en el hombro de Nick. "Estás loca. No vas a verte mejor ni siquiera con diez hechizos cosméticos."

"Vete al Giro," murmuré. "Francis me reconocerá. Necesito un amuleto."

Edden observó con interés. Sentía la presión de la adrenalina mientras buscaba un hechizo de vieja con mi mano buena. Finalmente dejé el bolso en el asiento, agarré el hechizo adecuado y lo invoqué. Me lo puse alrededor del cuello y Edden no podía creerlo. Su aprobación fue muy satisfactoria. El hecho de que hubiera aceptado mi amuleto al comienzo tuvo mucho que ver en mi decisión de quedarle debiendo un par de favores. Cada vez que un humano demostraba aprecio por mis hechizos, sentía un calorcito en el corazón. *Majadero*.

Metí todo en desorden dentro del bolso y salí de la camioneta.

"¿Listos?" dijo Jenks sarcásticamente. "¿No quieres peinarte antes?"

"Vete al diablo, Jenks" le dije a la vez que Nick me daba la mano. "Puedo bajar sola" agregué.

Jenks saltó desde Nick hacia mí para posarse en mi hombro. "Te ves como una vieja. Compórtate como una."

"Es una viejita," dijo Edden tomándome del hombro para evitar que cayera mientras que mis botas de vampiro tocaban el pavimento. "Me recuerdas a mi madre," dijo volteando los ojos y tapándose la nariz. "Inclusive, hueles igual."

"Ya cállense todos ustedes" dije. La falta de aire hizo que sintiera vértigo y el dolor que sentí al bajar del auto subió por mi columna vertebral hasta el cráneo con intención de quedarse ahí un buen rato. Estaba dispuesta a no dejarme vencer por la fatiga así que me solté de Edden y caminé tambaleandome hasta las puertas. Los dos hombres me siguieron tres pasos atrás. Me sentía como un marrano en mis jeans anchos y esa espantosa blusa escocesa. Además, la idea de ser una vieja tampoco me subía mucho el ánimo. Empujé las puertas pero no logré abrirlas. "¿Podría alguien abrirme la puerta?" Jenks rió.

Nick me tomó del brazo mientras que Edden abrió la puerta. Una oleada de aire caliente nos golpeó el rostro. "Ven," dijo Nick. "Apóyate en mí. Así pareces más vieja."

Podía aguantar el dolor. Era la fatiga lo que me golpeaba el orgullo y me obligaba a aceptar el brazo de Nick. O bien era eso o entraba gateando a la terminal.

Entré emocionada. Mis corazón se aceleró a medida que pasaba la mirada por la recepción en busca de Francis. "Ahí está" susurré.

Francis estaba casi totalmente oculto por una planta decorativa hablando con una chica joven que vestía el uniforme del municipio. El hechizo de Percy surtía su efecto acostumbrado pues ella parecía molesta. Había tres cajas a su lado sobre el mostrador y toda mi existencia dependía de ellas.

Nick me tiró suavemente del codo bueno. "Vamos mamá, vamos a sentarnos allá."

"Vuelve a llamarme así y me encargaré de tu planificación familiar," lo amenacé.

"Mamá," dijo Jenks lanzando oleadas de brisa sobre mi cuello con sus alas.

"Basta," dijo Edden serio y en voz baja. No le quitó la mirada a Francis ni un segundo. "Ustedes tres vayan a sentarse allá a esperar. Nadie se mueve a menos que Percy trate de escapar. Voy a cerciorarme de que esas cajas no sean cargadas en ningún autobús." Sin dejar de mirar a Francis, el capitán tocó el arma que llevaba debajo de la chaqueta dirigiéndose indiferentemente hacia el mostrador. Edden le sonrió a otra dependiente de lejos.

¿Sentarnos a esperar? Sí. Por qué no.

Tuve que ceder ante los suaves jalones de Nick y nos dirigimos hacia la fila de asientos. Eran anaranjados, como los de la AFE, y se veían igualmente incómodos. Nick me ayudó a sentarme en uno y él lo hizo en el de al lado. Se estiró y fingió dormir la siesta con los ojos entreabiertos observando a Francis. Me senté derecho con mi bolso sobre los muslos, aferrándome a él como lo hacen las viejitas. Y entendí por qué: todo me dolía y pensaba que si me acomodaba me desbarataría en pedazos.

De pronto gritó un niño y me sobresalté. Alejé la mirada de Francis que estaba muy ocupado haciendo el ridículo para fijarme en otras personas. Había una madre cansada con tres niños, uno de ellos aún con pañales, discutiendo con un empleado acerca de unos cupones. Un grupo de hombres de negocios absortos en sus cosas, caminando para arriba y para abajo dándose ínfulas, como si esta terminal fuera solo un mal sueño y no la realidad de su existencia. Un par de jóvenes caminando peligrosamente juntos, a lo mejor escapándose de sus padres. Vagos. Un viejo mal vestido que me hizo una seña con un ojo.

Me puse muy nerviosa. Aquí no estaba segura. La S.E. podía estar en cualquier lugar, lista a cazarme.

"Tranquilízate, Raque" dijo Jenks como si me hubiera leído la mente. "La S.E. no te va atrapar cuando el capitán de la AFE juega en tu mismo equipo."

"¿Cómo puedes estar tan seguro?" pregunté.

Sentí el viento producido por sus alas soplando en mi cuello.

"No lo estoy."

Nick abrió los ojos y se sentó derecho. "¿Cómo te sientes?" preguntó en voz baja.

"Yo estoy bien, gracias" dijo Jenks. "¿Sabías que un gigante de la AFE me arrancó una maldita ala? Mi mujer me va a matar."

Sonreí. "Con hambre" le respondí. "Agotada."

Nick me miró antes de volver los ojos hacia Francis. "¿Quieres algo de comer?"

En su bolsillo sonaron las monedas que habían sobrado del viaje en taxi hasta la AFE. "Aún te queda suficiente para comprar algo en esa máquina que está ahí."

Una leve sonrisa apareció en mis labios. Era agradable tener a alguien que se preocupara por mí. "Seguro. Gracias. ¿Qué tal algo con chocolate?"

"Chocolate" reiteró Nick poniéndose de pie. Miró a Francis al otro lado del recinto desde las máquinas con alimentos. El tonto estaba inclinado encima del mostrador, seguramente tratando de que la chica le diera su número telefónico. Nick se alejó. En realidad se movía con mucha gracia para ser tan delgado. ¿Qué habría hecho para que la AFE se lo llevara?

"Algo con chocolate," repicó Jenks en falsete. "¡Ohhhhh ... Nick, eres mi héroe!"

"Vete al infierno," le dije más por costumbre que otra cosa.

"¿Sabes una cosa Raque?" dijo Jenks mientras se acomodaba mejor sobre mi hombro. "Vas a ser la abuela más extraña que jamás haya visto."

Estaba demasiado cansada para responder. Respiré profundamente pero despacio para que no me doliera. Mis ojos saltaron de Francis a Nick. Sentí algo de emoción mirando la alta figura de Nick mientras compraba algo en la máquina con su cabeza inclinada mirando las monedas. "Jenks, ¿qué piensas de Nick?" El duende rebuznó, pero al ver que le hablaba en serio se calmó. "Está bien" dijo. "No te lastimará. Está con esa honda de complejo de héroe y tu pareces necesitar alguien que te rescate. Deberías haberle visto la cara cuando estabas tirada en el sofá de Ivy. Pensé que se iba a morir. Pero no esperes que piense lo mismo que tú sobre lo que está bien o está mal."

Alcé las cejas y me dolió la cara. "¿Magia negra?" susurré. "Por Dios Jenks, no me digas que la practica."

Jenks se rió fuertemente. "No. Me refiero a que no le importa robarse los libros de la biblioteca."

"Ahh" pensé de nuevo en su intranquilidad cuando estábamos en las oficinas de la AFE y luego en la camioneta. ¿Eso era todo? No podía ser. De todas formas, los duendes eran reconocidos por sus juicios de personalidad, no importa que tan sucios, excéntricos o bocones fueran. ¿Cambiaría la opinión de Jenks si le contaba lo de mi marca demoníaca? Me daba miedo preguntarle. Diablos, me daba mucho miedo mostrársela.

Alcé la mirada para ver a Francis riendo, escribiendo algo en un papel y pasándoselo a la chica detrás del mostrador. Se pasó la mano por debajo de la nariz y luego le hizo una sonrisa de ratón. "Buena chica," susurré cuando la arrugó y la lanzó por encima del hombro mientras Francis caminaba hacia la puerta.

Mi corazón pareció despertar. ¡Se dirigía hacia la puerta! *Maldición.*

Busqué ayuda. Nick estaba luchando con la máquina y me daba la espalda. Edden estaba conversando con un hombre vestido con el uniforme de las empresa de autobuses. El capitán tenía la cara roja y los ojos fijos en las cajas detrás del mostrador. "Jenks" dije suavemente. "Ve por Edden."

"¿Qué? ¿Quieres que vaya gateando tal vez?"

Francis iba a mitad de camino de la puerta. No confiaba

en Clayton. No era capaz de detener la orinada de un perro. Recé para que Edden se diera la vuelta pero no lo hizo. "¡Vé por él!" le dije sin importarme su desagrado, bajándolo de mi hombro al piso.

"¡Raquel!" gritó Jenks a medida que yo trataba de caminar tan rápido como me era posible para interponerme entre Francis y la puerta. Era muy lenta, pero Francis pasó delante mío.

"Disculpe, joven" gorgoteé con el pulso corriendo por el esfuerzo. "¿Podría decirme dónde está la zona de equipajes?"

Francis giró velozmente y yo traté de no manifestar mi temor de que me reconociera y viera el odio que sentía por lo que había hecho. "Esta es la terminal de autobuses, señora" dijo con su clásica cara de fastidio. "Aquí no hay zona de equipajes. Sus cosas están en el andén."

"¿Cómo dice?" pregunté, maldiciendo a Edden. *¿Dónde demonios estaba?* Agarré duro el brazo de Francis y se volteó a mirar mi mano arrugada por el hechizo.

"¡Está afuera!" gritó tratando de zafarse, sacudiéndose cuando sintió mi perfume.

Pero yo no lo soltaba. Pude ver de reojo a Nick que miraba atónito mi silla vacía. Su mirada recorrió a la gente hasta que finalmente me vio. Se alarmó y corrió hacia Edden.

Francis llevaba sus papeles debajo del brazo y con la otra mano trataba de zafarse de mis dedos que lo agarraban. "Suélteme, señora" dijo. "Aquí no hay zona de equipajes."

Sentí un calambre y él tiró con fuerza acomodándose la camisa. "Maldita vieja murciélago," dijo bufando. "¿Qué demonios es lo que hacen ustedes las ancianas? ¿Nadar en perfume?" Pero entonces se quedó con la boca abierta. "Morgan" pronunció mi nombre casi sin aire, reconociéndome. "Me dijo que estabas muerta."

"Lo estoy" repuse, y mis rodillas amenazaron con doblarse. Sólo me sostenía la adrenalina.

Su estúpida mirada me dijo que no tenía idea de lo que

estaba sucediendo. "Tú vienes conmigo. Denon me dará un ascenso cuando te vea."

Agité la cabeza. Tenía que hacer esto de acuerdo a la ley, de lo contrario Edden se iba a cabrear. "Francis Percy, bajo la autoridad de la AFE, te estoy acusando de conspirar voluntariamente para traficar drogas biológicas."

Su sonrisa desapareció y su cara se puso blanca bajo su horrible barbita. Dirigió la mirada por encima de mi hombro hacia el mostrador. "¡Mierda!" dijo, y dio media vuelta para salir corriendo.

"¡Alto!" gritó Edden, demasiado lejos para que sirviera. Salté sobre Francis agarrándolo por las rodillas. Los dos caímos pesadamente. Francis se retorció dándome una patada en el pecho tratando de escapar. Jadeé con dolor.

Un golpe de aire pasó por encima de nosotros y alcé la mirada. Yo veía las estrellas mientras Francis luchaba por soltarse.

No, pensé, al ver que una bola de fuego azul se estrellaba contra la pared del fondo. *Las estrellas eran de verdad.*

El suelo tembló con la fuerza del estallido. Las mujeres y los niños gritaban cayendo de espaldas contra las paredes. "¿Qué fue eso?" tartamudeó Francis. Se retorció debajo de mí y se quedó mirando boquiabierto por una fracción de segundo mientras que la llamarada azul golpeaba la horrible pared amarilla y giraba para desaparecer.

Asustada por primera vez, me di vuelta para ver a mis espaldas. Ahí había un hombre de pie, de baja estatura, bien vestido y que parecía muy seguro con una bola roja del más allá en una mano. Una mujer menuda vestida igual, sonriente, con una mano en la cintura, cubría la puerta principal. Había una tercera persona. Un tipo musculoso del tamaño de un Volkswagen parado junto al mostrador.

Parecía que la reunión anual de brujos y brujas en la costa oeste había terminado.

Grandioso.

Treinta y uno

Francis respiraba agitadamente. "¡Suéltame!" chilló temeroso con voz aguda y desagradable. "¡Suéltame Raquel! ¡Van a matarte!"

Le clavé los dedos mientras trataba de soltarse. Yo resoplaba de dolor pues su esfuerzo por librarse hacía que mis heridas se abrieran. La sangre empezó a salir. Busqué torpemente un amuleto en mi bolso mientras que la bola del más allá que sostenía el hombre de baja estatura comenzó a cambiar de rojo a azul. *Maldición*. Estaba invocando un hechizo.

"¡Esto es lo único que me faltaba!" murmuré furiosa encima de Francis tratando de retenerlo.

Ahora la gente corría. Desaparecían por los pasillos y salían al estacionamiento. Cuando los brujos combaten, sólo sobreviven los que corran más rápido. Tomé una bocanada de aire y vi que el hombre ya no movía los labios. Moviendo la mano hacia atrás lanzó el hechizo.

Jadeando alcancé a levantar un poco a Francis y lo puse frente a mí.

"¡No!" gritó. Estaba aterrado al ver que el hechizo venía directamente hacia él.

La fuerza del golpe nos lanzó por el suelo hasta las sillas. Francis clavó su codo en mi brazo herido y sentí mucho dolor. Su grito se apagó en un gorgoteo.

Mi hombro me estaba matando de dolor y traté de quitarme a Francis de encima. Cayó al piso sin conocimiento mientras yo retrocedí observándolo. Estaba cubierto por una delgada película azul que palpitaba. Tenía un poco en mi manga pero se escurrió sola para unirse con la que cubría a Francis. Estaba convulsionando envuelto en ella y de repente se quedó inmóvil.

Alcé la mirada. Los tres asesinos estaban hablando en latín y formaban extrañas figuras en el aire con las manos. Sus movimientos eran elegantes y deliberados.

"¡Raquel!" gritó Jenks a tres sillas de distancia. "Están fabricando una red. ¡Sal de ahí! ¡Tienes que salir de ahí!"

¿Salir? pensé mirando a Francis. El azul había desaparecido dejándolo tirado en el suelo con las piernas y los brazos abiertos en ángulos extraños. Me invadió el horror. Había hecho que Francis recibiera mi golpe. Fue un accidente. No fue mi intención matarlo.

Sentí náuseas y un nudo en el estómago. Dejé mi temor a un lado y me puse de pie con la fuerza que me infundía la rabia. Me aferré de una de las sillas anaranjadas y la acerqué tratando de levantarme. Habían logrado que usara a Francis como escudo. *Dios mío. Estaba muerto por mi culpa.*

"¿Por qué me hicieron hacer eso?" pregunté en voz baja mirando al hombre. Di un paso al frente sintiendo la tensión del ambiente. No estaba segura si lo que hice estuvo mal. Estaba viva, pero no quise hacerlo. "¿Por qué me hicieron hacer eso?" pregunté más fuerte. Sentía pinchazos por todo el cuerpo y pensé que era el comienzo de la red. No me importó. Tomé mi bolso y le di una patada a mi amuleto sin invocar.

El brujo de la línea ley abrió los ojos sorprendido cuando me acerqué a él. Con actitud decidida, empezó a invocar más fuerte. Podía escuchar a los otros dos susurrando como el viento. Era fácil moverse en el centro de la red, pero cuanto más me acercaba al borde más difícil me resultaba moverme. Estábamos parados dentro de un globo de aire azul. Del otro lado, Nick y Jenks empujaban tratando de entrar por la fuerza.

"¡Tú me hiciste hacerlo!" le grité.

Mi cabello se movió con una corriente del más allá. La red se volvió sólida. Con los dientes apretados, eché un vistazo a través de la bruma azul y pude ver los músculos del hombre fornido que ayudaba a sostener el globo al tiempo que lanzaba hechizos de líneas ley a los desaventajados oficiales de la AFE que llegaron corriendo. Ya no me importaba. Dos de los brujos estaba adentro conmigo y no irían a ninguna parte.

Estaba furiosa y frustrada. Estaba cansada de vivir escondida en una iglesia, cansada de esquivar plastas explosivas, cansada de lavar mi correspondencia en agua salada y cansada de vivir con miedo. Y, por culpa mía, Francis estaba tirado en el piso sucio de un asqueroso terminal de autobuses. Por más gusano que fuera, no merecía esto.

Caminé cojeando hasta el hombre y abrí mi bolso. Metí la mano para sentir las muescas de los hechizos de sueño. Llena de furia, lo froté contra mi cuello y lo dejé colgando de la cuerda. Empezó a mover los labios y sus manos comenzaron a dibujar patrones. Si me iba a lanzar un hechizo inmundo, me quedaban apenas cuatro segundos. Si era suficientemente fuerte para matarme, cinco segundos.

"¡Nadie!" exclamé avanzando sostenida por voluntad pura. Se asombró al ver mi marca demoníaca cuando cerré el puño. "¡Nadie me obliga a mí a matar a alguien!" le grité lanzando mi brazo.

Los dos tambaleamos. Mi puño aterrizó en su mandíbula. El dolor en mi mano fue tal que me hizo agachar. El hombre trastabilló hacia atrás pero logró equilibrarse y repentinamente dejó de concentrar su poder. Furiosa, apreté los dientes y lancé mi puño de nuevo. No esperaba que lo atacara físicamente—los brujos de líneas ley nunca lo esperaban—y alzó su brazo para detenerme. Le agarré los dedos doblándolos hacia atrás y creo que le rompí por lo menos tres.

Gritó de dolor y al mismo tiempo se escuchó el grito de incredulidad de la mujer al otro lado del vestíbulo. Ella se lanzó hacia adelante en carrera. Aún lo tenía agarrado de la mano. Levanté mi pierna y tiré de él hacia mí asestándole un buen golpe. Sus ojos dieron vueltas y cayó de espaldas agarrándose el estómago. Miró con ojos llorosos a alguien detrás mío. Aun sin respirar rodó hacia la derecha.

Yo caí jadeante al piso y rodé hacia la izquierda. Entonces se oyó una explosión que me erizó. Alcé la cabeza para ver una bola de más allá verde que se extendía por la pared y el vestíbulo. Giré. La mujer menuda seguía acercándose con la cara seria y los labios en permanente movimiento. En sus manos sostenía una bola roja del más allá que comenzaba a inflarse y a exhibir rayas verdes por el esfuerzo que hacía para doblarla a su voluntad.

"¿Quieres vértelas conmigo?" le grité desde el piso. "¿Sí?" Me levanté tambaleando con una mano en la pared para mantener el equilibrio. El hombre detrás de mí dijo una palabra pero no escuché. Era demasiado ajena a mi mente para poder entenderla pero logró infiltrarse en mi cabeza. Traté de buscarle sentido. Pero entonces mis ojos se abrieron y traté de gritar.

Me tomé la cabeza con las manos cayendo de rodillas, gritando. "¡No!" chillé, clavándome las uñas en el cuero cabelludo. "¡Fuera!" Azotes con sangre seca. Gusanos retorciéndose. Amargo sabor a carne podrida.

El recuerdo de ello abandonó mi subconsciente. Jadeando, levanté la mirada. Estaba agotada. Ya no había nada en mi cabeza. Mi corazón palpitaba. Veía puntos negros que bailaban ante mis ojos. Sentía la piel cosquilleandome, como si no fuera mía. *¿Qué diablos fue eso?*

El hombre y la mujer estaban juntos. Ella tenía la mano debajo de su codo ayudándolo mientras se retorcía encima de su mano rota. Sentían ira, pero se veían, seguros y satisfechos. Él no podía usar la mano, pero obviamente no la necesitaba para matarme. Con repetir esa palabra bastaría.

Estaba muerta. Una muerta fuera de lo común, pero arrastraría conmigo a uno de ellos.

"¡Ahora!" escuché débilmente a Edden que gritaba, como a través de una bruma.

Los tres nos pusimos en alerta cuando la red comenzó a descender. La sombra de bruma azul que cubría el aire desapareció. El brujo musculoso de afuera estaba ahora en el piso con las manos puestas detrás de la cabeza. Seis oficiales de la AFE lo tenían rodeado. Sentí una pizca de esperanza, aunque dolorosa.

Mis ojos se fijaron en una figura que corría. Nick. "¡Aquí!" grité, agarrando del suelo el hechizo de sueño que había invocado y agitándolo con la mano.

El asesino se dio la vuelta pero ya era tarde. Nick se lo puso a la mujer alrededor del cuello y retrocedió. Ella se dobló. El hombre corrió para sostenerla y ponerla en el suelo lentamente. Luego miró sorprendido alrededor de la terminal.

"¡Somos de la AFE!" gritó Edden. Se veía extraño con su brazo en el cabestrillo y su arma en la mano izquierda. "¡Ponga las manos detrás de la cabeza y deje de mover la boca o le volaré los sesos!"

El hombre parpadeó asombrado. Respiró profundo y luego empezó a correr.

"¡No!" grité. Aún tirada en el suelo, desocupé mi bolso. Tomé un amuleto, lo froté en mi cuello sangrante y se lo tiré a los pies. La mitad de mis hechizos estaban enredados por las cuerdas y salieron volando como una bala a la altura de sus rodillas envolviéndolo como quien le amarra las patas a una vaca. Tropezando, cayó pesadamente.

Los agentes de la AFE llovieron sobre él. Ahora yo solo podía observar y contener la respiración. Se quedó inmóvil. Mi hechizo lo hizo caer en un sueño profundo dejándolo indefenso.

El ruido del personal de la AFE me hizo dirigir la atención hacia Francis. Me acerqué a él gateando. Estaba tirado, solo, junto a los asientos. Temí lo peor y le di vuelta. Sus ojos sin movimiento miraban al techo fijamente. Me puse pálida. *Dios mío, no.*

De repente movió el pecho. Se sonrió estupidamente bajo

el sueño que estaba teniendo. Estaba vivo y respiraba bajo el efecto de un encantamiento profundo de línea ley. Sentí alivio. No lo había matado.

"¡Atrapado!" le grité en su delgada e inconsciente cara de ratón. "¿Me oíste saco de boñiga de camello? ¡Atrapado! ¡Caíste!" *No lo había matado*.

Los zapatos pardos rayados de Edden se detuvieron junto a mí. Estaba tensa y me limpié la sangre de la cara. *No había matado a Francis*. Con los ojos entreabiertos pasé la mirada por sus pantalones caqui y su cabestrillo. Tenía puesta la gorra y no pude alejar la mirada de las letras azules que decían AFE sobre el fondo amarillo.

Edden emitió un murmullo de satisfacción. Su gran sonrisa lo hacía verse como un gnomo. Entumecida, parpadeé. Me costaba un esfuerzo sobrenatural llenar de aire mis pulmones.

"Morgan" dijo el hombre alegremente extendiendo su mano gruesa para ayudarme a levantar. "¿Se encuentra bien?"

"No" refunfuñé. Estiré los brazos para aferrarme a él. Sentí que el suelo daba vueltas y vi a Nick que trataba de decir algo. Luego perdí el conocimiento.

Treinta y dos

"¡**E**scuchen!" gritó Francis escupiendo babitas con el fervor de sus palabras. "Les diré todo. Yo sólo tenía que hacer decomisos de azufre. Eso es todo. Pero descubrieron a uno y el Sr. Kalamack decidió cambiar los envíos. Me pidió que hiciera el cambio. ¡Eso es todo! Yo no soy un traficante de drogas biológicas. Por favor. ¡Tienen que creerme!"

Edden no respondió jugando al policía difícil sentado frente a mí. Los documentos de remisión que firmó Francis y que lo incriminaban estaban ahora en sus manos. Francis actuaba como un cobarde sentado a uno de los extremos de la mesa, dos sillas más allá. Estaba asustado y tenía los ojos bien abiertos. Se veía patético con esa camisa de colores y esa chaqueta de poliéster con las mangas subidas tratando de vivir su vida de sueños.

Yo estiré mi adolorido cuerpo lentamente con los ojos puestos en las tres cajas de cartón amontonadas al otro lado de la mesa. Sonreí levemente. Sobre mis muslos, debajo de la mesa, tenía un amuleto que le quité al asesino principal. Era de color rojo brillante, muy desagradable. Se volvería negro en caso de que yo muriera o pagara mi contrato. Yo pensaba dormir durante una semana tan pronto el infame se apagara.

Edden hizo que Francis y yo entráramos al cuarto de descanso de los empleados para evitar otro ataque de brujos.

Gracias a los noticieros locales, todo el mundo sabía donde estaba. Ahora esperaba el momento en que aparecieran hadas por las tuberías. Confiaba más en la manta que me envolvía que en los agentes de la AFE que rodeaban la habitación para que pareciera llena de gente.

Acomodé la manta mejor alrededor de mi cuello sintiendo su calor y la mínima protección que me ofrecía. Tenía una red tejida de pequeños hilillos de titanio que garantizaba la dilución de conjuros fuertes y rompía los más débiles. Los oficiales de la AFE usaban overoles hechos con esa misma tela y guardaba la esperanza de que a Edden se le olvidara pedírmela.

Mientras que Francis balbuceaba me dediqué a mirar las lúgubres paredes llenas de frases acerca de la alegría en el puesto de trabajo y cómo demandar al patrón. En una de las paredes había un horno de microondas y una nevera venida a menos. En otra una mesa con manchas de café. Tenían una decrépita máquina de dulces y sentí hambre otra vez. Nick y Jenks estaban en una esquina tratando de no entrometerse.

De repente se abrió la pesada puerta del cuarto. Entraron un oficial de la AFE y una mujer vestida con un provocativo vestido rojo. Llevaba un carné de identificación de la AFE alrededor del cuello. La gorra amarilla sobresalía como elemento ordinario. Adiviné que deberían ser Gerry y Briston, los del centro comercial. La mujer arrugó la cara y susurró burlonamente. "Perfume." Dejé escapar el aire. Me gustaría explicárselo, pero seguramente haría más mal que bien.

Los comentarios de los oficiales de la AFE me habían suministrado mi primera lección cuando me deshice del hechizo de disfraz y me convertí de viejita en mujer de veinte y tantos años de pelo ondulado rojo y con las curvas en su sitio, y uno que otro golpe. Me sentía como una semilla de maraca. Con mi cabestrillo, el ojo negro y envuelta en la manta me veía como un refugiado.

"¡Raquel!" gritó Francis con urgencia atrayendo mi atención. Su cara triangular estaba pálida y su pelo negro estaba hecho greñas. "Necesito protección. Yo no soy como tú. Kalamack va a matarme. ¡Haré lo que me pidan! Ustedes quieren a Kalamack. Yo quiero protección. Yo sólo me encargaba del azufre. No es mi culpa. ¡Raquel, tienes que creerme!"

"Sí, seguro." Estaba totalmente agotada. Respiré profundo y miré el reloj. Apenas habían transcurrido las doce de la noche pero a mí me parecía que ya iba a amanecer.

Edden sonrió. Su silla raspó el suelo cuando se levantó. Aferré bien el amuleto en mi mano y me incliné a mirar. Mi existencia dependía de aquellas cajas. Escuché el ruido de la cinta que se desprendía. Francis se limpió la boca observando con fascinación y miedo al mismo tiempo.

"Por amor a la Virgen" exclamó uno de los policías retrocediendo de la mesa tan pronto se abrió una de las cajas. "¡Son tomates!"

¿Tomates? Me puse de pie de un salto gruñendo de dolor. Edden saltó primero que yo.

"¡Están adentro!" balbuceó Francis. "Las drogas están adentro. Esconde las drogas en tomates para que los perros de la aduana no las detecten." Pálido tras su barbilla, se subió de nuevo las mangas. "¡Están ahí adentro! ¡Miren!"

"¿Tomates?" dijo Edden molesto. "¿Hace sus envíos en tomates?"

Cajas de tomates perfectos con tallos verdes. Quedé asombrada. Seguramente Trent introducía las ampollas durante el desarrollo de la fruta. Una vez maduros los tomates, las drogas ya estaban seguras adentro de un producto inofensivo que ningún humano se atrevía a comer.

"Ve allá Nick" demandó Jenks, pero Nick no se atrevió a moverse. Estaba pálido. Los dos policías que habían abierto las cajas se frotaban insistentemente las manos en el fregadero.

Como si se fuera a enfermar, Edden estiró la mano para agarrar un tomate y examinarlo. Su superficie era perfecta, sin un solo corte o rasguño. "Supongo que deberíamos abrir uno" dijo sin entusiasmo dejándolo sobre la mesa y limpiándose la mano en el pantalón.

"Yo lo haré," dije voluntariamente al ver que nadie se ofrecía. Alguien me pasó un cuchillo manchado. Lo agarré con la mano izquierda pero recordé que tenía la derecha en el cabestrillo. Busqué ayuda con la mirada pero ninguno de los policías de la AFE me miró a los ojos. Nadie estaba dispuesto a tocarlo. Alcé las cejas y dejé el cuchillo a un lado. "Está bien" dije. Alcé la mano y la dejé caer con fuerza sobre el tomate.

La camisa blanca de Edden quedó repentinamente salpicada de rojo. Su cara se tornó tan gris como su bigote y se escuchó un murmullo de desagrado entre los oficiales de la AFE. Alguno por poco vomita. Con el corazón palpitando, agarré el tomate con la mano y lo estrujé. La pulpa y las semillas corrieron entre mis dedos. De pronto mi respiración se detuvo al sentir un cilindro del tamaño de mi dedo meñique en la palma de la mano. Dejé caer la pulpa y agité mi mano. Hubo más murmullos de incredulidad al ver cómo se salpicaba la mesa con tomate. Era solo un tomate, pero por los ruidos de los musculosos y fuertes policías de la AFE, cualquiera creería que estaba estrujando un corazón putrefacto.

"¡Aquí está!" dije triunfalmente. Mostré en alto una ampolla de laboratorio cubierta de tomate. Nunca antes había visto drogas biológicas. Pensé que eran más impresionantes.

"Por todos los infiernos" dijo Edden muy suave tomando la ampolla con una servilleta. La satisfacción del descubrimiento pudo más que su aversión.

Francis estaba muy asustado. Su mirada pasó de las cajas a mí. "¿Raquel?" gimió. "Me protegerás de Kalamack, ¿verdad?"

Sentí que la rabia me recorría la columna vertebral. Me había traicionado y había traicionado todos mis principios por dinero. Me volví hacia él fijándole la mirada y acercándome a su cara. "Te vi donde Kalamack," le dije, y sus labios se pusieron tan blancos como un papel. Luego lo agarré de la colorida camisa dejándole una mancha roja. "Eres un traidor y te vas a podrir." Lo empujé de nuevo contra el espaldar del asiento y me senté con el corazón agitado por el esfuerzo, pero satisfecha.

"Bien, arréstenlo y léanle sus derechos."

Francis abrió y cerró la boca aterrado mientras que Briston sacó sus esposas de la cintura y se las puso alrededor de las muñecas. Me quité difícilmente mi brazalete hechizado de la mano mala y se lo lancé en caso de que Francis tuviera algo malévolo escondido bajo la manga. Edden dio su visto bueno y Briston se lo puso a Francis.

Los ojos de Francis estaban fijos en la ampolla. Creo que no escuchaba al hombre que estaba junto a él. "¡Raquel" gritó tan pronto le volvió la voz. "¡No dejes que me mate! ¡Me matará! ¡Yo te entregué a Kalamack! Ahora quiero un trato. ¡Quiero protección! Así funcionan estas cosas ¿verdad?"

Miré a Edden. Limpié lo que me quedaba de tomate con una servilleta de papel. "¿Tenemos que escuchar esto ahora?"

Edden sonrió maliciosamente. "Briston, mete a este costal de mierda en la camioneta. Registra su confesión por escrito y luego grábala. Léele sus derechos de nuevo. No quiero errores."

Francis se puso de pie y su silla raspó el sucio piso de baldosas. Su cara estaba demacrada y el pelo le caía sobre los ojos. "¡Raquel, diles que Kalamack me matará!"

Miré a Edden y apreté los labios. "Es verdad."

Francis comenzó a lloriquear al oír mis palabras. Sus ojos oscuros parecían embrujados, sin saber si debía estar contento o preocupado de que alguien tomara en serio sus temores.

"Dale una manta EAC" dijo Edden con desgano. "Cuídenlo."

Me sentí más tranquila. Francis estaría seguro cuanto más rápido lo sacaran de aquí.

Briston miró las cajas de tomates. "Capitán ¿y las cajas?"

Sonrió inclinándose sobre la mesa teniendo cuidado de no ensuciarse los brazos con el tomate derramado. "Vamos a dejar que las manejen los de pruebas."

Aliviada, Briston le hizo una señal a Clayton. "¡Raquel!" balbuceó Francis mientras se lo llevaban. "Vas a ayudarme ¿verdad? ¡Les diré todo!"

Cuatro policías de la AFE sacaron a Francis y los tacones de Briston sonaron musicalmente. La puerta se cerró y yo cerré los ojos agradeciendo el silencio. "Vaya noche," susurré.

La risa de Edden me hizo abrir los ojos. "Estoy en deuda contigo, Morgan" me dijo sosteniendo la ampolla blanca con tres servilletas de papel. "Después de verte luchar contra esos dos brujos no logro entender por qué Denon está tan obsesionado con hacerte desaparecer. ¡Eres un agente de todos los diablos!"

"Gracias" susurré al tiempo que suspiraba. Temblé recordando cómo me atreví a enfrentarme a dos brujos de línea ley al mismo tiempo. Estuve muy cerca. Si Edden no le hubiera roto la concentración al tercer brujo que sostenía la red, a lo mejor ahora estaría muerta. "Quiero darte las gracias por cubrirme la espalda" dije suavemente.

Una vez que se fueron los policías de la AFE, Nick salió de su esquina. Me dio un vaso con algo que alguna vez fue café. Lentamente se sentó en la silla junto a mí con la mirada puesta en las tres cajas que había en la mesa y el tomate desparramado. Parece que sintió más valor al ver a Edden tomarlo con la mano. Sonreí cansada y aferré el vaso de café para sentir el calor.

"Le agradecería que le informara a la S.E. que va a pagar mi contrato" le dije, "antes de poner un pie fuera de este cuarto" agregué, acomodándome mejor la manta EAC.

Edden dejó la ampolla con lentitud reverente. "Con la

confesión de Percy, Kalamack no podrá comprar su libertad." Ahora sonreía de oreja a oreja. Clayton me dijo que también decomisamos el azufre en el aeropuerto. Tal vez debería salir más en lugar de estar aquí detrás de este escritorio."

Tomé un sorbo de café. Su sabor amargo me llenó la boca y tragué sin ganas. "¿Y la llamada?" pregunté, dejando el café y observando el amuleto rojo sobre mis muslos.

Edden se sentó gruñendo y sacó un pequeño teléfono celular. Lo acunó en la mano y oprimió un sólo número con el dedo pulgar. Miré a Jenks para ver si estaba observando. Las alas del duende se agitaron. Impaciente, se deslizó sobre Nick y caminó sobre la mesa hasta mí. Yo lo alcé hasta mi hombro antes de que me lo pidiera. Jenks se paró junto a mi oído. "Tiene programado el número de la S.E."

"Qué tal eso," dije. La herida en mi frente me dolió cuando traté de alzar las cejas.

"Voy a exprimirle hasta la última gota de jugo a esta fruta" dijo Edden acomodándose atrás en su silla mientras timbraba el teléfono. La ampolla blanca estaba frente a él como un diminuto trofeo. "¿Denon? La próxima semana es luna llena. ¿Cómo estás?"

Quedé boquiabierta. No era el número de la S.E. Tenía programado el número de mi ex jefe. ¿Y seguía vivo? ¿El demonio no lo había matado? Seguramente consiguió a otra persona que le hiciera el trabajo sucio.

Edden me hizo un gesto sin entender por qué me sorprendía y regresó su atención al teléfono. "Magnífico," dijo interrumpiendo a Denon. "Escucha, quiero que canceles la orden que tienes contra una tal Srta. Raquel Morgan. ¿La conoces? Trabajaba para ti." Hubo una pausa y casi pudo descifrar lo que decía Denon pues hablaba muy fuerte. Jenks agitó las alas parado sobre mi hombro. Edden sonrió levemente.

"Ah, *sí* la recuerdas" dijo. "Magnífico. Retira a tu gente. Nosotros vamos a pagar." De nuevo una pausa y otra sonrisa.

"Denon, no sabes lo molesto que me siento. Ella no puede trabajar para la AFE. Haré la transferencia del dinero tan pronto abran los bancos por la mañana. Ah, y por favor, envía uno de tus furgones a la estación principal de autobuses. Tengo tres brujos para ser extraditados a la S.E. Estaban armando un escándalo y puesto que estábamos en los alrededores decidimos atraparlos por ustedes."

La conversación del otro lado de la línea no sonaba muy alegre y Jenks jadeó. "Ayyy Raquel," tartamudeó. "Está cabreado."

"No," dijo Edden serio sentándose derecho. "Obviamente lo disfrutaba." "No" dijo de nuevo haciendo una mueca. "Debiste pensarlo antes de mandarlos contra ella."

Las mariposas que tenía en el estómago estaban desesperadas por salir. "Dígale que tiene que disolver el amuleto principal que me enlaza" le dije colocándolo encima de la mesa para que lo viera brillar.

Edden cubrió la bocina con la mano. "¿El qué?"

Mis ojos se fijaron en el amuleto. Seguía brillando. "Dígale que quiero que disuelva el amuleto principal que me enlaza. Todos los grupos de asesinos que me buscan tienen un amuleto igual a este." Lo toqué con un dedo para cerciorarme si el cosquilleo que sentía era real o imaginario. "No se detendrán mientras brille."

Alzó las cejas. "¿Un amuleto que indica si aún estás viva?" me preguntó y yo asentí con una amarga sonrisa. Se trataba de un amable favor que se hacían los tríos de asesinos para que ninguno perdiera el tiempo planeando la muerte de alguien que ya estaba muerto.

"Ummm" dijo Edden acercando el teléfono al oído. "Denon," dijo amablemente. "Sé buen chico y apaga el hechizo que enlaza los signos vitales de Morgan para que pueda irse a dormir a casa."

La voz de Denon tronó en el pequeño parlante. Yo salté cuando oí reír a Jenks que hizo una voltereta para sentarse en mi arete. Pasé la lengua por los labios observando el amuleto deseando que se apagara. Nick me tocó el hombro y salté de nuevo pero seguí con la mirada clavada en el amuleto.

"¡Ya está!" exclamé al ver que titilaba y se apagaba. "¡Miren! ¡Desapareció!" Me latía el pulso y cerré los ojos pensando cómo se apagaban todos en la ciudad. Seguramente Denon tenía con él el amuleto maestro para ser el primero en enterarse de mi desaparición. Era un enfermo.

Lo levanté con dedos temblorosos y lo sentí pesado. Nick y yo nos miramos. Sentía tanto alivio como yo, y su sonrisa le llegaba hasta los ojos. Solté el aire recostándome en la silla mientras guardaba el amuleto en mi bolso. Había desaparecido la amenaza de muerte.

Denon enfadado preguntaba por el teléfono y Edden sonreía cada vez más. "Enciende tu televisión, Denon, buen amigo" dijo alejando el teléfono del oído un momento. "¡Dije que enciendas tu televisión! ¡Enciéndela!" Edden me miró. "Adiós Denon" le dijo en un falsete burlón. "Nos vemos en misa."

Edden colgó el teléfono. Se recostó en el espaldar de su silla y descansó su brazo bueno sobre el herido. Sonreía satisfecho. "Eres una bruja libre, Raquel. ¿Qué se siente regresar de la muerte?"

Mi cabello cayó hacia adelante al inclinarme para verme. Cada una de mis heridas reclamaba atención. Mi brazo palpitaba en el cabestrillo y me dolía la cara. "Maravilloso" repuse con una sonrisa. "Se siente maravilloso." Ahora podía regresar a casa y meterme debajo de las cobijas.

Nick se puso de pie con una mano en mi hombro. "Vamos Raquel. Te llevaremos a casa" dijo suavemente. Luego miró brevemente a Edden. "¿Puede completar los papeles mañana?"

"Seguro." Edden se levantó tomando cuidadosamente la ampolla entre los dedos dejándola caer en el bolsillo de la camisa. "Quisiera que estuvieras presente durante el interrogatorio del Sr. Percy, si puedes. Tienes un amuleto para detectar mentiras, ¿no es así?" Tengo curiosidad de compararlo con nuestros equipos electrónicos.

Sentía aturdida la cabeza y traté de acumular fuerzas para levantarme. No quise decirle a Edden el trabajo que se requiere para fabricar uno de esos amuletos y tampoco saldría a comprar hechizos por lo menos durante un mes. Tenía que dejar pasar un tiempo mientras que los amuletos dirigidos hacia mí salieran del mercado. Tal vez dos meses. Miré el amuleto negro sobre la mesa y controlé el temblor. *Tal vez nunca.*

De repente se escuchó un leve ruido de explosión y el piso tembló. Luego silencio absoluto y el sonido lejano de gente que gritaba a través de las paredes. Miré a Edden. "Eso fue una explosión" dijo, y mil ideas desfilaron por sus ojos. Pero sólo una me caló: *Trent.*

La puerta del cuarto se abrió súbitamente estrellándose contra la pared. Briston entró cayendo en el asiento que había ocupado Francis. "Capitán Edden" dijo jadeando. "¡Clayton! ¡Dios mío, Clayton!"

"Quédense con las pruebas" dijo, y salió disparado por la puerta casi tan rápido como un vampiro. Los gritos de la gente invadieron el recinto antes de que la puerta se cerrara. Briston estaba de pie con su vestido rojo y los nudillos de las manos blancos por la tensión de aferrarse a la silla. Agachó la cabeza pero pude ver cómo se le hinchaban los ojos de pesadumbre y frustración.

"Raquel" dijo Jenks tirando de mi oreja. "Levántate. Quiero ver qué sucedió."

"Fue Trent" susurré, sintiendo un nudo en las tripas. *Francis.*

"¡Levántate!" gritó Jenks como si pudiera alzarme de las orejas. "¡Arriba Raquel!"

Me levanté sintiéndome como un burro tirando de un arado. Me temblaba el estómago pero con la ayuda de Nick caminamos hacia el ruido y la confusión. Me envolví en la manta apretando mi brazo herido contra el cuerpo. Ya sabía lo que encontraría. Había visto a Trent matar a un hombre por lo menos. Pretender que se quedaría sentado con una soga legal alrededor del cuello era ridículo. Pero, ¿cómo se movilizó tan rápido?

El vestíbulo era un caos de vidrios rotos y un tropel de gente. El aire fresco de la noche penetraba por un agujero donde antes había vidrio. Había uniformes azules y amarillos de la AFE por todas partes y no precisamente para ayudar. Sentí el hedor a plástico quemado y veía el fuego negro y anaranjado que provenía del estacionamiento donde se quemaba la camioneta de la AFE. Luces rojas y azules se reflejaban contra las paredes.

"Jenks" dije sin aliento mientras que él me tiraba de las orejas para hacerme mover. "Deja de hacer eso o yo misma te destriparé."

"Entonces mueve tu trasero de brujita más rápido. No veo nada desde aquí."

Nick alejaba a los buenos samaritanos que se acercaban para ayudarme pensando que había sido herida por la explosión. Entonces cogió una gorra amarilla de la AFE y me la puso en la cabeza. Así nos dejaron tranquilos. Me sostuvo por la cintura con su brazo derecho a medida que caminábamos encima de los vidrios rotos. Ahora ya no estábamos iluminados por las luces amarillas de la estación sino por las luces titilantes de los autos de la AFE.

Afuera, los noticieros hacían su agosto desde un rincón. Sus gestos emocionados se iluminaban con las luces. Sentí un nudo en el estómago al caer en la cuenta de que su presencia fue la causa de la muerte de Francis.

Con los ojos entreabiertos por el calor, me acerqué donde estaba el capitán Edden parado en silencio, mirando, a diez metros del auto en llamas. Me detuve a su lado sin decir palabra. No me miró. Sopló el viento y el olor a plástico quemado me hizo toser. No había nada que decir. Francis estaba ahí adentro. Ahora estaba muerto.

"Clayton tenía un chico de trece años" dijo Edden con los ojos fijos en las nubes humo.

Sentí como si me hubieran dado un golpe en el estómago

y tuve que esforzarme para mantenerme en pie. Trece años. Mala edad para perder a su papá.

Edden respiró hondo. La fría expresión de su cara me heló. Las temblorosas sombras de las llamas hicieron resaltar las facciones de su cara. "No te preocupes, Morgan" dijo. "El trato es que me entregues a Kalamack y la AFE pagará tu contrato." Su cara estaba repleta de emociones pero no supe si eran de dolor o de rabia. "Tú me lo entregaste y yo lo dejé ir. Sin la confesión de Percy todo lo que tenemos es la palabra de una bruja muerta contra la suya. Para cuando obtenga una orden de allanamiento, los campos de tomates de Kalamack habrán desaparecido bajo la tierra. Lo siento. Se va a escabullir. Esto" dijo señalando el fuego, "esto no es tu culpa."

"Edden" comencé, pero levantó la mano.

Entonces se alejó caminando. "No quiero errores" se dijo a sí mismo. Estaba más golpeado que yo. Un oficial de la AFE de uniforme amarillo corrió a alcanzarlo, pero él no le prestó atención.

Volví los ojos hacia las llamas negras y doradas. Sentí enfermar. Francis estaba ahí adentro junto con mis hechizos. Parece que no traían tanta suerte después de todo.

"Esto no es tu culpa" dijo Nick sosteniéndome de nuevo con el brazo cuando mis rodillas flaqueaban. "Tú les advertiste. Hiciste todo lo que pudiste."

Me recosté en él antes de que cayera. "Lo sé" repuse secamente, convencida de que así era.

Un camión de bomberos se acercó en zigzag entre los autos estacionados, despejando la calle y atrayendo más gente con sus esporádicos sonidos de sirena. "Raquel" dijo Jenks jalando de nuevo.

"Ya déjame en paz, Jenks" le dije frustrada y amargada.

"Pues sacude tu escoba, brujita. Jonathan está del otro lado de la calle" repuso.

"¡Jonathan!" La adrenalina cruzó mi cuerpo adolorido y me solté de Nick. "¿Dónde?"

"¡No mires!" dijeron Nick y Jenks al unísono.

Nick me abrazó de nuevo y comenzó a dar la vuelta.

"¡Alto!" grité, ignorando el dolor tratando de ver a mis espaldas. "¿Dónde está?"

"Sigue caminando" dijo Nick secamente. "Tal vez Kalamack también te quiere ver muerta."

"¡Maldición! ¡Váyanse los dos al maldito Giro!" grité. "¡Quiero ver!" Empecé a resistirme para ver si lograba detener a Nick. Funcionó, pues logré soltarme y comencé a caminar.

Me di vuelta para explorar la calle de enfrente y me llamó la atención alguien que caminaba con paso rápido y familiar. Jonathan estaba mezclado entre el personal de emergencia y los fisgones. Era fácil ubicar a ese hombre alto y refinado que sobresalía sobre la muchedumbre. Estaba apurado, dirigiéndose hacia un auto estacionado frente al camión de bomberos. Observé con preocupación el largo auto negro pues sabía quién estaba adentro.

Manoteé a Nick para que me soltara cuando trató de enderezarme, maldiciendo a las personas y a los autos que se cruzaban en mi camino. La ventanilla de atrás bajó. Trent me miró a los ojos y contuve el aire. Las luces de los vehículos de emergencia me dejaron ver que su cara estaba herida y su cabeza cubierta de vendajes. El odio en sus ojos me apretó el corazón. "Trent" murmuré. Nick corrió para sostenerme pasando sus brazos debajo de los míos.

Nick se quedó quieto y los dos vimos cómo Jonathan se detuvo junto a la ventanilla. Se inclinó para escuchar a Trent. Mi pulso se aceleró al ver que el hombre alto se enderezó abruptamente para buscarme con la mirada. Temblé sintiendo el odio que emanaba de Jonathan.

Los labios de Trent se movieron y Jonathan saltó. Me dio un último vistazo y caminó tieso hacia la puerta del chofer. Luego escuché como tiraba la puerta.

No pude quitarle los ojos a Trent. Su expresión estaba llena de ira, pero sonrió y aquello me hizo pensar en la promesa que transmitía. La ventanilla subió y el auto se alejó lentamente.

No hice nada durante un instante. El pavimento estaba caliente. Si me levantaba tendría que moverme. Denon no mandó al demonio. Fue Trent.

Treinta y tres

Me agaché para recoger el periódico del último escalón de la iglesia. El olor a hierba recién cortada y el pavimento húmedo era como un bálsamo para mis sentidos. De pronto sentí que algo sucedía en la acera. En alerta, asumí mi posición de defensa. La niñita que montaba en su bicicleta rosada haciendo sonar la campanilla me hizo sentir como una tonta. Sus talones brillaban mientras pedaleaba tan rápido como si la persiguiera el mismo diablo. Sonreí golpeando el periódico contra la palma de mi mano y vi que daba la vuelta a la esquina. Me esperaba todas las tardes.

Había transcurrido una semana desde que la amenaza de muerte de la S.E. se había cancelado oficialmente. Pero yo seguía viendo asesinos. Claro que no sólo la S.E. quería verme muerta.

Exhalé ruidosamente y dejé que la adrenalina se asentara mientras cerraba la puerta de la iglesia a mis espaldas. El sonido del papel resonó en las pesadas vigas y paredes del santuario a medida que buscaba las páginas de avisos clasificados. Luego puso el resto debajo del brazo y me dirigí hacia la cocina mirando los avisos personales.

"Ya era hora de que te levantaras, Raque" dijo Jenks haciendo ruido con sus alas, volando en círculos por el estrecho pasillo. Jenks olía a jardín. Estaba vestido con ropas de trabajo y parecía un Peter Pan en miniatura con alas. "¿Vamos a ir por ese disco o no?"

"Hola Jenks" dije, sintiendo ansiedad y expectativa. "Sí, claro. Ayer solicitaron a un exterminador." Puse el periódico sobre la mesa del comedor empujando los mapas y colores de Ivy para hacer espacio. "Mira" le dije señalándole. "Encontré otro."

"A ver, déjame ver" exigió el duende aterrizando directamente encima del papel con las manos en la cintura.

Pasé los dedos por el aviso leyendo en voz alta. "TK busca reestablecer comunicación con RM, asunto: posible incursión de negocios." No había número telefónico pero era obvio quién lo había escrito: Trent Kalamack.

Con cierta preocupación me senté a la mesa. Miré hacia el jardín por encima de Don Pez, ahora en su nueva pecera de vidrio. Aun cuando mi contrato estaba pagado y la S.E. no era mayor amenaza, aún tenía que vérmelas con Trent. Sabía que producía drogas biológicas. Por eso, yo era una amenaza. Ahora él tenía paciencia, pero si yo no aceptaba trabajar para él me iba a poner bajo tierra.

Ahora ya no quería su cabeza. Quería que me dejara en paz. Chantajearlo era perfectamente aceptable y mucho más seguro que tratar de deshacerme de él en las cortes. Era un hombre de negocios y el lío para desembarazarse de un juicio era peor que su deseo de que trabajara para él o de verme muerta de una vez por todas. Necesitaba más que una simple hoja arrancada de su agenda. Hoy obtendría lo que necesitaba.

"Bonita pinta, Jenks" dijo Ivy desde el pasillo.

Salté asustada pero cambié mi actitud fingiendo acomodarme un mechón de cabello. Ivy estaba recostada contra el marco de la puerta. Parecía el espíritu de la muerte vestida con su bata negra. Se dirigió a la ventana para cerrar las cortinas y se recostó contra la mesa en la penumbra.

Mi silla chirrió al recostarme. "Te levantaste temprano."

Ivy se sirvió una taza de café frío del día anterior hundiéndose en el asiento frente a mí. Tenía ojeras y la bata mal amarrada a la cintura. Pasó los dedos con desgano por la hoja donde Jenks había dejado sus huellas de tierra. "Esta noche es luna llena. ¿Vamos hacerlo?"

Respiré rápidamente sintiendo que mi corazón golpeaba. Me puse de pie para botar el café viejo y preparar fresco antes de que Ivy se lo bebiera. Hasta yo tenía estándares más altos que ese. "Sí" repuse, sintiendo que me erizaba.

"¿Segura de que estás dispuesta a hacerlo?" preguntó fijando los ojos en mi cuello.

Me pareció sentir una punzada donde me miró, pero tal vez era mi imaginación. "Estoy bien" repuse, tratando de no taparme la herida con la mano. "Me siento mucho mejor. Me siento perfecta." Los pastelillos sin sabor de Ivy me produjeron hambre y náuseas al mismo tiempo y había recuperado la resistencia en tres días en lugar de tres meses. Matalina me había quitado los puntos del cuello que casi no dejaron cicatriz. Me preocupaba haberme recuperado tan rápido si tenía que pagar por ello más adelante, y de qué forma.

"¿Ivy?" pregunté mientras sacaba sobras del refrigerador. "¿De qué estaban hechos esos pastelillos?"

"Azufre."

Giré sorprendida. "¿Qué?" pregunté.

Jenks hizo una mueca e Ivy no me quitó la mirada de encima mientras se ponía de pie. "Estoy bromeando," dijo secamente. Me quedé mirándola. "¿No puedes aceptar una broma?" agregó caminando hacia el pasillo. "Dame una hora. Llamaré a Carmen para que se mueva."

Jenks saltó al aire. "Maravilloso" dijo agitando las alas. "Voy a despedirme de Matalina." El vuelo de Jenks produjo un haz de luz en la cocina cuando pasó en medio de las cortinas.

"¡Jenks! ¡No saldremos antes de una hora!" No necesitaba tanto tiempo para despedirse.

"¿A no?" escuché su voz lejana. "¿Acaso crees que mis hijos brotaron de la tierra?"

Me sonrojé y encendí la cafetera. Mis movimientos dejaban ver mi ansiedad y me detuve a pensar un instante. Había pasado la semana anterior planeando cuidadosamente con Jenks mi entrada donde Trent. Tenía un plan. También tenía un plan de apoyo. Tenía tantos planes que no entendía por qué no salían de mis orejas cuando me sonaba la nariz.

Mi ansiedad y el inevitable cumplimiento de horarios de Ivy nos colocaron exactamente una hora más tarde en la calle. Ivy y yo estábamos vestidas de cuero como motociclistas. Nuestra imagen no era precisamente la de un par de angelitos, especialmente la de Ivy. Escondidos alrededor del cuello llevábamos amuletos de esos que nos indicaban si estábamos bajo amenaza de muerte. Era mi plan de escape. Si me metía en problemas rompería el hechizo y el amuleto de Ivy se pondría rojo. Ella insistió, además de otras cosas que a mí me parecían innecesarias.

Subí al asiento del pasajero de la motocicleta de Ivy sin nada más que ese amuleto, un frasco de agua salada para romper el hechizo, una poción de visón y Jenks. Lo demás lo tenía Nick. Acomodé mi cabello en el casco y bajé la visera protectora y así comenzamos a movernos por Los Hollows cruzando el puente en dirección a Cincinnati. El sol de la tarde me calentaba los hombros. Hubiera querido que fuéramos de verdad tan sólo dos chicas en moto en plan de compras un viernes.

Pero en realidad nos dirigíamos hacia un estacionamiento para encontrarnos con Nick y la amiga de Ivy, Carmen. Ella tomaría mi lugar fingiendo ser yo durante el día, juntas de paseo por el campo. Me parecía una exageración, pero si con ello Ivy se sentía más tranquila, estaba bien.

Con ayuda de Nick me metería al jardín de Trent desde el estacionamiento. Él fingiría ser el tipo que extermina los insectos de los jardines, pues Jenks había infestado los preciados rosales de Trent el sábado anterior. Una vez adentro, lo demás sería fácil; eso, al menos es lo que yo me repetía constantemente.

Salí tranquila de la iglesia, pero cada cuadra que recorríamos hacia la ciudad era como un azote. Pensaba en mi plan una y otra vez analizando los defectos y los "qué tal si." Todo lo que habíamos diseñado parecía a prueba de errores visto desde la tranquilidad de nuestra cocina, pero dependía mucho de Nick e Ivy. Confiaba en ellos pero me sentía intranquila.

"Tranquilízate," gritó Ivy girando para salir de la ruidosa calle y entrando al estacionamiento junto a la plaza de la fuente. "Esto funcionará. Un paso a la vez. Eres una buena agente, Raquel."

Mi corazón dio un salto y asentí con la cabeza. Ivy no pudo ocultar la preocupación en su voz.

El estacionamiento estaba fresco y le dio la vuelta a la cerca para evitar pagar. Conduciría directo, como si estuviéramos en una calle. Me quité el casco al ver la camioneta blanca decorada con pasto verde y cachorros. No le había preguntado a Ivy dónde consiguió una camioneta de mantenimiento de jardines y tampoco lo haría ahora.

La puerta trasera se abrió mientras nosotros nos acercábamos. De la camioneta saltó la flaca amiga vampiro de Ivy vestida igual que yo con el brazo extendido para tomar mi casco. Se lo entregué al mismo tiempo que me bajé de la moto y ella tomaba mi lugar. Ivy nunca disminuyó la velocidad de la moto. Observé a Carmen metiendo su cabello rubio en el casco y aferrarse a la cintura de Ivy. ¿De verdad me veía yo así? No. Yo no era así de flaca. "Nos vemos esta noche, ¿ok?" dijo Ivy por encima del hombro siguiendo su camino.

"Entra" dijo Nick bajito, su voz opacada por el interior de la camioneta. Las miré una última vez y de un salto entré a la camioneta, cerrando la portezuela apenas entró Jenks.

"¡Por todos los diablos!" exclamó Jenks. "¿Qué demonios te hiciste?"

Nick dio media vuelta en el asiento del conductor. Sus dientes contrastaban muy fuerte sobre su piel maquillada de oscuro. "Mariscos," dijo dándose unas palmaditas en los ca-

chetes inflados. Su disfraz no era un hechizo. Se había teñido el pelo de negro metálico y con esa cara rechoncha no
parecía él. Era un buen disfraz y no activaba los detectores
de hechizos.

"Hola Raque Reque" me dijo con los ojos brillando.
"¿Cómo estás?"

"Estupendo," mentí nerviosa. No debí involucrarlo, pero
la gente de Trent conocía a Ivy. Además, él insistió. "¿Estás
seguro de que quieres hacer esto?"

Puso la camioneta en reverso. "Tengo un pretexto a
prueba de fuego. Mi tarjeta de marcar tiempo indica que estoy trabajando."

Lo miré con recelo mientras me quitaba las botas. "¿Estás
haciendo esto en tiempo de trabajo?"

"Nadie me está vigilando. Mientras cumpla con el trabajo, no les importa."

Lo miré con ironía. Estaba sentada encima de una lata
de insecticida y le dí una patada a mis botas para alejar-
las del camino. Nick había conseguido un trabajo limpiando
objetos en el Museo de Eden Park. Constantemente me sorprendía con su capacidad para adaptarse. En una semana
consiguió apartamento, lo amuebló, compró un camión des-
tartalado, consiguió trabajo y me invitó a salir—una invitación muy bonita incluyendo un tour por la ciudad en
helicóptero. Dijo que su antigua cuenta de banco le había
ayudado a organizarse de nuevo rápidamente. Seguramente
a los bibliotecarios les pagaban mucho más de lo que había
imaginado.

"Es mejor que te cambies," dijo casi sin mover los labios
mientras pagaba en la casilla automática y salíamos afuera.
"Llegaremos en menos de una hora."

Sentía mucha ansiedad y alcancé la bolsa blanca que tenía
el logotipo de la compañía de jardines. Allí metí unos zapatos livianos, mi amuleto indicador de seguridad y mi nuevo
traje de seda y nylon. Todo comprimido en una bolsa del tamaño de la palma de la mano. Hice campo para un visón y
un duende fastidioso y encima puse el overol de papel dese-

chable de Nick. Entraría como visón, pero por nada del mundo iba a quedarme así.

Mis hechizos brillaban por su ausencia. Sin ellos me sentía desnuda y si me atrapaba la S.E., lo máximo que podían imputarme era por violar la propiedad privada. Si portaba un sólo hechizo, inclusive uno que apenas produjera mal aliento, sería suficiente para que me acusaran de intentar lastimar a alguien. Eso era un delito grave y yo era un agente. Conocía la ley.

Me desvestí completamente atrás mientras Nick distraía a Jenks. Guardé toda posible prueba de mi presencia en la camioneta dentro de un tarro marcado SUSTANCIAS TÓXICAS y tomé la poción de visón. Apreté los dientes esperando el terrible dolor de la transformación. Jenks no dejó en paz a Nick cuando se enteró de que yo estuve desnuda. No quise anticipar que me iba a desnudar para no tener que aguantarme los chistes y comentarios de Jenks. Por eso tenía listo el vestido.

De ahí en adelante todo funcionó a tiempo.

Nick logró entrar al jardín sin problema pues lo esperaban. El verdadero servicio de jardines recibió mi llamada esa misma mañana cancelando la solicitud. Los prados estaban desocupados pues era luna llena y cerraban por mantenimiento general. Transformada en visón, correteé por los tupidos rosales que Nick debía rosear con un insecticida tóxico que en realidad era agua salada para transformarme de nuevo en persona. El amuleto, la ropa y los zapatos que me lanzó Nick fueron bienvenidos, especialmente teniendo en cuenta el comentario morboso de Jenks acerca de mujeres pálidas grandes desnudas mientras se balanceaba feliz en un tallo de rosa. Estaba segura de que el agua salada mataría las rosas en lugar de los furiosos insectos de Jenks. Pero eso también era parte del plan. Si por alguna razón me descubrían, Ivy entraría con un nuevo cargamento de plantas.

Jenks y yo pasamos la mayor parte de la tarde destripando insectos. Era mucho mejor que el agua salada para las rosas de Trent. Los jardines permanecían en silencio y los demás trabajadores siguieron las indicaciones de mantenerse a distancia que instaló Nick alrededor del rosal. Cuando finalmente salió la luna, yo estaba más tiesa que un gnomo virgen el día de su matrimonio, y el frío no ayudaba para nada.

"¿Ahora?" preguntó Jenks sarcásticamente. Sus alas parecían invisibles excepto por un ligero brillo plateado que le resplandecía de noche volando encima de mí.

"Ahora" repuse entre dientes a medida que avanzaba con mucho cuidado entre las espinas.

Jenks volaba en la vanguardia y así empezamos a merodear entre arbustos y árboles majestuosos. Finalmente entramos por una puerta trasera del comedor. De ahí al vestíbulo principal era cerca. Jenks ajustó las cámaras como de costumbre.

La nueva cerradura de la oficina de Trent nos dio más trabajo. Con el corazón palpitando, me moví intranquila junto a la puerta durante cinco minutos eternos que se demoró Jenks tratando de abrirla. Maldiciendo como de costumbre, finalmente me pidió ayuda para que sostuviera un interruptor con un papel sin doblar. Naturalmente, no se tomó la molestia de advertirme que estaba cerrando un circuito hasta que un corrientazo me hizo caer sentada en el trasero.

"¡Idiota!" susurré desde el piso mostrándole el puño en lugar de lanzárselo a las narices como hubiera querido. "¿¡Qué demonios crees que haces!?"

"No lo habrías hecho si te lo digo" repuso desde el techo.

Ignoré su estúpida justificación y empujé la puerta. Pensaba encontrarme con Trent esperándome y pude respirar tranquila al ver que no había nadie, sólo se veía la lucecilla del acuario detrás de su escritorio. Inmediatamente me dirigí agachada hasta el cajón de abajo y esperé a que Jenks me confirmara que no estaba con alarma. Contuve el aire y lo abrí. No había nada.

No me sorprendí y miré a Jenks encogiéndome de hombros. "Plan B" dijimos a un tiempo. Saqué un trapo del bolsillo y limpié todo. "A la oficina de atrás."

Jenks salió volando por la puerta y regresó. "Nos quedan cinco minutos. Tenemos que apurarnos."

Asentí con la cabeza mirando por última vez la oficina de Trent antes de seguir a Jenks. Zumbó delante de mí por el pasillo a la altura de mi pecho. Nerviosa, lo seguí a una distancia prudencial. Mis zapatos no hacían ruido sobre la alfombra a medida que trotaba por el edificio desocupado. El amuleto alrededor de mi cuello brillaba de un hermoso color verde.

Mi pulso se aceleró y sonreí al ver a Jenks parado frente a la puerta de la segunda oficina de Trent. Esto era lo que me hacía falta y la razón por la cual quería abandonar a la S.E.: la emoción, la lucha contra las adversidades. Quería demostrar que era más inteligente que los malos. Esta vez conseguiría lo que vine a llevarme. "¿Cuánto tiempo tenemos?" susurré frenando en seco sacándome un mechón de cabello de la boca.

"Tres minutos." Voló arriba y abajo. "No hay cámaras en su oficina privada. No está allí. Ya revisé."

Satisfecha, entré por la puerta y la cerré muy suave después que Jenks entró volando.

El olor del jardín era como un bálsamo. La luz de la luna entraba como si fuera la mañana. Me arrastré hasta el escritorio con una mueca irónica, pues ahora tenía la sensación de que estaba siendo utilizada. En segundos encontré el portafolio junto al escritorio. Jenks movió el cerrojo y yo lo abrí. Los dos suspiramos al ver los discos bien ordenados en filas. "¿Estás segura de que estos son?" musitó Jenks sobre mis hombros mientras que yo sacaba uno para meterlo en mi bolsillo.

Yo sabía que sí eran, pero apenas abrí la boca para responderle, sentimos que se rompía una rama en el jardín.

El corazón me latía aceleradamente y le hize a Jenks una señal con el dedo para que se escondiera. Voló en silencio hasta las luces. Yo contuve la respiración y me agaché detrás del escritorio.

Tenía la esperanza de que fuera un animal pero no fue así.

Pasos suaves primero que después se tornaron fuertes. Una sombra alta pasó segura del camino a la terraza. Dio tres pasos ágiles y mis rodillas flaquearon cuando reconocí la voz de Trent. Cantaba una canción que no pude reconocer mientras que se movía de tal forma que me producía escalofríos en la espalda. *Mierda,* pensé, tratando de acurrucarme más detrás del escritorio.

Trent estaba de espaldas buscando algo en el armario. Un incómodo silencio reemplazó su canto y se sentó en el borde de la silla entre la terraza y yo, mudándose de zapatos por una botas de montar. La luz de la luna hacía brillar su camisa blanca y parecía que la luz atravesara su chaqueta. Era difícil saberlo en la oscuridad, pero me pareció que su vestimenta inglesa de jinete era verde en lugar de roja. *Trent cría caballos,* pensé, *pero, ¿monta de noche?*

El golpe para acomodar sus talones en las botas sonó duro. Mi respiración comenzó a acelerarse al ver que se ponía de pie, pues se veía mucho más alto que de costumbre. La luz se opacó al paso de una nube frente a la luna y por poco no caigo en la cuenta de que estiró la mano debajo del asiento que había usado.

Con un movimiento suave sacó una pistola y me apuntó directamente. Sentí un nudo en la garganta.

"Puedo escucharla" dijo con voz firme. "Salga" "Ahora."

El escalofrío me recorrió de pies a cabeza y sentí agujas en las puntas de los dedos. Me acurruqué más debajo del escritorio pues no podía creer que me hubiera sentido. Pero me estaba mirando de frente, con las piernas bien abiertas y su sombra se veía formidable. "Baja el arma primero," susurré.

"¿Srta. Morgan?" dijo sorprendido como si esperara encontrar a otra persona. "¿Por qué debería bajarla?" preguntó con voz triste a pesar de la carga de amenaza que llevaba.

"Mi compañero le está apuntando con un hechizo en este momento" mentí. La sombra se movió y miró hacia el techo. "Luces, cuarenta y ocho por ciento" ordenó con voz gruesa. El cuarto se iluminó pero no lo suficiente para arruinar mi visión nocturna. Con mis rodillas convertidas en gelatina me levanté fingiendo que todo esto estaba planeado. Me apoyé en su escritorio con mi vestido apretado y crucé los tobillos.

Con la pistola en la mano, Trent me examinó con los ojos rápidamente. Se veía repugnantemente refinado e inteligente en su traje verde de montar. Me esforcé por no mirar el arma que me apuntaba a pesar de que tenía las tripas revueltas. "¿La pistola?" le dije confrontándolo y mirando hacia el techo donde estaba Jenks.

"¡Suelte el arma, Kalamack!" gritó Jenks desde una luz con sus alas zumbando en son de ataque.

Trent asumió una pose informal parecida a la mía. Le sacó las balas a la pistola y la tiró a mis pies. No la toqué pero sentí que mi respiración se normalizaba. Las balas sonaron al caer en un bolsillo de su chaqueta de montar. Con esta luz pude ver que sus heridas demoníacas habían sanado. Tenía un golpe amarillento en una mejilla y el extremo de un yeso sobresalía de la manga de la chaqueta. En la quijada mostraba un rasguño sanando. No pude evitar pensar que, a pesar de todo, aún se veía muy bien. No era normal que se sintiera tan seguro teniendo un hechizo mortal colgando sobre su cabeza.

"Me basta decir una palabra, y Quen llegará en tres minutos" dijo indiferentemente.

"¿Y cuánto tiempo necesita para morir?" amenacé.

Apretó los dientes con rabia. Así se veía más joven. "¿Vino para eso?"

"Si fuera así ya estaría muerto."

Acepté eso como verdad. Parado ahí, recto, vio su portafolio abierto. "¿Qué disco tomó?"

Fingiendo sentirme segura, me quité un mechón de pelo de los ojos. "Huntington. Si algo me sucede, este disco irá a seis diarios y tres canales de noticias, junto con la hoja que falta en su agenda." Di unos pasos para alejarme del escritorio. "Déjeme en paz" le dije en clara amenaza.

Se quedó parado con los brazos colgando a los lados, pero

su brazo roto haciendo un ángulo. Sentí aguijones en la piel y también que mi máscara de seguridad comenzaba a desaparecer. "¿Magia negra?" rió burlonamente. "Los demonios asesinaron a tu padre. Qué pena ver morir a la hija de la misma forma."

"¿Qué sabe usted de mi padre?" le pregunté asombrada.

Dirigió la mirada hacia mi muñeca, la que tenía la marca del demonio, y palidecí. Sentí un nudo en el estómago recordando cómo ese demonio me mataba lentamente. "Espero que lo haya lastimado" le dije sin importarme el temblor de mi voz. A lo mejor pensaría que era de rabia. "No entiendo cómo logró sobrevivir. Yo por poco no lo logro."

Trent se puso rojo y me apuntó con el dedo. Me gustaba verlo actuar como una persona normal. "Fue un error haber mandado a ese demonio a atacarme" dijo con decisión. "Yo no me meto con magia negra y tampoco permito que lo hagan mis empleados."

"¡Miserable mentiroso!" exclamé sin importarme si sonaba como una inmadura. "Recibió lo que merece. ¡Yo no empecé esto, pero seré maldita si no lo termino!"

"Yo no soy el que porta la marca demoníaca, Srta. Morgan" dijo fríamente. "¿Y además mentirosa? Decepcionante. Estoy pensando seriamente en retirarle mi oferta de trabajo. Espero que rece usted para que no sea así, pues no tengo por qué seguir tolerando sus actos."

Estaba furiosa. Respiré profundo para decirle que era un idiota, pero me detuve. Trent pensaba que yo había invocado al demonio que lo atacó. Estaba asombrada de lo que estaba pensando. Alguien había invocado dos demonios: uno para mí y otro para Trent, y seguro no había sido la S.E. Podía apostar mi vida. Con el corazón en la mano iba a explicarlo, pero cerré la boca.

Trent se veía preocupado. "¿Srta. Morgan?" dijo suavemente. "¿Qué idea acaba de filtrarse por esa cabeza suya?"

Moví la cabeza y pasé la lengua por mis labios a la vez que retrocedí unos pasos. Si Trent pensaba que yo hacía magia negra me dejaría en paz. Además, mientras que yo tuviera pruebas de su culpabilidad, no se arriesgaría a matarme. "No trate de acorralarme en una esquina" lo amenacé, "y no lo molestaré más."

Trent endureció su expresión. "Váyase" me dijo, moviéndose elegantemente por la terraza. Intercambiamos posiciones simultáneamente. "Voy a ser generoso con usted y le daré una buena ventaja para comenzar" dijo mientras alcanzaba su portafolio para cerrarlo. Su voz era oscura y tan pertinaz como hojas de arce descompuestas. "Me tomará diez minutos llegar hasta mi caballo."

"¿Cómo dice?" le pregunté confundida.

"No he perseguido a una presa con dos piernas desde que murió mi padre." Trent se ajustó su casaca verde de montar con un movimiento agresivo. "Es luna llena, Srta. Morgan," dijo con voz profunda y deseosa. "Los perros están sueltos. Usted es una ladrona. Según la tradición, es mejor que empiece a correr. ¡Rápido!"

Mi corazón pareció estallar y mi cara se puso pálida. Tenía lo que quería, pero no me servía de nada si no podía escapar. Había cincuenta kilómetros de bosques desde donde yo estaba y la ayuda más cercana. ¿A qué velocidad corría un caballo? ¿Cuánto podía correr antes de caer exhausta? Tal vez debí decirle que yo no había enviado al demonio.

El sonido distante de un corno atravesó la oscuridad y respondió una jauría. El temor me atravesó como un cuchillo. Era un temor viejo tan primario que nada podía aplacarlo. Ni siquiera sabía de dónde venía. "Jenks, ¡vámonos!"

"Aquí detrás tuyo, Raque" respondió desde el techo.

Corrí tres pasos y salté desde la terraza de Trent aterrizando sobre los helechos. Entonces escuché el estallido de un disparo y las hojas junto a mí quedaron destruidas. Salté hacia el huerto y corrí tan rápido como pude.

¡Bastardo! pensé. Mis rodillas temblaban. ¿Qué pasó con mis diez minutos?

Corrí dando tropezones buscando mi frasco de agua salada. Mordí la tapa e introduje mi amuleto. Titiló y se apagó, pero el de Ivy se encendería de color rojo. El camino era menos de un kilómetro y medio y allí estaba la reja de entrada. La ciudad estaba a cincuenta. ¿Cuánto demoraría en llegar Ivy?

"¿Qué tan rápido puedes volar Jenks?" le pregunté jadeando en mi carrera.

"Bastante rápido, Raque."

Me quedé en los senderos hasta alcanzar la pared del jardín. Uno de los perros ladró al verme trepar y otro le respondió. *Mierda.*

Mi respiración seguía el ritmo de mis zancadas. Crucé un prado perfecto y me introduje en un bosque macabro. Los ladridos quedaron a mis espaldas. Parece que la pared les estaba dando trabajo. Tendrían que dar la vuelta. Tal vez lograría salir de allí. "Jenks" dije jadeando a medida que mis piernas comenzaban a protestar. "¿Cuánto tiempo llevo corriendo?"

"Cinco minutos."

Dios me ayude, rogué en silencio. Las piernas me dolían.

Jenks iba adelante dejando caer polvillo de duende para indicarme el camino. Pasé por cientos de árboles mientras mis pies golpeaban el piso rítmicamente. Mis pulmones me dolían y mis costillas también. Si salía con vida de esta, me prometí correr cinco millas todos los días.

El ladrido de los perros cambió. Aun cuando los oía lejos, presentí que prometían darme alcance muy pronto. La sensación me golpeó como un aguijón. Pero acumulé fuerzas buscando voluntad para mantener mi ritmo.

Seguí corriendo. Tenía el pelo pegado en la cara. Espinas y zarzas me rasgaron la ropa y las manos. Los cornos y los perros se aproximaban. Fijé la mirada en Jenks que volaba adelante pero un fuego estalló en mis pulmones abrasándome el pecho. Detenerme sería morir.

Llegué a una quebrada que me pareció un oasis. Caí al

agua y me levanté jadeando. Mis pulmones hacía el esfuerzo máximo y me sequé el agua de la cara para poder respirar. Los latidos de mi corazón eran más fuertes que el áspero sonido de mi respiración. Los árboles hacían todo más macabro. Yo era la presa. Todos en el bosque observaban en silencio agradeciendo no estar en mi lugar.

Mi respiración carraspeaba oyendo a los perros. Estaban cerca. Oí el corno y me invadió el terror. No sabía cuál de todos los ruidos era peor.

"¡Levántate Raquel!" decía Jenks con urgencia. "Sigue la corriente."

Me levanté con mucho esfuerzo y seguí corriendo por los bajíos. El agua reduciría mi velocidad pero también a los perros. En cuestión de minutos Trent dividiría a la jauría para buscarme a ambos lados de la corriente. De esta no escaparía.

El ladrido de los perros cambió. Yo exploré la orilla con pánico. Habían perdido el rastro aun cuando estaban justo detrás de mí. La imagen de ser destrozada por perros casi me paraliza y apenas podía mover las piernas. Trent se pintaría la frente con mi sangre. Jonathan guardaría un mechón de mi pelo en un cajón de su armario. Debí decirle a Trent que yo no le había mandado a ese demonio. Pero ¿me habría creído?

El rugido de una motocicleta me hizo reaccionar. "Ivy," dije, tratando de apoyarme en un árbol. La carretera estaba cerca. Seguro que se había puesto en camino antes. "Jenks, no dejes que siga de largo" dije jadeando por un poco de aire. "Estaré detrás de tí."

"¡Listo!"

Salió disparado y yo comencé a moverme. Los perros aullaban, buscaban. Escuché voces que daban instrucciones y eso me hizo correr. Un perro ladró fuerte y claro. Otro respondió. La adrenalina me recorrió el cuerpo. Las ramas me golpeaban la cara y caí a la carretera. Las palmas de las manos laceradas me ardían pero no tenía aire para gritar. Me esforcé por levantarme. Temblando miré por la carretera y vi que me bañaba una luz blanca. El rugido de la moto fue como la bendición de un ángel. Ivy. Tenía que ser ella. Tenía que estar en camino antes de que activara mi amuleto.

Me puse de pie, lista, con los pulmones a punto de reventar. Los perros se acercaban y podía oír los pasos de los cascos de los caballos. Caminé dando tumbos, sacudiendo las manos frente a la luz blanca. De pronto se detuvo con un ruido atronador junto a mí.

"¡Súbete!" gritó Ivy.

Casi no podía levantar la pierna, así es que ella me jaló para sentarme. El motor retumbaba y me aferré a su cintura para no caer. Jenks se clavó en mi cabello. Casi no podía sentir sus manos. La moto giró, saltó y arrancó.

El cabello de Ivy flotó hacia atrás golpeándome en la cara. "¿Lo conseguiste?" gritó al viento.

No pude responderle. Estaba temblando por el susto. La adrenalina me había abandonado, pero luego sentiría las consecuencias. Veía pasar el pavimento y el viento se llevó el calor de mi cuerpo enfriando mi sudor. Luchando contra las náuseas, moví mis dedos entumecidos y sentí el disco en el bolsillo de adelante. Le di un golpecito en el hombro, incapaz de hablar. Sólo respiraba.

"¡Muy bien!" gritó.

Estaba exhausta y dejé descansar mi cabeza sobre la espalda de Ivy. Mañana me quedaría en la cama hasta que llegara el diario de la tarde. Creo que iba a estar demasiado adolorida para moverme. Mañana me pondría vendas en las heridas de ramas y espinas. Esta noche, era mejor no pensar nada sobre esta noche.

Sentí escalofrío. Al darse cuenta, Ivy giró la cabeza. "¿Te sientes bien?" gritó.

"Sí" le dije al oído para que pudiera oírme. "Estoy bien. Gracias por venir a buscarme." Me saqué su pelo de la boca y miré hacia atrás fijamente.

Tres jinetes estaban parados bajo la luna que alumbraba la carretera. Los perros giraban inquietos levantando el cuello alrededor de las patas de los caballos. Lo logré, pero sentí que se me heló hasta la médula cuando el jinete de la mitad me hizo un saludo con la frente.

De repente sentí una sensación particular. Lo había superado. Él lo sabía y tenía la nobleza de aceptarlo. ¿Cómo no sentirse impresionada por alguien tan seguro de sí mismo? "¿Qué diablos es Trent?" susurré.

"No lo sé" repuso Jenks parado en mi hombro. "No lo sé."

Treinta y cuatro

La música de jazz a media noche va bien con los grillos. En eso pensaba mientras le agregaba trozos de tomate a la ensalada. Tuve un momento de duda viendo los rojos pedazos entre las hojas verdes. Miré a Nick por la ventana frente a la parrilla. Saqué los trozos y revolví la lechuga de nuevo para ocultar lo que quedaba dentro. Nick no se daría cuenta. Además, no se iba a morir por eso.

Me sentí atraída por el sonido y el olor de la carne asada y me incliné encima de Don Pez para ver mejor. Nick llevaba puesto un delantal que decía: "No muerdas al cocinero. Bésalo." Se veía a gusto y tranquilo parado delante del fuego a la luz de la luna. Jenks estaba sobre su hombro y volaba hacia arriba como las hojas del otoño con el viento cuando saltaban las llamas.

Ivy estaba en la mesa. Tenía un aspecto lúgubre y trágico leyendo la última edición del diario de Cincinnati a la luz de una vela. Había niños duendes por todas partes con alas transparentes que lanzaban destellos de luz reflejada de la luna, ya tres días llena. Sus gritos persiguiendo a las luciérnagas rompían el sonido opaco del tráfico de Los Hollows. Era una combinación reconfortante. Era el sonido de la seguridad que me hacía recordar los días de asados con mi familia. Un vampiro, un humano, una manada de duendes, era una familia un tanto extraña, pero me sentía bien de estar viva esta noche junto a mis amigos.

Satisfecha, mezclé la ensalada con aliño y tomé salsa para carnes. Luego salí abriendo la puerta de anjeo con la espalda que se cerró con un golpe haciendo saltar a Jenks y los niños quienes se dispersaron por el cementerio. Ivy alzó la mirada del diario cuando puse la ensalada y las botellitas a su lado. "Oye, Raquel," me dijo. "Nunca me contaste dónde encontraste esa camioneta. ¿Tuviste problemas para devolverla?"

Alcé las cejas. "Yo no conseguí esa camioneta. Pensé que lo habías hecho tú."

Simultáneamente miramos a Nick parado frente a la parrilla dándonos la espalda. "¿Nick?" pregunté y él se puso un poco tenso. Me acerqué a él con la salsa para carnes en la mano. Manoteé a Jenks para que se fuera y pasé mi brazo por atrás de la cintura de Nick. Sonreí al ver que contenía sorprendido la respiración. *Qué diablos. Estaba bien para ser humano.* "¿Te robaste esa camioneta por mí?" le pregunté.

"La tomé prestada" repuso parpadeando, pero inmóvil.

"Gracias" dije sonriendo y le entregué la botellita de salsa.

"Oh, Nick" canturreó Jenks con su típico falsete burlón. "¡Eres mi héroe!"

Suspiré molesta soltando a Nick y dando unos pasos hacia atrás. Ivy resopló en señal de asombro y Jenks lanzaba besos al aire volando en círculos alrededor de nosotros.

Fastidiada, lancé la mano para golpear a Jenks.

Él saltó hacia atrás, quedándose estático en un punto, asombrado porque estuve a punto de alcanzarlo. "Qué romántico" concluyó antes de volar hasta donde Ivy para molestarla. "¿Y qué tal va tu nuevo trabajo?" dijo arrastrando las palabras aterrizando a su lado.

"¡Ya cállate Jenks!" amenazó.

"¿Trabajo? ¿Tienes una misión?" le pregunté a la vez que abría su periódico para esconderse tras él.

"¿No sabías?" preguntó Jenks alegremente. "Edden y el juez se pusieron de acuerdo para imponerle a Ivy trescientas horas de trabajo comunitario por dejar fuera de combate a medio departamento de policía. Ha estado trabajando toda la semana en el hospital."

Asombrada, me dirigí hacia la mesa del jardín. Una esquina del diario temblaba. "¿Por qué no me lo dijiste? le pregunté mientras doblaba las piernas para sentarme frente a ella en el estrecho banco.

"Tal vez porque se ve como un caramelo a rayas" exclamó Jenks. Nick y yo nos miramos sin entender. "Ayer la vi cuando se dirigía al trabajo. Tiene que vestirse con una pequeña falda de rayas blancas y rosadas y un blusa estampada" rió Jenks cayendo de mi hombro. "Y mallas ajustadas para taparse el animado trasero. Se ve bastante bien en la moto."

¿Un vampiro vestido a rayas? Me esforcé por visualizar esa imagen.

Nick soltó una carcajada que trató de convertir inmediatamente en tos. Los nudillos de los dedos de Ivy se tornaron blancos. Dada la hora y la atmósfera relajaba, no era difícil que decidiera arrastrar un aura, y ciertamente estos chistes no estaban teniendo un buen efecto.

"Está en el Centro Médico Infantil cantando y organizando té con galletas," siguió Jenks sin poder contener la risa.

"Jenks," susurró Ivy. El diario bajó lentamente y yo sentí ansiedad al ver que sus ojos comenzaban a tornarse negros.

Con las alas desplegadas, Jenks hizo una mueca y abrió la boca. Ivy enrolló el diario y trató de golpearlo más rápido que el sonido. El duende salió disparado hasta la copa del roble riendo.

De repente, todos giramos ante el chirrido de la reja de madera de adelante. "¿Hola? ¿Llego demasiado tarde?" dijo la voz de Keasley.

"¡Estamos acá atrás!" grité al notar la sombra lenta de Keasley sobre el prado cubierto de rocío y los arbustos y árboles silenciosos.

"Traje el vino" dijo tan pronto estuvo más cerca. "El rojo va con la carne, ¿correcto?"

"Gracias Keasley" dije recibiéndole la botella. "No debió molestarse."

Sonrió y trató de entregarme un sobre relleno que llevaba bajo el brazo. "Esto también es tuyo" dijo. "El cartero no quería dejarlo en la entrada, así que yo firmé."

"¡No!" gritó Ivy estirando el brazo desde el otro lado de la mesa para agarrar el sobre. Jenks también voló desde el roble agitando las alas. Ivy se lo arrebató de las manos.

Keasley la miró de mal humor y decidió hacerle compañía a Nick junto a la parrilla.

"Ya ha pasado más de una semana" le dije fastidiada a medida que me secaba la mano del sudor de la botella que trajo Keasley. "¿Cuándo me dejarás abrir mi correspondencia?"

Ivy no respondió. Acercó la vela de citronela al sobre para leer el nombre del remitente. "Tan pronto Trent deje de mandarte correo" dijo suavemente.

"¡Trent!" exclamé. Me acomodé el pelo detrás de la oreja pensando en la carpeta que le había entregado a Edden hacía dos días. Nick volteó la cabeza y se veía preocupado. "¿Qué quiere?" musitó.

Ivy miró a Jenks. "Está limpio. Ábrelo" dijo el duende.

"Por supuesto que está limpio," gruñó Keasley. "¿Acaso crees que le daría una carta hechizada?"

Tomé el sobre de las manos de Ivy. Se sentía liviano. Pasé nerviosamente una uña por debajo de la tapa para abrirlo. Adentro se sentía un bulto y sacudí el sobre encima de la mano.

Del sobre salió el anillo que usaba en el dedo meñique y lo atrapé con la mano. Quedé boquiabierta por la sorpresa. "¡Mi anillo!" dije. Con el corazón dando golpes, miré mi otra mano y vi que no lo llevaba puesto. Alcé la mirada para ver la sorpresa de Nick y la preocupación de Ivy. "Pero cómo…" tartamudeé, pues no recordaba haberlo perdido jamás. "¿Cuándo? ¿Jenks? No puede ser que lo haya perdido en su oficina, ¿o sí?"

El tono de mi voz era alto y sentí presión en el estómago

cuando agitó la cabeza negativamente y sus alas se tornaron oscuras. "Esa noche no llevabas ninguna joya. Debió tomarlo después."

"¿Hay algo más?" preguntó Ivy secamente.

"Sí" repuse poniéndome mi anillo. Al comienzo lo sentí extraño pero luego se fue acomodando. Con las manos heladas, saqué un papel grueso de lino con olor a pino y manzana.

"Srta. Morgan," empecé a leer lentamente. "Felicitaciones por su nueva independencia. Cuando se de cuenta de lo ilusoria que es, le mostraré la verdadera libertad."

Dejé caer el papel sobre la mesa. Aquella inquietante sensación que tuve de que él me había estado observando mientras dormía se deshizo cuando comprendí que tan sólo era eso. El chantaje había echado raíces. Funcionó.

Puse aliviada los codos sobre la mesa y la frente entre mis manos. Trent había tomado mi anillo por un motivo: para demostrarme que podía hacerlo. Yo me infiltré en su "casa" tres veces. Tal vez él no toleraba el hecho de que podía hacerlo y sintió la necesidad de responder para demostrar que era capaz de hacer lo mismo. Había logrado acorralarlo y con eso avanzaba mucho en el camino de liberarme de mi sentimiento de vulnerabilidad.

Jenks voló por encima de la carta. "Costal de babosas" dijo, dejando escapar polvillo de duende. "¡Logró evadir mi vigilancia!, lo logró. ¿Cómo diablos lo hizo?"

Levanté el sobre y vi que el sello postal tenía la fecha del día siguiente al que escapé de él y sus perros. El hombre se movía rápido. Tenía que darle crédito por ello. Entonces pensé si sería él o Quen el que hizo el robo, pero apostaría a que había sido Trent.

"¿Raque?" dijo Jenks aterrizando sobre mi hombro, tal vez preocupado por mi silencio. "¿Te sientes bien?"

Miré la cara de preocupación de Ivy pensando en alguna forma de reírme de esta situación. "Voy a ir tras él" dije en broma.

Jenks se alejó de mi volando alarmado, Nick se dio media

vuelta y Ivy se puso seria. "Espera un minuto," dijo mirando a Jenks.

"¡Nadie me hace esto a mí!" continué haciendo un esfuerzo por no reír para no arruinar el juego.

Keasley frunció el ceño y se sentó acomodándose bien.

Ivy se puso más pálida que de costumbre a la luz de la vela. "Más despacio Raquel" me advirtió. "Él no hizo nada. Sólo quería tener la última palabra. Déjalo de ese tamaño."

"¡Volveré!" grité, alejándome un poco en caso de que estuviera atrayéndola demasiado y decidiera venir por mí. "Yo le enseñaré" dije agitando un brazo. "¡Voy a entrar a escondidas para robarle sus malditos lentes y se los mandaré por correo el día de su maldito cumpleaños!"

Los ojos de Ivy se pusieron negros. "¡Si lo haces te matará!"

¿De verdad creía que regresaría? ¿Estaba loca? Mi boca temblaba pues yo hacía esfuerzos para no reír. Keasley se dio cuenta y comenzó a sonreír extendiendo el brazo para alcanzar la botella de vino aun cerrada.

Ivy giró con velocidad de vampiro. "¿De qué te ríes, brujo?" dijo inclinándose hacia adelante. "Se va a matar. Jenks, dile que se va a matar. No te dejaré hacerlo Raquel, te lo juro. ¡Te amarraré antes de permitir que regreses!"

Sus dientes brillaban bajo la luz de la luna y estaba a punto de estallar. Una palabra más y habría sido capaz de cumplir su amenaza. "Está bien" dije con indiferencia. "Tienes razón. Lo dejaré en paz."

Ivy se quedó inmóvil y Nick dejó escapar un gran suspiro desde la parilla. Keasley quitó lentamente la cubierta de la botella. "Vaya, vaya. Te engañó, Tamwood" dijo riendo con gusto. "Te engañó de lo lindo."

Ivy se quedó mirándome, su cara blanca y perfecta oculta tras la realidad de que la había engañado. El desconcierto inicial cambió en alivio y después en molestia. Respiró profundo y se puso seria. Con rabia, se sentó de golpe a la mesa y agitó el papel.

Jenks reía formando círculos de polvillo de duende que

caían como rayos de sol que brillaban sobre sus hombros. Me levanté con una sonrisa y me dirigí a la parrilla. Eso me había gustado de verdad, casi tanto como haber tomado el disco. "Oye, Nick" dije acercándome por detrás. "¿Ya está esa carne?"

Nick sonrió. "Ya está a punto, Raquel."

Bien. Luego pensaría en todo lo demás.

Las aventuras de Raquel Morgan continúan con...

EL REGRESO DE LOS MUERTOS VIVIENTES

A continuación presentamos un extracto de la segunda novela de Kim Harrison, *El Regreso de los Muertos Vivientes*.

Subí un poco más la correa de lienzo sobre mi hombro para acomodar la regadera y me estiré para alcanzar la planta que colgaba. El sol entraba a chorros y me calentaba a través de mi overol azul de jardinera. Al otro lado del vidrio de las ventanas había un patio pequeño rodeado de oficinas de funcionarios importantes. Con los párpados entreabiertos por el sol, apreté la manija de la manguera y sentí que pasaba el agua.

Sonaba el tableteo de los teclados de las computadoras, al tiempo que yo me movía de planta en planta. Las conversaciones telefónicas se filtraban desde las oficinas hasta el mostrador de la recepción, y también unas carcajadas que más parecían ladridos de perro: eran hombres lobos. Cuanto mayor era su jerarquía en la manada, más humanos parecían. Pero la risa siempre los delataba.

Seguí con la mirada la hilera de plantas colgantes frente a las ventanas, hasta que mis ojos se detuvieron en el acuario de peces detrás del escritorio de la recepcionista. Sí... sí. Aletas de color marrón claro. Una mancha negra del lado derecho. Era él. El señor Ray criaba pececillos koi para la exposición anual de peces de Cincinnati. El ganador del año anterior siempre estaba expuesto en la parte exterior de su oficina; pero esta vez había dos peces, y los Howler no tenían a su mascota. El señor Ray pertenecía a los muchachos Den, rivales del equipo de béisbol de Entremundos. No había que pensarlo demasiado para saber quienes se la habían llevado.

"Entonces . . ." dijo la mujer sonriendo detrás del escritorio mientras metía una resma de papel en el cargador de la impresora. "¿Mark está de vacaciones? No me lo había dicho."

Asentí con la cabeza mientras me movía otro metro arrastrando mi equipo de riego sin mirar a la secretaria que vestía un elegante sastre ejecutivo marrón. Mark estaba de "vacaciones" profundamente dormido en un agujero del edificio donde trabajó antes de venir a este sitio, gracias a una poción de sueño temporal. "Sí señora," repuse subiendo la voz y agregándole cierto ceceo. "Él me dijo qué plantas tenía que regar." Entonces escondí mis uñas pintadas de rojo debajo de las palmas de las manos antes de que las viera. No iban bien con la imagen de mujer jardinera trabajadora, aun cuando eso debí pensarlo antes. "Todas las plantas de este piso. Luego las del vivero del techo."

Ella sonrió dejando ver los dientes. Era una mujer lobo de alta jerarquía en la manada de la oficina. Lo supe por el esmalte. Además, el señor Ray no tendría a un perro de secretaria cuando podía pagar el salario de una loba. Despedía un ligero olor de almizcle que no era del todo desagradable. "¿Le habló Mark del ascensor de servicio en la parte de atrás del edificio?" preguntó de forma servicial. "Es mucho más cómodo que tirar esa carretilla por las escaleras."

"No señora" respondí, ajustándome mejor la fea gorra con el logotipo de jardinería. "Tal vez quiere complicarme las cosas para que no le invada su territorio." Sentí que mi pulso se aceleraba y decidí empujar la carretilla de Mark más lejos con sus podadoras, su fertilizante y su sistema de riego. Yo sí conocía la existencia del ascensor, de las seis salidas de emergencia, de los pulsadores de alarma y del lugar donde guardaban las rosquillas.

"Hombres," dijo ella girando los ojos antes de sentarse de nuevo frente a su pantalla. "¿Acaso no se dan cuenta de que nosotras podríamos regir el mundo si quisiéramos?"

Aprobé evasivamente y rocié la siguiente planta con un poco de agua. Yo creía que lo regíamos ya.

De pronto escuché un zumbido sobre el ruido de la impresora y el suave parloteo de la oficina. Era Jenks, mi socio, que venía desde la oficina del jefe volando hacia mí de mal humor. Sus alas de libélula estaban rojas de agitación y dejaban caer polvillo de duende como rayos de sol. "Ya terminé con las plantas de allá adentro" dijo hablando duro mientras aterrizaba sobre el aro de la matera frente a mi. Se paró con las manos en la cintura, como un Peter Pan medieval, pero vestido de overol azul, como un basurero. Su esposa le había tejido una gorra que hacía juego con ese color. "Sólo necesitan agua. ¿Necesitas ayuda aquí afuera o puedo irme a dormir en la camioneta?" agregó mordazmente.

Me quité el tanque de la regadera y lo bajé para destornillar la tapa. "Necesito una bolita de fertilizante" le dije. Quería averiguar qué era lo que le molestaba.

Jenks voló hacia la camioneta refunfuñando y comenzó a escular. Por todos lados volaron estacas, tiras de pH y cintas verdes. "Lo encontré" dijo, y me trajo una bolita blanca tan grande como su propia cabeza. La dejó caer adentro del tanque y de inmediato sonaron burbujas. No era una bolita de fertilizante sino un oxigenador y potenciador para producir limo. Vaya con Jenks.

"Oh no, Raquel" susurró aterrizando en mi hombro. "Es poliéster. ¡Estoy vestido con poliéster!"

Me tranquilicé al ver qué era lo que le producía ese mal humor. "Vas a estar bien."

"¡Voy a quitarme esta cosa!" repuso, rascándose agitadamente debajo del cuello. "No puedo vestirme con poliéster. Los duendes somos alérgicos. Mira. ¿Lo ves?" Inclinó la cabeza para que su rubia cabellera descubriera el cuello; pero estaba muy cerca y no pude verlo bien. "Verdugones... ¡y apestan! Puedo oler el petróleo. Estoy vestido de dinosaurio muerto. No puedo vestirme de animales muertos. Es una locura, Raquel."

"¿Jenks?," le dije, mientras enroscaba de nuevo la tapa de

la regadera y la colgaba a mis espaldas, dándole un empujoncito de paso. "Yo también llevo puesto lo mismo. Ya cállate."

"¡Pues apesta!"

Lo vi frente a mi suspendido en el aire. "¿Por qué no encuentras algo que podar?" le dije apretando los dientes.

Me despidió con un gesto de la mano y se alejó volando
hacia atrás. En fin. Toqué el bolsillo trasero de mi espantoso
overol azul para tomar las podadoras. Mientras que señorita
secretaria escribía diligentemente una carta, yo coloqué un
taburete y me subí para podar las hojas de la planta que colgaba junto a su escritorio. Jenks me ayudaba y pasados algunos minutos respiré. "¿Todo listo allá adentro?"

Me dijo sí con la cabeza y con los ojos fijos en la puerta
de la oficina del señor Ray. "La próxima vez que revise su
correo electrónico, todo el sistema de seguridad de Internet
se va a caer. Si sabe algo de informática, lo arreglará en
cinco minutos. Si no, le tomará horas."

"Sólo necesito cinco minutos" respondí. El sol que entraba por la ventana me hacía sudar. Adentro olía a jardín…
un jardín con un perro mojado que jadeaba ahí tirado encima
de las frías baldosas.

Mi pulso se aceleró y me moví hasta la planta siguiente.
Ya estaba detrás del escritorio y la mujer estaba nerviosa.
Invadí su territorio, pero tendría que aguantarme. Yo era la
chica del agua. Tuve la esperanza de que ella relacionara mis
nervios con el hecho de que estábamos tan cerca, y seguí
trabajando. Tenía una mano en la tapa del tanque de la regadera. Con un solo giro quedaría abierta. Otro giro más y quedaría cerrada

"¡Vanessa!," sonó un grito airado desde la oficina de atrás.

"Aquí vamos" dijo Jenks volando hasta las cámaras de
seguridad del techo.

Me di la vuelta y ví a un hombre furioso que asomaba
medio cuerpo, un lobo según deduje por su estatura y com-
plexión pequeñas. "Otra vez" dijo. Su cara estaba roja y se
aferraba con fuerza al marco de la puerta. "Odio a estos aparatos. ¿Que tiene de malo el papel? Me gusta el papel."

La secretaria hizo una sonrisa profesional. "Señor Ray, no me diga que volvió a gritarle. Ya se lo dije. Las computadoras son como las mujeres. Si se les grita o se les piden demasiadas cosas al mismo tiempo, se bloquean y no obtendrá nada."

El hombre masculló alguna respuesta y desapareció otra vez en su oficina sin caer en la cuenta de que ella lo había amenazado. Mi corazón dio un brinco mientras que colocaba el taburete junto al tanque de la regadera.

Vanessa suspiró. "Que Dios lo ayude," murmuró al tiempo que se ponía de pies. "Ese hombre es capaz de fracturarse las bolas con la lengua" dijo con una mirada desesperada. Entonces entró en la oficina marcando el paso con sus tacones. "No toque nada. Ya regreso," me dijo en voz alta.

Respiré hondo. "¿Las cámaras?"

Jenks se posó sobre mí. "Diez minutos. Campo despejado." Entonces voló hasta la puerta principal y se acomodó en marco, arriba, para vigilar el corredor de afuera. Sus alas se movieron veloces y me hizo una señal de aprobación con sus diminutos pulgares.

La ansiedad me tensó la piel. Levanté la tapa del acuario y saqué la red verde que llevaba en el bolsillo de adentro del overol. Me paré en el taburete, enrollé la manga hasta el codo y metí la red en el agua. Los dos pececillos nadaron como relámpagos para esconderse atrás.

"Raquel," susurró Jenks de repente. "Todo va bien. Apenas está llegando."

"Vigila las puertas Jenks," le dije mordiéndome los labios con los dientes. *¿Cuánto tiempo toma atrapar a un pez?* Empujé una piedrita para atrapar al que estaba escondido detrás, pero nadaron hacia el frente.

De pronto sonó el teléfono. "Jenks…contesta," le dije tranquilamente mientras colocaba la red en ángulo para acorralarlos contra una esquina. "Te tengo…."

Jenks voló desde la puerta y cayó encima del botón rojo. "Oficina del señor Ray…espere por favor" dijo con voz de falsete.

"Maldición," dije, al ver que uno de los peces se me escapaba aleteando por el borde de la red. "Vamos...tan solo quiero llevarte a casa...especie de cosa resbalosa," amenacé apretando los dientes. "Casi...casi." Lo tenía entre la red y el vidrio. Si tan sólo se quedara quieto...

"¡Oiga!" dijo una voz gruesa que provenía del pasillo.

La adrenalina me hizo levantar la cabeza. Un hombre pequeño, de barbita bien cortada y con una carpeta llena de papeles debajo del brazo, estaba ahí parado en el pasillo que conducía a las otras oficinas. "¿Qué hace?" me preguntó agresivo.

Miré el tanque con mi brazo sumergido y la red vacía. El pez se había escapado. "Eh...dejé caer mis tijeras" repuse.

Un taconeo de zapatos y la voz de Vanessa llegaron de la oficina. "¡Señor Ray!"

Diablos. Hasta aquí llegó la forma sencilla de hacer esto. "Jenks, plan B" le dije gruñendo mientras tomaba el borde de arriba del acuario y tiraba de él.

Vanessa gritó en el otro cuarto cuando 25 galones de agua sucia de peces cayeron como una cascada sobre su escritorio. El señor Ray estaba a su lado. Yo salté del taburete empapada de la cintura hasta los pies. Nadie se movió. Estaban paralizados mientras yo examinaba el piso. "¡Te tengo!" grité, fijándome que tenía el que necesitaba.

"¡Quiere llevarse el pez!" gritó el hombrecito y el pasillo empezó a llenarse de gente. "¡Atrápenla!"

"¡Corre!" gritó Jenks. "Yo me encargo de quitártelos de encima."

Jadeando, caminé encorvada en zigzag tratando de sostenerlo sin lastimarlo. Se contorneaba y retorcía hasta que al fin logré asegurarlo entre mis dedos. Luego lo metí en la regadera, cerré bien la tapa y levanté la cabeza.

Jenks parecía una luciérnaga infernal volando de un lobo al otro, esgrimiendo lápices y lanzándolos en lugares sensibles: un duende de 10 centímetros conteniendo a tres hombres lobo. No me sorprendí. El señor Ray miraba conformado hasta caer en la cuenta de que yo tenía uno de sus peces. "¿Qué demonios hace usted con mi pez?" dijo rojo de ira.

"Estoy de salida" repuse. Entonces se abalanzó contra mí con sus manos gruesas. Yo, encantada, lo agarré del brazo tirándolo hacia adelante contra mi pie. Luego retrocedió tomándose el estómago con los brazos.

"¡Deja ya de jugar con esos perros!" le grité a Jenks mientras buscaba alguna manera de escapar. "Tenemos que irnos."

Entonces tomé el monitor de la computadora de Vanessa y lo lancé contra el vidrio. Hace tiempos que quería hacer lo mismo con el de Ivy. Quedó hecho trizas y la pantalla se veía extraña sobre el césped. Llovieron lobos furiosos a la sala que dejaban escapar su almizcle. Agarré el tanque y me lancé por la ventana. "¡Tras ella!" gritó alguien.

Caí de hombros sobre el césped bien cortado, y luego de rodar me puse de pies. "¡Arriba!" dijo Jenks. "¡Por allá!"

Cruzó el pequeño patio encerrado y yo lo seguí cargando la pesada regadera a mis espaldas. Con las manos libres pude trepar por el enrejado. Las espinas me rasgaron la piel pero no le presté atención.

Apenas llegué arriba jadeando respiré de nuevo, pero el sonido de ramas rotas me anunció que venían siguiéndome. Subí por el borde del techo y corrí. El aire estaba caliente y la silueta de los edificios de Cincinnati apareció ante mí.

"¡Salta!" me dijo Jenks tan pronto llegué al borde.

Confiaba en él. Salté corriendo del techo agitando las manos. Sentí una explosión de adrenalina y un vacío en el estómago: ¡un estacionamiento! ¡Me hizo saltar del techo para aterrizar en un estacionamiento!

"¡Yo no tengo alas Jenks!" grité. Apreté los dientes y doblé las rodillas.

El dolor me invadió apenas golpeé el pavimento. Caí hacia adelante raspándome las palmas de las manos y el tanque con el pececillo sonó y cayó al romperse la correa. Yo rodé para absorber el impacto.

El tanque de metal también salió rodando y yo salí corriendo tras él a pesar del dolor. Mis dedos lo alcanzaron a rozar, pero quedó debajo de un auto. Maldije mi suerte y me tiré de estómago sobre el piso, estirándome para alcanzarlo.

"¡Ahí está!" gritaron.

Sentí un ruido metálico en el auto junto a mi, y luego otro más. El pavimento a mi lado de repente tenía un agujero y me rosearon pedacitos de metralla. ¿Me disparan?

Gruñendo, me escurrí debajo del auto y tiré el tanque. Luego lo tomé entre los brazos y retrocedí. "¡Escuchen!," les grité quitándome el pelo de la cara. "¿Que demonios están haciendo? ¡Es tan solo un pez...y ni siquiera es suyo!"

Los tres lobos parados en el techo me miraban. Uno se rascó la cara con el revólver.

Yo di media vuelta y comencé a correr. Esto ya no valía la pena por quinientos dólares. Cinco mil, tal vez. *La próxima vez voy a averiguar los pormenores antes de cobrar la tarifa básica,* pensé mientras corría detrás de Jenks.

"¡Por aquí!" chilló Jenks. Trocitos de pavimento saltaban golpeándome al tiempo que sonaban los disparos. El estacionamiento no tenía rejas y con las piernas temblando por la adrenalina, corrí a meterme entre los peatones. El corazón me latía fuerte y me detuve un instante para verlos ahí junto a la silueta de los edificios. No habían saltado. No necesitaban hacerlo. Dejé sangre por todo el enrejado, pero no pensé que fueran a seguirme la pista. No era su pez. Era el de los Howler. Además, el equipo de béisbol de Entremundos pagaría mi arriendo del mes.

Mis pulmones trabajaban agitados mientras trataba de igualar mi paso con el de la gente que me rodeaba. Hacía calor y sudaba bajo mi costal de poliéster. Seguramente Jenks me cubría la espalda, así es que me metí en un callejón para cambiarme. Dejé a los peces en el piso y recosté la cabeza contra la fresca pared de un edificio. Lo había logrado. Ya podía pagar otro mes de arriendo.

Me levanté para quitarme el amuleto de disfraz que llevaba alrededor del cuello. De inmediato me sentí mejor, pues la apariencia de mujer oscura de pelo marrón y nariz grande desapareció, revelando mi ondulado pelo rojo hasta los hombros y mi piel pálida. Miré mis palmas raspadas y las froté con cuidado. Podría haber comprado un amuleto para el dolor, pero no quería portar muchos por si acaso me atrapaban y la "intención de robar" se cambiaba por "intención de lastimar físicamente." De la primera podía escabullirme, pero de la segunda tendría que defenderme. Yo era agente y conocía la ley.

El aire de septiembre se sentía bien a la sombra. Me acomodé la blusa, alcé el tanque y caminé bajo el sol sintiéndome yo de nuevo. Le puse mi gorra a un chico en la cabeza que se quedó mirándola, sonrió, y me hizo un tímido saludo mientras que su mamá se agachaba para preguntarle dónde la había encontrado. Estaba en paz con el mundo y comencé a caminar por el andén. Mis tacones sonaban y me solté el pelo. Iba en dirección de *Fountain Square* para tomar el autobús. Había olvidado ahí mis lentes oscuros esa mañana y con algo de suerte los encontraría. Ay dios, cómo disfrutaba de la independencia.

Habían transcurrido casi tres meses desde que perdí la paciencia por los casos de pacotilla que me confiaba mi antiguo jefe de Seguridad Entremundos. Me sentía utilizada y subvalorada, así que decidí romper el acuerdo verbal y dejar la S.E. para comenzar mi propia agencia. En ese momento me pareció que era una buena idea hacerlo. Luego, sobreviví a la amenaza de muerte cuando no pude pagar el soborno por incumplir mi contrato con la S.E.. Pero eso me abrió los ojos; y jamás lo habría logrado sin la ayuda de Ivy y Jenks.

Curiosamente, ahora que empezaban a conocerme, las cosas se ponían más difíciles en lugar de ser más fáciles. Claro que ahora le estaba dando buen uso a mi grado profesional fabricando los hechizos que antes compraba, algunos de los cuales nunca había podido costear. Pero el dinero era un problema real. No es que no pudiera conseguir trabajos: es que el dinero no duraba mucho en el jarrón de galletas encima de la nevera.

Lo que me gané probando que una pandilla trataba de in-

culpar a un zorro de la pandilla rival, se fue en pagar la reno-
vación de mi licencia de bruja. Antes la pagaba la S.E.
Luego encontré al familiar perdido de un aprendiz de brujo;
pero el dinero lo usé para pagar la cláusula adicional de mi
seguro de salud. Yo no sabía que a los agentes libres no nos
cubría. La S.E. me daba un carné que había usado antes.
Después le tuve que pagarle a un tipo para que neutralizara
los hechizos mortales que le lanzaron a todas mi pertenen-
cias y que aun estaban metidas en un depósito; comprarle a
Ivy una nueva levantadora de seda porque estropeé la suya;
y de paso, comprarme algo de ropa, pues tenía que mantener
mi buena reputación.

Pero el verdadero desagüe de mis finanzas eran los taxis.
Casi todos los conductores de autobuses de Cincinnati me
reconocían al verme y no me recogían. Por eso, Ivy tenía
que recogerme para llevarme a casa. Era injusto. Ya había
pasado casi un año desde que accidentalmente les hice caer
el cabello a todos los pasajeros de un autobús cuando trataba
de atrapar a un lobo.

Estaba aburrida sin dinero. Por lo menos ahora tenía algo
por recuperar las mascotas de los Howler. Era lo de un mes.
Además, los lobos no me perseguirían, pues no eran sus peces. Si querían hacer un reclamo en la S.E., tendrían que ex-
plicar dónde los obtuvieron.

"Oye Raque," dijo Jenks descendiendo desde quién sabe
donde. "Tu espalda está fuera de peligro. ¿Cuál es el plan B?"

Alcé las cejas y lo miré con sorna mientras volaba a mi
lado, justo a mi paso. "Tomar a los peces y correr como el
demonio."

Jenks rió y aterrizó en mi hombro. Había tirado su diminuto uniforme y ahora se veía normal con su camisa verde
de seda de manga larga y pantalón. Llevaba una pañoleta
roja amarrada a la cabeza como señal para otros duendes y
hadas de que no estábamos invadiendo sus territorios. Sus
alas lanzaban destellos donde aun quedaba el polvillo de
duende que lanzó durante la confusión de mi escapada.

Disminuí el ritmo a medida que nos aproximábamos a

Fountain Square. Busqué a Ivy pero no la encontré. Ya más tranquila, me senté del lado seco de la fuente mientras jugaba con mis lentes de sol en la mano. Ya vendría. Esa mujer vivía pendiente de los horarios.

Mientras Jenks pasaba debajo del rocío para quitarse el "hedor a dinosaurio muerto," yo abrí los lentes y me los puse. Mis ojos descansaron apenas se oscureció el brillo de esa tarde de septiembre. Estiré mis largas piernas y me quité el amuleto de olor que llevaba alrededor del cuello para lanzarlo al agua. Los lobos siguen pistas por el olor, y si se decidían perseguirme, la pista terminaría en este lugar tan pronto me subiera al auto de Ivy y nos largáramos.

Con la esperanza de que nadie hubiera caído en la cuenta, eché un vistazo por encima de la gente a mi alrededor: ví a un vampiro lacayo, anémico y nervioso, realizando el trabajo diurno de su amante; a dos humanos que susurraban y se reían de verle las heridas del cuello; a un brujo cansado…no…un aprendiz de brujo, pues no olía a secoya, sentado en una banca vecina comiendo panecillos; y yo. Respiré lento para recuperarme. Tener que esperar a que alguien te recoja es un anticlímax.

"Me gustaría tener un auto," le dije a Jenks mientras ponía entre mis piernas el tanque con los peces. Diez metros más allá se veía el movimiento del tráfico. Había más autos, de modo que pensé que serían pasadas las dos de la tarde. Era el momento en que empezaban a coexistir humanos y Entremundos en este pequeño y reducido espacio. Pero las cosas se hacían más fáciles cuando bajaba el sol y casi todos los humanos se retiraban a sus hogares.

"¿Y para qué quieres un auto?" preguntó Jenks parado sobre mis rodillas al tiempo que sacudía sus alas de libélula con grandes brazadas. "Yo no tengo auto. Nunca he tenido uno y me movilizo bien. Los autos son un problema" dijo. Yo ya no lo escuchaba. "Tienes que ponerles gasolina, mantenerlos y perder el tiempo lavándolos. Además, necesitas un lugar para guardarlos. ¿Y el dinero que gastas en ellos? ¡Son peor que tener novia!"

"No me importa" repuse moviendo repetidamente mis pies para irritarlo. "Me gustaría tener un auto." Seguí mirando a la gente. "James Bond nunca tiene que esperar el autobús. He visto todas sus películas y jamás tiene que esperar por el autobús." Lo miré con ojos entreabiertos. "Le haría perder...clase."

"Eh...sí," repuso con la atención fija en lo que sucedía a mis espaldas. "Y, además, resulta más seguro. ¡Lobos, a las once!"

Comencé a respirar más rápido a medida que giraba para verlos. De nuevo sentí tensión. "¡Mierda!" susurré, alzando el tanque. Eran esos tres de nuevo. Lo supe por su estatura y la manera como respiraban profundamente. Apreté los dientes y me puse de pies. *¿Dónde estaba Ivy?*

"¿Raque?" preguntó Jenks. "¿Por qué te persiguen?"

"No lo se." Pensé en mi sangre que quedó en aquellas rosas. Si no rompía la pista de olor me seguirían hasta la casa. Pero...¿por qué? Tenía la boca seca y me senté dándoles la espalda segura de que Jenks los vigilaba. "¿Ya me vieron?" le pregunté.

Jenks salió volando y regresó un segundo más tarde. "No. Tienes una ventaja de media cuadra, pero es mejor que te muevas."

Me moví un poco y evalué el riesgo de quedarme quieta esperando a Ivy, o moverme y que me vieran. "¡Maldición! Ojalá tuviera un auto" murmuré. Me incliné hacia la calle para intentar ver el techo azul de algún autobús, un taxi, cualquier cosa. *¿Dónde demonios estaba Ivy?*

OTROS LIBROS INTERESANTES...

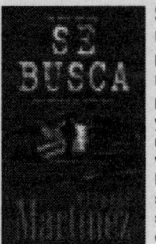

SE BUSCA
Una Novela de Suspenso
Michele Martinez
ISBN: 0-06-083752-7 (libro de bolsillo)

Melanie Vargas es madre soltera con una vida de hogar caótica y una carrera prometedora en la procuraduría federal. Una noche de verano, mientras pasea por las calles de Nueva York, ve como la casa de un rico y poderoso ex procurador arde en llamas mientras que su dueño torturado y asesinado yace en su interior. Melanie sabe que un caso tan prominente —como seguramente lo será éste— sería bueno para la trayectoria de su carrera y decide tomar el caso. Pero esta oportunidad podría llegar a costarle más aun ya que tendrá que descubrir al culpable antes de que el asesino la encúentre a ella.

LA AMANTE PERFECTA
Stephanie Laurens
ISBN: 0-06-083751-9 (libro de bolsillo)

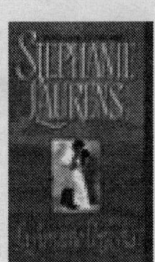

Por fin en español, una novela de romance por Stephanie Laurens, autora best seller en el *New York Times* y a nivel internacional.

¿Qué harías tú para seducir a *La Amante Perfecta*? Simón Cynster ha decidido encontrar la pareja ideal —alguien que sea una perfecta dama de día y una amante ardiente de noche. Jamás se imaginó que Portia Ashford, a quien conoce desde la infancia, sería la mujer que le provocaría una irresistible atracción, hasta que un beso apasionado le hace cambiar de parecer para siempre. Pero a medida que él y Portia comienzan a explorar las profundidades de la arrebatadora pasión que comparten, sucede algo terrible...algo que pone a Portia en peligro mortal, forzando a Simón a proteger a su adorada amante perfecta.

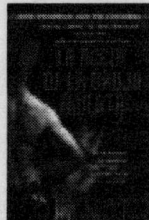

LA NOCHE DE LA BRUJA MUERTA
Kim Harrison
ISBN 0-06-083750-0 (libro de bolsillo)

Los vampiros son los reyes de la noche en un mundo de despiadados predadores, poblado de peligros inimaginables... Y Rachel Morgan es quien tiene la difícil tarea de asegurarse que ese mundo se mantenga civilizado. Ella es una bruja, una cazarrecompensas irresistible y atractiva que se asegurará de encontrarlos a todos... ya sea vivos o muertos.

La Noche de la Bruja Muerta es una novela de fantasía llena de magia, acción, romance y misterio, una lectura divertida e ideal para los amantes de lo supernatural.

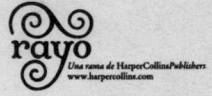